Handbook Series in Occupational Health Sciences

Series Editors

Kevin Daniels
Norwich Business School
University of East Anglia
Norwich, UK

Johannes Siegrist
Centre for Health and Society
Faculty of Medicine, Heinrich-Heine-Universität Düsseldorf
Düsseldorf, Germany

The Handbook Series in Occupational Health Sciences offers a unique opportunity to get acquainted with robust updated evidence on specific topics of key interest in occupational health research and practice. The series provides a venue for the large amount of significant recent scientific advances in research on occupational health due to the overriding importance of work and employment in developed and rapidly developing countries. The series is interdisciplinary, encompassing insights from: occupational medicine, epidemiology, ergonomics, economics, occupational health psychology, health and medical sociology, amongst others. Volumes in the series will cover topics such as socioeconomic determinants of occupational health; disability, work and health; management, leadership and occupational health; and health implications of new technologies at work and of new employment-related global threats. With a broad scope of chapters dealing with in-depth aspects of the volume's themes, this handbook series complements more traditional publication formats in the field (e.g. textbooks; proceedings), using a new system of online updating and providing explanatory figures and tables. Written by an international panel of eminent experts, the volumes will be useful to academics, policy researchers, advanced students and high-level practitioners (e.g. consultants, government policy advisors).

More information about this series at http://www.springer.com/series/15678

Ute Bültmann • Johannes Siegrist
Editors

Handbook of Disability, Work and Health

With 51 Figures and 46 Tables

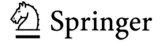

Editors
Ute Bültmann
Department of Health Sciences,
Community and Occupational Medicine
University of Groningen, University
Medical Center Groningen
Groningen, The Netherlands

Johannes Siegrist
Centre for Health and Society
Faculty of Medicine, Heinrich-Heine-
Universität Düsseldorf
Düsseldorf, Germany

ISBN 978-3-030-24333-3   ISBN 978-3-030-24334-0 (eBook)
ISBN 978-3-030-24335-7 (print and electronic bundle)
https://doi.org/10.1007/978-3-030-24334-0

© Springer Nature Switzerland AG 2020
This work is subject to copyright. All rights are reserved by the Publisher, whether the whole or part of the material is concerned, specifically the rights of translation, reprinting, reuse of illustrations, recitation, broadcasting, reproduction on microfilms or in any other physical way, and transmission or information storage and retrieval, electronic adaptation, computer software, or by similar or dissimilar methodology now known or hereafter developed.
The use of general descriptive names, registered names, trademarks, service marks, etc. in this publication does not imply, even in the absence of a specific statement, that such names are exempt from the relevant protective laws and regulations and therefore free for general use.
The publisher, the authors, and the editors are safe to assume that the advice and information in this book are believed to be true and accurate at the date of publication. Neither the publisher nor the authors or the editors give a warranty, expressed or implied, with respect to the material contained herein or for any errors or omissions that may have been made. The publisher remains neutral with regard to jurisdictional claims in published maps and institutional affiliations.

This Springer imprint is published by the registered company Springer Nature Switzerland AG
The registered company address is: Gewerbestrasse 11, 6330 Cham, Switzerland

Series Preface

The Handbook Series in Occupational Health Sciences offers a unique opportunity to get acquainted with robust updated evidence on specific topics of key interest in occupational health research and practice. The series provides a venue for the large amount of significant recent scientific advances in research on occupational health due to the overriding importance of work and employment in developed and rapidly developing countries. The series is interdisciplinary, encompassing insights from: occupational medicine, epidemiology, ergonomics, economics, occupational health psychology, health and medical sociology, among others. Volumes in the series will cover topics such as socioeconomic determinants of occupational health; disability, work, and health; management, leadership, and occupational health; and health implications of new technologies at work and of new employment-related global threats. With a broad scope of chapters dealing with in-depth aspects of the volume's themes, this handbook series complements more traditional publication formats in the field (e.g., textbooks, proceedings), using a new system of online updating and providing explanatory figures and tables. Written by an international panel of eminent experts, the volumes will be useful to academics, policy researchers, advanced students, and high-level practitioners (e.g., consultants, government policy advisors).

Volume Preface

This volume is the first one of a new series of handbooks on Occupational Health Sciences. The start of this new series represents a timely response to a growing body of scientific evidence on relationships between occupational conditions and health in times of far-reaching global changes of employment and work. Research in this field can no longer be restricted to one single discipline, but requires trans-disciplinary approaches from biomedical, behavioral, social, and economic sciences. This series of handbooks sets out to offer updated, comprehensive high-quality scientific information on major topics of occupational health research. The knowledge provided by an international panel of eminent experts is available to a specialized and non-specialized readership committed to understanding and improving the complex associations of occupational life with health and well-being.

In this book, major links between work, health, and disability are explored by a variety of scientific approaches. In the recent past, these links received growing attention by the international research community, not least in view of rapidly aging populations and a related increase of persons with disabilities. Moreover, with the endorsement of the United Nations' Convention on the Rights of Persons with Disabilities in 2007, disability became an issue of increasing policy relevance, calling for innovative scientific analysis and evaluation. Here, the associations between work, health, and disability are analyzed in two directions represented in two main sections of the book that complement each other. Chapters in the first section summarize current knowledge on adverse effects of distinct occupational hazards, both material and psychosocial, on working people's physical or mental health that may result in functional impairment, disability, and early exit from the labor market. Importantly, several chapters deal with options of reducing this burden by targeted programs of prevention and rehabilitation, supported by national social and labor policies. In the second section, crucial socioeconomic and psychosocial aspects of persons living and working with a disability are addressed, emphasizing opportunities and restrictions of sustainable (re)employment. Models of good practice and innovative rehabilitation strategies inform readers about most recent developments. As a unique feature, this collection of chapters provides available research evidence on return to work for eight different conditions of disability or chronic disease, thus offering in-depth knowledge to health-care professionals and other stakeholders who deal with the treatment and rehabilitation of persons with disability.

An introductory chapter provides readers with a summary of major insights delivered by the books' 34 chapters, and each single chapter may serve as a key resource of reference on its topic. Taken together, this book represents a pathbreaking synthesis of robust cross-disciplinary knowledge with rich implications for practice and policy. We hope that its content will be useful to graduate/postgraduate students, occupational health professionals, researchers, experts/consultants, and stakeholders/policy makers in occupational health institutions, in the business sector, and in public administrations, including governments and non-governmental organizations. Through the diffusion and implementation of its knowledge, it may be instrumental in promoting health-conducive working conditions, in preventing work-related disability risks, and in improving access or return to work, rehabilitation, and social integration.

We, the Editors, are very grateful to the authors who, as outstanding scientists, devoted their unique expertise by contributing their chapters to this book. We are convinced that, by doing so, they provided invaluable new insights and offered promising solutions to challenging problems. We also want to thank Pia Schneider for her excellent support in preparing final text versions of the chapters, and we are grateful for a constructive and successful collaboration with the team from Springer Nature that was involved in the production of this book.

June 2020   Ute Bültmann
                                                                                                      Johannes Siegrist

Contents

1 Two Perspectives on Work, Disability, and Health:
   An Overview 1
   Ute Bültmann and Johannes Siegrist

Part I Occupational Hazards, Impaired Health, and Disability Risk 15

2 The Changing Nature of Work and Employment in
   Developed Countries 17
   Werner Eichhorst

3 Trends in Work and Employment in Rapidly Developing
   Countries 33
   Martin Hyde, Sobin George, and Vaijayanthee Kumar

4 Concepts and Social Variations of Disability in Working-Age
   Populations 53
   Johannes Siegrist and Jian Li

5 Trajectories from Work to Early Exit from Paid Employment ... 71
   Alex Burdorf and Suzan Robroek

6 Policies of Reducing the Burden of Occupational Hazards and
   Disability Pensions 85
   Espen Dahl and Kjetil A. van der Wel

7 Burden of Injury Due to Occupational Exposures 105
   Jukka Takala

8 Occupational Causes of Cancer 127
   Jack Siemiatycki and Mengting Xu

9 Respiratory Work Disability in Relation to Occupational
   Factors 153
   Paul D. Blanc and Kjell Torén

10	**Occupational Determinants of Musculoskeletal Disorders** . . . . Alexis Descatha, Bradley A. Evanoff, Annette Leclerc, and Yves Roquelaure	169
11	**Occupational Determinants of Cardiovascular Disorders Including Stroke** . . . . Töres Theorell	189
12	**Occupational Determinants of Affective Disorders** . . . . Reiner Rugulies, Birgit Aust, and Ida E. H. Madsen	207
13	**Occupational Determinants of Cognitive Decline and Dementia** . . . . Claudine Berr and Noémie Letellier	235
14	**Work-Related Burden of Absenteeism, Presenteeism, and Disability: An Epidemiologic and Economic Perspective** . . . . Marnie Dobson, Peter Schnall, Ellen Rosskam, and Paul Landsbergis	251
15	**Surveillance, Monitoring, and Evaluation** . . . . Stavroula Leka and Aditya Jain	273
16	**Promoting Workplace Mental Wellbeing** . . . . Angela Martin, Clare Shann, and Anthony D. LaMontagne	289
17	**Reducing Inequalities in Employment of People with Disabilities** . . . . Ben Barr, Philip McHale, and Margaret Whitehead	309

Part II Access/return to Work of Persons with Disabilities or Chronic Diseases **329**

18	**A Human Rights Perspective on Work Participation** . . . . Jerome Bickenbach	331
19	**Regulatory Contexts Affecting Work Reintegration of People with Chronic Disease and Disabilities** . . . . Katherine Lippel	347
20	**Employment as a Key Rehabilitation Outcome** . . . . Kerstin Ekberg and Christian Ståhl	365
21	**Personal and Environmental Factors Influencing Work Participation Among Individuals with Chronic Diseases** . . . . Ranu Sewdas, Astrid de Wind, Femke I. Abma, Cécile R. L. Boot, and Sandra Brouwer	385
22	**Cancer Survivors at the Workplace** . . . . Anja Mehnert-Theuerkauf	399

23	Return to Work After Spinal Cord Injury	417
	Marcel W. M. Post, Jan D. Reinhardt, and Reuben Escorpizo	
24	Coronary Heart Disease and Return to Work	431
	Angelique de Rijk	
25	Return to Work After Stroke	451
	Akizumi Tsutsumi	
26	Common Mental Disorders and Work	467
	Silje Endresen Reme	
27	Work-Related Interventions to Reduce Work Disability Related to Musculoskeletal Disorders	483
	Dwayne Van Eerd and Peter Smith	
28	Addictive Disorders: Problems and Interventions at Workplace	505
	Clemens Veltrup and Ulrich John	
29	Factors of Competitive Employment for People with Severe Mental Illness, from Acquisition to Tenure	525
	Marc Corbière, Élyse Charette-Dussault, and Patrizia Villotti	
30	Concepts of Work Ability in Rehabilitation	551
	Kari-Pekka Martimo and Esa-Pekka Takala	
31	Facilitating Competitive Employment for People with Disabilities	571
	Gary R. Bond, Robert E. Drake, and Jacqueline A. Pogue	
32	Implementing Best Practice Models of Return to Work	589
	Vicki L. Kristman, Cécile R. L. Boot, Kathy Sanderson, Kathryn E. Sinden, and Kelly Williams-Whitt	
33	IGLOO: A Framework for Return to Work Among Workers with Mental Health Problems	615
	Karina Nielsen, Joanna Yarker, Fehmidah Munir, and Ute Bültmann	
34	Shifting the Focus from Work Reintegration to Sustainability of Employment	633
	Monika E. Finger and Christine Fekete	
35	Investing in Integrative Active Labour Market Policies	661
	Finn Diderichsen	
Index		675

About the Series Editors

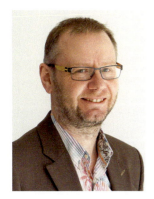

Kevin Daniels is Professor of Organizational Behaviour at the University of East Anglia, United Kingdom. He has a Ph.D. in Applied Psychology (1992), is a Fellow of the British Psychological Society, and a Fellow of the Academy of Social Sciences. His research covers approaches to health, safety, and well-being, originally with particular focus on the psychology of job design and more latterly an interest in multidisciplinary approaches to well-being. He has authored or co-authored over 85 peer-reviewed journal articles, 25 book chapters, and 15 books or major reports. From 2015 to 2021, he was lead investigator for evidence program on work and well-being, one of the foundational research programs of the UK's What Works Centre for Wellbeing. From 2015 to 2019, he served as editor of the *European Journal of Work and Organizational Psychology* and also in associate editor positions at the *British Journal of Management*, *Human Relations*, and *Journal of Occupational and Organizational Psychology*.

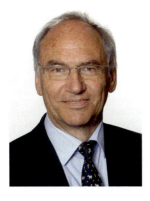

Johannes Siegrist is currently Senior Professor of work stress research at Heinrich Heine University Duesseldorf in Germany. He received his Ph.D. in Sociology from the University of Freiburg i. Br. in 1969, and he held professorships for medical sociology at the Universities of Marburg and Duesseldorf from 1973 to 2012. He was visiting professor at the Johns Hopkins University (USA) (1981) and at Utrecht University (NE) (1994). With his long-standing research on health-adverse psychosocial work environments and social inequalities in health, he has published more than 500 papers and book chapters and has written or edited several international books. In addition to his collaboration in distinct European research networks, he served as a consultant to the World Health Organization, and he chaired several national and international academic societies. Among other distinctions, he is a member of Academia Europaea (London) and a corresponding member of the Heidelberg Academy of Sciences.

About the Editors

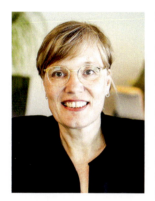

Ute Bültmann is full Professor of Work and Health in the Department of Health Sciences, Community and Occupational Medicine at the University Medical Center Groningen/University of Groningen in the Netherlands. She completed both her M.Sc. and Ph.D. at Maastricht University, the Netherlands. From 2003 until 2007, she worked at the National Institute of Occupational Health in Copenhagen, Denmark. Her research includes the epidemiology of work and (mental) health and the measurement of health-related functioning at work. In addition to collaborative work and health research in Canada, she is affiliated with the National Research Centre for the Working Environment in Copenhagen (DK) and the Karolinska Institutet in Stockholm (SE). She is Vice-President of the European Public Health Association (EUPHA) Section "Social Security, Work and Health." She (co-)authored more than 200 scientific publications. Her current research activities focus on work and health research from a life-course perspective with strong policy and practice links. She is a VICI laureate of the Netherlands Organisation for Scientific Research (NWO) for her research on "Today's youth is tomorrow's workforce: Generation Y at work."

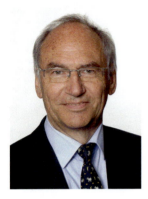

Johannes Siegrist is currently Senior Professor of work stress research at Heinrich Heine University Duesseldorf in Germany. He received his Ph.D. in Sociology from the University of Freiburg i. Br. in 1969, and he held professorships for medical sociology at the Universities of Marburg and Duesseldorf from 1973 to 2012. He was visiting professor at the Johns Hopkins University (USA) (1981) and at Utrecht University (NE) 1994). With his long-standing research on health-adverse psychosocial work environments and social inequalities in health, he has published more than 500 papers and book chapters and several international books. In addition to his collaboration in distinct European research networks, he served as a consultant to the World Health Organization, and he chaired several national and international academic societies. Among other distinctions, he is a member of Academia Europaea (London) and a corresponding member of the Heidelberg Academy of Sciences.

Contributors

Femke I. Abma Department of Health Sciences, Community and Occupational Medicine, University of Groningen, University Medical Center Groningen, Groningen, The Netherlands

Birgit Aust National Research Centre for the Working Environment, Copenhagen, Denmark

Ben Barr Department of Public Health and Policy, University of Liverpool, Liverpool, UK

Claudine Berr Neuropsychiatry: Epidemiological and Clinical Research, INSERM U1061, University of Montpellier, Montpellier, France

Centre Mémoire Ressources et Recherche, Hôpital Gui de Chauliac, Montpellier, France

Jerome Bickenbach University of Lucerne and Swiss Paraplegic Research, Nottwil, Switzerland

Paul D. Blanc Division of Occupational and Environmental Medicine, Department of Medicine, University of California San Francisco, San Francisco, CA, USA

Gary R. Bond Westat, Lebanon, NH, USA

Cécile R. L. Boot Department of Public and Occupational Health, Amsterdam Public Health Research Institute, Amsterdam UMC, VU University, Amsterdam, The Netherlands

Sandra Brouwer Department of Health Sciences, Community and Occupational Medicine, University of Groningen, University Medical Center Groningen, Groningen, The Netherlands

Ute Bültmann Department of Health Sciences, Community and Occupational Medicine, University of Groningen, University Medical Center Groningen, Groningen, The Netherlands

Alex Burdorf Department of Public Health, Erasmus University Medical Center, Rotterdam, The Netherlands

Élyse Charette-Dussault Department of Psychology, Université du Québec à Montréal, Montréal, QC, Canada

Marc Corbière Department of Education, Career Counselling, Université du Québec à Montréal (UQAM), Montréal, QC, Canada

Centre de Recherche de l'Institut Universitaire en Santé Mentale de Montréal (CR-IUSMM), Research Chair in Mental and Work, Foundation of IUSMM, Montréal, QC, Canada

Espen Dahl Oslo Metropolitan University, Oslo, Norway

Angelique de Rijk Department of Social Medicine, Care and Public Health Research Institute (CAPHRI), Faculty of Health, Medicine and Life Sciences, Maastricht University, Maastricht, The Netherlands

Astrid de Wind Department of Public and Occupational Health, Amsterdam Public Health Research Institute, Amsterdam UMC, VU University, Amsterdam, The Netherlands

Alexis Descatha INSERM, U1085, IRSET (Institute de recherché en santé, environnement et travail), ESTER Team, University of Angers, Angers, France

University of Versailles Saint-Quentin-en-Yvelines, Versailles, France

INSERM, UMS 011 UMR1168, Villejuif, France

AP-HP, Occupational Health Unit, Raymond Poincaré University Hospital, Garches, France

Inserm U1085-Unité de santé professionnelle AP-HP UVSQ, Garches, France

Finn Diderichsen Department of Public Health, University of Copenhagen, Copenhagen, Denmark

Marnie Dobson Center for Occupational and Environmental Health, University of California, Irvine, CA, USA

Robert E. Drake Westat, Lebanon, NH, USA

Werner Eichhorst IZA and University of Bremen, Bremen, Germany

Kerstin Ekberg Community Medicine, Department of Health, Medicine and Caring Sciences, Linköping University, Linköping, Sweden

Reuben Escorpizo Department of Rehabilitation and Movement Science, University of Vermont, Burlington, VT, USA

Bradley A. Evanoff Division of General Medical Sciences, School of Medicine, Washington University in St. Louis, St. Louis, MI, USA

Christine Fekete Swiss Paraplegic Research, Nottwil, Switzerland

Department of Health Sciences and Medicine, University of Lucerne, Lucerne, Switzerland

Monika E. Finger Swiss Paraplegic Research, Nottwil, Switzerland
Department of Health Sciences and Medicine, University of Lucerne, Lucerne, Switzerland

Sobin George Centre for Study of Social Change and Development, Institute for Social and Economic Change, Banglore, India

Martin Hyde Centre for Innovative Ageing, Swansea University, Swansea, UK

Aditya Jain Management Division, Nottingham University Business School, University of Nottingham, Nottingham, UK

Ulrich John University Medicine Greifswald, Institute of Community Medicine, Greifswald, Germany

Vicki L. Kristman EPID@Work Research Institute, Department of Health Sciences, Lakehead University, Thunder Bay, ON, Canada

Vaijayanthee Kumar Indian Institute of Management, Indore, MP, India

Anthony D. LaMontagne Determinants of Health Domain, Institute for Health Transformation, Deakin University, Geelong, VIC, Australia

Paul Landsbergis SUNY Downstate School of Public Health, Brooklyn, NY, USA

Annette Leclerc INSERM, UMS 011 UMR1168, Villejuif, France

Stavroula Leka Department of Marketing and Management, Cork University Business School, University College Cork, Cork, Ireland
School of Medicine, University of Nottingham, Nottingham, UK

Noémie Letellier Neuropsychiatry: Epidemiological and Clinical Research, INSERM U1061, University of Montpellier, Montpellier, France

Jian Li Department of Environmental Health Sciences, Fielding School of Public Health; School of Nursing, University of California, Los Angeles, CA, USA

Katherine Lippel Faculty of Law (Civil Law Section), Canada Research Chair in Occupational Health and Safety Law, University of Ottawa, Ottawa, ON, Canada

Ida E. H. Madsen National Research Centre for the Working Environment, Copenhagen, Denmark

Kari-Pekka Martimo Ilmarinen Mutual Pension Insurance Company, Helsinki, Finland

Angela Martin Menzies Institute for Medical Research and Tasmanian School of Business and Economics, University of Tasmania, Hobart, TAS, Australia

Philip McHale Department of Public Health and Policy, University of Liverpool, Liverpool, UK

Anja Mehnert-Theuerkauf Department of Medical Psychology and Medical Sociology, University Medical Center Leipzig, Leipzig, Germany

Fehmidah Munir Loughborough University, Loughborough, UK

Karina Nielsen Institute for Work Psychology, University of Sheffield, 8Sheffield, UK

Jacqueline A. Pogue Westat, Lebanon, NH, USA

Marcel W. M. Post Center of Excellence for Rehabilitation Medicine, UMC Utrecht Brain Center, University Medical Center Utrecht and De Hoogstraat Rehabilitation, Utrecht, The Netherlands

Department of Rehabilitation Medicine, University of Groningen, University Medical Center Groningen, Groningen, The Netherlands

Jan D. Reinhardt Institute for Disaster Management and Reconstruction, Sichuan University and Hong Kong Polytechnic University, Chengdu, China

Swiss Paraplegic Research, Nottwil, Switzerland

Department of Health Sciences and Health Policy, University of Lucerne, Lucerne, Switzerland

Silje Endresen Reme University of Oslo, Oslo, Norway

Suzan Robroek Department of Public Health, Erasmus University Medical Center, Rotterdam, The Netherlands

Yves Roquelaure INSERM, U1085, IRSET (Institute de recherché en santé, environnement et travail), ESTER Team, University of Angers, Angers, France

Ellen Rosskam Center for Social Epidemiology, Los Angeles, CA, USA

Reiner Rugulies National Research Centre for the Working Environment, Copenhagen, Denmark

Department of Public Health, University of Copenhagen, Copenhagen, Denmark

Department of Psychology, University of Copenhagen, Copenhagen, Denmark

Kathy Sanderson EPID@Work Research Institute, Faculty of Business Administration, Lakehead University, Thunder Bay, ON, Canada

Peter Schnall Center for Occupational and Environmental Health, University of California, Irvine, CA, USA

Ranu Sewdas Department of Public and Occupational Health, Amsterdam Public Health Research Institute, Amsterdam UMC, VU University, Amsterdam, The Netherlands

Clare Shann University of Tasmania, Hobart, TAS, Australia

Shann Advisory, Preston, Geelong, VIC, Australia

Determinants of Health Domain, Institute for Health Transformation, Deakin University, Geelong, VIC, Australia

Johannes Siegrist Centre for Health and Society, Faculty of Medicine, Heinrich-Heine-Universität Düsseldorf, Düsseldorf, Germany

Jack Siemiatycki École de santé publique, Université de Montréal, Montreal, QC, Canada

Université de Montréal Hospital Research Centre, (CRCHUM), Montreal, QC, Canada

Kathryn E. Sinden EPID@Work Research Institute, School of Kinesiology, Lakehead University, Thunder Bay, ON, Canada

Peter Smith Institute for Work and Health, Toronto, ON, Canada

Christian Ståhl Unit of Education and Sociology, Department of Behavioural Sciences and Learning, Linköping University, Linköping, Sweden

Esa-Pekka Takala Finnish Institute of Occupational Health, Helsinki, Finland

Jukka Takala International Commission on Occupational Health, ICOH, Rome, Italy

Töres Theorell Stress Research Institute, Stockholm University, Stockholm, Sweden

Kjell Torén Department of Occupational and Environmental Medicine, Sahlgrenska Academy, University of Gothenburg, Gothenburg, Sweden

Akizumi Tsutsumi Department of Public Health, Kitasato University School of Medicine, Sagamihara, Japan

Kjetil A. van der Wel Oslo Metropolitan University, Oslo, Norway

Dwayne Van Eerd Institute for Work and Health, Toronto, ON, Canada

Clemens Veltrup Fachklinik Freudenholm Ruhleben, Ploen, Germany

Patrizia Villotti Department of Education, Career Counselling, Université du Québec à Montréal (UQAM), Montréal, QC, Canada

Margaret Whitehead Department of Public Health and Policy, University of Liverpool, Liverpool, UK

Kelly Williams-Whitt Dhillon School of Business, University of Lethbridge, Calgary, AB, Canada

Mengting Xu École de santé publique, Université de Montréal, Montreal, QC, Canada

Université de Montréal Hospital Research Centre, (CRCHUM), Montreal, QC, Canada

Joanna Yarker Birkbeck, University of London, London, UK

Two Perspectives on Work, Disability, and Health: An Overview

Ute Bültmann and Johannes Siegrist

Contents

Part I 3
Part II 7
References 13

Abstract

This introductory chapter presents "Two perspectives on work, disability and health." With the first perspective, the contribution of occupational hazards and stressful working conditions to the burden of chronic disease and disability is illustrated, by reviewing and discussing evidence related to leading disorders and impairments. Moreover, options of reducing this burden by worksite health promotion and by targeted social policies are presented. With the second perspective, the socioeconomic and psychosocial aspects of persons living with a disability are explored, with special emphasis on (re)employment opportunities or restrictions. Models of good practice and innovative rehabilitation strategies inform readers about most recent developments. Both perspectives complement each other, and they offer new knowledge that may be instrumental in strengthening efforts of professional and other stakeholders to promote health-conducive working conditions, to prevent work-related disability risks, and to improve access or return to work, rehabilitation, and social integration. The two

---

U. Bültmann (✉)
Department of Health Sciences, Community and Occupational Medicine, University of Groningen, University Medical Center Groningen, Groningen, The Netherlands
e-mail: u.bultmann@umcg.nl

J. Siegrist
Centre for Health and Society, Faculty of Medicine, Heinrich-Heine-Universität Düsseldorf, Düsseldorf, Germany
e-mail: Johannes.Siegrist@med.uni-duesseldorf.de

© Springer Nature Switzerland AG 2020
U. Bültmann, J. Siegrist (eds.), *Handbook of Disability, Work and Health*, Handbook Series in Occupational Health Sciences, https://doi.org/10.1007/978-3-030-24334-0_35

perspectives on work, disability and health, are illustrated by 34 chapters in Part I and Part II.

Keywords

Work · Occupation · Health · Disability · Prevention · Labour market · Return to work

This book provides readers with a summary of research evidence on links between work, health, and disability. There are several reasons for a growing importance of these links. First, in times of rapid growth of aging populations, in developed as well as in rapidly developing countries, the prevalence of disability within total populations has been increasing, given its strong dependence on the aging process (OECD 2010). Second, as a consequence of population aging, the dependency ratio of labor market participation has been steadily increasing, at least in high-income countries, urging national pension systems to extend the life span of active work by postponing the statutory eligibility age for full pension. With larger proportions of older workers participating in paid employment, a substantial burden of disease and disability motivated employers as well as health and social protection systems to strengthen worksite health promotion and return to work activities. Third, within the last few decades, the nature of work, employment, and labor markets underwent profound changes, as explained below, thus challenging traditional patterns of dealing with occupational health and disease, and of offering social protection to workers. Last, but not least, the way of conceptualizing disability underwent a profound change, specifically with the affirmation and endorsement of the United Nations' Convention on the Rights of Persons with Disabilities (United Nations 2007), enabling persons with disability to become more fully integrated into societal life, including paid employment (WHO 2011).

While becoming an issue of increasing policy relevance, the links between work, health, and disability also received growing attention by the international research community. During recent decades, the number of empirical studies addressing these links has risen dramatically. Despite the many systematic reviews and meta-analyses, it seems almost impossible to overview this rich body of findings. In part, this difficulty is due to the heterogeneity of research approaches and designs, the lack of standardized measurement methods, and an underdeveloped theoretical analysis. Additionally, research on these links often needs to crosscut disciplinary boundaries, integrating social and behavioral sciences with biomedical sciences. This may add to the difficulties of developing a clear-cut view of the state of the art.

With this book, we set out to provide readers with a systematic, though selective, representation of relevant research achievements in this interdisciplinary field. By the term "systematic," we mean that the body of knowledge is presented along two major perspectives. The first perspective deals with those aspects of the working life that ultimately contribute to the development of functional impairment and disability. Many answers to this question depend on findings from longitudinal epidemiological studies of employed populations. Therefore, in the first part of this volume, the contribution of occupational hazards and stressful working conditions to the burden of chronic disease and disability is illustrated, by reviewing and discussing evidence related to leading disorders and impairments. Moreover, several chapters deal with options of reducing this burden by worksite health promotion and by targeted social policies. With the second perspective, we explore the socioeconomic and psychosocial aspects of persons living with a disability, with special emphasis on (re)employment opportunities or restrictions. Cross-sectional and longitudinal studies highlight the relevance of improved coping with functional limitations and of appropriate societal efforts toward full social participation. Models of good practice and innovative rehabilitation strategies inform readers about most recent developments.

Both perspectives complement each other, and they offer new knowledge that may be instrumental in strengthening efforts of professional and other stakeholders to promote health-conducive working conditions, to prevent work-related disability risks, and to improve access or return to work, rehabilitation, and social integration. As mentioned, these two perspectives are represented in the two main sections of the book. Part I is concerned with occupational hazards, impaired health, and disability risk, whereas Part II deals with access/return to work of persons with disabilities or chronic diseases. In this introductory chapter, we give a brief account of essential insights provided by each chapter along these two perspectives.

Part I

The three chapters of the *first part* of this section introduce some general issues and challenges. *Werner Eichhorst* describes major changes of work and employment in a globalized economy, driven by technological progress and economic constraints. These changes affect workers in positive as well as negative ways. Job loss, growth of nonstandard employment including job instability, work intensification, and increased pressure of training and reskilling provide new challenges. The author concludes that distinct social and labor market policies need to be strengthened to prevent an increased burden of work-related disease and disability and a widening of social inequalities. While the first chapter deals mainly with developed countries, *Martin Hyde, Sobin George, and Vaijayanthan Kumar*, in the second chapter, address the quality of work and employment in rapidly developing countries. They illustrate the severe threats of high unemployment rates, highly prevalent informal (or even unpaid) work, and low availability of occupational safety and health services and measures with reference to six developing countries, India, China, Brazil, Mexico, Indonesia, and the Russian Federation. The fact that 75% of the global workforce is exposed to these threats underlines the importance of a global strategy toward providing sustainable working and living conditions. The different concepts of disability and the social variations of functional impairment in working-age populations define the content of the chapter written by *Johannes Siegrist and Jian Li*. With the Convention on the Rights of Persons with Disabilities (United

Nations 2007) and the WHO's International Classification of Functioning, Disability and Health (ICF) (WHO 2001), a landmark step of promoting equal rights to persons with disability was achieved, with improved options of full social participation. Yet, two distinct interpretations of disability, the "minority approach" and the "universal approach," dominated the professional discourse, resulting in different definitions of the target populations. At the level of labor market participation, persons with disability are still less frequently active, and there is a clear social gradient, with lower participation among those with low socioeconomic status. Based on recent findings from longitudinal data, the chapter demonstrates this social gradient for early exit from paid work as well. It ends by discussing policy implications for attempts toward reducing these inequalities. The trajectories from work to early exit from labor market are explained in more detail in the following chapter by *Alex Burdorf and Suzan Robroek*. These trajectories are complex, given the two directions of effects between work and health. On one hand, adverse work increases the probability of developing disability and of early exit from labor market. On the other hand, poor health and impairment acts as an important determinant of employability. The authors conclude that special preventive efforts should be directed at vulnerable groups, i.e., people with high risk of unemployment and with limited work ability. Extending this scope to the level of national policies, *Espen Dahl and Kjetil A. van der Wel* in their chapter argue that effective policies of enhancing labor market participation of disabled people should include investments into improved quality of work and employment and an extension of programs based on supported employment programs. These efforts, rather than financial incentives or legal sanctions, would not only increase employability but also reduce the burden of financial hardship related to disability.

The *second part* of Part I demonstrates research evidence on the main health consequences of occupational hazards and stressors. It starts with an informed overview of the burden of injury due to occupational exposures by *Jukka Takala*. While the incidence of fatal and nonfatal occupational injuries was substantially reduced in high-income countries, mainly due to technological progress, reduction of hazardous jobs, and improved occupational safety and health measures, it continues to be a major concern in the less developed parts of the world. Despite the uncertainties of estimates based on administrative data, there is reason to believe that, globally, 7,500 people die every day due to occupational injuries and work-related disorders, such as cancer and cardiovascular and respiratory diseases. Adding nonfatal injuries and work-related disability to this burden results in a substantial amount of economic costs for every country. The author rightly calls for concerted policy efforts to strengthen prevention at work. Occupational causes of cancer are the topic of the chapter by *Jack Siemiatycki and Meng Zing Xu*. According to current scientific knowledge, there are some 50 definite occupational carcinogens, resulting in the fact that between 4% and 14% of all male cancer deaths in the different countries are attributable to occupational exposures. Among working women the proportion is much lower. Main occupational exposures are asbestos, night shift work, mineral oils, solar radiation, silica, and diesel engine exhaust. For reasons of compensation and prevention, detailed monitoring and continued preventive action are required to tackle this challenge. *Paul A. Blanc and Kjell Toren* shed light on the bidirectional associations of respiratory disorders and occupational conditions. On the one hand, specific occupational exposures are risk factors of respiratory disorders. The impact of mining on lung fibrosis is a well-known example. On the other hand, workers suffering from respiratory disorders such as chronic obstructive pulmonary disease or asthma experience increased risks of job change or job loss, long-term absenteeism, but also presenteeism. The authors discuss the multiple manifestations of "respiratory work disability" in occupational life, and they point to the need of a more comprehensive scientific approach toward this relevant problem.

Occupational factors are particularly important for the development of several additional, widely prevalent chronic disorders. Musculoskeletal disorders (MSD) are the first one of four disorders discussed in this context, given the fact that they are the leading cause of work disability in developed countries. *Alexis Descatha, Bradley A Evanoff, Annette Leclerc, and Yves Roquelaure* argue that MSD mainly result from non-traumatic injury of soft-tissue structures due to biomechanical factors, such as long-term, repetitive hand movements or hand-arm elevations, static work in awkward positions, or unhealthy ways of sitting. Continued muscular tension or strain contributes to regional upper-body pain as well as low-back pain. Increased muscular force production has also been observed under conditions of chronic psychosocial stress at work, thus calling for an interdisciplinary study of the complex links between work and MSD. In today's working life, many job tasks contribute to the burden of this range of disorders (e.g., widely prevalent computer-based jobs). Their human and economic costs underline again the need for far-reaching measures of worksite health promotion. Cardiovascular disorders (CVD), and in particular coronary or ischemic heart disease (IHD), are a second widespread chronic disease where adverse working conditions play an important role. In his comprehensive review, *Töres Theorell* identifies three types of occupational determinants. Traditionally, research focused on physical and chemical risk factors, such as heavy physical activity, noise, heat, carbon monoxide, plumb, and other substances, but these conditions only account for a limited part of the variance. A second line of research showed that work time arrangements, specifically shift work and long working hours, make a significant contribution to the development of CVD. More recently, a third line of research was concerned with a health-adverse psychosocial work environment and its stress-physiological effects on the cardiovascular system. Strong evidence on its role was contingent on the availability of results from occupational cohort studies and the use of theoretical models of stressful work, such as demand-control (or job strain), effort-reward imbalance, or organizational injustice. This knowledge has now direct impact on measures of primary and secondary prevention. Along similar lines, *Reiner Rugulies, Birgit Aust, and Ida E.H. Madsen* demonstrate that the adverse psychosocial working conditions mentioned increase the risk of depressive disorders to a significant extent, both among working men and women. This rather consistent evidence is based on more than two dozens of prospective investigations and is supported by experimental or quasi-experimental studies on potential psychobiological pathways. The authors conclude that future research should examine the health effects of theory-based interventions and explore the links between work and nonwork determinants of depression, preferably in a life course perspective. Cognitive decline and dementia define the fourth condition of ill health as related to occupational life. *Claudine Berr and Noemie Letellier* argue that cognitive aging is a lifelong process that might be accelerated by distinct adverse working conditions. Among these, neurotoxic substances inherent in a variety of job task profiles contribute to cognitive decline. For instance, exposure to pesticides and lead was associated with an increased risk of Parkinson's disease, and exposure to organic solvents, such as benzene and chlorinated solvents, was related to elevated levels of cognitive impairment. Additionally, psychosocial job characteristics seem to contribute to cognitive aging in two directions. While jobs defined by task complexity and challenging demands requiring responsibility are protective as they strengthen workers' cognitive reserve, passive jobs (low demands, low control) that lack cognitive stimulation promote cognitive impairment in midlife and early old life.

The occupational exposures as well as the chronic disorders mentioned in these chapters point to a common underlying pattern, their consistent social stratification. Workers with lower skill level or with lower occupational position are more often exposed to adverse working conditions, and they suffer more often from the disorders discussed than their better educated or higher-ranked colleagues. This significant pattern of social inequality calls for structural approaches toward worksite health promotion and prevention. The *third part* of Part I deals with this challenge. Focusing on the broader context of work and health in the United States of America (USA), *Marnie Dobson, Peter Schnall, Ellen Rosskam, and Paul Landsbergis* emphasize the large impact of adverse working conditions on workers', employers', and society's costs in terms of disability pensions, absenteeism, presenteeism, and incident nonfatal and fatal stress-related diseases. In the United States, societal safety nets to mitigate this adversity are relatively weak. Poor coverage of universal healthcare access, restricted availability of state disability pensions, underdeveloped occupational health and safety services and related legislation, and a major responsibility of employers and business organizations for the costs of work-related illnesses are some of the reasons for this critical situation that affects most strongly vulnerable socioeconomic groups. The US conditions of work, disability, and health are in sharp contrast to those of Northern and Western European countries where comprehensive social and labor policies contribute to a reduction of the burden of work-related illnesses. Regulatory and voluntary approaches on health, safety, and well-being are an important component of such policies, as explained in the next chapter by *Stavroula Leka and Aditya Jain*. This holds particularly true for employed persons with disability. These two lines of protection complement each other. Regulations are legally binding conventions imposed by the International Labour Organization to all countries that have adopted their ratification. Up to now, some 40 conventions have been implemented in an attempt to strengthen occupational health and safety globally. Voluntary approaches are realized in two ways. First, they indicate the commitment of business organizations to comply with distinct quality standards of health-protecting procedures at work set by international standardization bodies.

These commitments are maintained without external sanctions. The same holds true for the second approach, i.e., agreements between social partners (employer organizations and trade unions). For instance, at the level of European organization, agreements on telework, work-related stress, and inclusive labor market were enacted. Available instruments of surveillance, monitoring, and evaluation support this implementation process. What are the models of best practice to promote healthy work at the level of companies and organizations? The chapter by *Angela Martin, Clare Shann, and Anthony D. LaMontagne* offers a partial answer to this question by presenting the results of a rapid review of recent intervention research on promoting mental well-being at work. Based on findings from randomized controlled trials and other well-controlled study designs, the available scientific evidence suggests that harm can be prevented and well-being can be promoted by measures at the individual and organizational level. Individual-focused approaches include the prevention of depression, suicide, and bullying, whereas organization-based interventions reduce work-related stress by improving work time control, autonomy, support, and reward at work. With the availability of online interventions (e.g., mindfulness, resilience, relaxation, physical activity), the implementation of workplace mental health programs can be accelerated. According to authors, such acceleration is needed in order to cope with a pressing problem of occupational public health. The final chapter of Part I, written by *Ben Barr, Philip McHale, and Margaret Whitehead*, is concerned with ways of reducing the large employment gap between people with and without disability, a gap that is most obvious when comparing low-skilled manual occupations with more privileged occupations and professions. To this end, the authors develop a typology of active labor market policies in high-income countries, with a focus on measures to integrate sick and disabled people into work. This can be achieved by promoting disability-friendly work environments and/or by strengthening individual employability. Examples from the United Kingdom, Sweden, Denmark, and Canada indicate that a mix of these two strategies is most likely to reduce this gap and the associated poverty rate. Although measures in the welfare benefit system to counteract disincentives to work are welcome, they were shown to be rather ineffective in case of disability. Therefore, to reduce social inequalities in employment access and level of income among persons with disability, targeted, well-balanced approaches toward increasing their employability need to be designed.

Part II

The second perspective of analysis within this book concerns the socioeconomic and psychosocial aspects of persons living with a disability. Here, opportunities of integration into the labor market are of primary interest. This is not the first volume dealing with this topic, as documented by two important books published in the past decade, i.e., the *Handbook of Work Disability* (Loisel and Anema, 2013) and the *Handbook of Return to Work* (Schultz and Gatchel 2016). However, different from these volumes, our book addresses determinants and outcomes of access or return to work in a broad spectrum of major disabilities or chronic diseases, with special attention to the specific characteristics of each single health condition. By doing so, the knowledge offered by these chapters should be of particular interest to health-care professionals who deal with the treatment and rehabilitation of patients with specific disabilities or diseases. Part II again contains three parts. In the *first* part, key ethical, legal, and socioeconomic questions related to disability are analyzed. The *second* – and main – part presents research evidence on return to work for eight different conditions of disability or chronic disease. In the *third* part, rehabilitation strategies and policy challenges are discussed in a broader framework, integrating promising approaches from different countries.

The first chapter of this section presents a human rights perspective on social participation in disability. *Jerome Bickenbach* argues that access to work is central to full social participation, and as a source of material and psychological well-being, it represents a basic human right. As the proportions of unemployment or underemployment are disproportionally high among persons with mental or physical disability, these societal groups deserve special policy support to reduce their social exclusion and discrimination. With the United Nations' Convention on the Rights of Persons with Disabilities, such policy support has become manifest at global level (United Nations 2007). In particular, Article 27 declares access to work among persons with disability an important human right, with implications for practical empowerment (e.g., accessibility) and of accommodation (e.g., provision of medical and vocational rehabilitation, of health and insurance coverage). Despite this landmark policy document, much needs to be done in practice to meet this basic human right among the many underserved disabled people around the world. In her comprehensive overview, *Katherine Lippel* provides an international perspective on regulatory issues that determine the context in which work reintegration of people with chronic disease and disabilities takes place. First, the relevance of legal rules for the science of work disability prevention is addressed. To this end, the chapter underlines the importance of local regulatory protections and processes when developing measures that aim to predict return to work, and examining the ways in which the legal rules affect the behavior of participants in the work reintegration processes. Second, the chapter presents categories of legal rules that have an impact on different key stakeholders involved in the return to pre-injury employment or reentrance of the labor market (e.g., rules on workers' compensation and sickness insurance). The author argues that, as the economic value of the disabled worker is key to the return to work incentives, current regulatory models may systemically exclude those in greatest need of support. Is "employment" a key rehabilitation outcome? The chapter *by Kerstin Ekberg and Christian Stahl* illustrates that the commonly used outcome measures of return to work interventions capture only part of the process leading to sustainable participation in the labor market. If work disability policies restrict benefits for the sick-listed and unemployed in favor of active work reintegration, they may run the risk of increasing the inequality gap in the labor market, since these policies focus on individual responsibilities and agency rather than on resource-generation. Dynamic developments at the labor markets and at work may create new challenges for work disability prevention research and practice. The authors propose that the notion of equality needs to be reconsidered. Rather than focusing on the aim of returning to any job, they maintain that the quality of jobs also needs to be taken into account to enable sustainable participation in the labor market. In the final chapter of the first part, *Ranu Sewdas, Astrid de Wind, Femke Abma, Cécile Boot, and Sandra Brouwer* provide an informed state-of-the-art overview on the personal and environmental factors that influence work participation among individuals with chronic disease. Instead of disease-specific factors, the authors identify disease-generic factors. In particular, lower-educated, older women with chronic disease seem to be vulnerable for work participation. To increase return to work, strong psychological resources, a supportive social and work environment, and organizational policies aiming at an open communication need to be strengthened. In line with the above chapters, the authors argue that all stakeholders involved in this process should deal with new developments at work, such as increasing demands to work longer and to be more flexible.

The *second* – and main – part of this section presents detailed research evidence on return to work for eight different conditions of disability or chronic disease, i.e., cancer, spinal cord injury, coronary heart disease, stroke, common mental disorders, musculoskeletal disorders, addictive disorders, and severe mental illness. Returning to working life is playing an increasingly important role for cancer patients through improved survival rates, but whether patients succeed in working with and after cancer depends on a variety of societal, economic, and individual medical and psychosocial factors. The chapter by *Anja Mehnert-Theuerkauf* shows that while many cancer patients have a high motivation to return to work, they also experience persisting health problems, mainly due to multimodal cancer therapies during cancer survivorship. Prevalent health problems in cancer survivors that adversely impact work include psychological distress, pain, fatigue, and depression. Factors identified as barriers for return to work are low socioeconomic status and heavy physical work, whereas options of flexible working time arrangements and available social support at work facilitate reintegration. Cancer survivorship programs and self-management interventions need to address these persisting health problems to facilitate retaining or returning to work. The author concludes that interdisciplinary, occupational intervention programs involving physical, psychosocial, and occupational components are effective for return to work. *Marcel Post, Jan Reinhardt, and Reuben Escorpizo* follow up with a chapter on spinal cord injury, a seriously disabling condition. This chapter summarizes the evidence on work participation and vocational rehabilitation of people with spinal cord injury. Many non-modifiable and modifiable determinants of work participation are presented. While non-modifiable determinants include age, sex, ethnicity, and type of spinal cord injury, modifiable factors primarily concern functional ability, motivation, and the availability of workplace accommodations and vocational rehabilitation services. The authors also introduce vocational rehabilitation. They advocate that vocational rehabilitation ideally starts early after the onset of spinal cord injury and should be tailored to the individual needs. In conclusion, current evidence on specific vocational rehabilitation intervention outcomes is sparse, but some beneficial effects of Individual Placement and Support programs have been reported. In the following chapter on coronary heart disease and return to work, *Angelique de Rijk* provides a comprehensive review of the literature. After a cardiac event, up to 80% of employees return to work within 1 year. Cardiac rehabilitation, which focuses on the physical, psychological, and social functioning, contributes to faster return to work. The author argues that specific attention to work-related risk factors might improve the return to work rate and success. The chapter reviews, first, workplace risk factors for cardiac patients; second, factors that prolong sickness absence in cardiac patients; and, third, the effectiveness of return to work interventions for cardiac patients. Many factors are identified, and positive effects of interventions are found for comprehensive rather than unidimensional interventions. The author concludes with a set of key recommendations derived from scientific evidence and expert advice. The chapter by *Akizumi Tsutsumi* sheds light on return to work after stroke, recognized as the single largest cause of severe disability worldwide. The author reports that approximately 40–55% of patients with stroke need active rehabilitation and 60% of stroke survivors need job modification after stroke. Factors associated with return to work include functional recovery, extent of higher brain dysfunction, employer flexibility, and support from family or co-workers. While rehabilitation techniques have been improved and some rehabilitation programs have been shown to be effective, there is a paucity of studies on vocational outcomes after stroke. The author argues that the system of return to work for workers with disabilities, such as disease treatment (including rehabilitation), workplace accommodation, and cooperation and coordination among stakeholders, should be consolidated. Common mental disorders, such as anxiety and depression, are responsible for a significant loss of work capacity. The chapter by *Silje Endresen Reme* takes a close look at barriers and opportunities for work among people with common mental disorders. The chapter starts with describing the consequences of not working and the benefits of staying at or returning to work. Significant barriers and opportunities of return to work from various perspectives are presented, including the individual, health-care, workplace, and societal perspective. The author emphasizes that work (dis)ability is a complex phenomenon that calls for integrated and interdisciplinary solutions. For instance, health-care interventions with an explicit focus on work are crucial, as well as multicomponent interventions that include contact with the workplace. Also, the larger societal context the individual is a part of has a substantial impact on opportunities and barriers for work, particularly the compensation system. The author concludes that legislative changes, as well as larger structural interventions to improve opportunities for work among people with common mental disorders, are not adequately addressed, neither in practice nor in research. In the following chapter, *Dwayne van Eerd and Peter Smith* provide an extensive overview of work-related interventions designed to reduce the burden of work disability due to musculoskeletal disorders. To date, musculoskeletal disorders cause considerable disability and lost productivity in many economic sectors worldwide. The authors also point to some salient topics needing more research, such as the role of sex and gender, or the options of sitting and standing at work. The overview suggests that the seven return to work principles established some years ago continue to be supported by current scientific literature. In particular, consistent support for employers providing work accommodations and communication between health-care providers and the workplace has been found. The authors call for more high-quality studies, given the restricted evidence regarding interventions to reduce the work disability caused by musculoskeletal disorders.

In their chapter on addictive disorders, *Clemens Veltrup and Ulrich John* illustrate the severe consequences of problematic substance use at work, with a particular focus on alcohol intoxication and alcohol dependence. The consequences of problematic substance use for work are mental and physical health problems, but substance misuse may additionally contribute to job loss. The chapter sheds light on organizational, social, and individual risk factors that contribute to the development of addictive disorders. Workplace interventions may help to cope with addictive behavior. To this end, they should include (1) psychosocial interventions concerning substance use problems, (2) substance use-related brief interventions, (3) peer-supported interventions, (4) web-based interventions, (5) mandatory screening, and (6) general health promotion programs. Finally, the chapter points to the important distinction between acute and post-acute treatment programs that support individuals to return to their workplace or to find a new job. In the final chapter of the second part, *Marc Corbiere, Élyse Charette-Dussault, and Patrizia Villotti* provide a comprehensive review of factors for competitive employment for people with severe mental illness. People with severe mental illness face numerous obstacles to obtain and sustain employment in the regular labor market. With work as the cornerstone of recovery, the literature highlights a ceiling effect of job acquisition and brief job tenure for most people with severe mental illness, regardless of the length of follow-up and the number of jobs obtained. Despite the many factors expected to open the doors to the world of work and employment for people with severe mental illness, such as legislation, pension benefits in support of disabled persons, advancement in treatment efficacy, or development of vocational services and programs, these factors did not result in expected success rates, according to the authors' judgment. Job acquisition and job tenure remain major challenges for people with severe mental illness, and these challenges have to be addressed by integrated efforts from all involved stakeholders.

The third and last part of Part II starts with a chapter by *Kari-Pekka Martimo and Esa-Pekka Takala* on the concepts of work ability in rehabilitation. The authors argue that the understanding of work ability exerts an impact on a) what kind of rehabilitation activities are implemented and b) which aspects of these rehabilitation activities are emphasized. In this chapter, eight concepts of work ability are presented and discussed in detail. While in the medical concept of work ability, rehabilitation focuses on restoring health with medical care, the employability concept of work ability includes all actions that help the person to access work, retain employment, and advance in the work career. Alongside the different concepts, work ability can also be viewed as a social construct based on negotiations of different societal levels. Interestingly, emerging integrative concepts emphasize processes of individual and contextual factors that define a person's *capability* to work. The authors conclude that in rehabilitation, a comprehensive concept of work ability should be shared by all stakeholders to develop optimal rehabilitation processes aiming at a common goal. How to facilitate competitive employment for people with disabilities? *Gary Bond, Robert Drake, and Jacqueline Pogue* provide a scholarly review of the history, effectiveness, and current use of Individual Placement and Support, also called IPS-supported employment, with various disability groups. Positive outcomes in improving employment and (cost-)effectiveness have been demonstrated across a variety of clinical, demographic, and socioeconomic groups of people with serious mental illness. IPS is a flexible approach, consisting of eight principles, to helping unemployed people with disabilities gain employment. All involved stakeholders, i.e., clients, practitioners, and program leaders, understand the IPS principles and find them appealing. Recent research on other disability groups, including people with anxiety, depression, posttraumatic stress disorder, developmental disabilities, substance use disorder, and spinal cord injury, has shown promise. The authors recommend that IPS should be offered to all people with serious mental illness and to veterans with posttraumatic stress disorder who want to work competitively. In the following chapter, *Vicki Kristman, Cecile Boot, Kathy Sanderson, Kathryn Sinden, and Kelly Williams-Whitt* develop a new practice-based model of return to work implementation, compare it to existing practice-based models, demonstrate the application of the new model using a case scenario, and indicate how the new model fits with recommendations for best practices from those engaged in return to work on a daily basis. The authors introduce a "Best Practices for Return to Work Implementation Model" that has a holistic approach and consists of three stages involved in best practices for return to work: stay at work and early and prolonged return to work. For all three stages, the authors describe the role of the involved stakeholders; and the workplace's organizational culture and structure are also taken into account. The authors maintain that the model has the capacity to be of value to both researchers and practitioners focusing on the return to work process, regardless of reasons for employee absence or jurisdiction. *Karina Nielsen, Joanna Yarker, Fehmidah Munir, and Ute Bültmann* introduce the IGLOO (Individual, Group, Leader, Organizational and Overarching) contextual factors framework for return to work among workers with mental health problems. The authors identify resources, i.e., factors that facilitate return to work at five levels: the individual (e.g., beliefs about being able to manage a successful return to work, health behaviors), the group (work groups, friends, and family), the leader (line managers and health-care providers who take the lead in supporting workers' return), and the organizational (human resource policies and external organizations) and the overarching context (social security systems). While resources that pertain to the work and nonwork context are discussed, the authors also highlight the importance of understanding how the resources are applied at the different levels. Finally, the authors argue that there is a need to understand how societal factors, such as legislation, culture, and national policies, impact in particular sustainable return to work outcomes. In the following chapter by *Monika Finger and Christine Fekete*, the shift from work reintegration to sustainability of employment is described and illustrated by the case of spinal cord injury (SCI) and acquired brain injury (ABI). While there is an impressive body of research on factors related to return to work after SCI and ABI, evidence on sustained employment applying a life course approach is scarce and mainly available from qualitative research. The authors argue that long-term work trajectories of persons with SCI and ABI are complex and that sustainability may depend on various factors, such as motivation, new employment identities, and supporting family members, employers, and co-workers. On an organizational level, flexible work schedules, adapted task profiles, an accessible workplace, and technical devices were reported as facilitators for sustained employment. The authors conclude that a continuous "person-job-match" monitoring is recommended to properly accommodate the changing abilities after the initial return to work period and to prevent premature labour market exit. The final chapter of this part, written by *Finn Diderichsen*, demonstrates the increasing relevance of investing in integrative, active labour market policies (ALMP) in European countries. The chapter illustrates policy entry points in a model based on the WHO's International Classification of Functioning, Disability and Health (ICF), it describes different profiles of ALMP in European countries, and it presents recent developments that favor activation and motivation rather than protection. ALMP aim at reconciling both the supply with the demand of the labor market and the workplace demands with the employee's work abilities. Several tools are applied by ALMP to increase motivation, qualification, socialization, and networking. The chapter describes tools aiming at the combination of different types of flexibility and security, including "flexicurity." Despite the advantages of ALMP, the challenge remains to enhance individual choice while at the same time to maintain adequate social protection, healthy workplaces, and incentives to work there.

In summary, this book offers a uniquely comprehensive review of current knowledge on the intertwined processes between work and disability. With its many examples of models of good practice, and with its evidence-based policy recommendations, it may help those who are engaged in preventive and rehabilitative efforts to promote employability and sustainable work participation for persons with disability, and to strengthen healthy work in general. With its call for more in-depth knowledge and with its demonstration of controversial topics, it may motivate those who are committed to research to find new solutions to open questions.

References

Loisel P, Anema JR (eds) (2013) Handbook of work disability. Prevention and management. Springer, New York
OECD (2010) Sickness, disability and work: breaking the barriers. A synthesis of findings across OECD countries. Paris. https://doi.org/10.1787/9789264088856-en
Schultz IZ, Gatchel RJ (eds) (2016) Handbook of return to work. From research to practice. Springer, New York
United Nations (2007) Convention on the rights of persons with disabilities. G.A. Res. 61/106. Available from: http://www.un.org/esa/socdev/enable/rights/convtexte.htm
World Health Organization (2001) International classification of functioning, disability and health. WHO, Geneva
World Health Organization (2011) World report on disability. WHO, Geneva

Part I

Occupational Hazards, Impaired Health, and Disability Risk

The Changing Nature of Work and Employment in Developed Countries

Werner Eichhorst

Contents

Introduction	18
Future Trends	18
Job Characteristics, Tasks, and Skill Requirements	19
Forms of Work and Forms of Flexibility	23
Designing Good Institutions	25
The Role of Labor Market Institutions	25
General Principles and Policy Implications	25
Education	26
Labor Market Regulation	28
Social Protection and Active Labor Market Policies	29
Conclusion	30
Cross-References	30
References	31

Abstract

The current public debate about the future of labor in developed countries is characterized by the role of human work in the course of globalization and vast technological changes. While the severe extent of automation is not observed by empirical studies, there probably will be significant changes in the structure of jobs and strengthened inequalities between socioeconomic groups. In this regard, public policy is of decisive importance to shape the quality of jobs and to encounter possible aberrations. The institutions should be aimed at allowing an appropriate balance between flexibility and security as well as achieving a fair distribution of opportunities and risks in the labor market and access to employment. It is essential to focus on the protection of workers instead of jobs themselves and to develop both superior contractual and social protection for

---

W. Eichhorst (✉)
IZA and University of Bremen, Bremen, Germany
e-mail: eichhorst@iza.org

non-standard workers. Additionally, investments in human capital for all types of education and in continuous training are the foundation for future employability.

> **Keywords**
>
> Employment changes · Human work · Polarization · Non-standard employment · Future employability · Active labor market policies · Labor market institutions · Social protection

Introduction

The world of work and employment is constantly changing; however, over the last years, and in the face of a new wave of technological innovation, this long-standing issue has started to attract renewed and additional attention both in the academic and policy community. Against this backdrop, this introductory chapter assesses the recent and expected changes in work and employment, starting from the joint influence of technological progress and globalization but addressing also issues of institutional flexibility and an increasingly diverse workforce. It will then continue to discuss the main policy areas that shape the functioning of labor markets before outlining policy reforms that might be needed and implemented in order to be better prepared for the requirements of the future. The chapter argues for policies that can combine flexibility and security through different mechanisms of protection against labor market risks, rebalancing the role of employment protection, unemployment benefits, active labor market policies, and training. As policy reforms depend on the capacities to adopt and deliver, the paper discusses the preconditions of successful institutional change in a "progressive" direction.

Future Trends

The future of employment is influenced by four main factors that interact with each other: globalization, technology, demographic change, and labor market institutions. Through these factors, future potentials for productive engagement, economic growth, and societal wealth are given, implying also further rises of standards of living, productivity, and good quality jobs. However, there are also risks involved, in particular an increase in inequality or polarization in the world of work as some groups will find it easier to benefit from these opportunities than others. Hence, from a policy point of view, creating or maintaining and adapting inclusive labor markets that provide for access to quality employment are crucial. Taking a broader perspective, one has to acknowledge that despite progressive global economic integration and technological innovation acting as universal driving forces, distinct regional, sectoral, and occupational differences in employment continue to exist. We see specific patterns of diversity in employment patterns, job characteristics, and job quality. The challenges implied by this from the point of view of policymaking are to keep pace with potentially deep and accelerating structural changes in economic activities, with implications also for global value chains and more complex divisions of labor, both locally and globally, and to prepare labor market institutions in a way that they can contribute to positive socioeconomic outcomes. However, specific national circumstances and starting conditions have to be taken into account.

Job Characteristics, Tasks, and Skill Requirements

Technological progress leading to ever-increasing opportunities for automation as well as the global economic integration questions the future existence of routine jobs both in manufacturing and services, i.e., jobs that can easily be automated with available technology or relocated (see in particular Frey and Osborne 2013; Arntz et al. 2016; Nedelkoska and Quintini 2018). This is not only a question of blue collar manufacturing jobs or elementary occupations in some services, but this can also affect medium-skilled white collar work to the extent that available technologies allow for automation and/or relocation to countries with lower costs at given skill levels. Hence, in this segment of employment, either capital will substitute for labor, in particular in high-income countries, or jobs will continue to be relocated to places with lower wages. In other areas there are still good reasons to rely on human work in developed countries (Fig. 1).

As regards high-income countries, these developments imply a continued growth of jobs (and the respective shares of employment) in areas and occupations that are less likely to be automated or offshored to low-wage countries. This is relevant for all jobs that are dominated by tasks that continue to require human abilities such as

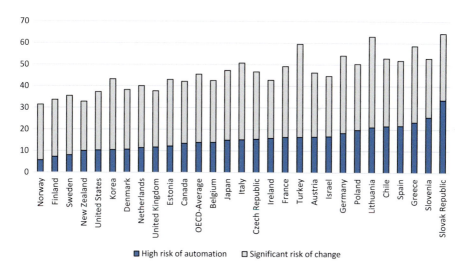

Fig. 1 The automatability potential in OECD countries. (Source: own figure, based on Nedelkoska and Quintini (2018, Fig. 4.2, p. 49))

creativity, social intelligence, judgment, and manual flexibility. This holds for jobs that are mainly characterized by innovation and creativity, coping with complex information and decision-making under conditions of uncertainty as well as interactions between human beings (Brynjolfsson and McAfee 2014; Berger and Frey 2016). These are core human competences that are not likely to be replaced by machines, and stable direct employment will continue to be an option, in particular if high productivity based on specific skills and experiences is required. In general, employment prospects are favorable where human capacities and skills are complementary to technological possibilities. This has specific consequences for skills needed, i.e., the acquisition of skills through different stages of education from general initial education to vocational and tertiary education but also formal and informal learning on the job. Furthermore, companies will have to adjust the organization of work so that skills can be used in the most effective and productive way.

These changes are not something entirely new, and even the potentially disruptive character of digital technologies often assumed has yet to be shown. For the time being, we can rather expect a more evolutionary development along the lines that can already be observed in empirical studies covering the last decades. These studies highlight the growth of knowledge-intensive work, in particular in science, research, and development or creative occupations as well as employment in health, education, and social services, where a strong interactive component is present. In many of these occupations, additional jobs have been created, and working conditions, not least earning potentials, have increased over the last years. The current employment situation is shaped, and the future development will likely continue to be characterized by a strong premium on the capacity to cope with complexities and uncertainty, to innovate, create, and interact, as well as on speedy adjustment or even first-mover advantages. Growth of highly skilled and oftentimes highly paid jobs tends to lead to increased inequality in labor markets. This distinguishes the development in this segment of the labor market from medium-skilled jobs with a predominantly routine-oriented task content which tends to exhibit employment and wage stagnation due to stronger technological rationalization as well as competition from outside. At the same time, more elementary occupations in the service sector that are difficult to automate or offshore due to their personal and local nature can still expand, albeit with less attractive or declining working conditions. Hence, in a stylized fashion, polarization of labor markets results (Autor et al. 2003; Goos et al. 2014). However, polarization is anything but uniform as there are marked differences between countries and periods studied, pointing at the crucial role of the macroeconomic environment on the one hand and institutions on the other hand (Fig. 2).

Taking a global perspective, the positive employment and income situation of the highly skilled in developed countries go along with a stagnation or decline of the economic prospects of the low- and medium-skilled segment of the labor force in high-income countries (Milanovic 2016). At the same time, in many medium-income economies, a new middle class has emerged due to the integration of their countries into the global division of labor.

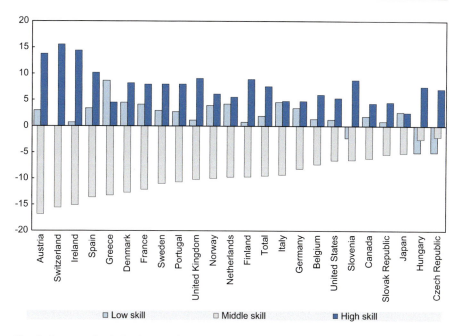

Fig. 2 Patterns of polarization: employment changes in OECD countries, 1995 to 2015. (Source: OECD (2017, Fig. 3.A1, p. 121). Note: percentage point changes in total employment in the respective clusters of ISCO-88 major occupational groups)

Hence, in a situation of increasing technological penetration of production processes in manufacturing and services, we can expect the labor market of the future to rather be dominated by tasks and therefore related job profiles that are characterized by specific human capacities which cannot easily be replaced by technological solutions – at least for the foreseeable future which will, however, still be characterized by a continuing race with or against the machines. Hence, human work that is complementary to technological solutions or is performed in areas quite remote from automatability will become most important. That also means that future jobs, generally speaking, will be more and more shaped by the individuals performing them so that individual skills, capacities, motivation, and experiences are of crucial importance for high productivity, high performance, and effective use of skills (see, e.g., also OECD 2016).

Going beyond these general trends, we can expect that not all sectors and world regions will be affected by the use of the latest technology at the same time and at the same speed as observable in the most advanced sectors, firms, or countries. In fact, there is some room for variation of change and delay as regards the diffusion of technology. Some countries or regions embark on this path somewhat later, and some sectors and firms within sectors are more advanced than others. While this means that first or early mover advantages will not be realized under such circumstances, the asynchronical, significantly delayed implementation of latest technologies gives some time to adjust and catch up. Yet, there is also a risk that the first movers and the regions that agglomerate the most "modern" jobs and firms benefit from the technological opportunities in a disproportionate manner so that others are left behind.

Despite all of this emphasis on productivity increases driven by technological innovations, there is no substantial hint at a structural decline of paid work at a global scale, not even in world regions with high levels of technological penetration. Rather, technological progress that leads to higher productivity, fewer jobs, and lower production costs in highly automatable areas tends to create positive demand effects as well as positive spillover effects in other sectors so that employment grows (Gregory et al. 2019).

Hence, the hypothesis of massive technology-induced net job losses or a new era of mass unemployment due to technological change and automation has still to be proven and will probably not pass the test. For the time being, it seems more plausible to expect continuous change and "creative destruction" with some jobs disappearing, others undergoing more or less fundamental change, and new jobs emerging. That means that if markets and firms can adapt as regards their products and services as well as operational processes and workers' skills can be updated to the demands of the near future, this transformation can be managed successfully. Hence, while changes in employment will occur and are not only inevitable but create new opportunities, the paths labor markets will take can be shaped by policy action (Fig. 3).

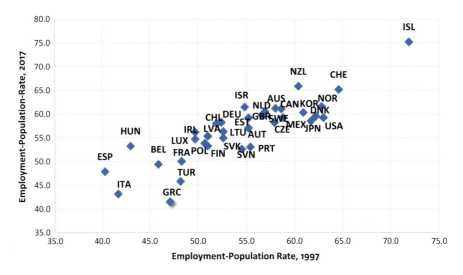

Fig. 3 Long-term developments of employment rates, 1997 and 2017. (Source: own figure, based on ILO (2018))

Forms of Work and Forms of Flexibility

It seems fair to say that modern technologies reducing communication and coordination costs in conjunction with open borders can deepen both global competition and collaboration at the same time. Global integration, technological solutions, but also institutional changes allowing for flexible employment tend to lead to ever more diverse types of employment and a further "fissuring" (Kalleberg et al. 2003) of work as it is organized within and between firms. Current trends in terms of flexible forms of work within and at the margin of firms tend to dissolve clear-cut borders of firms through the emergence of a more flexible workforce that is in one way or another linked to firms, but not integrated fully and permanently while firm staff itself is working in a more flexible manner. This can be observed both in the local context and also at a global scale with more and more elaborate forms of contracting, implying also longer and more complex value chains.

Flexible forms of work will be used when available in order to shift risks and costs of adaptation. This holds for established types of flexible or non-standard employment (ILO 2016; OECD 2015; Kalleberg 2009, 2018; Eichhorst and Marx 2015) such as fixed-term contracts, temporary agency work, but also on-call work or "zero-hour contracts" as well as different types of work performed outside dependent employment such as self-employment with or without employees, freelance work, project-based collaboration, "crowdworking," or even more casual or informal types of work. The latter are still dominant in many low- and medium-income countries, while non-standard forms of work are relevant to a varying degree in developed countries. The use of specific forms of highly fluid or flexible employment options depends on a number of factors such as the labor market regulation in place and the level of economic development but also on labor demand and supply patterns that differ across sectors, countries, and regions. Long-lasting direct, dependent, and formal employment, which is still taken as a benchmark in many contexts due to its above-average working conditions and social protection, will still be a realistic option if skill needs are specific, with experience, motivation, and loyalty being of crucial importance to employers and their business models (Eichhorst and Marx 2015). Staff able to perform such high performance, often demanding jobs is not easily to be found on the external labor market, and these types of tasks cannot be easily outsourced or automated.

In principle, new phenomena such as "crowdworking" using online platforms as intermediaries can question the viability of direct (formal) dependent employment as the dominant category of work in developed countries if one assumes that more and more jobs or tasks can be assigned to providers using online platforms with a global reach. However, to date this phenomenon has only played a minor role, with limited relevance in some professional and service activities, often performed in addition to traditional dependent or self-employed work (see, e.g., Berg 2016; Harris and Krueger 2015; Katz and Krueger 2016; Huws et al. 2018) (Fig. 4).

But employment relations do not only become more diverse as regards the formal contractual status; even with permanent and directly employed staff, intra-firm or internal flexibility is on the increase. This holds for flexible remuneration and

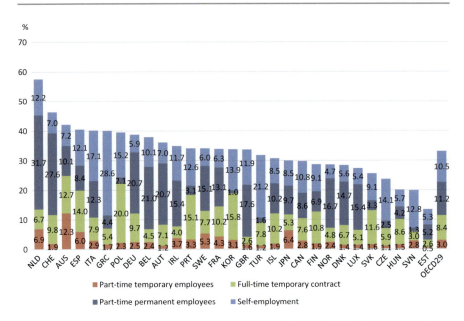

Fig. 4 Non-standard employment by type, in % of total employment, 2013. (Source: own figure, based on OECD (2015, Fig. 4.1, p. 140))

working time and mobile working but also more performance-oriented, project-based work in the framework of stable employment relationships. Apart from this more or less advanced polarization of the labor market, associated with employment opportunities and job quality in terms of pay and employment stability, new risks emerge at workplaces in modern economies. While traditionally, accidents and occupational diseases resulted from physical hazards in sectors such as manufacturing, the highly flexible and productive world of work growing in developed economies exhibits new risks due to intense or even excessive psychosocial demands, resulting in mental health issues if the work environment is not supportive. If work is not organized in sustainable ways, negative side effects of work in terms of psychosocial disorders might become more prevalent in the future (see, among others, Siegrist and Wahrendorf 2016).

This can be monitored using indicators on job quality developed by the OECD addressing job strain that emerges if job demands are excessive and not appropriately balanced by job-related resources (see Cazes et al. 2015; cf. also Eurofound 2016). Hence, given the differences in skills, we will also see a tendency toward inequality in access to good jobs, with some groups being confined to less attractive types of work regarding lower job stability, low pay, or lack of social protection. Again, with well-designed policies, inequalities can be mitigated.

Designing Good Institutions

The Role of Labor Market Institutions

Despite technological innovations and global economic interactions, labor market institutions will continue to play a crucial role. In fact, they will shape the functioning of labor markets also in an era of technological progress and global economic integration. The impact of technology, globalization, and other factors on employment will be mediated through institutions, as this has been the case in the past. In particular, the institutional arrangements of labor markets impact on the directions employment can take, referring to the channels of adjustment via types of employment, working time and wage flexibility, and the skill profiles of the workforce or firm organization, to name just a few. Hence, the quantity and the quality of future jobs depend on institutional conditions, and the better they are suited to future requirements, the better the chances of creating more and better jobs. This is far from uniform. Different national and sectoral employment models have emerged in the past, and in a modified form that is suitable to the current and expected challenges, these paths will be relevant for the future (see, e.g., Amable 2003; Hall and Soskice 2001; Estevez-Abe et al. 2001; Thelen 2014). Of course, path dependency is ambivalent. On the one hand, it makes fundamental changes more difficult; on the other hand, mutually supporting elements can create opportunities that would not be available otherwise.

General Principles and Policy Implications

What can "social progress" mean in the context of the future of work? What would a "progressive" design of labor market institutions and reforms look like? From the point of view adopted in this chapter, this means developing institutions in a way so that "good jobs for all" become more realistic. But what are good jobs? What is a well-designed set of labor market institutions? Good jobs are free of major characteristics of precariousness, such as a lack of stability and a high risk of job loss, a lack of safety measures, and an absence of minimal standards of employment protection; they enable working persons to exert some control on matters such as the place and the timing of work and the tasks to be accomplished, and these jobs place appropriately high demands on the working person, without overtaxing their resources and capabilities and without harming their health; they provide fair employment in terms of earnings and of employers' commitment toward guaranteeing job security; they offer opportunities for skill training, learning, and promotion prospects within a life course perspective, thereby sustaining work ability and stimulating individual development; they prevent social isolation and any form of discrimination and violence;

and they aim at reconciling work and extra-work demands by implementing appropriate rules in day-to-day practices (Eichhorst et al. 2018).

In line with this, good labor market institutions should be able to balance flexibility and security and achieve a fair distribution of opportunities and risks in the labor market and access and mobility to employment. In particular, they should aim at reducing additional layers of polarization and segmentation induced by labor market institutions so that some segments of the labor market enjoy certain privileges and are relatively closed, whereas other employment types are of low job quality, effectively separated by barriers in mobility to good jobs for some groups or establishing labor market segments that do not offer opportunities. Hence, well-designed institutional arrangements should be capable of preparing everyone to participate successfully in the labor market and to achieve a reasonable, acceptable job quality at least at a minimum level, with a realistic chance to move beyond.

While such criteria for good jobs and good institutions can be formulated at a very general level at the global scale, they need to be substantiated in more concrete forms, addressing relevant policy issues and feasible solutions in the respective economic and institutional context.

There are three main areas of intervention in favor of social progress along the lines defined above: (a) education, (b) the regulation of labor markets, and (c) social protection and active labor market policies. These policy areas and potential solutions in these fields are not necessarily new, but there is need and scope for further reform in most countries as regards an updating and modernization of existing routines and rules to match the requirements of a changing world of work.

Education

The first core area of public policy is education. Investment in human capital is of utmost importance when it comes to creating good jobs and ensuring individual employability and productivity in the future. This holds for all types of education and training over the different stages of the life course. From a policy angle, ensuring both the best quality available and universal access, not sacrificing one objective for the other is a major issue in most countries. The main orientation should be to provide, first, a basic skill foundation for everyone to ensure employability in the labor markets of the future and then to provide education that makes the most out of individual potentials to progress further so that tasks that are essential for future non-routine jobs can be performed. In the context of European and other developed countries, this is often described as a "social investment" approach (Hemerijck 2015), pointing at the "investive" character of human capital formation.

1. Quality-oriented early childhood education can provide the basic foundation for benefiting from further education and training, and it has been shown that the cost/benefit balance is particularly positive at this stage, making a case for strong investment in this phase of life (Cunha et al. 2006). As regards schooling, a reliable base of general education is crucial for further skill developments later in life.

2. Vocational education and training can provide an effective pathway from school to work at the upper secondary level (below higher education). The combination of structured learning in firms with more general education in schools helps avoid situations of high youth unemployment and protracted trajectories of transition into the labor market (Eichhorst 2015; Eichhorst et al. 2015). However, it is important to keep vocational training attractive to both apprentices and employers in order to avoid a long-term decline of this medium segment of qualification. This calls for a regular adjustment of occupational profiles and curricula, a viable reconciliation of general and specific skills, as well as for pathways to and combinations with higher education and continuous education to upgrade and update skills acquired via vocational training while also opening up professional careers beyond the medium range.
3. Tertiary education has a particular role, as many of the dynamically growing occupations characterized by creative, innovative, interactive, and analytical features require a high level of qualification, both with professional and general competences. This calls for a sufficiently large academic sector, where access is not limited to privileged groups, and for an articulation of higher education and the world of work.
4. Continuous vocational education and training will be important not just for high-skilled and younger workers that often benefit from employer-led initiatives in this field. Rather, all in the labor force will need a timely adjustment and updating of their skills. Given observable deficits in access of workers to further education in many countries currently, this would involve some systematic engagement of employers, social partners, and the public side (Fig. 5).

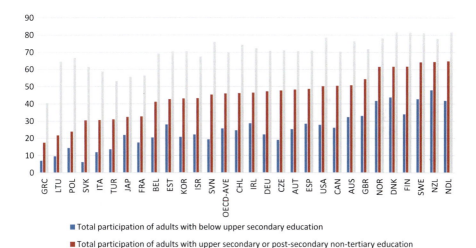

Fig. 5 Participation in continuous training, 2012. (Source: own figure, based on OECD (2018a, Table A7.3, p. 146). Note: reference year for a few countries is 2015)

Labor Market Regulation

Labor market regulation can create an additional, institutionally induced layer of labor market segmentation, resulting in a compartmentalization of employment systems and barriers to mobility. To facilitate mobility and a fair distribution of labor market risks, a balance between flexibility and security is desirable from a social progress point of view. This means moving from protecting (existing) jobs to protecting workers by providing access to good jobs and ensuring a chance for making "good" transitions, i.e., not getting stuck in vulnerable types of employment (Boeri 2011; Scarpetta 2014).

More concretely, as regards the regulation of contract types, this means questioning strict dismissal protection for those on open-ended contracts and developing better protection of those on the different forms of non-standard contracts. While there are substantial reasons for flexible types of employment such as short-term, temporary contracts or agency work, the risks involved with these types of jobs can be minimized by appropriate models of regulation.

It makes sense to smoothen the transition from an entry position, often used to screen workers, into a more stable employment relationship, avoiding one critical moment when employers have to decide on the establishment of a fully protected open-ended contract. This would mean a step-by-step phasing in of employment protection (severance pay) in line with tenure. Irrespective of the existence of both fixed-term and open-ended contracts or if there is only one type of contract, workers with short tenure would acquire some minimum severance pay entitlement, and if employment continues, they would accumulate further entitlements. Overly rigid protection in case of very long tenure can be avoided by introducing a maximum threshold of severance pay after some years of service. Reducing regulatory gaps and differential treatment of contracts will then reduce incentives for contractual arbitrage based on different regulatory requirements and resulting variation in nonwage labor costs. A similar argument can be made about incentives to create formal employment relationships. Reducing the administrative costs of formalization and designing benefits only available in case of formal employment can set incentives to formalize jobs and businesses, making formal employment more attractive to market actors.

Also in the future, some of the new forms of work such as freelance, self-employment, and own-account work will operate outside labor legislation that focuses on the protection of dependent workers. However, some principles of worker protection should also apply to them, in particular in the realm of social protection (rather than labor law) such as unemployment insurance, old age, and disability pensions. This is less clear with regard to typical labor law regulations applying only to dependent employees such as working time and minimum wages (see, e.g., Harris and Krueger 2015).

Last but not least, balancing different aspects of flexibility regarding the organization of work within firms is a core parameter of productive and sustainable employment in the future. This holds for aspects such as working time, availability, and mobile working. In general, these areas require some agreements at the firm level or in relevant subgroups, but there is some scope for broader frameworks set by legislation and/or collective agreements. To create good or better working environments, incentives to firms that care about their employees and limit negative external effects in terms of a termination of employment due to sickness or disability (or in case of dismissals for economic reasons) might be considered (see, e.g., De Groot and Koning 2016; Koning 2016).

Social Protection and Active Labor Market Policies

Unemployment benefits and active labor market policies can be a superior tool compared to employment protection as they protect workers rather than jobs and facilitate a more dynamic employment regime with higher mobility between jobs and between occupations and sectors rather than trying to stabilize existing jobs (Scarpetta 2014).

Unemployment benefit can smooth individual income during phases out of work and stabilize aggregate income in times of recession. If too generous and long lasting, incentives to reenter employment might be weakened, in particular after longer phases out of work. Most developed countries have some system of unemployment benefits in place. Large variations in terms of accessibility, generosity, and availability criteria exist. Furthermore, coverage is far from universal. The situation is even more diverse when looking around the globe. In this policy area, improving legal and actual coverage and establishing a reasonable generosity of unemployment benefits both for short-term and long-term unemployed are part of the policy package that also needs to comprise effective and well-targeted active labor market policies.

When employment protection is eased, hiring and firing of (permanent) staff are potentially encouraged. In such a case, severance pay and/or experience-rated employer contributions to unemployment insurance could act as a layoff tax (Blanchard and Tirole 2007), encouraging a reasonable level of flexibility within the firms over hiring and firing or temporary layoffs and recalls which would lead to external effects to the detriment of unemployment insurance schemes. Hence, in such a model, contributory systems could set incentives for sustainable employment practices favoring internal adjustment and continuous training. The same logic applies to short-time work schemes (i.e., a partial unemployment benefit covering hours not worked and paid) that help stabilize employment relations for a certain period in a situation of a temporary labor demand slump.

As a general principle, social protection via contributory schemes should be extended to all types of workers, not only to certain types of jobs or categories of workers (see OECD 2018b). Of course, this also requires a regular liability to pay taxes and social security contributions by workers (and their employers or clients), irrespective of the type of earnings. A particular challenge arises when it comes to extending benefit coverage in legal and actual terms to workers that are typically not or only partially covered. This holds for non-standard workers in the formal sector when their employment spells are too short to accumulate sufficient entitlements to unemployment insurance benefits, for many forms of self-employed workers or freelancers that operate outside a dependent employment, and for informal workers who still represent a major category of employment in developing and emerging economies. Also in these cases, it makes sense to open up access to contributory unemployment insurance schemes and to means-tested income support funded through taxes. In case of self-employed, freelancers, and crowdworkers using online platforms, there is no employer but clients or intermediaries that should take part of the responsibility to contribute to the insurance fund. This would not only improve the protection side of these workers but also establish a level playing field between firms employing dependent staff and (networks of) freelancers.

A major insight from policy reforms and empirical research over the last decades is that benefit access of working-age people should not be unconditional but depend on the availability for work and participation in active labor market policy measures that can facilitate the (re)entry into work (Martin 2015). The evidence available shows that supportive programs need to be targeted and that in many cases training (of the unemployed, but also those at risk) can generate positive medium- and long-term effects (see Card et al. 2015a, b for overview papers). For more vulnerable people, job search assistance and monitoring are not sufficient.

Conclusion

While change is a permanent feature of work and employment, the current situation is characterized by a massive attention and increasing concerns about the future of work performed by humans in developed countries. Yet, fears of human labor becoming extinct obviously lack backing by empirical studies. However, what is most relevant for shaping the future is to take into account the continuous, incremental, but eventually fundamental change in actual task and job structures. In the future, human work will be characterized by an ever stronger role of interaction, creativity, judgment, and related core human abilities. From an institutional and policy point of view, creating an environment that helps develop and apply these competencies effectively is most crucial for a positive employment scenario. Most importantly, potential divides between socioeconomic groups that can benefit from this change and those unable to cope with these changes should be mitigated by a reconfiguration of labor market institutions and related practices at sectoral or firm level.

Cross-References

- ▶ Investing in Integrative Active Labour Market Policies
- ▶ Trajectories from Work to Early Exit from Paid Employment
- ▶ Trends in Work and Employment in Rapidly Developing Countries

References

Amable B (2003) The diversity of modern capitalism. Oxford University Press, Oxford

Arntz M, Gregory T, Zierahn U (2016) The risk of automation for jobs in OECD countries: a comparative analysis. OECD social, employment and migration working papers 189. OECD Publishing, Paris

Autor DH, Levy F, Richard JM (2003) The skill content of recent technological change: an empirical exploration. Q J Econ 118(4):1279–1334

Berg J (2016) Income security in the on-demand economy: findings and policy lessons from a survey of crowdworkers. ILO conditions of work and employment series 74. ILO, Geneva

Berger T, Frey CB (2016) Structural transformation in the OECD: digitalisation, deindustrialisation and the future of work. OECD social, employment and migration working papers 193. OECD Publishing, Paris

Blanchard OJ, Tirole J (2007) The optimal design of unemployment insurance and employment protection: a first pass. J Eur Econ Assoc 6(1):45–77

Boeri T (2011) Institutional reforms and dualism in European labor markets. In: Ashenfelter O, Card D (eds) Handbook of labor economics, vol 4b. Elsevier, Amsterdam

Brynjolfsson E, McAfee A (2014) The second machine age: work, progress, and prosperity in a time of brilliant technologies. W. W. Norton, New York

Card D, Kluve J, Weber A (2015a) Active labour market policy evaluations: a meta-analysis. Econ J 120(548):452–477

Card D, Kluve J, Weber A (2015b) What works? A meta analysis of recent active labor market program evaluations. IZA discussion paper 9236. IZA, Bonn

Cazes S, Hijzen A, Saint-Martin A (2015) Measuring and assessing job quality: the OECD job quality framework. OECD social, employment and migration working papers 174. OECD Publishing, Paris

Cunha F, Heckman JJ, Lochner L, Masterov DV (2006) Interpreting the evidence on life cycle skill formation. In: Hanushek E, Welch F (eds) Handbook of the economics of education, vol 1. Elsevier, Amsterdam

De Groot N, Koning P (2016) Assessing the effects of disability insurance experience rating: the case of the Netherlands. IZA discussion paper 9742. IZA, Bonn

Eichhorst W (2015) Does vocational training help young people find a (good) job? IZA world of labor 2015-112. IZA, Bonn

Eichhorst W, Marx P (eds) (2015) Non-standard employment. Edward Elgar, Cheltenham

Eichhorst W, Rodriguez-Planas N, Schmidl R, Zimmermann KF (2015) A road map to vocational education and training in industrialized countries. ILR Rev 68(2):314–337

Eichhorst W, Portela de Souza AP et al (2018) The future of work: good jobs for all? The IPSP chapter on employment. In: Rethinking society for the 21st century: report of the International Panel on Social Progress, vol 1. Cambridge University Press, Cambridge

Estevez-Abe M, Iversen T, Soskice D (2001) Social protection and the formation of skills: a reinterpretation of the welfare state. In: Hall PA, Soskice D (eds) Varieties of capitalism: the institutional foundations of comparative advantage. Oxford University Press, Oxford

Eurofound (2016) 6th European working conditions survey. Publications Office of the European Union, Luxembourg

Frey CB, Osborne MA (2013) The future of employment: how susceptible are jobs to computerisation? University of Oxford working paper. Oxford Martin Programme on Technology and Employment, Oxford

Goos M, Manning A, Salomons A (2014) Explaining job polarization: routine-biased technological change and offshoring. Am Econ Rev 104(8):2509–2526

Gregory T, Salomons A, Zierahn U (2019) Racing with or against the machine? Evidence from Europe. IZA discussion paper 12063. IZA, Bonn

Hall PA, Soskice D (2001) An introduction to varieties of capitalism. In: Hall PA, Soskice D (eds) Varieties of capitalism: the institutional foundations of comparative advantage. Oxford University Press, Oxford

Harris SD, Krueger AB (2015) A proposal for modernizing labor laws for twenty-first-century work: the 'independent worker'. The Hamilton Project discussion paper 2015–10. Brookings, Washington, DC

Hemerijck A (2015) The quiet paradigm revolution of social investment. Soc Polit 22(2):242–256

Huws U, Spencer NH, Syrdal DS (2018) Online, on call: the spread of digitally organized just-in-time working and its implications for standard employment models. N Technol Work Employ 33(2):113–129

ILO (2016) Non-standard work around the world: understanding challenges, shaping prospects. ILO, Geneva

ILO (2018) Employment-to-population ratio: ILO modelled estimates, May 2018 on ILOSTAT. ILO, Geneva

Kalleberg AL (2009) Precarious work, insecure workers: employment relations in transition. Am Sociol Rev 74(1):1–22

Kalleberg AL (2018) Precarious lives: job insecurity and well-being in rich democracies. Polity, Cambridge

Kalleberg AL, Reynolds J, Marsden PV (2003) Externalizing employment: flexible staffing arrangements in U.S. organizations. Soc Sci Res 32(4):525–552

Katz LF, Krueger AB (2016) The rise and nature of alternative work arrangements in the United States, 1995–2015. NBER working paper series 22667. NBER, Cambridge

Koning P (2016) Privatizing sick pay: does it work? IZA world of labor 2016–324. IZA, Bonn

Martin JP (2015) Activation and active labour market policies in OECD countries: stylised facts and evidence on their effectiveness. IZA J Labor Policy 4(4):1–29

Milanovic B (2016) Global inequality: a new approach for the age of globalization. Harvard University Press, Cambridge

Nedelkoska L, Quintini G (2018) Automation, skills use and training. OECD social, employment and migration working papers 202. OECD Publishing, Paris

OECD (2015) In it together: why less inequality benefits all. OECD Publishing, Paris

OECD (2016) OECD employment outlook 2016. OECD Publishing, Paris

OECD (2017) OECD employment outlook 2017. OECD Publishing, Paris

OECD (2018a) Education at a glance 2018. OECD Publishing, Paris

OECD (2018b) The future of social protection: what works for non-standard workers? OECD Publishing, Paris

Scarpetta S (2014) Employment protection. IZA world of labor 2014–12. IZA, Bonn

Siegrist J, Wahrendorf M (eds) (2016) Work stress and health in a globalized economy: the model of effort-reward imbalance. Springer International Publishing, Cham

Thelen K (2014) Varieties of liberalization and the new politics of social solidarity. Cambridge University Press, Cambridge

Trends in Work and Employment in Rapidly Developing Countries

3

Martin Hyde, Sobin George, and Vaijayanthee Kumar

Contents

Introduction	34
Labor Force Trends	35
Trends in Unemployment	37
Structural Transformation of the Workforce	38
Declining Employment in Agriculture	39
A Stagnant Industrial Sector?	39
The Growing Service Sector	41
The Growth of Vulnerable Employment	42
Informal Work	46
Conclusion	49
Cross-References	50
References	50

Abstract

Over the few decades, we have seen significant changes in the global economy and, correspondingly, to the nature of work. The emergence of a number of middle-income countries (MICs), such as China and India, on to the global economic stage has drawn millions of workers into the global labor market. Yet the rapid economic growth of these MICs raises a number of questions about type and quality of employment that is being created in these countries and what this

M. Hyde (✉)
Centre for Innovative Ageing, Swansea University, Swansea, UK
e-mail: martin.hyde@swansea.ac.uk

S. George
Centre for Study of Social Change and Development, Institute for Social and Economic Change, Banglore, India
e-mail: sobing@gmail.com

V. Kumar
Indian Institute of Management, Indore, MP, India
e-mail: vaijayanthee86@gmail.com

© Springer Nature Switzerland AG 2020
U. Bültmann, J. Siegrist (eds.), *Handbook of Disability, Work and Health*, Handbook Series in Occupational Health Sciences, https://doi.org/10.1007/978-3-030-24334-0_2

means for the health and well-being of those living and working there. The aim of this chapter is to explore the trends in work and employment in the rapidly developing MICs (Brazil, China, India, Indonesia, Mexico, and the Russian Federation). The data show we can see a number of common trends across the MICs. All have undergone some form of structural transformation which has seen employment in agriculture decline and employment in the service sector grow. However, this has not necessarily led to the growth of good quality jobs. Indeed, the data point to rising unemployment in some MICs and the persistence of a high rate of employment in the informal sector. Moreover, there are worrying signs that gender inequalities in labor market participation are widening in a number of MICs. There are concerns that these trends could lead to an increase in work-related disability and poor health across the developing countries.

Keywords

Developing countries · Labur market · Structural transformation · Informal work · Vulnerable employment

Introduction

Over the few decades, we have seen significant changes in the global economy and, correspondingly, to the nature of work. The emergence of a number of middle-income countries (MICs), such as China and India, on to the global economic stage has drawn millions of workers into the global labor market and shifted the poles of global economy away from its traditional centers in the Global North. Yet the rapid economic growth of these MICs raises a number of questions about type and quality of employment that is being created in these countries and what this means for the health and well-being of those living and working there (Hyde and Theorell 2018). Understanding the nature of employment and work in these countries is essential if we are to ensure that economic growth does not come at the cost of human health and disability. As the WHO Commission on Social Determinants of Health (CSDH) has clearly stated, the creation of fair employment and decent work are key factors for reducing inequalities in health both within and between nations (CSDH 2008). This goal has been enshrined in the UN's Sustainable Development Goals which have identified the need to "Promote sustained, inclusive and sustainable economic growth, full and productive employment, and decent work for all" for all countries. Encouragingly there is also evidence that there is now greater awareness about occupational health and safety risks in developing countries (Kortum and Leka 2014). However, many workers in these countries do not have decent work and face serious threats to their health and an increased risk of work-related disability as a consequence. Hence the aim of this chapter is to provide an overview of the trends in employment and work in the rapidly developing MICs in order to better grasp the occupational health and psychosocial work environment challenges that these workers face.

Most developing countries have pursued some form of development model based around economic growth. These models vary due to the incorporation of different approaches, such as the degree of openness or closeness to globalization, opportunities for regional integration, reliance on the private sector or state sector as the key driver for growth, use of technology, and more recently, changes in social policy and the creation of a more flexible labor market. All these factors have had both positive and negative effects on occupational structures. These differences notwithstanding, we can see a number of common trends across the MICs. All have undergone some form of structural transformation which has seen employment in agriculture decline and employment in the service sector grow. However, the proportions employed in industry have remained relatively stable, leading to concern that a number of countries are undergoing "premature deindustrialization" (Kuhn et al. 2018). In addition, there are fears that the types of jobs that are being created in these countries, especially in the service sector, are characterized by less contract duration and job security, more irregular working hours (both in terms of duration and consistency), increased use of third parties (temporary employment agencies), growth of various forms of dependent self-employment (like subcontracting and franchising), and also bogus/informal work arrangements (i.e., arrangements deliberately outside the regulatory framework of labor, social protection, and other laws) (Quinlan 2015). Consequently, a large share of the labor force remains employed in low productivity activities in the informal sector or is trapped in vulnerable forms of employment. Many are self-employed, work in a household enterprise without outside workers, or work in a family business without pay. Low labor participation rates and high unemployment are also issues of concern; women, in particular, are less likely to enter the labor force, while in many countries, a growing number of youth are filling the ranks of the unemployed. In addition, with the exception of a minority of formal sector workers, most workers are vulnerable to abuse, poor working conditions, risk of exploitation, and lack of income protection (Cho et al. 2012).

Labor Force Trends

About 75% of the global labor force lives and works in developing countries. This figure has remained remarkably stable over the past few decades. However, this apparent stability masks some regional and international variation within the developing economies (Kuhn et al. 2018). This is to be expected as developing countries are not a homogenous group but are divided by geography, demography, culture, political systems, and income level. To address this heterogeneity, most analyses focus on clusters or groups of developing countries. The most common approach is to group together countries by region, e.g., Asia, Latin America and the Caribbean, etc. This is quite a natural approach as it fits with the way most of us are taught to see the world, e.g., as continents on maps. However, relying simply on geographical proximity is problematic as countries within a region may still differ in terms of their economic growth, labor market composition, and employment policies. To avoid this issue, we have decided to use the World Bank's schema for country classifications by income level. More precisely we have taken the middle-income countries (MICs) as our base, as these are the countries that have seen the greatest economic growth within the developing world. The World Bank classifies lower middle-income economies as those with a GNI per capita between $1,026 and $4,035; upper middle-income economies are those with a GNI per capita between $4,036 and $12,475; high-income economies are those with a GNI per capita of $12,476 or more. However, even within this group, there are wide disparities in the rates of growth. Over the past decade, a number of alternative classifications have emerged to try to capture these emerging or newly industrializing countries, such as BRIC (Brazil, Russia, India, and China), BRICS (BRIC + South Africa), MINT (Mexico, Indonesia, Nigeria, and Turkey), and CIVETS (Colombia, Indonesia, Vietnam, Egypt, Turkey, and South Africa) (Frank 2013; Reuters Staff 2010). However, for the purposes of this chapter, we have taken an empirical approach and will focus, when possible, on the six countries which have had the greatest increase in GDP between 1991 and 2017. These are Brazil, China, India, Indonesia, Mexico, and the Russian Federation, which, reassuringly, are the countries that tend to feature in these other schemata.

As Table 1 shows, in contrast to the aforementioned stability of the MICs as a whole, we can see quite wide disparities in the change in the size of the labor market between these six emerging economies. Here we can see that the Russian Federation experienced an actual decrease in their labor force, while in Mexico the labor force almost doubled in size over this 27-year period.

However, the key issue is not the size of the labor force but the rate of labor market participation in the population, specifically the extent to which there are any gender inequalities in participation. In many developing countries, women often work on farms or in other family enterprises without pay, and others work in or near their homes, mixing work and family activities during the day. Even in the MICs, access to well-paid jobs for women remains unequal. Hence, female labor market participation is often seen as good indicator of the development of a country and its commitment to addressing gender inequalities. Moreover, a low female participation rate drives adult employment rates down and keeps an important source of human capital idle. However, as we can see from the data in Fig. 1, although labor market participation has improved for women in some of the rapidly developing countries

Table 1 Size of the labour market in rapidly developing countries 1991–2017

	1991	2017	Change 1991–2017 (%)
Brazil	61,720,617	104,278,222	68.95
China	648,168,644	786,738,207	21.38
India	335,309,031	520,194,130	55.14
Indonesia	76,000,177	127,110,965	67.25
Mexico	31,461,036	58,072,901	84.59
Russian Federation	76,344,438	75,638,703	−0.92

Source: ILOSTAT

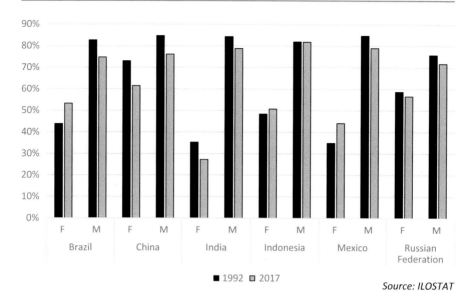

Fig. 1 Labour force participation rates for men and women in rapidly developing countries. (Source: ILOSTAT)

since the early 1990s, e.g., Brazil and Mexico, it is still way below than the rate for men. More worrying is that in a number of the countries, notably India which was already at a low level in 1992, the rate has actually fallen over the past few decades.

Trends in Unemployment

Despite showing signs of recovering from the impact of the global financial crisis, MICs have experienced a significant increase in unemployment rates between 2014 and 2017. This has again been driven by major economic downturns, in part due to the commodity price slump in many large economies, such as Brazil and the Russian Federation (Kuhn et al. 2018). Here it appears that the faster growing economies have been harder hit. By 2017 the unemployment rate had risen to 6.3% in the upper MICs, while it has remained relatively stable at around 4.5% in the lower MICs since 2010. Within the rapidly developing economies, we can see that there are very different trends and levels in the rate of unemployment (see Fig. 2). While unemployment rates in India and China have remained very stable, at around 4–5%, unemployment rates have been much more volatile in other countries. The mid-1990s was a notable period of high unemployment in the Russian Federation with rates near 14%. However, by 2017 these were just slightly higher than those in China. Conversely the rates in Brazil have dramatically shot up, nearly doubling from around 7% in 2014 to 13% in 2017. Clearly this poses issues for those seeking employment in this country.

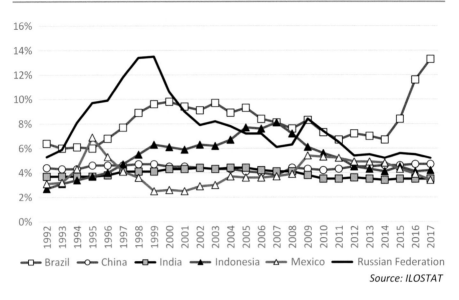

Fig. 2 Trends in the unemployment rate in rapidly developing counties 1992–2017. (Source: ILOSTAT)

This is especially so as unemployment may be linked to an increase in informal employment and vulnerable employment in developing countries. In a situation of job scarcity, workers may be forced to accept informal, precarious, or dangerous jobs. Hence, unemployment rates can impact on overall employment quality and the presence of informal work arrangements, within which workers typically lack adequate social protection, are generally paid less, and have poor working conditions (Janta et al. 2015).

Structural Transformation of the Workforce

Over the last few decades, the adoption of various models of development, technological advancements, and industrial changes have all reshaped the landscape of labor and led to a structural transformation of the economies in the rapidly developing MICs. The process of structural transformation is typically characterized by the gradual reallocation of production factors from traditional activities (e.g., agriculture and low value-added manufacturing) to modern activities (e.g., high value-added manufacturing and services). This shift from primarily mining, forestry, and agricultural economies to industrial economies with a growing service sector has modified the composition and profile of the labor force and led to a redefinition of the labor market. At the same time, they have spurred changes in the structure and composition of the workforce, in the organization of work, as well as in labor relations, and they have further given rise to a new international division of labor. Across all income groups, an ever-increasing number of workers in the MICs are projected to be employed in the service sector, while the employment share in agriculture is set to continue its long-term downward trend. Furthermore, the share of manufacturing employment is expected to continue its decline in upper MICs and to grow only marginally in lower middle-income ones, raising concerns about "premature deindustrialization," in which the MICs are seeing declining shares of industrial employment at earlier stages of economic development compared to the high-income countries. For the MICs as a whole, the proportion of the workforce employed in agriculture has fallen from 51% of the workforce in 1991 to 27% in 2017. Conversely the proportions employed in the service sector have grown from 27% in 1991 to 48% in 2017. However, the proportions employed in industry have remained relatively constant over the period at between one-fifth and one-quarter of the workforce. There are concerns that rather than leading to the growth of higher quality, stable employment in the formal sector, as happened in the high-income countries, this process of premature deindustrialization could lead to the growth of informal and vulnerable employment in the developing economies (World Employment and Social Trends 2018).

Declining Employment in Agriculture

However, as Fig. 3 shows, these aggregate figures mask wide international variations. Although all countries have seen a decline in the proportion of those employed in agriculture, the relative size of the agricultural workforce remains higher in India (42%) and Indonesia (31%) than the average for the MICs. Conversely rates started low and remained low in Russia, falling from 10% to 7% over 27 years. Among the most rapidly growing countries, China has experienced the fastest fall in the relative size of the agricultural workforce. In 1991 rates were close to those in Indonesia, but by 2017 they had fallen to the same level of Mexico and Brazil.

In many respects this is seen as a good news story for worker's health. Agricultural work is often very physically demanding and dangerous. The rate of fatal occupational accidents is generally higher in the agricultural sector than in the industrial or service sectors in the lower and middle income countries (Hämäläinen et al. 2017). Those employed in this area can be at risk of exposure to chemicals and other toxins (Abhilash and Singh 2009) as well as living in poor conditions and can have higher rates of poor health behaviors (Roy and Chowdhury 2017).

A Stagnant Industrial Sector?

There was concern throughout the 1990s that through the process of economic globalization, multinational corporations would shift their manufacturing capacity from the developed economies to the developing economies in order to capitalize on lower wages and weaker employment protection in those countries (Ahasan 2001; Dicken 2007; Kamuzora 2006). The extent to which this was actually borne out in practice is still being debated. However, these debates highlight the fact that the

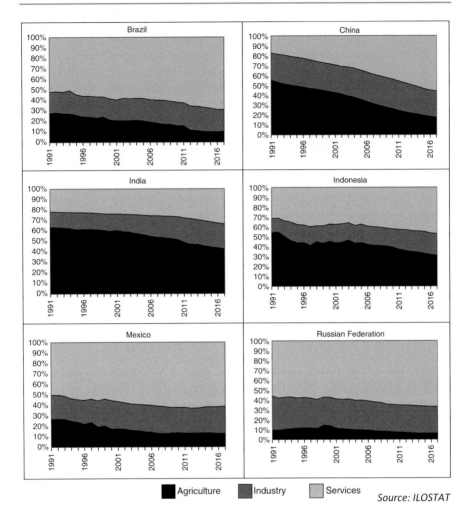

Fig. 3 Employment in agriculture, industry, and services in rapidly developing middle-income countries 1991–2017. (Source: ILOSTAT)

process of industrialization of the developing economies took place within a radically different world than that of the higher income countries. The process of structural change followed by many developing countries has often differed significantly from the path taken by developed countries over the past century. In particular, compared to developed countries, the majority of developing countries, especially those in Latin America and Africa, have witnessed contracting shares of both employment and output in the manufacturing sector at relatively lower levels of income per capita (Rodrik 2016). This phenomenon of "premature deindustrialization" has been found to have important consequences for both the speed of development and the type of employment created.

As already noted when we look at the MICs as a whole, it appears as if the relative size of the industrial workforce has remained quite stable across the 27-year period. However, when we look at the trends for the individual countries in Fig. 3, we can see that this appearance of stability belies a great deal of individual variation. There has been a notable convergence to the mean among the individual countries. For example, 34% of Russian workers were employed in industry in 1991 compared to 15% in India. By 2017 the figures were 27% and 24%. Hence the extent to which these countries are experiencing premature deindustrialization differs widely. However, this does not mean that all the jobs that are created in these emerging industrial sectors are good quality jobs. Figures from India show that while the incidence of fatal as well as nonfatal accidents has declined from 65.59 per 1000 persons in 1980 to 0.90 in 2011, the proportion of fatal injuries has increased from 0.2% in 1980 to 5.4% in 2006 and 10% in 2011. Also, while relatively few studies have reported statistics on occupational diseases, figures that exist show that between 38 and 55% of workers in slate pencil and precious/semiprecious stone manufacturing suffer from silicosis, 30–49% of workers in textile and jute manufacturing report byssinosis, and the prevalence of asbestosis has been reported to be 3–9% among workers involved in its manufacture (Suri and Das 2016). A key reason for the persistence of these hazardous jobs in developing countries is that liberalized trade has come together with a transfer of obsolete and hazardous technologies and machinery; relocation of occupational hazards, such as hazardous chemicals, new work, and organizational processes; and an increase in assembly line, low-quality and precarious jobs (Kortum et al. 2010).

The Growing Service Sector

While employment in agriculture is falling and employment in industry is stagnant or only slowly expanding, the picture is reversed when we look at the relative growth of employment in the service sector (Fig. 3). There is a clear group of countries, Russia, Brazil and Mexico, which already had a relatively well-established service sector in 1991. Still, all three countries saw an increase, and, for example, by 2017 almost 70% of the workforce in Brazil was employed in this sector. However, although all countries saw an expansion of this sector, the growth was much faster in China which went from having the lowest level of service sector (17%) in 1991 to having rates comparable to Mexico, Russia, and Brazil by 2017 (56%). At the other end of the scale, the relative size of the service sector in India has remained stable, and, as a consequence, it is falling behind the wider group of MICs.

This shift from employment in agriculture to services is often heralded as a positive development both for the wider economy, leading to the growth of productive jobs in the services sector, and for workers escaping the back-breaking work in the countryside. However, for many developing and emerging countries, this shift has been associated with employment growth in the low-productivity services sectors, such as the retail trade, often as informal own-account workers or casual workers, where working conditions are often poor (Cho et al. 2012; Kuhn et al. 2018). Perhaps the clearest example of this has been the growth in call centers throughout the MICs. These have been called "electronic sweatshops" due to limited task variety, little control over when to take calls and how long to spend on them, and other restricting circumstances (Lin et al. 2009; Sprigg and Jackson 2006; Sprigg et al. 2003, 2007). These conditions have been shown to lead to inadequate sleep, job stress, and poor physical health among Indian call center workers (Rameshbabu et al. 2013).

Hence, although these figures point to a trend toward the structural transformation of these rapidly developing MICs, with a shift from largely agrarian economies to a growing service sector, we must take into account the impact on forms of employment and working conditions. Such a transformation will only lead to improvements in living standards if it can generate more and better jobs. However, as we have seen the rapid growth of ICT services in recent years in some emerging countries, notably India has not generated sustainable employment opportunities or high-quality jobs for the large majority of the population (Kuhn et al. 2018).

The Growth of Vulnerable Employment

Across the globe, millions are trapped in vulnerable employment positions due to the sociopolitical and economic status of the country. Although precarious employment helps deal with the growing issue of unemployment, it leaves the "vulnerable" workers suffering from uncertainty and often deplorable working conditions. The ILO (2018b) defines vulnerable workers as "Own-account workers and contributing family workers [who] have a lower likelihood of having formal work arrangements, and are therefore more likely to lack elements associated with decent employment, such as adequate social security and a voice at work." Lack of a decent job with a decent wage, security, health and safety, and access to fundamental rights are becoming universally distressing issues that demand urgent attention. Beyond this, a vulnerable worker is likely to experience job insecurity and/or find themselves caught in a series of ambiguous employment relationships. They also lack access to social protection and benefits usually associated with employment. They also suffer from low pay and face substantial legal and practical obstacles to joining a trade union and bargaining collectively. Finally, such workers do not get regular jobs even after years of service and acquiring skills, and they end up being unable to escape temporary work (Zhou 2006).

The progress toward reducing vulnerable employment across the world has stalled since 2012. In 2017, around 42% of workers worldwide are estimated to be in vulnerable forms of employment. This rate is expected to remain particularly high in the developing and emerging countries, at above 76% and 46%, respectively. Of greater concern, there are fears that this trend might go into reverse with the number of people in vulnerable employment projected to increase by 17 million per year in 2018 and 2019. Workers in vulnerable forms of employment are typically subject to high levels of precariousness, in that they are more likely to be informally employed, have fewer chances to engage in social dialogue, and are less likely to benefit from job security, regular incomes, and access to social protection than their wage and salaried counterparts (Kuhn et al. 2018).

The proportion of male workers who can be classified as in vulnerable employment has fallen across the middle-income countries as a whole over the past 28 years. However, the rates are still very high, and nearly every second male worker was still in vulnerable employment in 2017. Moreover, these average rates mask wide international variations among the fastest-growing middle-income countries. It is clear from the figures that the levels of vulnerable employment are much higher in India and have not changed much over 1991, remaining at around 80% of the male workforce. At the other end of the scale, the rates of vulnerable employment are lowest in Russia, and, although there has been a slight increase, it has remained under 10% of the workforce. The levels and trends for women are very similar to those for men (Fig. 4). Overall the rates have fallen since 1991 in all countries except Russia.

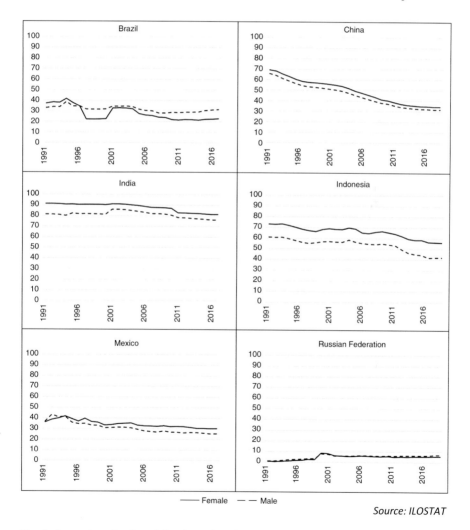

Source: ILOSTAT

Fig. 4 Proportion of male and female workers in vulnerable employment in rapidly developing countries 1991–2017. (Source: ILOSTAT)

However, the rates remain alarmingly high in India (81%) and Indonesia (56%). As the term suggests, these workers are very often found in the lowest level of the occupational hierarchy with appalling conditions at work and limited or no access to social security (see Box A for a more detailed review of vulnerable employment in India).

These poor working conditions coupled with being in a weak bargaining position mean that many vulnerable workers face exposure to occupational health hazards (Quinlan 2015).

Box A. Vulnerable Employment in India

One of the most significant challenges faced by India is of growing incidences of precarious employment across many sectors (Sapkal and Sundar 2017). Although neoliberal economists argue that precarious jobs can act as a springboard for economic growth, however, it has proven to be a great risk to the nation's economic growth and development (Sundar 2012). As nonstandard forms of employment, including contract labor, informal employment, and involuntary temporary and involuntary part-time work, continue to rise in India, fundamental questions about the social costs of economic growth are being asked.

With a rapid wave of liberalization and privatization beginning in the 1990s, India witnessed the entry of MNC's and accelerated globalization which created a boom in vulnerable jobs. It is well documented that nearly 81% of all employed Indians earn their living by working in the informal sector, with only 6.5% in the formal sector and 0.8% in the household sector (International Labour Organization 2018c). In fact, the ILO report suggests that the Asia-Pacific region will add 23 million jobs between 2017 and 2019, aided by employment growth in South Asian nations, especially India; however, a lot of jobs being created are of poor quality despite strong economic growth, and some 77% of workers in India will have vulnerable employment by 2019 (Kuhn et al. 2018).

The vast majority of workers in India represent the informal/unorganized sector. The shift from agricultural jobs has not brought any respite as most of the workers moved to the industries such as construction and manufacturing in the recent years, which is propelled by the high rates of internal migration in India (Agrawal and Chandrasekhar 2015). According to latest National Sample Survey Office (NSSO) estimates, the construction sector is one of the most predominant sectors employing labor migrants and is also a sector which has seen a rapid increase in employment in the recent years (Srivastava and Sutradhar 2016). What is appalling is that most of the new jobs being created in the formal sector are actually informal because the workers do not have access to employment benefits or social security (ILO Country Office for India 2016). In India, evidence shows people enter the informal economy not by

(continued)

choice but because of lack of opportunities in the formal economy and the absence of other means of livelihood (Woetzel et al. 2017). Moreover, the numbers stuck in precarious work in the Indian public sector are far higher than in the private sector. This raises the question why the Indian government has not taken action on this vital issue to protect the "have not" workers.

Vulnerable employment and informal jobs often intersect with other forms of disadvantage posing even greater threats to health and well-being. Studies show that women and children employed in manufacturing suffer from lower wages, less control over decision-making, and the risk of sexual harassment (Mandal 2009; Saiyed and Tiwari 2004). Children engaged in the manufacturing sector often work for 6 h or more per day in poorly ventilated, dark, unhygienic, and dusty conditions (Tiwari and Saha 2014). Exposure to such hazardous conditions, especially for those so young, is a cause for concern in a country that already has a high level of work-related disease and injury. It is estimated that the annual incidence of occupational disease in India is between 924,700 and 1,902,300 and results in around 121,000 deaths (Leigh et al. 1999). The rates of occupational injury are even higher. Based on the survey of agriculture injury incidence, Mohan and Patel (1992) estimated annual incidence of 17 million injuries per year (two million of which were moderate to serious) and 53,000 deaths per year in agriculture alone.

The union and the state governments in India engage in labor regulation and follow established labor laws. However, most labor laws save a few like the Minimum Wages Act of 1948, cover workers in the organized sector, that is, workers in the industrial establishments, shops, and commercial establishments employing 10 or more workers (Papola et al. 2008). The Indian Planning Commission has proposed several measures to enhance the welfare of workers in the area of occupational safety and health (Joseph et al. 2009). However, in spite of this, the intricacies of labor laws are more than often used by the rich and the powerful to either hinder welfare measures or else prolong adjudication to the detriment of vulnerable workers like contract and informal workers who are underprivileged and insecure (Kumar 2015).

It is time to expose the deplorable situation of vulnerable workers. The laws and regulations need rethinking and reforms to adequately address the present and emerging employment challenges ensuring basic fairness and security to workers and balancing the interests of workers and employers.

For example, many farmers in Latin America and the Caribbean combine subsistence production with temporary wage labor in more developed enterprises. However, these jobs tend to be characterized by hazardous working conditions and low pay. Hence, even though, as we have seen earlier in the chapter, the proportion of those employed in agriculture countries like Brazil and Mexico have declined, these new working patterns have led to a change in the epidemiological profiles of agricultural laborers and subsistence farmers. Nowadays traditional health risks such as malnutrition, parasitism, and endemic diseases are found side by side with new problems such as occupational cancers and musculoskeletal diseases (Pan American Health Organization Program on Workers' Health 2001). In addition to this, the high level of job insecurity and weaker bargaining power among vulnerable workers has also encouraged widespread presenteeism in many countries, both sickness presenteeism (when workers go to work when ill) and long hour presenteeism (when additional unpaid hours are worked because it is "expected" or workers fear losing their job) (Cooper and Lu 2016; Evans-Lacko and Knapp 2016; Quinlan 2015). This is a concern as studies have shown that presenteeism increases the risks of poor health for the worker (Lu et al. 2013; Wang et al. 2010) and also can also have wider health effects, e.g., transmitting infections and illnesses to other employees or customers.

Informal Work

The ineffectiveness of the global economy to create high-quality jobs has led to the rapid growth of the informal employment in developing (and increasingly in developed) countries. The informal economy comprises more than 60% of the global labor force and more than 90% of micro and small enterprises (MSEs) worldwide. However, this is a very diverse "economy" which manifests itself in a variety of forms across and within economies. According to the ILO, informal work refers to all economic activities by workers and economic units that are not covered or insufficiently covered by formal arrangements either in law or in practice. Hence, as minimum standards for working conditions tend to be defined only for the formal sector, those working in the informal sector are not protected by any national labor laws. They also do not receive employer-based health insurance or pensions. The International Conference of Labour Statisticians (2003) defines informal workers as (1) own-account workers and employers in their own informal sector enterprises; (2) contributing family workers; (3) members of informal producers' cooperatives; and (4) employees holding informal jobs. Across the developing countries there appears to have been a steady rise in the informal labor market.

Developing countries have higher shares of informal employment than developed countries. Although they represent 82% of world employment, 93% of the world's informal employment is in developing countries. More than two-thirds of the employed population in developing countries are in informal employment, while less than one-fifth of the employed population are in developed countries (International Labour Organization 2018b). In sub-Saharan Africa, the informal sector is growing. Around 60% of the working population in Africa are in the informal sector. However, this varies widely across the continent from 34% in South Africa to around 90–95% in Benin, Chad, and Mali (Eijkemans 2001). Across Latin America and the Caribbean, the incidence of informality also remains high. The mean share of informal employment in total employment across countries in the region is around 58%, ranging from 25% in Uruguay to over 83% in Bolivia. This share is also high in countries with relatively higher levels of income, such as Chile, Brazil, and Argentina, where it stands above 40%, exceeding 53% in Mexico and 60% in Colombia. In addition, in some countries, including Mexico, Paraguay, and, to a lesser extent, Brazil, the incidence of informal jobs is also significant among formal enterprises (Kuhn et al. 2018; Quinlan 2015). Similar trends are evident in the Russian Federation where temporary employment rose from around 2% in 1992 to over 14% in 2008, though it then declined to 8% in 2011. However, much of this temporary employment is informal. In 2002, 65% of all informal employees were employed on a fixed-term, project-based, or casual basis although this had fallen marginally to 59%. In 2002, (International Labour Organization 2016). Overall, the data on trends over time for selected MICs (Fig. 5) show that the rates of informal employment have remained relatively stable over the past decade. Only in Vietnam has there been a discernible fall, but this has merely returned the rate to what it was before the global financial crisis.

It needs to be noted that there is a high degree of overlap between informal, precarious, and vulnerable employment (International Labour Organization 2016; Quinlan 2015). For example, even if there are fewer women than men in informal employment, women in the informal economy are more often found in the most vulnerable situations, for instance, as domestic workers, home-based workers, or contributing family workers, than their male counterparts (Kuhn et al. 2018).

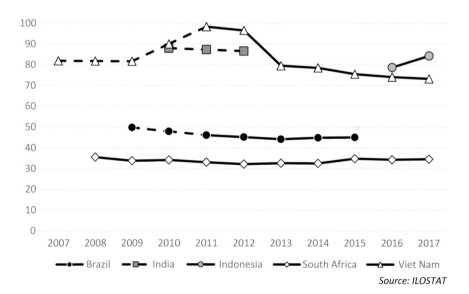

Fig. 5 Informal employment as a percent of employment for selected middle-income countries (%). (Source: ILOSTAT)

Box B. Informal Work in India

The informal sector is an integral part of Indian economy. It generates about 60% of the national income, and of 88 million women workers, only 4.5 million work in the organized sector. The informal economy and employment in the informal sector have been growing in India, and several studies have indicated the expansion of informal employment in India and growing informality of work in both formal and informal sectors subsequent to the introduction of labor market flexibilization policies, which are part of the economic reform project in India (George 2016; Ghosh 2008; Goldar and Aggarwal 2010; Maiti and Mitra 2010).

Recent NSSO data on employment and unemployment (2012–2013) show that only 13% of the Indian workforce had minimum social security entitlements such as provident funds, pension, gratuity, health care, and maternity benefit. We can, hence, comfortably, say that as much as 83% of the Indian workforce is in the category of informal workers. The sectors, which have the highest share of informal employment, were construction (99%); agriculture, accommodation, and food service activities (98%); and allied activities (96%). The extent of informality could be understood from the share of workers who did not have any social security entitlements and other statutory benefits. As the data shows, nearly 72% of the Indian workforce did not have any social security benefits, and their share was 80% rural and 63% in urban India (see George and Sinha 2018). Similarly, George and Sinha (2018) noted that 85% of workers in rural and 72% in urban India did not receive formal employment contracts; 70% did not have paid leaves, and 32% in rural and 12% of workers in urban areas had daily basis wages. Most unfortunately there is a substantial wage gap between regular and casual workers in both rural and urban India (Papola and Kannan 2017). Precarious and atypical employment increased in formal sector as well. As per the data presented by Papola and Kannan (2017) based on the NSSO surveys, informal employment in formal sector was nearly 51% of the formal sector in 2009–2010, which increased to 56% in 2012. Similarly, unionization declined in India (George and Sinha 2018). According to the Ministry of Labour, only 1% of the Indian workforce is unionized, and about 97% of the membership is in the formal sector. The presence of trade unions or other forms of workers collective is minimal in the informal sector, where labor right violations are rampant (George and Sinha 2018).

We have also examined the health protection schemes available to the workers to shed light on the direct interconnectedness of informality and health protection. Nearly 77% of workers in rural and 72% in urban areas are not covered under any health insurance scheme. While employees in the organized sector were covered under the employer's health insurance scheme, public sector continues to be the major provider of health insurance in the informal sector. However, as already indicated, the coverage is lower (20%).

Conclusion

The vast majority of occupational health and work environment research has been undertaken in the high-income countries of the developed world. However, nearly three-quarters of the global workforce are in the developing countries. The Chinese workforce alone exceeds that of the European Union. The rapid economic growth that these countries have experienced has the potential to lift millions out of poverty and to create decent jobs for the growing global workforce. However, until relatively recently, tackling psychosocial risks in the workplace and occupational health has not been a priority in developing countries because of competing social, economic, and political challenges (Nuwayhid 2004). Therefore, if we are to successfully meet the UN Sustainable Development Goal to "Promote sustained, inclusive and sustainable economic growth, full and productive employment, and decent work for all," we need to better understand and engage with the labor market and employment conditions in the developing countries.

What the figures in this chapter show is that there has been a significant growth in the size of the labor market across the rapidly developing MICs. This could in part be due to the structural transformation that has occurred throughout the developing world as more and more people are leaving agricultural work to find work in the industrial and, rapidly expanding, service sector. However, this has not necessarily led to the growth of good quality jobs. Indeed, the data point to rising unemployment in some MICs, notably Brazil, and the persistence of a high rate of employment in the informal sector. Moreover, there are worrying signs that gender inequalities in labor market participation are widening in a number of MICs. Also, although we have presented the data for the different dimensions of employment separately, in the real world, there are significant intersections between them. It is those who are the most disadvantaged, often women and children, who will be most likely to engage in informal and/or hazardous work, which, in turn, is likely to cause injury and/or disease and will, consequently, most likely lead to increased poverty, creating a vicious cycle. On the basis of these trends, it is possible that we are facing a real epidemic of occupationally related health and disability across the developing countries.

It is encouraging that there is a growing awareness of the threats to health posed by working conditions in the developing countries. Organizations such as the ILO and Women in Informal Employment: Globalizing and Organizing (WIEGO) have an active presence in many countries and are working with employers, policy makers, and workers to improve working conditions. However, more needs to be done. In many countries, there are neither the resources nor the institutional structure to deal with the control of occupational hazards. Services are also scarce because many managers and employers have failed to recognize the relationship between the workplace, health, and development. We also face a huge data deficit in these countries, many of whom do not regularly collect data on working conditions. In order to better advocate for improvements in the quality of work, we need the sort of robust data and analyses that has been carried out in the high-income countries over the past few decades. Without this hard evidence, it will be a challenge to convince policy makers and practitioners to take action.

Cross-References

▶ Investing in Integrative Active Labour Market Policies
▶ Policies of Reducing the Burden of Occupational Hazards and Disability Pensions
▶ The Changing Nature of Work and Employment in Developed Countries

References

Abhilash P, Singh N (2009) Pesticide use and application: an Indian scenario. J Hazard Mater 165(1–3):1–12

Agrawal T, Chandrasekhar S (2015) Short term migrants in India: characteristics, wages and work transition. Retrieved from Mumbai, India: https://EconPapers.repec.org/RePEc:ind:igiwpp:2015-007

Ahasan R (2001) Legacy of implementing industrial health and safety in developing countries. J Physiol Anthropol Appl Hum Sci 20(6):311–319

Cho Y, Margolis D, Newhouse D, Robalino D (2012) Labor markets in low and middle income countries: trends and implications for social protection and labor policies. World Bank social protection discussion papers, 67613. World Bank, Washington, DC

Cooper C, Lu L (2016) Presenteeism as a global phenomenon: unraveling the psychosocial mechanisms from the perspective of social cognitive theory. Cross Cult Strateg Manag 23(2):216–231

CSDH (2008) Closing the gap in a generation: health equity through action on the social determinants of health. Final Report of the Commission on Social Determinants of Health. Geneva, World Health Organization

Dicken P (2007) Global shift: mapping the changing contours of the world economy. Sage, London

Eijkemans G (2001) WHO-ILO joint effort on occupational health and safety in Africa. WHO, Geneva

Evans-Lacko S, Knapp M (2016) Global patterns of workplace productivity for people with depression: absenteeism and presenteeism costs across eight diverse countries. Soc Psychiatry Psychiatr Epidemiol 51(11):1525–1537

Frank WP (2013) International business challenge: does adding South Africa finally make the BRIC countries relevant? J Int Bus Res 12(1):1

George S (2016) Work and health in informal economy: linkages from export oriented garment sector in Delhi. Daanish Books, New Delhi

George S, Sinha S (2018) Labourcape and labour space in India: critical reflections. In: George S, Sinha S (eds) Redefined labour spaces: organising workers in post liberalized India. Routledge, London/New York, pp 17–43

Ghosh B (2008) Economic reforms and trade unionism in India-A macro view. Indian J Ind Relat 43:355–384

Goldar B, Aggarwal SC (2010) Informalization of Industrial Labour in India: Are labour market rigidities and growing import competition to blame? Institute for Economic Growth, New Delhi, Manuscript

Hämäläinen P, Takala J, Kiat TB (2017) Global estimates of occupational accidents and work-related illnesses 2017. Retrieved from Singapore:

Hyde M, Theorell T (2018) Work environment, health and the international agenda. In: Hyde M, Chungkham HS, Ladusingh L (eds) Work and health in India. Policy Press, Bristol, pp 45–66

ILO Country Office for India (2016) Indian labour market update. Retrieved from New Delhi: http://www.ilo.org/wcmsp5/groups/public/%2D%2D-asia/%2D%2D-ro-bangkok/%2D%2D-sro-new_delhi/documents/publication/wcms_496510.pdf

ILO (2018) World Employment and Social Trends. ILO, Geneva

International Labour Organisation (2003) Report of the Conference No ICLS/17/2003/R, 24 Nov.–3 Dec 2003. Paper presented at the seventeenth international conference of labour statisticians, Geneva

International Labour Organisation (2016) Non-standard employment around the world: Understanding challenges, shaping prospects. ILO, Geneva

International Labour Organisation (2018) Women and men in the informal economy: a statistical picture. Retrieved from Genva:

International Labour Organization (2018b) Definitions and metadata. Retrieved from http://www.ilo.org/wesodata/definitions-and-metadata/vulnerable-employment

International Labour Organization (2018c) Women and men in the informal economy. a statistical picture, 3rd edn. International Labour Organization, Geneva

Janta B, Ratzmann N, Ghez J, Khodyakov D, Yaqub O (2015) Employment and the changing labour market. Global societal trends to 2030: Thematic report 5. Rand, Santa Monica

Joseph B, Injodey J, Varghese R (2009) Labour welfare in India. J Work Behav Health 24(1–2):221–242

Kamuzora P (2006) Non-decision making in occupational health policies in developing countries. Int J Occup Environ Health 12(1):65–71

Kortum E, Leka S (2014) Tackling psychosocial risks and work-related stress in developing countries: the need for a multilevel intervention framework. Int J Stress Manag 21(1):7–26. https://doi.org/10.1037/a0035033

Kortum E, Leka S, Cox T (2010) Psychosocial risks and work-related stress in developing countries: health impact, priorities, barriers and solutions. Int J Occup Med Environ Health 23(3):225–238

Kuhn S, Milasi S, Yoon S (2018) World employment social outlook: trends 2018. ILO, Geneva

Kumar P (2015) Who benefits from the law? Reminisces from fieldwork on contract (agency) workers in India. Paper presented at the labour law research network conference Amsterdam. http://www.labourlawresearch.net/sites/default/files/papers/LLRN%20paper-%20Who%20benefits%20from%20the%20law-Pankaj%20Kumar,%20JNU,%20India%20(1)%20copy.pdf

Leigh J, Macaskill P, Kuosma E, Mandryk J (1999) Global burden of disease and injury due to occupational factors. Epidemiology (Baltimore) 10(5):626–631

Lin Y-H, Chen C-Y, Lu S-Y (2009) Physical discomfort and psychosocial job stress among male and female operators at telecommunication call centers in Taiwan. Appl Ergon 40(4):561–568

Lu L, Lin HY, Cooper CL (2013) Unhealthy and present: motives and consequences of the act of presenteeism among Taiwanese employees. J Occup Health Psychol 18(4):406

Maiti D, Mitra A (2010) Skills, inequality and development. Retrieved from New Delhi: http://www.iegindia.org/upload/publication/Workpap/wp306.pdf

Mandal AK (2009) Strategies and policies deteriorate occupational health situation in India: a review based on social determinant framework. Indian J Occup Environ Med 13(3):113

Mohan D, Patel R (1992) Design of safer agricultural equipment: application of ergonomics and epidemiology. Int J Ind Ergon 10(4):301–309

Nuwayhid IA (2004) Occupational health research in developing countries: a partner for social justice. Am J Public Health 94(11):1916–1921

Pan American Health Organization Program on Workers' Health (2001) Regional plan on workers' health. Retrieved from Washington, DC: http://www.who.int/occupational_health/regions/en/oehamregplan.pdf

Papola T, Kannan K (2017) Towards an India wage report. International Labour Organization

Papola TS, Pais J, Sahu PP (2008) Labour regulation in indian industry: labour regulation in Indian industry: towards a rational and equitable framework. Bookwell Publishers, New Delhi

Quinlan M (2015) The effects of non-standard forms of employment on worker health and safety. ILO, Geneva

Rameshbabu A, Reddy DM, Fleming R (2013) Correlates of negative physical health in call center shift workers. Appl Ergon 44(3):350–354

Reuters Staff (2010) After BRICs, look to CIVETS for growth – HSBC CEO. Retrieved from https://www.reuters.com/article/hsbc-emergingmarkets/after-brics-look-to-civets-for-growth-hsbc-ceo-idUSLDE63Q26Q20100427

Rodrik D (2016) Premature deindustrialization. J Econ Growth 22(1):1–33

Roy SK, Chowdhury TK (2017) Health status and lifestyle of the Oraon tea garden labourers of Jalpaiguri district, West Bengal. In: Hyde M, Chungkham HS, Ladusingh L (eds) Work and health in India. Policy Press, Bristol, pp 179–192

Saiyed HN, Tiwari RR (2004) Occupational health research in India. Ind Health 42(2):141–148

Sapkal RS, Sundar SKR (2017) Determinants of precarious employment in India: an empirical analysis. In: Kalleberg AL, Vallas SP (eds) Precarious work. Research in the sociology of work, vol 31. Emerald Publishing Limited, Bingely, pp 335–361

Sprigg CA, Jackson PR (2006) Call centers as lean service environments: job-related strain and the mediating role of work design. J Occup Health Psychol 11(2):197

Sprigg CA, Smith PR, Jackson PR (2003) Psychosocial risk factors in call centres: an evaluation of work design and well-being. HSE. London

Sprigg CA, Stride CB, Wall TD, Holman DJ, Smith PR (2007) Work characteristics, musculoskeletal disorders, and the mediating role of psychological strain: a study of call center employees. J Appl Psychol 92(5):1456

Srivastava R, Sutradhar R (2016) Labour migration to the construction sector in india and its impact on rural poverty. Indian J Hum Dev 10(1):27–48

Sundar SKR (2012) The contract labour in India: the battle between flexibility and fairness. In: Sundar SKR (ed) Contract labour in India: issues and perspectives. Daanish Books, New Delhi, pp 5–24

Suri S, Das R (2016) Occupational health profile of workers employed in the manufacturing sector of India. Natl Med J India 29(5):277

Tiwari R, Saha A (2014) Morbidity profile of child labor at gem polishing units of Jaipur, India. Int J Occup Environ Med 5(3):125–129

Wang J, Schmitz N, Smailes E, Sareen J, Patten S (2010) Workplace characteristics, depression, and health-related presenteeism in a general population sample. J Occup Environ Med 52(8):836–842

Woetzel J, Madgavkar A, Gupta S (2017) India's labour market – a new emphasis on gainful employment. Retrieved from New York: https://www.mckinsey.com/~/media/McKinsey/Featured%20Insights/Employment%20and%20Growth/A%20new%20emphasis%20on%20gainful%20employment%20in%20India/Indias-labour-market-A-new-emphasis-on-gainful-employment.ashx

Zhou J-P (2006) Reforming employment protection legislation in France. International Monetary Fund, Paris

Concepts and Social Variations of Disability in Working-Age Populations

4

Johannes Siegrist and Jian Li

Contents

Introduction	54
Understanding Disability: A Minority Perspective or a Universal Perspective?	55
Analyzing Disability in Working-Age Populations	56
Prevalence and Social Distribution of Disability	58
Consequences of Disability for Health-Related Work Exit	61
A Synthesis	63
Implications for Policy	65
References	67

Abstract

Disability has been conceptualized in different ways, either as a notion confined to a minority group characterized by permanent bodily impairment and social exclusion or as a universal human condition of functional decline that is becoming more prevalent with increasing age. This latter notion seems more appropriate if applied to working-age populations, in particular as disability is analyzed on a continuum of varying severity and duration. This chapter deals with the prevalence and social distribution of disability in middle-aged to early-old-age working populations in modern societies, using evidence from three cohort studies, the Health and Retirement Study (USA), the English Longitudinal Study of Ageing, and the Survey of Health, Ageing and Retirement in Europe. It demonstrates consistent social gradients of disability, leaving those with lower socioeconomic

---

J. Siegrist (✉)
Centre for Health and Society, Faculty of Medicine, Heinrich-Heine-Universität Düsseldorf, Düsseldorf, Germany
e-mail: Johannes.siegrist@med.uni-duesseldorf.de

J. Li
Department of Environmental Health Sciences, Fielding School of Public Health; School of Nursing, University of California, Los Angeles, CA, USA
e-mail: jianli2019@ucla.edu

© Springer Nature Switzerland AG 2020
U. Bültmann, J. Siegrist (eds.), *Handbook of Disability, Work and Health*, Handbook Series in Occupational Health Sciences, https://doi.org/10.1007/978-3-030-24334-0_36

positions at higher risk. Moreover, we analyze consequences of disability for health-related work exit, most often in terms of disability retirement. Again, social disparities are observed, and adverse physical and psychosocial work environments contribute to an accumulation of disadvantage. The chapter concludes with a discussion of policy implications of available knowledge, pointing to different entry points for interventions that aim at promoting health and improving the quality of work and employment.

Keywords

Disability · Work ability · Social inequalities · Adverse working conditions · Disability retirement · Activity limitations · Cohort studies

Introduction

Disability has been conceptualized in different ways, and the social norms, attitudes, and practices toward people with disabilities underwent profound changes in history (Stiker 1999). In modern societies, a major shift occurred during the second half of the twentieth century. Disability has no longer been viewed as an individual's impairment that evokes societal reactions of social deviance, exclusion, or even discrimination, denying basic human rights to them. Rather, it has now been conceived as the result of "complex interactions between health conditions and features of an individual's physical, social, and attitudinal environment that hinder their full and effective participation in society" (Officer and Groce 2009, p. 1795). In terms of human rights, societies are now obliged to offer equal opportunities of participation in social life to people with disabilities, and these rights have been advocated and contested by civil rights movements, most successfully in the United States and in Europe. As a result, since the early 2000s, these rights have been affirmed and endorsed in the United Nations' Convention on the Rights of Persons with Disabilities (United Nations 2007), and many national legal developments as well as social, labor, and health policy initiatives since resulted in successful strategies to improve the lives of people with disabilities (WHO 2011).

At the same time, physicians and other health professionals started to broaden their view of disability that traditionally was dominated by an overly medicalized model of impairment and capacity limitation, largely ignoring socio-structural and psychosocial aspects. Most importantly, with the publication and implementation of the World Health Organization's International Classification of Functioning, Disability and Health (ICF), a universal descriptive tool of classification for data collection and clinical practice has been established that analyzes disability along three interconnected areas of human functioning within distinct social, natural, and built environments: (1) bodily functions and structures, (2) human activities, and (3) social participation (WHO 2001). Moreover, with its distinction between a person's capacity to perform actions and the actual performance of activities, the ICF emphasizes the important role of environmental barriers against full social participation among people with disabilities. Despite this comprehensive approach with its focus on the lived experience of persons, at least two different, far-reaching interpretations of disability seem to prevail up to now, both in the medical world and in those parts of everyday life that are influenced by medical knowledge and practice. In a recent seminal paper, these interpretations were labeled the "minority approach" and the "universal approach" (Bickenbach et al. 2017).

Starting with a short description of these two interpretations, this chapter will analyze disability within a restricted frame of reference, dealing with its occurrence, social distribution, and consequences for labor market participation among working-age populations in modern Western societies. Finally, we discuss some policy implications of the main finding of this review, i.e., the prevalence of consistent social inequalities of disabilities and their consequences for labor market participation.

Understanding Disability: A Minority Perspective or a Universal Perspective?

Is disability recognized as a universal human condition occurring in all populations, specifically with increasing age, or is its notion confined to a minority group within total populations, characterized by a permanent and severe bodily impairment and restricted social participation? Answers to this question matter because of the different societal and political strategies related to either definition. If considered a universal phenomenon reflecting a basic vulnerability of the human body and a lack of control over health shocks and injuries, disability manifests itself as a continuum with varying severity, duration, or course of progression and with varying options of reducing bodily impairment and functional decrement. In fact, major disabilities occurring among old-age populations are defined by these features. Being a universal phenomenon as part of the human condition, disability requires universal social and health-related policies that are applicable to everyone experiencing this condition. If considered a permanent and severe bodily impairment, disability mainly concerns a minority group of people whose life is characterized by distinct limitations of functioning and restrictions of social participation. As argued by Bickenbach et al. (2017), disability in this perspective is conceived as a dichotomy, distinguishing those with disability from those without this experience. Accordingly, as these restrictions contradict basic human rights, the primary policy goal for persons with disability is advocacy for legal and social change, aiming at reducing discrimination and increasing participation in social life.

It is evident that estimates of the prevalence of disability greatly vary according to the underlying definition. For instance, the World Report on Disability, applying the minority perspective, maintains that some 15% of the population in each country are persons with disabilities (WHO 2011). In contrast, at least in rapidly aging societies, much larger proportions of the population are experiencing disability to some extent (Lopez et al. 2006). The minority perspective of disability has also been useful in developing an advocacy agenda calling for rights and against social disadvantage and discrimination. Along these lines the World Report on Disability argues that persons with disabilities "face widespread barriers to accessing services, and experience poorer health outcomes, lower education achievement, less economic participation and higher rates of poverty than people without disabilities" (Bickenbach et al. 2017, p. 544). Therefore, the primary focus is on policies that improve the conditions of a disadvantaged minority rather than on efforts to promote health and reduce disabilities among total populations, within and beyond the range of health-care services (Lollar and Crews 2003). Historically, the minority perspective has been highly successful in promoting the rights of persons with disabilities and extending their opportunities of social participation, by removing barriers and by modifying societal attitudes and practices (United Nations 2007). Yet, despite its merits, this minority approach may not be the leading perspective of dealing with functional limitations, its determinants, and its consequences in a longer-term perspective, given an increase in chronic diseases and unhealthy aging (Zola (1989). As Bickenbach et al. (2017) argue, "a universal policy would match the level of resource, service, or support to the level of need, recognizing that impairments, though dynamic over the life course, tend...to be increasing in both number and severity" (p. 547). Therefore, it seems justified to adopt a universal perspective of disability, without disregarding the special needs and priorities of a minority group with enduring acquired or developmental disabilities. Specifically, with a focus on adult populations, the prevalence of mild to moderate disabilities resulting from age-related functional decline and spread of chronic diseases is increasing, calling for its analysis as conditions that vary on a continuum of severity, duration, and activity limitations.

Analyzing Disability in Working-Age Populations

Different approaches were used to assess the prevalence of disability in working-age populations. One such approach is based on administrative data of the frequency of chronic diseases with impact on work ability, resulting in longer-term sickness absence, use of rehabilitation services, or assignment of disability pension (OECD 2013). However, given the diversity of frequency and severity of chronic diseases, and given the variation of statutory regulations of access to sick pay, rehabilitation, and disability pension between different national health and social policies, any estimate of disability frequency based on administrative data remains highly uncertain (OECD 2013). Another approach is based on primary data collected in longitudinal cohort studies on aging, where the occurrence of disability is measured by established indicators of reduced physical and cognitive functioning and where its major determinants and its further consequences (e.g., morbidity, early exit from labor market, mortality) are analyzed. Here, we restrict the analysis to a review of major findings on the prevalence and social distribution of disability derived from primary data of three large epidemiologic cohort studies on middle-aged to early-old-age working populations in modern Western societies. We explore what is known about the prevalence and social distribution of disability and the consequences of disability for continued labor force participation. The three studies cover populations from the United States (Health and Retirement Study (HRS, Juster and Suzman 1995)) and from Europe (English Longitudinal Study on Ageing (ELSA, Marmot et al. 2003) and Survey of Health, Ageing and Retirement in Europe (SHARE, Börsch-Supan et al. 2005)). At its onset, this latter study included 11 European countries (Sweden, Denmark, the Netherlands, Belgium, France, Germany, Austria, Switzerland, Spain, Italy, Greece), but their number was increased in later waves. Importantly, the investigators of these three studies harmonized their measurement to some extent, thus enabling several comparisons across countries.

HRS is one of the earliest panel studies on middle-aged and elderly persons with regular survey intervals, at least in the United States (Juster and Suzman 1995). It started in 1992, with a sample of 18,496 participants aged 51 onward, with regular 2-year survey intervals, collecting rich data on work and employment, health, healthcare utilization, income and wealth, pension, and family and social relationships. The assessment of disability in HRS is complex, reflecting major changes in conceptualizing disability, such as the move from a traditional disablement model to the more comprehensive ICF model (Agree and Wolf 2018). The most often used measures include the activities of daily living (ADL) and the instrumental activities of daily living (IADL) list of items, complemented by a set of items on physical functioning (mobility restrictions). This information relies on self-reports and does not address issues of dependency on help from another person. To reduce heterogeneity of responses to these items, anchoring vignettes on disability were introduced more recently, and detailed measures of cognitive functioning and of social participation were included in an attempt to reflect core ICF dimensions of disability (Agree and Wolf 2018).

ELSA contains a representative sample of the community-dwelling English population aged 50 and over. Starting in 2002 with a total sample of 12,100 participants, it covers a broad range of topics on living and working conditions of individuals and households, assessed in interviews, and it additionally collects data from distinct tests of functioning (Marmot et al. 2003). More recently, biomedical data and detailed tests of functioning were included. The data collection is repeated on a 2-year interval, as is the case with HRS. At baseline, the measurement of disability was restricted to physical function (ADL, IADL, mobility measures related to the leg and arm, walking speed, falls) and cognitive function (memory, executive function, and a summary index).

SHARE is the first cross-national investigation of work, health, retirement, and socioeconomic conditions of elderly people (50 years and older) in Europe, largely based on measurements included in HRS and ELSA. It started in 2004 with a baseline sample of 32,442 participants, and data collection has been repeated in a 2-year interval. In 2008, extensive life history micro data were additionally collected (SHARELIFE), covering core domains of the life course: children, partners, employment, health, and accommodation (Börsch-Supan et al. 2011). Disability was assessed with a broad range of measures, including ADL, IADL, Global Activity Limitation Indicator (GALI), mobility limitations, grip strength, walking speed, balance, and cognitive tests (Börsch-Supan et al. 2005). As in the previous studies, different operational definitions of disability are used in scientific publications, but the relatively highest consistency and comparability were achieved with regard to ADL and IADL (Chan et al. 2012). It is of interest to note that one study developed a measure of disability that distinguished impairment from restriction in activity and participation, in line with the ICF model. Based on confirmatory factor analysis, two scales measuring "impairment" and "activity and participation limitations," respectively, were developed (Reinhardt et al. 2013).

The next section reviews major findings on the prevalence of disability and its social distribution in the three studies. This section is followed by a summary of findings on the impact of disability on early exit from labor market, mainly assessed by assignment of a disability pension.

Prevalence and Social Distribution of Disability

Given a relatively long observation period of HRS, the prevalence and time trend of disability have been extensively analyzed. For instance, the prevalence of disability remained at a low level from 2001 to 2009, ranging from 10% to 12% of any ADL disability and from 7% to 9% of any IADL disability (Verbrugge and Liu 2014). This phenomenon was in accordance with an earlier investigation of HRS for a similar observation time (Freedman et al. 2013). Though the overall prevalence of disability remained stable, one study indicated an increase in the age group 53–64 years, distinct from older groups. Here, significant increases on ADL/IADL limitations, mobility, large muscle, and gross motor function indices were observed (Chen and Sloan 2015). Education was examined in several studies in its association with disability. In an observational study from 1994 to 2010, there was a strong negative correlation of education with the prevalence of disability, including minor and major ADL and IADL limitations (Rehkopf et al. 2017), and longitudinally, educational attainment was an important predictor of disability changes (Chen and Sloan 2015) as well as accelerated disability onset (Latham 2012; see also Verbrugge et al. 2017). These latter findings are in line with the observation of Stenholm et al. (2014) that low education is associated with poorer levels of physical functioning. In a study by van Zon et al. (2016) with HRS longitudinal data, similar results were observed using wealth as an indicator of socioeconomic position. As efforts toward reducing the prevalence and the social inequality of early-old-age disability may be compromised by the US health-care system that disadvantages socioeconomically deprived population groups, it is of interest to compare the situation in the United States with the one in Europe where universal access to health care is common in a large majority of countries. What is the prevalence and social distribution of disability in England and in continental Europe, as represented by ELSA and SHARE?

In baseline data from *ELSA*, the prevalence of disability in terms of one or more difficulties in ADL was about 10% in the age group 50–59. Yet, clear social variations were observed as this prevalence was 17.8% among participants in routine and manual occupational classes as compared to 7.7% among those in managerial and professional occupational classes. Similar social inequalities were observed for IADL. Concerning difficulty with mobility, 50.3% of routine and manual workers in this age group reported some difficulty, compared to 35.1% among managers and professionals. A further disability indicator, the mean summary index of cognitive function, was calculated for women and men in this age group (ranging from 5 to 55, with higher scores reflecting better function). Overall, this score was 37.7, but among those with higher education, including degrees, it was as high as 41.0, whereas it reached 33.6 among those with low or no qualification (Marmot et al. 2003). Another study used data from wave 6 (2012–2013), where disability was defined as having limitation in one or more activities, including ADL and IADL. The prevalence in this sample (mean age 66 years) was 20.9%, and disabled persons were significantly poorer, had a weaker social network, and suffered three times more often from depressive symptoms than those without disability (Lustosa Torres et al. 2016). Availability of data from multiple waves allows a dynamic analysis of processes between socioeconomic, behavioral, and psychosocial factors and the incidence of disability. One such study reported an incident disability rate between any two out of five consecutive waves of 20.3%, defined as one or more IADL limitations. This incidence was associated with lower socioeconomic position, lack of labor market participation, and poorer physical and social activities (d'Orsi et al. 2014). Finally, an important recent investigation compared wealth-associated disparities of incident disability over 10 years between the United States (HRS) and England (ELSA), where disability was defined as experiencing one or more ADL activity limitations (Makaroun et al. 2017). In the age group 54–64 years, the gradient of cumulative incidence of the first ADL difficulty according to wealth quintiles was steeper in the United States than in England, and it was also steeper than the gradient observed in the older-age group. Importantly, in the age group 54–64, 48% of those in the lowest wealth quintile were at risk of developing disability within 10 years, compared to 15% among those in the highest wealth quintile. Detailed comparative results between the two studies are given in Fig. 1 (Makaroun et al. 2017).

Information from *SHARE* indicates that, at baseline, 9.2% and 11.8% of men reported one or more ADL and IADL difficulties, respectively, and these figures were 12.5% and 21.1% among women. As expected, there was a pronounced age gradient in all measures of disability. Lower socioeconomic status was consistently associated with more functioning limitations, where similar contributions of education and income (as two main indicators of socioeconomic status) were observed. For instance, odds ratios of one or more IADL limitations for those in the lower two quintiles of income distribution compared to those in the upper two quintiles were 1.70 (95% CI 1.45; 2.00) among men and 1.46 (95% CI 1.30; 1.65) among women. Similar findings are reported for mobility limitations, eyesight problems, grip strength, and fear of falling (Börsch-Supan et al. 2005). Furthermore, the social distribution of activity limitations was obvious from longitudinal analyses on incident functional limitations long before retirement age (Nilsson et al. 2010).

Another analysis based on the ICF model of disability compared the variation of mean impairment scores and mean activity and participation scores according

Fig. 1 Cumulative incidence of the first ADL difficulty by wealth quintile. ADL indicates activity of daily living; ELSA, the English Longitudinal Study of Ageing. (Source: Makaroun et al. 2017; printed with copyright permission from JAMA Internal Medicine)

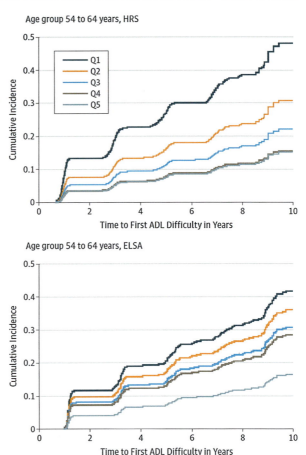

to income (as the main indicator of socioeconomic status) in the eleven countries under study, where three groups of high, medium, and low income were distinguished. With regard to impairment, income differences were particularly large in Spain, France, and Germany, and overall levels were lowest in Switzerland, Sweden, and Denmark. Concerning activity and participation limitation, income differences were largest in Spain and Belgium, and overall levels were lowest in Switzerland and Greece. Across all countries, education and income (three groups each) were associated with significantly increased incidence rate ratios of the two disability measures between wave 1 and wave 2. For instance, the incidence rate ratio of activity and participation limitation was 2.02 (95% CI 1.45; 2.80) for the lowest education group and 1.93 (95% CI 1.42; 2.62) for the medium education group compared to the highest educational group. A similar pattern was observed for income. These findings indicate a higher burden of disability among older employed men and women in lower socioeconomic positions (Reinhardt et al. 2013).

There is limited information available comparing socioeconomic inequalities of disability across populations of the three studies HRS, ELSA, and SHARE. In an analysis of two measures of disability, mobility limitations and IADL limitations, assessed in 48,225 adults aged 50–85 years, associations of wealth with disability according to age were analyzed using fractional polynomials of age and controlling for sociodemographic characteristics and important risk factors (Wahrendorf et al. 2013). Wealth was measured as household total net worth (accumulated savings), adjusted for household size, categorized into country-specific tertiles. In each country or region, wealth was significantly associated with both indicators of disability, but gradients in working-age populations were steeper in the United States and in England than in the countries of continental Europe. The discrepancy between low and high wealth was highest in case of mobility limitation in the US sample. A further investigation of a large US sample of men and women aged 55–64 confirmed this steep social gradient, with particular reference to income (Minkler et al. 2006). Those below the administrative poverty line were six times more likely to experience functional limitations compared to the wealthiest group, but a gradient along all income categories was documented. These findings indicate that social inequalities of disability do exist in countries with universal access to health care as well as in the United States with its restricted health-care system, although to a lesser extent. Therefore, extending access to health care, while important, may not be sufficient to reduce the social gradient of limitations of activity and social participation among middle-aged and early-old-age populations (see below). Obviously, these consistent social inequalities have their roots in differential health-related, behavioral, psychosocial, and socioeconomic vulnerability in earlier stages of life (e.g., Landös et al. 2018). While it is beyond the current contribution to analyze these risk and protective factors, the question of interest here concerns the longer-term consequences of incident midlife disability for work ability and premature exit from labor market.

Consequences of Disability for Health-Related Work Exit

Disability pension (DP) is an established measure of social protection in advanced societies, and its regulations vary widely between the different countries (OECD 2013). Generally, DP is based on a medically certified diagnosis that indicates the inability to continue regular work as previously, due to a physical or mental impairment. DP provides some compensation of income loss in case of early exit from the labor market, either on a temporary or permanent basis. The frequency of receiving a DP and the level of compensation heavily depend on institutional characteristics of national pension systems, the demographic composition of the workforce, and the economic performance of a country. Overall, work inability due to long-standing ill health or disability defines the major pathway of early exit from labor market, but several other determinants were documented (Carr et al. 2018). Among these, adverse physical and psychosocial working conditions and socially disadvantaged living circumstances seem to play a prominent role. What is known from the three aging studies about the interplay of reduced health, adverse work, and low socioeconomic position as determinants of early exit from paid work?

Researchers dealing with *HRS* so far mainly preferred to analyze associations of disabling health conditions with early exit from paid work rather than the role of adverse working conditions or low socioeconomic position in the pathways triggering premature retirement. There is now robust evidence that poor health at baseline increases the risk of health-related exit from work, whether measured as self-rated general or physical poor health, as prevalence of multiple chronic conditions, or as severe insomnia (McDonough et al. 2017; Roy 2018; Dong et al. 2017). Some of these studies controlled for the effect of sociodemographic or work-related factors, whereas other reports found independent effects of socioeconomic or work-related conditions. For instance, in an analysis of trajectories from employment to work disability among women, higher risks of being work-disabled were observed among black and Hispanic women, compared to white women, and these risks were associated with social disadvantage in earlier stages of the life course (Brown and Warner 2008). Long-term effects of adverse socioeconomic and psychosocial childhood conditions on elevated occurrence of health-related work exit were found for men and women in the context of HRS (Bowen and González 2010). A further investigation showed that recurrent work-to-family conflicts increased disability risks over an observation period of 10 years (Cho and Chen 2018). Yet, a particularly strong impact of low education and low occupational position on elevated risks of DP comes from a recent longitudinal analysis comprising seven aging studies, including HRS. In the US sample, low occupational position and low level of education were associated with a twofold risk of DP both among men and women (Carr et al. 2018).

Several European studies on aging put special emphasis on the combined effects of disabling health- and work-related factors on early exit from work. In *SHARE*, in addition to poor self-rated health, lack of physical activity and having a job with low control or with an imbalance between high efforts spent and low rewards received in turn predicted an increased risk of DP (Robroek et al. 2013). High demand in combination with low control at work (or "job strain") is a stress-theoretical model of health-adverse job characteristics that has been related to a broad range of ill health outcomes (Karasek and Theorell 1990; Theorell et al. 2015). As a complementary theoretical model, effort-reward imbalance defines health-adverse employment conditions where effortful jobs are not adequately compensated by rewards in terms of material, status-related, nonmaterial, and socioemotional rewards (Siegrist 1996). Again, this model was shown to predict a range of health outcomes, including health-related work exit (Siegrist and Wahrendorf 2016). These factors of a stressful psychosocial work environment were observed in relation to DP in an earlier report from SHARE (van den Berg et al. 2010). It is of interest to note that the prevalence of low job control and effort-reward imbalance follows a social gradient in SHARE, such that lower occupational positions are associated with a higher level of work-related stress (Wahrendorf et al. 2013). Along these lines, two findings from *ELSA* deserve attention. One finding indicates that adverse working conditions, in terms of low control at work (a component of the demand-control model) and low recognition (a component of the effort-reward imbalance model), predict early exit from paid work (Carr et al. 2016). The other finding confirms a significantly elevated risk of being granted a DP among English working men and women with low educational level or low occupational position (Carr et al. 2018). For instance, the hazard ratio of disability retirement among employed older men and women in the lowest of three occupational categories compared to those in the highest occupational group is 2.38 (95% CI 1.48; 3.81) and 2.04 (95% CI 1.36; 3.07), respectively, if adjusted for self-rated health and birth cohort (Carr et al. 2018).

These results indicate that social inequalities in the consequences of disabling health resulting in early exit from paid work are a robust fact across different countries. A research network in Scandinavian countries contributed additional insights into the interplay of poor health, adverse work, low socioeconomic position, and early retirement. For instance, according to a register linkage study from Finland, the risk of disability retirement was particularly high if persons suffered from cardiovascular disease and were simultaneously located in a low socioeconomic position (Virtanen et al. 2017). Further investigations showed that associations of low socioeconomic status with DP varied by type of disabling disease, with strongest relationships for musculoskeletal disorders and cardiovascular diseases but weaker association with depression (Polvinen 2016, Leinonen et al. 2011, Pietiläinen et al. 2018). These associations were largely mediated by adverse physical working conditions, in particular if DP was granted due to musculoskeletal disorders or injuries. However, complementary studies from Finland demonstrate that adverse psychosocial working conditions are important predictors of DP as well, for general DP (such as low job control, Knardahl et al. 2017) and for DP due to depression (Juvani et al. 2018). In this latter case, the study linked three theoretical concepts of psychosocial stress at work, assessed in 2008 among 41,862 employees, to national records of disability pensions until 2011: job strain, effort-reward imbalance, and organizational injustice. Compared to employees without exposure to any of these stressors, those exposed to all three stressors simultaneously had a 4.7-fold increased risk of disability pension from depressive disorders. Moreover, this risk was particularly high among employees aged 35–50 if they simultaneously suffered from job strain and effort-reward imbalance. The study also documented significantly elevated risks of DP due to musculoskeletal disorders and all-cause DP among employees experiencing a clustering of work stressors (Juvani et al. 2018).

A Synthesis

This contribution supports the argument that disability is best conceptualized as a universal human condition rather than a phenomenon defining specifically those minority groups within total populations that are characterized by a permanent and severe bodily impairment and restricted social participation. Although ensuring rights and extending social participation among these latter groups remains an important policy aim, disability, defined as the result of widespread functional limitations starting in midlife and culminating among the oldest groups, has to be addressed at the level of total populations. A brief summary of results from cohort studies in modern Western societies has shown that the frequency of restrictions in basic everyday activities varies between 10% and 20% in early old age, with an even higher percentage in case of mobility limitations. The consequences of disabling health conditions are particularly severe among employed men and women in midlife and early old age. We learned that the risk of early exit from paid work is critically elevated in persons with poor health, including limitations of physical or mental functioning. Despite the fact that disability pensions to some extent compensate for work-related income loss, for many of those people, a premature exclusion from the labor market is associated with multiple socioeconomic and psychosocial disadvantages.

Conceptualizing disability as a universal human condition has enabled researchers to study human life within an extended perspective of functioning, as defined by the World Health Organization's ICF classification. Accordingly, disability is analyzed along three interconnected areas of human functioning within distinct social, natural, and built environments: bodily functions and structures, human activities, and social participation. The combined study of these areas has produced a wealth of new knowledge. For instance, in the context of working life, it became evident that impaired bodily functioning can adversely affect cognitive and affective functioning, reduce commitment to work and work ability, and increase the risk of social isolation and exclusion. Or take the case of organizational measures of enhanced employability where people with disability can maintain their jobs, thus avoiding exclusion from the labor market. The far-reaching impact of environmental factors on the development and course of disability has been illustrated above with our main focus on social inequality.

Prospective findings indicate that people who live and work in less advantaged conditions have a higher probability of developing disabling functional limitations and that such limitations manifest themselves at an earlier stage in life compared to people who live in more privileged circumstances. Although a potential influence of social selection cannot be ruled out – claiming that persons with poorer health are more likely to suffer from downward social mobility, thus clustering in low socioeconomic positions, – it is more likely that adverse socioeconomic conditions play an important role in causal pathways leading to increased disability risks. Two complementary explanations developed in the frame of life course research support this notion. The "pathway" model posits that children born and growing up in families with restricted socioeconomic and psychosocial resources may perform less successfully in their educational attainment, thus having fewer options of accessing a high-quality job. Once this pathway into a lower occupational position has been achieved, there are limited chances of upward mobility, and continued exposure to a physically strenuous or psychologically demanding job in the long run will impair physical functioning and promote ill health. The model of "cumulative disadvantage" claims that the restricted socioeconomic and psychosocial resources of parents are transmitted to and "embodied" by their children during the process of socialization, rendering them more vulnerable when coping with the challenges of life in early adulthood and placing them more often in less advantaged social positions. These lower social positions are often associated with more physical or psychosocial stressors that in turn increase people's vulnerability. Thus, chains of stressful experiences accumulate in these people, increasing their risk of functional impairment and ill health (Graham and Power 2004). The model of cumulative disadvantage may also help explain why people in lower socioeconomic positions who once developed a disability are at higher risk of suffering from more serious consequences, e.g., in terms of early health-related exit from work. Successful coping with disability requires a strong mobilization of personal and socio-environmental protective factors. These protective factors may be available to a lesser extent in socially deprived groups, thus aggravating their burden of coping and its adverse consequences for health and well-being. To conclude, both models, "differential pathways" and "cumulative disadvantage," help in explaining the socially unequal burden of disability, its antecedents, and its consequences.

Implications for Policy

Given a robust basis of evidence on social inequalities in the prevalence and further course of disability, and given a relevant role of working conditions in associations of socioeconomic positions with disabilities, are there obvious policy implications of this scientific knowledge? As these inequalities result from processes occurring in a life course perspective, it is difficult to decide when and where to intervene. However, at least the following three entry points offer some opportunity of change. First, the observation of a higher prevalence and earlier onset of functional limitations among working people with lower socioeconomic positions calls for intensified efforts of providing worksite medical screening and company-based monitoring of health-damaging working conditions as part of occupational health and safety programs. To avoid potential discrimination, these measures should be offered to all employees in respective organizations but should be stratified according to need. By strictly observing data protection regulations, the screening and monitoring data obtained from occupational health and safety officials could be used to identify groups of employees with the highest need of support in terms of promoting their health and of reducing the adversity at their work, and respective programs could then be implemented. Obviously, this strategy requires the establishment of well-equipped occupational health and safety services as well as the existence of national regulations prescribing routine monitoring of quality of work and employment. Unfortunately, in a majority of countries, these requirements are currently far from being met. Yet, models of good practice are offered by several European countries, in particular Scandinavian countries, the Netherlands, France, and the United Kingdom, and by Australia, Japan, and Canada. Even within these countries, there seems to be a preference of offering worksite health promotion programs to better educated groups of employees. For instance, a meta-analysis of health effects of randomized controlled worksite interventions revealed that twice as many of the 40 reports included in this review were conducted in higher-skilled occupational groups than was the case in lower-skilled groups. This holds particularly true for interventions addressing overweight, musculoskeletal pain, and stressful working conditions (Montano et al. 2014). Thus, the double burden of poorer quality of work and higher risk of ill health among less-privileged occupational groups has not yet been adequately addressed. This conclusion is supported by a study forecasting the impact of disability on labor force development in the United States (Rehkopf et al. 2017). The authors argue that early support of socially disadvantaged working groups, specifically those with certain types of functional limitations, is needed, both in terms of providing health services and offering improved work environments to ensure a sustainable aging workforce in the near future.

A second opportunity of intervention concerns the improvement of work ability among all those middle-aged or early-old-age employed people who suffer from some manifest disability. Rather than excluding them from paid work by granting a disability pension – a procedure that is still common in a number of countries – comprehensive programs of medical and vocational rehabilitation should be put in place to improve health status and work ability. The German system is a well-known example of this approach.

Germany offers extensive medical rehabilitation services to all persons covered by the national statutory pension insurance following onset of a medically certified disabling condition or chronic disease. These services are offered in specialized rehabilitation clinics or in out-hospital training and treatment settings for several weeks, and costs are covered by the national pension funds. The underlying argument maintains that costs of rehabilitation are by far less expensive than costs of long-term provision of disability pensions, given the evidence of increased rates of successful return to work. As an example, a large study of cancer patients undergoing medical rehabilitation in Germany demonstrates that three quarters of all patients were able to return to work within 6 weeks following completion of the rehabilitation program (Mehnert and Koch 2013). Again, investments in comprehensive rehabilitation and reintegration services require an active national labor and social policy that is currently realized in a minority rather than a majority of countries.

The scientific reports mentioned above document a relevant impact of adverse physical and psychosocial working conditions on the development of disability and on elevated risks of early health-related exit from paid work. These conditions are not randomly distributed across working populations, but tend to cluster among groups with lower levels of skills and among those in low-ranking positions within occupational hierarchies. Therefore, a third entry point of interventions relates to policies that address social inequalities in exposure to health-adverse working conditions. These policies are best realized in the frame of national worksite health promotion programs enforced by legislation and adopted by employer organizations. During the past decades, in economically advanced societies, progress was achieved in reducing occupational diseases and occupational injuries, but, despite a solid scientific knowledge base, the burden of stressful psychosocial work environments has not yet received similar attention. As the prevalence of this burden follows a social gradient, with higher levels among those with lower positions (Wahrendorf et al. 2013), additional labor policies need to be implemented that address the special needs of socially disadvantaged workers. As an example, distinct integration policies were developed in some countries that provide training skills and continued education and supported employment or access to less physically demanding jobs and provision of incentives (e.g., more equitable wages and salaries) to those with the highest need. In Europe, Denmark, Sweden, the Netherlands, Germany, and Switzerland are countries with advanced levels of labor market integration policies. A comparative study analyzing the social gradient of stressful psychosocial work environments according to the extent of implementation of these integration policies documented that this gradient was steepest in countries with a weak integration policy and least pronounced in countries with strong respective developments (Lunau et al. 2015). Although these findings should be interpreted with caution, they point to smaller educational inequalities in the burden of work-related stress among working populations of countries with well-developed active labor market programs.

These three entry points of interventions toward improving the work ability and toward reducing the burden of disability in an aging workforce are far from being sufficient in view of persisting social inequalities of working people's health. In times of a globalized economy, restrictions of policies to the national context need to be overcome by establishing effective supranational regulations that ensure an extension of health-conducive work across all occupational groups.

References

Agree EM, Wolf DA (2018) Disability measurement in the Health and Retirement Study. Forum for Health Economics and Policy: 20170029

Bickenbach J, Rubinelli S, Stucki G (2017) Being a person with disabilities or experiencing disability: two perspectives on the social response to disability. J Rehabil Med 49:543–549

Börsch-Supan A, Brugiavini A, Jürges H, Mackenbach J, Siegrist J, Weber G (eds) (2005) Health, ageing and retirement in Europe – first results from the survey of health, ageing and retirement in Europe. MEA, Mannheim

Börsch-Supan A, Brandt M, Hank K, Schröder M (eds) (2011) The individual and the welfare state. Life histories in Europe. Springer, Berlin

Bowen ME, González HM (2010) Childhood socioeconomic position and disability in later life: results of the health and retirement study. Am J Public Health 100(1):197–203

Brown TH, Warner DF (2008) Divergent pathways? Racial/ethnic differences in older women's labor force withdrawal. J Gerontol B Psychol Sci Soc Sci 63(3):S122–S134

Carr E, Hagger-Johnson G, Head J, Shelton N, Stafford M, Stansfeld S, Zaninotto P (2016) Working conditions as predictors of retirement intentions and exit from paid employment: a 10-year follow-up of the English Longitudinal Study of Ageing. Eur J Ageing 13(1):39–48

Carr E, Fleischmann M, Goldberg M, Kuh D, Murray ET, Stafford M, Stansfeld S, Vahtera J, Xue B, Zaninotto P, Zins M, Head J (2018) Occupational and educational inequalities in exit from employment at older ages: evidence from seven prospective cohorts. Occup Environ Med 75 (5):369–377

Chan KS, Kasper JD, Brandt J, Pezzin LE (2012) Measurement equivalence in ADL and IADL difficulty across international surveys of aging: findings from the HRS, SHARE, and ELSA. J Gerontol B Psychol Sci Soc Sci 67B:121–132

Chen Y, Sloan FA (2015) Explaining disability trends in the U.S. elderly and near-elderly population. Health Serv Res 50(5):1528–1549

Cho E, Chen TY (2018) The effects of work-family experiences on health among older workers. Psychol Aging 33(7):993–1006

D'Orsi E, Junqueira Xavier A, Steptoe A, de Oliveira C, Ramos LR, Orrell M, Demakakos P, Marmot MG (2014) Socioeconomic and lifestyle factors related to instrumental activity of daily living dynamics: results from the English Longitudinal Study of Ageing. J Am Geriatr Soc 62:1630–1639

Dong L, Agnew J, Mojtabai R, Surkan PJ, Spira AP (2017) Insomnia as a predictor of job exit among middle-aged and older adults: results from the Health and Retirement Study. J Epidemiol Community Health 71(8):750–757

Freedman VA, Spillman BC, Andreski PM, Cornman JC, Crimmins EM, Kramarow E, Lubitz J, Martin LG, Merkin SS, Schoeni RF, Seeman TE, Waidmann TA (2013) Trends in late-life activity limitations in the United States: an update from five national surveys. Demography 50 (2):661–671

Graham H, Power C (2004) Childhood disadvantage and adult health: a lifecourse framework. Health Development Agency, London

Juster ET, Suzman R (1995) An overview of the Health and Retirement Study. J Hum Resour 30 (Suppl):7–56

Juvani A, Oksanen T, Virtanen M, Salo P, Pentti J, Kivimäki M, Vahtera J (2018) Clustering of job strain, effort-reward imbalance, and organizational injustice and the risk of work disability: a cohort study. Scand J Work Environ Health 44(5):485–495

Karasek R, Theorell T (1990) Healthy work. Stress, productivity, and the reconstruction of working life. Basic Books, New York

Knardahl S, Johannessen HA, Sterud T, Härmä M, Rugulies R, Seitsamo J, Borg V (2017) The contribution from psychological, social, and organizational work factors to risk of disability retirement: a systematic review with meta-analyses. BMC Public Health 17:176

Landös A, von Arx M, Cheval B, Sieber S, Kliegel M, Gabriel R, Orsholits D, van der Linden BWA, Blane D, Boisgontier MP, Courvoisier DS, Guessous I, Burton-Jeangros C, Cullati S (2018) Childhood socioeconomic circumstances and disability trajectories in older men and women: a European cohort study. Eur J Pub Health. https://doi.org/10.1093/eurpub/ckyl66

Latham K (2012) Progressive and accelerated disability onset by race/ethnicity and education among late midlife and older adults. J Aging Health 24(8):1320–1345

Leinonen T, Pietiläinen O, Laaksonen M, Rahkonen O, Lahelma E, Martikainen P (2011) Occupational social class and disability retirement among municipal employees – the contribution of health behaviors and working conditions. Scand J Work Environ Health 37(6):464–472

Lollar DJ, Crews JE (2003) Redefining the role of public health in disability. Annu Rev Public Health 24:195–208

Lopez AD, Mathers CD, Ezzati M, Jamison DT, Murray CJL (2006) Global and regional burden of disease and risk factors, 2001: systematic analysis of population health data. Lancet 367 (9524):1747–1757

Lunau T, Siegrist J, Dragano N, Wahrendorf M (2015) The association between education and work stress: does the policy context matter? PLoS One 10(3):e0121573

Lustosa Torres J, Lima-Costa MF, Marmot M, de Oliveira C (2016) Wealth and disability in later life: the English longitudinal study of ageing (ELSA). PLoS One 11(11):e0166825

Makaroun LK, Brown RT, Grisell Diaz-Ramirez L, Ahalt C, Boscardin WJ, Lang-Brown S, Lee S (2017) Wealth-associated disparities in death and disability in the US and England. JAMA Intern Med 177(12):1745–1753

Marmot M, Banks J, Blundell R, Lessof C, Nazroo J (eds) (2003) Health, wealth and lifestyles of the older population in England. The 2002 English Longitudinal Study of Ageing. The Institute for Fiscal Studies, London

McDonough P, Worts D, Corna LM, McMunn A, Sacker A (2017) Later-life employment trajectories and health. Adv Life Course Res 34:22–33

Mehnert A, Koch U (2013) Predictors of employment among cancer survivors after medical rehabilitation-a prospective study. Scand J Work Environ Health 39(1):76–87

Minkler M, Fuller-Thomson E, Guralnik JM (2006) Gradient of disability across the socioeconomic spectrum in the United States. N Engl J Med 355:695–703

Montano D, Hoven H, Siegrist J (2014) A meta-analysis of health effects of randomized controlled worksite interventions: does social stratification matter? Scand J Work Environ Health 40 (3):230–234. https://doi.org/10.5271/sjweh.3412

Nilsson CJ, Avlund K, Lund R (2010) Mobility disability in midlife: a longitudinal study of the role of anticipated instrumental support and social class. Arch Gerontol Geriatr 51(2):152–158

OECD (2013) Pensions indicators. Organisation for Economic Co-operation and Development, Paris

Officer A, Groce NE (2009) Key concepts in disability. Lancet 374:1795–1796

Pietiläinen O, Laaksonen M, Lahelma E, Salonsalmi A, Rahkonen O (2018) Occupational class inequalities in disability retirement after hospitalization. Scand J Public Health 46:331–339

Polvinen A (2016) Socioeconomic status and disability retirement in Finland. Causes, changes over time and mortality. Academic dissertation, University of Helsinki, Helsinki, Finland

Rehkopf DH, Adler NE, Rowe JW (2017) The impact of health and education on future labour force participation among individuals aged 55–74 in the United States of America: the MacArthur Foundation Research Network on an Aging Society. Ageing Soc 37(7):1313–1337

Reinhardt JD, Wahrendorf M, Siegrist J (2013) Socioeconomic position, psychosocial work environment and disability in an ageing workforce: a longitudinal analysis of SHARE data from 11 European countries. Occup Environ Med 70:156–163

Robroek SJ, Schuring M, Croezen S, Stattin M, Burdorf A (2013) Poor health, unhealthy behaviors, and unfavorable work characteristics influence pathways of exit from paid employment among older workers- a four-year follow-up study. Scand J Work Environ Health 39(2):125–133

Roy SB (2018) Effect of health on retirement of older Americans: a competing risks study. J Lab Res 39(1):56–98

Siegrist J (1996) Adverse health effects of high effort-low reward conditions at work. J Occup Health Psychol 1(1):27–43

Siegrist J, Wahrendorf M (eds) (2016) Work stress and health in a globalized economy: the model of effort-reward imbalance. Springer International Publications, Cham

Stenholm S, Westerlund H, Salo P, Hyde M, Pentti J, Head J, Kivimäki M, Vahtera J (2014) Age-related trajectories of physical functioning in work and retirement: the role of sociodemographic factors, lifestyle and disease. J Epidemiol Community Health 68(6):503–509

Stiker H (1999) A history of disability (trans: Sayers W). University of Michigan Press, Ann Arbor

Theorell T, Hammarström A, Aronsson G, Träskman Bendz L, Grape T, Hogstedt C, Marteinsdottir I, Skoog I, Hall C (2015) A systematic review and meta-analysis of work environment and depressive symptoms. BMC Public Health 15:738

United Nations (2007) Convention on the rights of persons with disabilities. G.A. Res. 61/106. Available from: http://www.un.org/esa/socdev/enable/rights/convtexte.htm

van den Berg T, Schuring M, Avendano M, Mackenbach J, Burdorf A (2010) The impact of ill health on exit from paid employment in Europe among older workers. Occup Environ Med 67:845–852

van Zon SK, Bültmann U, Reijneveld SA, de Leon CF (2016) Functional health decline before and after retirement: a longitudinal analysis of the Health and Retirement Study. Soc Sci Med 170:26–34

Verbrugge LM, Liu X (2014) Midlife trends in activities and disability. J Aging Health 26 (2):178–206

Verbrugge LM, Latham K, Clarke PJ (2017) Aging with disability for midlife and older adults. Res Aging 39(6):741–777

Virtanen M, Lallukka T, Ervasti J, Rahkonen O, Lahelma E, Pentti J, Pietiläinen O, Vahterade J (2017) The joint contribution of cardiovascular disease and socioeconomic status to disability retirement: a register linkage study. Int J Cardiol 230:222–227

Wahrendorf M, Reinhardt JM, Siegrist J (2013) Relationships of disability with age among adults aged 50 to 85: evidence from the United States, England and continental Europe. PLoS One 8 (8):e71893

World Health Organization (2001) International classification of functioning, disability and health. WHO, Geneva

World Health Organization (2011) World report on disability. WHO, Geneva

Zola IK (1989) Toward the necessary universalizing of a disability policy. Milbank Q 67:401–418

Trajectories from Work to Early Exit from Paid Employment

5

Alex Burdorf and Suzan Robroek

Contents

Introduction	72
Selection and Causation Hypotheses	73
Interplay Between Work and Health	73
Selection Hypothesis	73
Causation Hypothesis	76
A Working Life Course Perspective	77
Trajectories During Working Career	77
The Impact of Working Careers on Health After Retirement	79
Vulnerable Groups	80
Challenges and Conclusions	81
Cross-References	82
References	82

Abstract

Work and health are closely related. Unemployed individuals have both a poorer physical and a poorer mental health compared to employed individuals. This chapter presents evidence for the two mechanisms underlying the associations between unemployment and poor health. The selection mechanisms state that poor health increases the likelihood of exit from paid employment. The causation mechanism posits that unemployment is a risk factor for poor health. Both mechanisms will play a role during working careers, and, thus, a working life perspective is advised to capture how health will influence

---

A. Burdorf (✉) · S. Robroek
Department of Public Health, Erasmus University Medical Center, Rotterdam, The Netherlands
e-mail: a.burdorf@erasmusmc.nl; s.robroek@erasmusmc.nl

© Springer Nature Switzerland AG 2020
U. Bültmann, J. Siegrist (eds.), *Handbook of Disability, Work and Health*, Handbook Series in Occupational Health Sciences, https://doi.org/10.1007/978-3-030-24334-0_3

working capacity over the work life and how paid employment will influence health during working age and thereafter. Vulnerable groups are identified that will experience difficulties in prolonging their working lives in good health. In the existing socioeconomic inequalities in health, the ability to have access to paid employment is a critical factor. Likewise, inequalities in health and underlying causes will have a profound impact in educational differences in labor market attainment. It is advised to further develop the working life perspective in new metrics, such as working life expectancy and working years lost, and in new methods to decompose these new metrics into underlying causes of loss of work capacity.

Keywords

Employment transitions · Vulnerable groups · Socioeconomic inequalities · Health

Introduction

The rapid growth in life expectancy by almost 5 years in the past 25 years in most European countries demonstrates that population health is better than ever before. Although it is debated whether years in good health have increased more rapidly than years with health impairments (Deeg et al. 2018), the higher life expectancy has profound implications for the workforce. In recent years many countries have enacted policies to increase labor force participation and to extend the statutory retirement age to 67 years and beyond. Since the likelihood of health problems increases with age, it may be questioned whether most workers will be able to work longer in good health. There is increasing empirical evidence that poor health decreases the employability of older workers and that poor health plays an important role in premature displacement from the labor market (Van Rijn et al. 2014). In this respect, it is important to know how work will impact health and how work conditions will affect the ability of workers with health problems to remain in paid employment. A linked issue is how extended working careers will influence health and longevity thereafter. Thus, health will not only determine whether a person is able to work longer, but working longer will also affect a person's health.

In order to better understand the interplay between work and health, this chapter describes the theoretical framework of selection and causation mechanisms. These mechanisms act from the start of working careers; thus, a working life perspective is needed to better appreciate the influence of work on health and health on work during the entire working career. Some groups will require special attention when it comes to being able to work longer, most notably disabled workers and workers with chronic diseases. The chapter will end with current challenges in research and policies to prolong working careers in good health.

Selection and Causation Hypotheses

Interplay Between Work and Health

Work and health are closely related. Numerous studies have shown that individuals without a paid job have both a poorer physical and a poorer mental health compared to employed individuals (Bartley et al. 2004; Wanberg 2012). In the explanation of this health inequality, two important questions have to be answered: (1) Do workers with health problems drop out of paid employment? And (2) is loss of paid employment bad for your health?

The first question refers to the selection hypothesis: poor health acts as a barrier to enter and maintain paid employment; hence, in an aging workforce, the more healthy workers will survive. The healthy worker selection effect has been acknowledged for many decades, but empirical evidence on how this selection process operates exactly is from more recent years. The second question concerns the causation hypothesis: involuntary loss of paid employment will deteriorate an individual's health, especially mental health. In research these two hypotheses are difficult to disentangle and therefore require cautious scrutiny.

Selection Hypothesis

Health-Driven Exit from Paid Employment

The selection hypothesis is composed of two mechanisms that ensure that the working population is healthier than the general population: (1) workers with a poor health are more likely to be displaced from paid employment and (2) persons with health problems experience less opportunities to (re-) enter paid employment.

A recent meta-analysis on 29 longitudinal studies showed that health problems are an important barrier for maintaining paid employment – and thus for trajectories out of paid employment during the working life course through disability benefits, unemployment, and, to a lesser extent, early retirement (Van Rijn et al. 2014). Interestingly, the strength of the pooled association between health problems and exit from paid employment differed between specific measures of poor health. Self-rated poor health was a risk factor for transition into disability benefits (relative risk (RR) 3.61; 95% CI 2.44 to 5.35), unemployment (RR 1.44; 95% CI 1.26 to 1.65), and early retirement (RR 1.27; 95% CI 1.17 to 1.38). The presence of a chronic disease was a more modest risk factor for disability benefits (RR 2.11; 95% CI 1.90 to 2.33) and unemployment (RR 1.31; 95% CI 1.14 to 1.50), but not for early retirement. Among studies there was a large heterogeneity, suggesting that the influence of poor health on the ability to work will not only depend on nature and severity of health problems but also on individual, organizational, and national factors. A comparative study in 11 European countries nicely demonstrated the importance of these factors. The influence of self-rated health on becoming unemployed was stronger among higher educated persons than among those with a low education (Schuring et al. 2007). This may indicate that among highly educated workers, their health is one of the most important assets to maintain employability, whereas among low-educated workers, many other factors, such as economic developments and changes in required skills, play an important role. Indeed, the likelihood of becoming unemployed was much larger among low-educated than among high-educated workers, which will have masked the influence of poor health on exit from paid employment. Likewise, the association between poor health and becoming unemployed increased with lower unemployment rate at national level. It may be hypothesized that in countries with a booming labor market, job opportunities are plentiful and that only persons with severe health limitations are not absorbed into the workforce.

Specific Health Problems

The association between health problems and exit from paid employment will differ across types of health problems, and by pathway of exit from paid employment. In a Dutch longitudinal study, over 8000 employees between age 45 and 64 years were followed for 3 years to investigate the influence of chronic health problems on exit for paid employment through disability benefits, unemployment, and early retirement. Severe headache, diabetes mellitus, and musculoskeletal, respiratory, digestive, and psychological health problems predicted an increased risk of disability benefits (hazard ratios (HR) varying between 1.78 and 2.79). Circulatory (HR = 1.35) and psychological health problems (HR = 2.58) predicted unemployment, but other chronic diseases had no influence. Musculoskeletal disorders (HR = 1.23) and psychological health problems (HR = 1.57) were also associated with early retirement. Thus, all chronic diseases increased the likelihood on a disability benefit, but for other exit routes, the importance of specific chronic diseases differed. Psychological problems were a risk factor for any exit route from paid employment. A subsequent analysis showed an interaction between a chronic health problem and work conditions on the probability of receiving a disability benefit. Psychosocial work-related factors modified the influence of health problems on disability benefits. Specifically, among workers with health problems, higher autonomy, higher support, and lower psychological job demands reduced the risk of disability benefits by 82%, 49%, and 11%, respectively (Leijten et al. 2015). This study demonstrated that most workers with a chronic disease continued in paid employment, but that for some workers their disease in combination with the job requirements was too strenuous to remain a productive worker. Hence, the trajectory of workers with chronic health problems must be seen in the light of interference of work conditions with health.

For specific diseases, this process of interference has been studied in greater detail. There is clear evidence of an interaction effect of occupational exposure and respiratory disease on ability to work. In the European Community Respiratory Health Survey (ECRHS) among 11 European countries, subjects who reported physician-diagnosed asthma and held jobs with regular exposure to biological dusts, gases, or fumes had a 3.5 times higher likelihood of job change due to respiratory health problems during 7 years of follow-up (Toren et al. 2009). A later study showed that these associations were specifically observed among workers with less controlled asthma, indicating that some workers with asthma were able to cope with allergens in their working environment through medication, whereas for others survival in their job was not possible (Le Moual et al. 2014). In line with this finding, a recent study among 300 adults with asthma showed that workers with uncontrolled asthma had substantially higher sickness absence and lower productivity while at work (presenteeism) than workers with asthma under control by medication. Interestingly, the presence of psychological distress at work increased the negative influence of asthma on work performance (Moullec et al. 2015).

These studies illustrate that we need more insight into the complex interaction between disease and the work environment. The traditional focus in occupational health is on identifying risk factors for the onset of work-related disease, but we need a shift towards understanding which factors at work may lead to worsening of prognosis and lack of symptom control and even displacement from paid employment. Since work-related factors are in essence modifiable, they should not only be primary targets for intervention programs at the workplace but also be addressed in individual treatment plans.

Reentering Paid Employment

The selection hypothesis also asserts that persons with health problems will experience less opportunities to (re-)enter paid employment. This mechanism was demonstrated in a prospective study with 10 years follow-up in a representative sample of the Dutch working population with over 15,000 workers (Schuring et al. 2013). Workers with poor self-rated health had a reduced likelihood to return to paid employment after a period of unemployment. The effect of poor health on losing paid employment (hazard ratio 1.89) was larger than the effect of poor health as barrier to reenter paid employment (hazard ratio 1.33). The reentry curve into paid employment showed that the likelihood of entering paid employment decreased sharply over time; approximately 65% returned in a paid job within 2 years, and in the next 8 years, this likelihood increased by just another 20%. This suggests that the window of opportunity in rehabilitation in the Netherlands is relatively short and that re-employment services should be offered promptly.

In an attempt to further elucidate the mechanism on how poor health acts as a barrier for reentering paid employment, a longitudinal study with 6-month follow-up was conducted among 500 long-term unemployed persons (Carlier et al. 2014). Persons with a self-rated poor health had an approximately twofold lower likelihood to find a paid job than those in good health. Unemployed persons in poor health were less likely to actively search for a job, primarily due to attributing less value to having a job, opinions of close relatives that job search was not important, and also less reliance in their own ability to find a job. The mediation analysis showed that about 33% of the reduced likelihood on re-employment could be attributed to job search cognitions and behavior. In short, the labor market offers less opportunities for persons with a poor health, and these persons themselves exhibit less active behavior to find a job. This will lead to a vicious circle that may be difficult to be broken without explicit behavioral training (Brenninkmeijer and Blonk 2012).

The aforementioned complex interaction between disease and the work environment on health-driven exit from the labor market is also present for reentering paid employment after contracted a serious disease. A register-based study in Germany among more than 70,000 patients attending rehabilitation clinics showed that workers were less likely to return to their former job when those with mental illnesses had emotionally demanding labor and those with musculoskeletal diseases had physically strenuous jobs (Wiemer et al. 2017). For other diseases specific working conditions had less influence, but limited information on other strenuous factors at work may have hampered the researchers in identifying other meaningful associations.

Causation Hypothesis

The opposing mechanism of selection is causation. The causation theory stipulates that unemployment per se is a cause of poor health. Causation can act through two different pathways: (1) involuntary loss of paid employment may have a negative influence on health, whereas (2) gaining paid employment after being out of the workforce for some time may have a positive influence on health.

The first mechanism can be best studied when involuntary job loss can be considered to be completely exogenous to the individual. Such a condition is plant closure, which will not be determined by characteristics of individuals. A study on the long-term consequences of exogenous job loss found that men were more likely to be depressed and women reported poorer general health, more chronic conditions, and also poorer physical health (Schröder 2013). A register-based linkage study in Sweden identified job losses due to all establishment closures in Sweden in 1987 or 1988. During a subsequent 12-year period, the job loss increased the risk of hospitalization due to alcohol-related conditions, among both men and women, and due to traffic accidents and self-harm, among men only (Eliason and Storrie 2009).

When unemployment is a cause for deterioration of health, one would also expect that re-employment will improve health. However, this is difficult to demonstrate since entering paid employment cannot be considered a completely exogenous event. It can be expected that those who gained paid employment probably differed in (un)observed factors from those who remained unemployed, which would bias the estimates of the effect of re-employment on health. An alternative approach is to use a fixed-effects model whereby each individual serves as his or her own control, thus focusing on within-individual changes in health. This will eliminate any potential bias of time-invariant causes, whether measured or unmeasured. An extension is the recently developed hybrid method, where entering paid employment can be analyzed as within-individual associations, whereas factors that determine selection of person into the labor force can be analyzed as between-individual associations. This approach was taken in a recent Dutch study among 749 long-term unemployed persons with common mental disorders, as diagnosed by a physician in the past 12 months (Schuring et al. 2017). Entering paid employment resulted in substantial improvements in mental health (mean of 16 points on the mental health scale 0–100 of the Short-Form 12) and in physical health (mean of 10 points on the physical health scale 0–100 of the Short-Form 12). Among intermediate- and high-educated persons, entering paid employment had significantly larger effects on mental health than in low-educated persons. The study also showed that those in better health were more likely to gain paid employment.

This novel evidence for causal inference that work can be good for health reflects findings from observational studies in the past. The sociologic theory of latent functions by Jahoda (1982) posits that work contributes to personal identity and self-esteem and provides opportunities for social contacts and collective experiences, which may have direct and indirect effects on health. The vitamin model by Warr expands this theory by emphasizing the potential health benefits of skills use, social support, and motivation derived from work (Warr 1987). In the past years, several studies have shown that transiting from nonemployment to employment was associated with short-term improvements in mental health (Thomas et al. 2005, Schuring et al. 2011), social functioning, role limitations, and physical functioning (Schuring et al. 2011) and quality of life (Carlier et al. 2013). Yet, there is considerable debate as to who will benefit from moving into paid employment and the quality of the job needed to bestow positive health effects (Butterworth et al. 2011).

The emerging strong evidence on the causation mechanism that entering paid employment will improve health has important consequences. First, in treatment of persons with mental disorders, gaining work should be integrated as an essential part in the treatment protocol. Second, instead of focusing on inability to work when one has health problems, employers, healthcare professionals, and the general public should be made aware that work is in general good for health.

A Working Life Course Perspective

Trajectories During Working Career

So far, this chapter has presented information on health and work, derived from cohort studies with usually limited follow-up. These studies cannot describe the long-term course of diseases and associated displacement from the labor market over long periods, let alone working life. Järvholm et al. (2014) have demonstrated the long-term consequences of becoming too disabled to remain in the workforce. In a large construction cohort with almost 30 years of follow-up, profound differences were observed among 22 occupational groups for risk of disability pension, varying from a relative risk (RR) of 2.16 for rock workers to 0.54 for salaried workers compared to the reference group comprised of electricians. In an additional step, the total working time lost due to premature exit from paid employment during the working age was estimated. This showed a substantial number of working years lost due to disability pension before the age of 65 within these occupational groups: 3.2 years for rock workers, 1.4 years for electricians, and 0.7 years for salaried workers. Most working years were lost after the age of 50, predicting that an increase of the statutory retirement age from 65 to 67 years will imply that in some occupational groups, a substantial part of all workers will spend these additional years in disability (Järvholm et al. 2014).

This approach can be extended to estimation of the relative contribution of particular risk factors to working years lost due to premature displacement from the workforce through different exit routes. In the Survey on Health, Ageing and Retirement in Europe (SHARE), we have studied the effect of strenuous working conditions and self-rated poor health on early exit from the labor market through unemployment and early retirement. The longitudinal analysis showed clear associations of various lifestyle factors and working conditions with early retirement (odds ratios between 1.12 and 1.39) and unemployment (odds ratios between 1.05 and 1.71). An interesting finding was that the combined influence of lifestyle factors was of similar magnitude as the effects of adverse working conditions. Self-rated poor health remained a separate risk factor after adjustment for lifestyle factors and working conditions. In a multistate Markov model with population attributable fractions for lifestyle and working conditions, the impact of working conditions and unhealthy behaviors on working careers could be estimated. Under the assumption of elimination of work-related risk factors, working careers could be extended by at least 4 months. Similarly, poor lifestyle contributed about 4 months to working careers as well. Prevention of self-rated poor health would extend working careers on average by 6 months (Burdorf 2006). This new approach shifts the attention from risk estimates to working years lost during the working age and, as such, presents a life course perspective that illustrates the profound importance of timely interventions at the workplace in order to increase labor force participation among (elderly) workers.

In recent years new metrics have been developed to capture the working life course perspective. A key metric is working life expectancy (WLE) that expresses, in analogy to life expectancy, the number of years that a person is expected to spend in paid employment until he or she finally leaves the labor force for statutory retirement (Pedersen and Bjorner 2017). As linked measure, the working years lost (WYL) has been introduced, reflecting the working time lost due to premature exit from paid employment. A recent study in the Netherlands used WLE to evaluate changes in working careers over a 20-year period (Van der Noordt et al. 2019). During this period for a worker at age 58 in paid employment, total WLE increased from 3.7 to 5.5 years. However, for workers who experienced functional limitations in daily activities for more than 3 months, the WLE at age 58 increased only from 0.8 to 1.5 years. Expressed alternatively, workers with functional limitations will lose at least 4 years of being in paid employment in the 10 years before the statutory retirement age. A Danish study on workers aged 55–65 years reported that those in poor health at age 55 on average lost 1.3 working years before the age of 65 years. Interestingly, workers with access to an early retirement scheme retired about 2.5 years earlier than workers without access and in both groups of workers poor health had a similar detrimental effect of duration of working careers (Pedersen and Bjorner 2017).

This life course perspective of the workforce, captured in WLE and health-related WYL, offers new opportunities for research, for example, it can be used to evaluate long-term consequences of policy changes in labor legislation and to provide insight into socioeconomic inequalities during the working life course.

The Impact of Working Careers on Health After Retirement

An emerging topic is how working careers will influence morbidity and mortality after retirement. As described above, most studies have focused on the influence of working conditions and lifestyle behaviors on health and subsequent consequences for labor force participation in the workforce. It is well acknowledged that work-related morbidity and mortality will also arise after working life. Likewise, it is of interest to better understand how working careers will influence health after retirement. A linked issue is the current debate that if strenuous work has adverse effects on health, especially at older age with declining physical and cognitive function, then timely retirement may be health-preserving. In essence, when is retirement good for your health (Burdorf 2010)?

Addressing this question is important in view of the fact that many countries implement policy reforms to increase retirement age. Current studies present contradictory results. For example, in the French Gazel cohort, retirement at age 57 coincided with decreases in prevalence of self-rated health, depressive symptoms, and physical and mental fatigue (Westerlund et al. 2009), but no changes were observed for physician-diagnosed diseases, such as diabetes and coronary heart disease (Westerlund et al. 2010). The Whitehall II study reported that for many British civil servants, self-rated health improved after retiring, but for those with a high position job, their health deteriorated (Mein et al. 2003). A study in the European workforce provided a detailed analysis of health trajectories before, during, and after employment transitions. It was shown that among low-educated workers, self-rated poor health partly prompted their voluntary labor force exit through early retirement and becoming economically inactive, but thereafter these exit routes seemed to prevent further deterioration of their health. In contrast, among higher educated workers, early retirement had an adverse effect on their self-rated health. The findings suggest that retirement may have both adverse and beneficial effects on health, and these effects differ across educational level of individuals. National policies to increase labor force participation at an older age should acknowledge that health inequalities may increase when every person is required to be in paid employment until the same age before being able to retire (Schuring et al. 2015).

There is an abundance of literature on the effects of unemployment on later-life mortality. A meta-analysis on 42 studies with more than 20 million persons provided a pooled hazard ratio of 1.63 for mortality, after adjustment for age and additional covariates. The mean effect was larger among men than women. The detrimental effect of unemployment on late-life mortality seemed dependent on the period during life with unemployment. Increased mortality risk for unemployment was largest for persons in their early and middle careers and lowest for those in their late career (Roelfs et al. 2011). An ecological study on inequalities in healthy life years in 25 European countries confirmed the importance of paid employment for healthy life expectancy. For every 1% increase in unemployment rate, the healthy life expectancy at 50 years of age dropped by almost 0.7 years among men (Jagger et al. 2008). Thus, health is important for a good working career, and a good working career is important for quality of life and life expectancy.

Vulnerable Groups

With respect to prolonged working lives, there are several vulnerable groups at increased risk for early exit from paid employment, most notably persons with chronic diseases and workers with lower socioeconomic position. As described earlier, health problems are important reasons for exit from work. In several patient groups, the affected trajectories through working careers have been reported, most often describing the proportion of patients still in paid employment after a certain number of years after diagnosis. There are few studies that capture a working life perspective in a summary measure as working life expectancy. An illustrative example is presented by Lacaille and Hogg (2001), who estimated that in Canada, patients with arthritis or rheumatism had a reduced WLE among men of 4.2 years and among women of 3.1 years.

In recent years attention has grown for the role of work in socioeconomic health inequalities (Burdorf 2015). Two distinct patterns can be distinguished: educational attainment as determinant of labor market position and educational differences in working conditions, lifestyle, and health as underlying causes for educational differences in exit from the labor market. With regard to the first pattern, in a pooled analysis across 7 studies with almost 100,000 workers, those with lower educational attainment were consistently more likely to experience a health-related exit from paid employment (Carr et al. 2018). A recent Swedish report estimated a WYL gap across occupational class due to disability benefits of 2.0 among women and 2.3 among men at age 35 (Kadefors et al. 2019). Comparable results were published in Finland where male and female manual workers at age 50 were expected to work 3.6–3.7 fewer years than workers in the highest occupational class. A large proportion of this WYL gap could be attributed to health-related disability benefits (Leinonen et al. 2018).

These descriptive studies are very valuable, but they lack insight into underlying causes of these inequalities. Hence, there is a need for studies addressing the second distinct pattern. Our own studies have shown that lower educated workers were more likely to exit paid employment through disability benefits, unemployment, and economic inactivity. Self-rated poor health, unhealthy lifestyle, and unfavorable working conditions were associated with higher likelihood on disability benefits and unemployment and unhealthy lifestyle with economic inactivity. Educational differences in disability benefits were explained for 40% by health, 31% by lifestyle, and 12% by work characteristics. For economic inactivity and unemployment, up to

14% and 21% of the educational differences could be explained, particularly by lifestyle-related factors. The educational inequalities in working careers seem specifically due to a higher occurrence of adverse working conditions, unhealthy lifestyle, and poor health among low-educated workers compared to high-educated workers. The association between these risk factors and labor force participation did not systematically differ across educational groups (Robroek et al. 2015).

Vulnerable groups have an increased risk of exit from paid employment. The current evidence implies that policies to extend working life should provide institutional support for those with poor health.

Challenges and Conclusions

Most studies on the influence of health on early exit from paid employment rely on presenting risk estimates to demonstrate the importance of being in good health for a prolonged working career. In this chapter we argue that this information will insufficiently present insight into the cumulative loss of work capacity during working life. A life course perspective on the workforce is needed. Working life expectancy and working years lost due to prematurely quitting active work force participation may provide important summary metrics that capture entire trajectories in work status during working careers.

It is of great importance to gain more insight into the relative contribution of poor health, adverse working conditions, and unhealthy behaviors to loss of work capacity during working life. In fact, there is a concerning lack of evidence over which individual-, work-, and disease-related factors play a role in premature displacement from paid employment and what interventions are needed to counteract the adverse consequences of disease for labor force participation. This evidence is crucial for identifying persons and groups at risk for dropping out of the labor market. A linked issue is that there is a clear need for research aiming to develop strategies to support the ability to work for vulnerable groups, such as workers with chronic diseases and workers in low socioeconomic position with often strenuous working conditions.

This knowledge is also required for designing better preventive measures against work- and health-related exit from paid employment. Current interventions seldom take into account how diseases and working conditions will interact upon the ability of (older) workers to remain in paid employment until statutory retirement age. These preventive measures should also be guided by insight whether the majority of working years are lost by a limited number of rather young persons or many older persons who leave working life a few years before eligibility for old age retirement. In the first situation, measures to find and try to increase the work ability of susceptible individuals may be the preferred solution (selective prevention), while in the latter case, measures directed at the work environment may have a higher priority (universal prevention). Evidence-based policies and programs that promote working longer in good health should make amends for a tailored approach that acknowledges individual differences in health, working conditions, and health behaviors.

Cross-References

▶ Concepts and Social Variations of Disability in Working-Age Populations
▶ Policies of Reducing the Burden of Occupational Hazards and Disability Pensions
▶ Reducing Inequalities in Employment of People with Disabilities

References

Bartley M, Sacker A, Clarke P (2004) Employment status, employment conditions, and limiting illness: prospective evidence from the British household panel survey 1991–2001. J Epidemiol Community Health 58:501–506

Brenninkmeijer V, Blonk R (2012) The effectiveness of the JOBS program among the long-term unemployed: a randomized experiment in the Netherlands. Health Promot Int 27:220–229

Burdorf A (2006) The contribution of occupational hygiene to public health: new opportunities to demonstrate its importance. J Occup Environ Hyg 3:D120–D125

Burdorf A (2010) Is early retirement good for your health? BMJ 341:c6089

Burdorf A (2015) Understanding the role of work in socio-economic health inequalities. Scand J Work Environ Health 41:325–327

Butterworth P, Leach LS, Strazdins L et al (2011) The psychosocial quality of work determines whether employment has benefits for mental health: results from a longitudinal national household panel survey. Occup Environ Med 68:806–812

Carlier BE, Schuring M, Lötters FJB et al (2013) The influence of re-employment on quality of life and self-rated health, a longitudinal study among unemployed persons in the Netherlands. BMC Public Health 13:503

Carlier BE, Schuring M, Lenthe van FJ, Burdorf A (2014) Influence of health on job-search behavior and re-employment; the role of job-search cognitions and coping resources. J Occup Rehab 24:670–679

Carr E, Fleischmann M, Goldberg M et al (2018) Occupational and educational inequalities in exit from employment at older ages: evidence from seven prospective cohorts. Occup Environ Med 75:369–377

Deeg DJH, Comijs HC, Hoogendijk EO et al (2018) 23-year trends in life expectancy in good and poor physical and cognitive health at age 65 years in the Netherlands, 1993–2016. Am J Public Health 108:1652–1658

Eliason M, Storrie D (2009) Job loss is bad for your health – Swedish evidence on cause-specific hospitalization following involuntary job loss. Soc Sci Med 68:1396–1406

Jagger C, Gillies C, Moscone F et al (2008) Inequalities in healthy life years in the 25 countries of the European Union in 2005: a cross-national meta-regression analysis. Lancet 372:2124–2131

Jahoda M (1982) Employment and unemployment: a social psychological analysis. Cambridge University Press, New York

Järvholm B, Stattin M, Robroek SJW et al (2014) Heavy work and disability pension – a long term follow-up of Swedish construction workers. Scand J Work Environ Health 40:335–342

Kadefors R, Nilsson K, Östergren PO et al (2019) Social inequality in working life expectancy in Sweden. Z Gerontol Geriat 52 Suppl 1:52–61

Lacaille D, Hogg RS (2001) The effect of arthritis on working life expectancy. J Rheumatol 28:2315–2319

Le Moual N, Carsin AE, Siroux V et al (2014) Occupational exposures and uncontrolled adult-onset asthma in the European Community Respiratory Health Survey II. Eur Respir J 43:374–386

Leijten FRM, de Wind A, van den Heuvel SG et al (2015) The influence of chronic health problems and work-related factors on loss of paid employment among older workers. J Epidemiol Community Health 69:1058–1065

Leinonen T, Martikainen P, Myrskylä M et al (2018) Working life and retirement expectancies at age 50 by social class: period and cohort trends and projections for Finland. J Gerontol B Psychol Sci Soc Sci 73:302–313

Mein G, Martikainen P, Hemingway H et al (2003) Is retirement good or bad for mental and physical health functioning? Whitehall II longitudinal study of civil servants. J Epidemiol Community Health 57:46–49

Moullec G, FitzGerald JM, Rousseau R et al (2015) Interaction effect of psychological distress and asthma control on productivity loss? Eur Respir J 45:1557–1565

Pedersen J, Bjorner JB (2017) Worklife expectancy in a cohort of Danish employees aged 55–65 years – comparing a multi-state Cox proportional hazard approach with conventional multi-state life tables. BMC Public Health 17:879

Robroek SJW, Rongen A, Arts CH et al (2015) Educational inequalities in exit from paid employment among Dutch workers: the influence of health, lifestyle and work. PLoS One 10: e0134867

Roelfs DJ, Shor E, Davidson KW et al (2011) Losing life and livelihood: a systematic review and meta-analysis of unemployment and all-cause mortality. Soc Sci Med 72:840–854

Schröder M (2013) Jobless now, sick later? Investigating the long-term consequences of involuntary job loss on health. Adv Life Course Res 18:5–15

Schuring M, Burdorf A, Kunst A et al (2007) The effects of ill health on entering and maintaining paid employment: evidence in European countries. J Epidemiol Community Health 61:597–604

Schuring M, Mackenbach J, Voorham T et al (2011) The effect of re-employment on perceived health. J Epidemiol Community Health 65:639–644

Schuring M, Robroek SJW, Otten FWJ et al (2013) The effect of ill health and socioeconomic status on labour force exit and re-employment: a prospective study with ten years follow up in the Netherlands. Scand J Work Environ Health 39:134–143

Schuring M, Robroek SJW, Lingsma HF et al (2015) Educational differences in trajectories of self-rated health before, during, and after entering or leaving paid employment in the European workforce. Scand J Work Environ Health 41:441–450

Schuring M, Robroek SJ, Burdorf A (2017) The benefits of paid employment among persons with common mental health problems: evidence for the selection and causation mechanism. Scand J Work Environ Health 43:540–549

Thomas C, Benzeval M, Stansfeld SA (2005) Employment transitions and mental health: an analysis from the British household panel survey. J Epidemiol Community Health 59:243–249

Torén K, Zock JP, Kogevinas M et al (2009) An international prospective general population-based study of respiratory work disability. Thorax 64:339–344

Van der Noordt M, Van der Pas S, van Tilburg TG et al (2019) Changes in working life expectancy with disability in the Netherlands, 1992–2016. Scand J Work Environ Health 45:73–81

Van Rijn R, Robroek SJW, Brouwer S et al (2014) Influence of poor health on exit from paid employment: a systematic review. Occup Environ Med 71:289–294

Wanberg CR (2012) The individual experience of unemployment. Annu Rev Psychol 63:369–396

Warr P (1987) Work, unemployment and mental health. Clarendon Press, Oxford

Westerlund H, Kivimaki M, Singh-Manoux A et al (2009) Self-rated health before and after retirement in France (GAZEL): a cohort study. Lancet 374:1889–1896

Westerlund H, Vahtera J, Ferrie JE et al (2010) Effect of retirement on major chronic conditions and fatigue: French GAZEL occupational cohort study. BMJ 341:c6149

Wiemer A, Mölders C, Fischer S et al (2017) Effectiveness of medical rehabilitation on return-to-work depends on the interplay of occupation characteristics and disease. J Occup Rehabil 27:59–69

Policies of Reducing the Burden of Occupational Hazards and Disability Pensions

6

Espen Dahl and Kjetil A. van der Wel

Contents

Introduction	86
Disability and Poverty	87
Labor Force Participation Among Disabled People	88
Receipt of Disability Benefits	90
Disability and Working Conditions in the Postindustrial Labor Market	90
Disability Policies	92
Prevention	92
Compensation/Integration	93
Social Regulation	94
What Works?	95
Summary and Conclusion	99
Cross-References	100
References	101

Abstract

In this chapter we describe policy initiatives to enhance labor force participation among disabled people and assess their merits. One key message is that there is no easy or simple way to improve labor market participation and hence reduce poverty and receipt of disability benefit among disabled. If the aim is to further employment and economic well-being among disabled people, it is evident that much of the most popular disability policies pursued today, such as emphasis on work incentives, strict enforcement of conditionalities and sanctions, and focus on supply-side measures, employment quotas, and anti-discrimination legislation, do not have the desired effects. Some of them may even be counterproductive. Research evidence suggests, however, that interventions that improve the work environment, as well as programs based on supported employment approaches, are promising avenues for future policy development. As poverty is still a major

E. Dahl (✉) · K. A. van der Wel
Oslo Metropolitan University, Oslo, Norway
e-mail: espendah@oslomet.no; kjetil.wel@oslomet.no

© Springer Nature Switzerland AG 2020
U. Bültmann, J. Siegrist (eds.), *Handbook of Disability, Work and Health*, Handbook Series in Occupational Health Sciences, https://doi.org/10.1007/978-3-030-24334-0_4

85

challenge associated with disability, disability policies must still strive to ensure sufficient livelihood and economic independence for people with disabilities – with or without earnings from paid work.

Keywords

Disability policy · Working conditions · ALMP · Supported employment

Introduction

Welfare states in Europe and in the OECD face financial challenges due to aging populations and long-standing low fertility (Esping-Andersen 1999; OECD 2017). In addition, disability and sickness rolls have been on rise in many countries. In relation to this, a key policy advice from the OECD (2010) has been to improve the labor market integration of disabled people by strengthening economic incentives for sick workers, employers, benefit authorities, and service providers and increase employment expectations, responsibilities, and support among doctors and employment service caseworkers. Sick worker's partial work capacity needs to be assessed and made use of, according to the OECD, and employers need to get a "much more prominent role," supported by an employment-oriented occupational health service. These strategies are broadly in line with what has been become known as the "social investment" welfare state, particularly concerning young people with disabilities (Van Kersbergen and Hemerijck 2012).

However, the motivation to integrating disabled people in work is not purely financial but also mirrors a fundamental change in the notions of "the disabled person" and what having a disability entails in terms of work capacity. Social movements arguing for the "social model of disability" have contributed to this change (Owens 2015). The social model of disability opposes the biomedical view, which places the disabling condition – the impairment – at the level of the individual. Rather, the social model sees disability as a social construct: Impairment may become disability through the experience of "structural oppression; cultural stereotypes, attitudes, bureaucratic hierarchies, market mechanisms, and all that is pertaining to how society is structured and organized" (Thomas 2010). Being defined as "disabled" may thus in itself be a barrier to work.

The social model of disability is also underpinned by wider ideas about social justice, active citizenship, and realizing individual's capabilities (Halvorsen et al. 2017b). These perspectives are at the heart of the UN Convention on the Rights of Persons with Disabilities which aims to "promote, protect and ensure the full and equal enjoyment of all human rights and fundamental freedoms by all persons with disabilities, and to promote respect for their inherent dignity" (Article 1). The Convention further specifically addresses work and employment opportunities. Persons with disabilities have a right to work "on an equal basis with others; this includes the right to the opportunity to gain a living by work freely chosen or accepted in a labour market and work environment that is open, inclusive and accessible to persons with disabilities" (Article 27). Most of the EU and OECD countries have ratified the Convention and committed themselves to promote employment opportunities through prohibiting discrimination and providing rehabilitation, vocational training, and reasonable accommodation and ensuring safe and healthy working conditions.

In practice, disability policies have been directed toward at least three areas: (1) reducing the incidence of disability that results from injuries and hazardous working conditions in working life; (2) welfare arrangements and services that provide practical and economic support and enable participation in working life for people with varying levels of disability; and (3) securing social, legal, regulatory, and economic frameworks that protect against discrimination and promote stable employment among disabled people (including hiring and firing rules, workplace accommodation, universal access, etc.). Böheim and Leoni (2018) distinguish between the policy objectives prevention, activation, and protection, but it is not clear whether employment protection rules, accommodation, and universal access are included. Halvorsen et al. (2017b), in their analytical framework, separate between three subsystems in disability policy systems: a cash transfer system, a service delivery system, and a social regulation system. However, here the efforts to promote health and hinder impairments in the workforce are not captured. OECD (2010) offers a useful conceptual distinction between policies that pursue income compensation and policies that aim at actively integrating disabled into the labor market. The point is how these two dimensions work in combination. In this chapter, we combine these approaches into three policy objectives, *prevention*, *compensation/integration*, and *social regulation*, respectively.

In the following, we will present an overview of disability policies within these areas, critically discuss recent developments and trends, and assess consequences of this variety of policies for labor market outcomes among disabled people, before we sum up and conclude. We start, however, with a brief investigation of the empirical patterns of economic well-being, work, disability benefit receipt, and labor market trends.

Disability and Poverty

The overall aim of disability policy is to secure sufficient living standards and the economic resources to participate in society on an equal footing with everyone else, either through self-provision in the market or through social protection schemes. Hence, the investigation of poverty rates among disabled people is an excellent overall assessment of whether disability policies are effective. The development in poverty among the disabled and non-disabled population in Europe can be seen in Fig. 1. Disability is measured by limitations in activity.

Figure 1 shows, firstly, that poverty rates among disabled people lie consistently above those of the non-disabled. Secondly, there is a steady increase in poverty among disabled and non-disabled, in particular from 2009. Among disabled people this growth is significant as the poverty rate rose from 19% in 2005 to almost 24% in

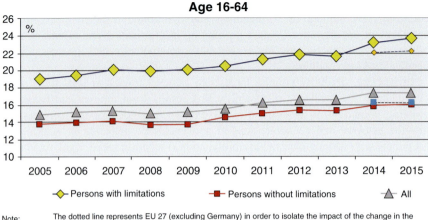

Fig. 1 Risk of poverty by disability status and year in the EU countries. Working age population. (Source: Grammenos 2018)

2015. Thirdly, the rise in poverty is somewhat more pronounced among disabled than non-disabled, resulting in a widening poverty gap between the two groups. It should also be mentioned that the poverty levels among disabled people most certainly are underestimated. Disabled people's needs are higher due to enhanced costs as well as extra costs (MacInnes et al. 2014). A similar development in poverty can be observed in the USA. In 2016, the percentage of disabled people who lived beyond the poverty line was 27. Eight years earlier it was 25% (http://www. disabilitystatistics.org/reports/acs.cfm?statistic=7). As we show below, the poverty rates may be linked to educational attainment, work opportunities, and welfare benefits.

Labor Force Participation Among Disabled People

The "labor force participation" of disabled people has different aspects. The disability employment rate tells us the extent to which people with disabilities have access to employment. However, from a social justice point of view, the disability employment gap, i.e., the difference in the employment rates for disabled and non-disabled people, may be more relevant.

Figure 2 displays both measures for the working age population in European countries. Most Northern European countries have high disability employment rates and low disability employment gaps, while Southern and many Eastern European countries combine low employment rates and large disability employment gaps. In general, there is a large degree of agreement between the two measures, but with a couple of exceptions: Norway has a higher disability

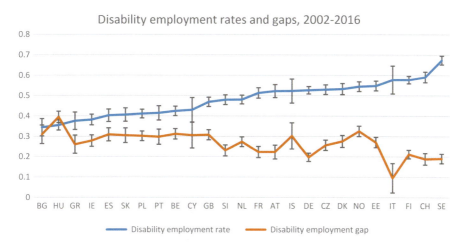

Fig. 2 Disability employment gaps and disability employment rates in European countries with 95% confidence intervals. Pooled data from round 1 to 8 of the European Social Survey (ESS), age 25–65, authors' calculations

employment gap than expected, and the Netherlands does less well than the other Northern European countries with regard to its disability employment rate. Italy seems to be an outlier, perhaps due to the few observations available in the ESS. Sweden, Switzerland, and Finland perform well on both indices, while Bulgaria, Hungary, and Greece have the lowest disability employment and high disability employment gaps.

While there is a dearth of international trend studies on disability employment, some indications exist. Holland et al. (2011) investigated trends in social inequalities in disability employment in five countries between the mid-1980s and 2003/2005. Disability was measured by limiting long-standing illness. In all countries, there was a clear decrease in employment among disabled persons with low education. For those with higher education, the picture was less clear. Lowest levels of employment among disabled people with low education were found in Canada and the UK, while the rates were higher in the Scandinavian countries. In a more recent study using a similar measure of disability and covering 25 European countries in the European Social Survey 2002–2012, Geiger et al. (2017) found on average increasing disability employment (7.6%) and decreasing disability employment gaps (4.9%). The countries contributing most to increase disability employment were Germany, Poland, the Czech Republic, and Belgium. No countries had a statistically significant reduction of the disability employment rate. Both studies focused on the working age population. In the USA, employment rates among disabled have declined recently, from 40% in the year 2008 to 36% in 2016 (http://www.disabilitystatistics.org/reports/acs.cfm?statistic=7).

According to the OECD (2010), people with disabilities have marked lower levels of educational attainment. Twice as many of the disabled have less than upper secondary education compared to the general population. However, a recent study indicates that it is more important to lift the educational level from primary to secondary education, than from secondary to tertiary (Bliksvaer 2018).

Receipt of Disability Benefits

On average around 6% of the working age population received a disability benefit in the OECD countries in 2008. There are, however, rather large differences between the countries. In Hungary, Norway, and Sweden, about 10% of those in their working ages received disability benefits (or long-term sickness benefits). At the other extreme, in Japan, Korea, and Mexico, only about 2%, or even fewer, went on disability benefit. In 11 OECD countries, there were a growing number of disability benefit recipients (OECD 2010).

Disability and Working Conditions in the Postindustrial Labor Market

Since disability is the product of the interaction between individual impairment and the demands of the working life, it is of interest to review some of the labor market changes that have taken place over the past decades. During the last half century, major labor market changes have occurred related to technological developments, upskilling, new modes of organization, shifting employment relations, and the global division of labor. These changes can be subsumed under the term "post-industrialization" (Bell 1973). According to Bell's ideal typical forecast, the transition to the "postindustrial society" is recognized by increased centrality of theoretical knowledge and the use of it for commerce, political, administrative, and strategic purposes; intellectual technology such as computing; an emerging knowledge class; a change from goods to services, also reflected in the occupational structure and the characteristics of work; increased labor market participation among women; and meritocracy. Many similar declarations of "epochal transformations" exist, although controversial (Doogan 2009).

The consequences of the postindustrial labor market for low-skilled workers and workers with disabilities in terms of long-term unemployment, poverty risk, and precariousness have been widely acknowledged (Esping-Andersen 1999; Standing 2011; Taylor-Gooby 2004). Although evidence exists on weakening labor market opportunities of low-skilled people with disabilities during the 1980s and early 1990s (Bartley and Owen 1996; Holland et al. 2011; van der Wel et al. 2010), the trend does not seem to be continuing (Geiger et al. 2017). Although expansion of high-skilled jobs has happened at the expense of low-skilled jobs, European countries have largely escaped massive unemployment or inactivity among low-skilled workers, unlike the US, according to Oesch (2015). (The study included Switzerland, Germany, Denmark, Spain, and the UK.) This is because there has been a simultaneous growth in education in most European countries, which has significantly reduced the number of low-skilled workers. Oesch (2015) further reports that employment rates among low-skilled workers were either stable or increased in the countries included in the study.

Furthermore, in the latest report from the European Working Condition Survey (EWCS), which covers the 28 EU countries, we observe little change in the share having fixed term contracts or being self-employed, indices of precarious work, between 2005 and 2015 (Eurofound 2017). Similarly, no dramatic change could be seen in the share reporting that they might lose their job in the next 6 months. There was an increase in decision latitude and in the skills discretion of European workers in the same period. These results do not suggest an escalation in "postindustrial" working conditions in the latter decade, which add to the doubts concerning this hypothesis expressed by studies using data from the 1980s (Burchell and Fagan 2004; Greenan et al. 2007). The overall picture in the report from the sixth EWCS (Eurofound 2017) is somewhat complex as some indices show progress, whereas others show deterioration. For example, the physical environment index, which captures a number of physical risks (e.g., biological and chemical), shows a small increase in exposure since 2005. The work intensity index, which measures exposure to work demands, shows a slight reduction in work intensity between 2005 and 2015. Working time quality also improved.

Nevertheless, as working conditions are closely linked to specific tasks and modes of work organizations in different industries, occupation is still a strong determinant of inequalities between workers. Overall, manual and low-skilled jobs expose workers to a number of physical hazards that are detrimental to health (Bambra 2011). Many low-skilled jobs, e.g., in the service industry, induce psychosocial stress through high demands/low decision latitude (Karasek 1979) or through an imbalance in rewards and efforts, in particular if combined with an orientation of overcommitment (Siegrist and Wahrendorf 2016). Workers in less-skilled occupations report significant poorer well-being and satisfaction with their working conditions. They also report higher levels of time pressure at work and a higher number of health problems and are less likely to stay in the job until old age.

Thus, the rather pronounced inequalities in poor working conditions in European working life and the lack of improvement on a number of indicators suggest that work characteristics have the potential to generate ill-health and disability. As employment prospects of disabled people are often in peripheral segments of working life (Roulstone 2012), characterized by low-skilled tasks and precariousness, the work environment may serve as barriers to enter work for people with impairments.

This perspective should not, however, overshadow the possibility that work also may be healthy and promote recovery. Only recently, researchers and politicians alike have directed attention to the possible salutogenic aspects of work (Waddel and Burton 2006). Furthermore, the availability of part-time jobs and opportunities for self-employment may help (older) disabled workers maintain employment (Jones and Latreille 2011; Pagan 2012).

Disability Policies

Prevention

Sound and safe working conditions in all segments of working life are a precondition for a healthy work force and an inclusive labor market. Physical, chemical, psychosocial, ergonomic, and organizational aspects of work may produce disability (Bambra 2011) and represent barriers to work for people with disabilities, as argued above. Preventive measures include work environment legislation, control and sanctioning, information to employers and employees, systematic workplace monitoring of occupational risk, and work place interventions. Work place interventions may be directed at the workplace as a whole (primary prevention), at specific target groups (secondary prevention), or directly toward sick or disabled employees (tertiary prevention) (Joyce et al. 2016). These include measures to improve time organization, enhance worker control or physical activity, or provide various forms of therapy (Bambra 2011; Goldgruber and Ahrens 2010; Joyce et al. 2016).

Since the 1989 Safety and Health Work Directive, numerous EU directives on working conditions have been passed (see https://ec.europa.eu/social/main.jsp?catId=706&langId=en). The EU has regulatory efforts in the areas of working time, temporary work, pregnant workers, and much more. Furthermore, in 2019, a European Labour Authority will be up and running as part of the European Pillar of Social Rights (https://ec.europa.eu/social/main.jsp?catId=1414&langId=en). The EU directive on the safety and health of workers places some general obligations on the employers. The first of these is that "the employer shall take the measures necessary for the safety and health protection of workers, including prevention of occupational risks and provision of information and training, as well as provision of the necessary organization and means" (https://eur-lex.europa.eu/legal-content/EN/TXT/HTML/?uri=CELEX:31989L0391&from=EN).

The obligations of the employer are further to avoid risks; to evaluate the risks which cannot be avoided, adapting the work to the individual and alleviating monotonous work and work at a predetermined work rate; and to develop a coherent prevention policy which covers technology, organization of work, working conditions, and social relationships. National work environment regulation has been in place for decades in most advanced capitalist countries (Bambra 2011, pp. 164–165) and with important legal steps taken during the 1970s (e.g., the 1975 Health and Safety at Work Act in the UK, the 1970 Occupational Safety and Health Act in the US, the 1977 Working Environment Act in Norway and Sweden, etc.).

While work environment legislation at the national and supranational levels is important, they need to be linked to action, knowledge, routines, and preventive measures at the level of the workplace and with information, control, and law enforcement at the national level, in order to be effective. Inspections and appropriate sanctions against employers are important and necessary measures in order to secure the implementation of health and safety regulation (Bambra 2011, p. 165).

Compensation/Integration

The main bulk of disability policies aim to provide practical and economic support and to enable participation in working life for people with varying levels of disability, i.e., compensation and integration (OECD 2010). However, in line with the biomedical model of disability, compensatory measures, like disability benefits, rehabilitation, and sheltered employment, have been the prevailing approach. In 2010, OECD wrote: "Public spending on disability is still dominated by 'passive' payments of benefits. Investment in employment support and vocational rehabilitation – 'active' spending – is generally small. This is despite the recent shifts in policy orientation from passive to active measures in most countries" (OECD 2010, p. 2). This shift in orientation could be seen in 20 OECD countries that introduced reforms that made their benefit systems stricter in terms of, e.g., more objective medical criteria, more rigorous vocational criteria, stricter sickness absence monitoring, and stronger work incentives. Less than a handful of countries registered an increase in benefit generosity and then from a low level. The OECD (2010) further notes that integration policies, such as improved incentives for employers and supported employment, were strengthened in all countries.

In the same, influential, report OECD recommends that in order to expand employment opportunities, financial incentives need to be strengthened for all actors involved. OECD is also an advocate for the introduction or honing of behavioral conditionality for disability benefit claimants. Activity requirements and (harsh) sanctions seem to be spreading to more nations and from social assistance to disability benefit recipients. Recently, Geiger (2017) has explored how these kinds of policies have diffused in seven OECD countries. He concludes that behavioral requirements now are widespread but that sanctioning is rare.

An updated study using the OECD conceptual framework indicates that countries have pursued different types of reforms since 1990 (Böheim and Leoni 2018). The study examines the extent to which sickness and disability policies at different time points can be characterized as oriented toward compensation or integration. The integration dimension includes "among other things, the complexity and consistency of benefits and support systems, the degree of employer obligation towards their employees, the timing and extent of vocational rehabilitation and the existence of work incentives for beneficiaries" (ibid., p. 169). Examples of the ten subcomponents of the OECD integration dimension are employer obligations, supported employment, subsidized employment, benefit suspension option, and work incentives. The compensation dimension, on the other hand, covers "the coverage and level of disability benefits, the minimum degree of incapacity needed for benefits and full benefit entitlement, the type of medical and vocational assessment, as well as information on sickness benefits" (ibid.). The authors show that the more recent reforms have led to the emergence of a distinct cluster of Northern and Continental European countries, the "social democratic" cluster, characterized by a combination of strong employment-oriented policies and comparatively high social protection levels. They also identify a "liberal" cluster, consisting of countries oriented toward low compensation and who, during the period, became increasingly oriented toward policies in the integration dimension, most notably work incentives, benefit suspension, and supported employment. Finally, the study identified a "residual" cluster consisting of countries with low reform activity and intermediate values on the two dimensions.

A new "paradigm" is emerging within both "liberal" and "social democratic" integrative measures, which fall between the compensation/integration and the social regulation areas in our overview. This paradigm may be dubbed a "support-side" policy, which distinguishes itself from the traditional supply-side and demand-side approaches (Frøyland et al. 2019). Compared with the traditional active labor market policies (train-then-place), this new paradigm focuses on working life as the arena for work inclusion (place-then-train), i.e., "support-side" policies "more proactively support client and collaborate closer with employers" (ibid., p. 195). These approaches further include financial incentive, cooperative action, and professional, long term if necessary, follow-up and are based on voluntary agreements and commitments encouraging a corporate culture that promotes diversity through progressive recruitment and accommodation measures within the workplace. Incentives are measures that aim to reduce the assumed risks connected to employing workers perceived to be high-risk recruits, such as the need for extended follow-up in the workplace. Support-side approaches rest on an assumption that even jobless disabled individuals have a work capacity that can be made use of when stigmatizing prejudice is removed and reasonable accommodation is undertaken. Examples of support-side measures are Supported Employment and Individual Placement and Support (Nøkleby et al. 2017).

Social Regulation

The social regulation subsystem of disability policies includes laws and policies aimed at changing the behavior of employers to facilitate and protect employment opportunities for disabled people. These policies can be hard, e.g., laws against discrimination or the use of employment quotas in combination with strict enforcement, or they can be soft, e.g., economic incentives or strategies to inform and support employers. While compensatory measures aim at redistribution in the face of markets failing to provide equal opportunities, regulatory measures aim at *remedying* market failure by influencing how markets work (Halvorsen et al. 2017b). The social regulatory system may include legislative means, financial incentives or persuasion through information, and appeals to actor's social conscience. Many of these strategies are included in place-then-train policies presented above. These different strategies presuppose that actors may be either forced, economically encouraged, or morally convinced to adhere to societal norms and expectations.

Supranational organizations have played a key role in developing regulatory policies. The European Union's Employment Equality Directive from 2000 contributed to "address areas which had not previously been regulated in most Member countries" (Waddington and Lawson 2009). A European comparative study reports that anti-discrimination legislation has been transposed in all 28 member countries

(Chopin and Germaine 2017). The report concludes that EU efforts in this area have "immensely enhanced legal protection against discrimination on the grounds of racial or ethnic origin, religion or belief, age, disability and sexual orientation across Europe" (p. 128). Most member states even provided further protection compared to the requirements of EU law, and many shortcomings have been remedied as a consequence of infringements proceedings by the European Commission or after pressure from stakeholders.

The UN Convention on the Rights of Persons with Disabilities (CRPD) probably served to give the EU stronger momentum in their efforts to implement the Employment Equality Directive (Halvorsen et al. 2017a). There is however much national variation in how anti-discrimination policies have been implemented in Europe, for instance, whether the private sector is covered and whether social – not only biomedical – definitions are included (Chopin and Germaine 2017; Sainsbury et al. 2017). The US has had one of the most extensive disability rights acts in the world, the 1990 Americans with Disabilities Act (Bambra 2011).

Many other social regulation measures exist. Some countries, like Germany, Italy, Czech Republic, Ireland, Poland, Luxembourg, Serbia, and Spain, use employment quotas which require 2–5% of a company's workforce to have a disability or a chronic condition (Bambra 2011; Sainsbury et al. 2017). Sometimes these quota requirements are coupled with financial incentives to encourage compliance. In the Czech Republic, companies can instead make payments to support employment of disabled people elsewhere (Sainsbury et al. 2017). Wage subsidies for employers are used in, for instance, Norway and Sweden as part of their regulatory approaches.

Finally, the broader employment protection legislation in a country may affect the opportunities for disabled people to retain work and their likelihood of getting work (Heggebo 2016; Reeves et al. 2014). A prominent example is the Danish "flexicurity" model which has been celebrated for creating high employment and low unemployment in the general working age population. The model combines three key elements, a flexible labor market legislation, generous unemployment insurance, and active labor market policy. In the next section, we will address the model's merits regarding the employment opportunities for people with health problems.

What Works?

While there is strong evidence that the work environment is related to health (Bambra 2011; Bonde 2008; Fletcher et al. 2011; Stansfeld and Candy 2006), causal inference is often difficult (Barnay 2016; Bonde 2008). Nevertheless, the studies that do exist seem to favor the idea that there is a true effect of work on health (Barnay 2016; Landsbergis et al. 2014). Improving working conditions in general thus should be high on the preventive policy agenda. Joyce et al. (2016) reviewed primary, secondary, and tertiary preventive workplace intervention and their effects on common mental disorders. Primary prevention interventions, which correspond to our prevention dimension, that increase worker's control and physical activity had modest effects on depression and anxiety. Cognitive behavioral therapy-based measures were related to better outcomes in both secondary prevention and tertiary prevention. In addition, exposure therapy had effect on both mental health and occupational outcomes in tertiary prevention. Primary prevention aimed at helping individuals seems to be more effective than interventions that target the work force as a whole, as were combined approaches (Goldgruber and Ahrens 2010).

Vooijs et al. (2015) carried out a systematic review of nine reviews of interventions to enhance labor market participation among people with chronic illness. Five medium quality reviews were retrieved. One of these reported inconclusive evidence for policy-based return-to-work programs. The others described interventions focused on changes at work, such as changes in work organization, working conditions, and work environment. Three of these reported positive effects of the intervention on work participation. The evidence reviewed indicated that work-oriented interventions could be effective for people with variety of chronic illnesses.

Van (according to APA rules) Oostrom and Boot (2013) conducted a systematic review of workplace interventions aiming at return to work and identified nine studies that met their inclusion criteria. They focused on people with musculoskeletal illness and mental health problems. The authors concluded that "workplace interventions are effective to reduce sickness absence among workers with musculoskeletal disorders when compared to usual care" (p. 352). This review confirmed and strengthened the evidence produced by an earlier review. Another important finding of the review was that abovementioned positive effects did not apply to health outcomes, as they were unaffected by the work place interventions. Given the aim of the intervention, i.e., to reduce barriers to work, this came as little surprise. There was a lack of studies of work place interventions for people with mental health problems and other health conditions. Hence, no conclusions could be drawn in this respect (van Oostrom and Boot 2013).

Clayton et al. (2012) undertook a systematic review of evaluations of interventions directed at the employers aimed at helping chronically ill or disabled people into work. The literature search included Canada, Denmark, Norway, Sweden, and the UK. Thirty studies were identified. The main findings of the review can be summed up in five points. Workplace adjustments seem to have a positive impact on employment among people with poor health, but such adjustments only apply to a minority. The reviewed evidence further suggests that financial incentives such as wage subsidies can have a positive impact given that they are sufficiently generous. However, unintended side effects are also reported. Moreover, involving employers in return-to-work planning can reduce later sick leave, but such policy often fails to have the level of intensity that is likely to make a difference. Some interventions increase social inequalities as they favor the more advantaged disabled people, e.g., those with higher education. Regarding anti-discrimination legislation the authors conclude that it is hard to detect a positive effect on employers' propensity to recruit disabled employees.

The other main regulative approach (in addition to anti-discrimination laws) to enhance disability employment is quotas. Assessments of this policy measure conclude that research on the effectiveness of quotas is limited (Delsen 1996) but that: "In a cross country perspective higher employment rates of persons with disabilities are not systematically correlated with employment quotas" and "According to available data quota systems only lead to small net employment gains" (Fuchs 2014, p. 5). This result is probably due to windfall gains, squeeze out, and substitution effects (Fuchs 2014).

Several comparative studies have investigated how more specific policies or policy packages are related to employment opportunities and disability benefit claim among people with impairment and long-standing illness. In a comparative analysis of 17 OECD countries, Morris (2017) found, first, that in countries with more employer responsibilities and stricter definitions of disability, there was a reduced likelihood of going on disability benefits. Secondly, and contrary to common belief, he showed that comprehensive rehabilitation systems and strong work incentive rules were unrelated to the likelihood of going on long-term disability cross-nationally. As two of the most widely used forms of employment policies for disabled, these null findings are worth highlighting. It is likely, however, that "rehabilitation systems" in this study mostly refer to provision of supply-side services which are proven to have limited employment effects. Another point is that it is rather common to use (reduction in) disability benefit caseload as an indicator of "successful" disability policies. We would argue that this is a misconception which is based on the assumption that reduced caseloads are equivalent to increased labor force participation. This assumption is, however, not supported by empirical evidence. In the OECD area, there is virtually no association between benefit receipt rates and employment rates among disabled people or changes over time in these phenomena (MacInnes et al. 2014: Figs. 5.1 and 5.2). Furthermore, improving work incentives by cutting benefits may have other unintended consequences. One recent study indicates that generous sick leave arrangements may constitute a source of resilience for workers, as the mental health of workers with the harshest working conditions was significantly better in countries with more generous sick pay arrangements (van der Wel et al. 2015). Another recent study even found that cuts in sickness benefit provision, although related to short-term gains, were related to *higher* sickness absence in the longer run (Sjoberg 2017). These results throw some doubt on the validity of OECD's recommendations to strengthen work incentives and expand traditional rehabilitation efforts to deal with the disability challenge.

In a study of the Scandinavian countries, Heggebo (2016) found that the Danish "flexicurity" model, described above, seems to stimulate on average better employment opportunities among disabled people. However, this turns out to be true only for individuals with higher education, whereas people with health problems and low education were "punished" in terms of labor market participation. Furthermore, the study indicated no particular benefit in terms of the overall disability employment rate. A comparative study by McAllister et al. (2015) by and large supports this. The authors stated that policies with higher employment protection and higher economic security, like the Swedish, were more beneficial for those with short education and health problems. Reeves et al. (2014), in a multi-country comparison, found that employment protection may reduce the risk of job loss among disabled women but only in countries that were moderately hit by the Great Recession. Employment protection legislation may also interact with the benefit system (Biegert 2017). Finally, econometric evidence on job satisfaction suggests that it is better to have a fixed term contract and high subjective job security than to have a permanent job and low job insecurity (Origo and Pagani 2009).

An increasingly popular policy nationwide is the use of benefit conditionalities and sanctions imposed on non-complying people with impairment or long-standing health problems. This policy option is part of the OECD integration dimension aiming at influencing the labor market behavior of the disabled and is recommended by the organization. An overview and assessment of six well-conducted studies from different countries conclude that only one study (from Norway) demonstrated a clear positive effect. The others show null or negative results. Two studies indicate that the stronger forms of disability conditionality are counterproductive as they show a reduction of labor force attachment among disabled people and detrimental effects on mental health (Geiger 2017, p. 120). Other studies corroborate these findings. In Finland, Malmberg-Heimonen and Vuori (2005) find absence of positive mental health effect of program participation among long-term unemployed if participation was enforced as well as lower reemployment rates. Davis (2018), in an analysis of data from the USA, demonstrates that harsher sanctions and stricter job search requirements affect mental health negatively among low-educated single mothers. Research findings like these are important in light of OECDs recommendation from 2010 to enforce conditionality in member states' disability policies. At that time, OECD's advice was not backed up by direct empirical evidence (Geiger 2017, p. 108) and still fails to gain support from empirical research.

Whereas supply-side (e.g., counseling) and demand-side approaches (e.g., wage subsidies) have proven to render limited impact on labor market participation among disadvantaged groups, "support-side" approaches that are based on place-then-train strategies and provision of long-term quality support at the workplace appear far more promising (Frøyland et al. 2019). Support-oriented programs such as Supported Employment and Individual Placement and Support (IPS) seem to outperform supply-side programs (Nøkleby et al. 2017). However, although many carefully conducted RCTs of IPS programs indicate a good effect on labor market participation among the target groups, the implementation of such programs in the real world is a somewhat different matter. A review of facilitators and barriers linked to the implementation of IPS programs identifies a number of barriers at different levels (Bonfils et al. 2017). This literature review points out influential factors at the level of the context, organization, cooperation/teamwork, and the individual. For example, an important facilitator is the adoption of a fidelity scale to measure quality and that the local leaders and IPS specialists are adequately educated and skilled. Barriers at the contextual level are present when the national employment policy contradicts the IPS program. At the local level, barriers are related to mental health professionals' negative attitudes toward IPS. Difficulties in implementing IPS in the real world suggest that if rolled out on a large scale, expectations as to the effectiveness of IPS schemes should be somewhat tempered. Furthermore, job quality is essential. Disabled people seem to more often occupy peripheral positions in the labor market (Roulstone 2012), which may also entail higher job insecurity and poorer working conditions.

Summary and Conclusion

Over the past decades, we have witnessed a radical shift in the perspective on the role disabled people have in relation to the labor market. Many disabled people want to work, are able to work, and lawfully have the right to work. Nonetheless, low employment rates and high poverty rates among disabled people persist, and this is despite the numerous policy initiatives that have been launched aiming at rising employment levels in many countries over the past few decades. We have seen policy reforms in the areas of prevention, compensation, and integration policies and in the regulation of the labor market. In the foregoing section, we have attempted to appraise how several of these policy initiatives and interventions have affected the labor market outcomes among chronically ill and impaired people.

Working conditions are a likely cause behind sickness absence and disability, and large differences exist between social and occupational groups (Eurofound 2017). Although legal frameworks exist to protect the health of workers, much can still be done to enforce compliance. Furthermore, examples of successful workplace interventions exist to increase workers' control and physical activity and hence their health and resilience. Improving working conditions in general may also ease the integration of disabled people into work. Prevention in terms of improving the work environment is and still should be an important priority.

Compensation and integration measures represent the main social policy tools to improve labor market participation and economic well-being among disabled people. Improving work incentives for beneficiaries, restricting eligibility criteria, enforcing activity requirements, and expanding costly training and rehabilitation schemes have been popular strategies, often advocated by the OECD (e.g., OECD 2010). However, doubts about the effectiveness of these approaches have emerged.

The underlying philosophy of such supply-side policies has been that the disabled person is lacking something that he or she needs for successfully entering the labor force and that jobs are in fact available (Frøyland et al. 2019). These assumptions have been dubious, as evidenced by available literature reviews referred to above. Furthermore, reduced benefit generosity combined with insufficient integration measures is hardly a good mix as evidenced by persistent or increasing poverty rates and no or negligible improvement in labor market participation in many countries among disabled persons. Reliance on work incentives and/or reduced benefit generosity are likely to be inefficient, may increase poverty and sickness absence, and may severely affect the mental health of disadvantaged workers, rather than generating higher employment rates among disabled people (Geiger et al. 2017; Lindsay et al. 2015; Sjoberg 2017; van der Wel et al. 2015).

Bridging between integration measures and social regulation, "support-side" approaches (place-then-train) focus on engaging, incentivizing, and supporting employers to take on disabled people. Although we have insufficient knowledge of large-scale implementation of such approaches, experimental evidence is highly promising. Programs that employ supported employment (e.g., Individual Placement and Support, IPS) have been shown to be effective in bringing people with severe health problems such as poor mental health into work (Nøkleby et al. 2017). Since mental health challenges are on the rise as a major reason for disability in many countries (Vornholt et al. 2018), this way of addressing the work issues among disabled people looks very promising, compared with existing alternatives which traditionally are supply-side oriented.

Regulative approaches, such as employment quotas and anti-discrimination legislation, do not seem to receive much empirical support, but it seems obvious that national and supranational legal frameworks have played an important role in defining the now broadly acknowledged aim of improving participation, economic well-being, and labor market opportunities of disabled people. Furthermore, employment protection legislation provides an important context in which other integrative efforts exist, and may affect labor market outcomes. Research reviewed here indicates that flexible hire-and-fire labor markets may come with costs in terms of mental health and social inequalities among disabled workers (Heggebo 2016; Origo and Pagani, 2009; Barnay 2016).

One key message that emanates from this analysis is that there is no easy or simple way to improve labor market participation and hence reduce poverty and receipt of disability benefit among disabled. It is hard to assess the employment effects of all the reviewed policies, reforms, and interventions in a rigorous and comprehensive way, so robust conclusions are not warranted. Yet, if the aim is to further employment and economic well-being among disabled people, available evidence indicates that much of the most popular disability policies pursued today, such as emphasis on work incentives, strict enforcement of conditionalities and sanctions, focus on "traditional" integration measures, employment quotas, and anti-discrimination legislation, do not have the desired effects, and some of them may even be counterproductive. Research evidence suggests, however, that interventions that improve the work environment, as well as programs based on supported employment approaches, are propitious avenues for future policy development.

Cross-References

- ▶ Investing in Integrative Active Labour Market Policies
- ▶ Reducing Inequalities in Employment of People with Disabilities
- ▶ Work-Related Burden of Absenteeism, Presenteeism, and Disability: An Epidemiologic and Economic Perspective

Acknowledgments A preliminary version of this chapter was presented at the expert group meeting in January 2019 of the research project "INTEGRATE" funded by the Norwegian Research Council (Project no 269298).

References

Bambra C (2011) Work, worklessness, and the political economy of health. Oxford University Press, Oxford

Barnay T (2016) Health, work and working conditions: a review of the European economic literature. Eur J Health Econ 17:693–709. https://doi.org/10.1007/s10198-015-0715-8

Bartley M, Owen C (1996) Relation between socioeconomic status, employment, and health during economic change, 1973–93. BMJ 313:445–449

Bell D (1973) The coming of post-industrial society: a venture in social forecasting. Basic Books, New York

Biegert T (2017) Welfare benefits and unemployment in affluent democracies: the moderating role of the institutional insider/outsider divide. Am Sociol Rev 82:1037–1064. https://doi.org/10.1177/0003122417727095

Bliksvaer T (2018) Disability, labour market participation and the effect of educational level: compared to what? Scand J Disabil Res 20:6–17. https://doi.org/10.16993/sjdr.3

Böheim R, Leoni T (2018) Sickness and disability policies: reform paths in OECD countries between 1990 and 2014. Int J Soc Welf 27:168–185. https://doi.org/10.1111/ijsw.12295

Bonde JPE (2008) Psychosocial factors at work and risk of depression: a systematic review of the epidemiological evidence. Occup Environ Med 65:438–445. https://doi.org/10.1136/oem.2007.038430

Bonfils IS, Hansen H, Dalum HS, Eplov LF (2017) Implementation of the individual placement and support approach – facilitators and barriers. Scand J Disabil Res 19:318–333. https://doi.org/10.1080/15017419.2016.1222306

Burchell B, Fagan C (2004) Gender and the intensification of work: evidence from the European working conditions surveys. East Econ J 30:627–642

Chopin I, Germaine C (2017) A comparative analysis of non-discrimination law in Europe 2017. European Commiesion, Brussels

Clayton S et al (2012) Effectiveness of return-to-work interventions for disabled people: a systematic review of government initiatives focused on changing the behaviour of employers. Eur J Pub Health 22:434–439. https://doi.org/10.1093/eurpub/ckr101

Davis O (2018) What is the relationship between benefit conditionality and mental health? Evidence from the United States on TANF policies. J Soc Policy 48:1–21. https://doi.org/10.1017/S0047279418000363

Delsen L (1996). Employment opportunities for the disabled) In: Schmid G, O'Reilly J, Schömann K (eds) International handbook of labour market policy and evaluation. Edward Elgar, Cheltenham, pp 520–550

Doogan K (2009) New capitalism? Polity Press, Malden

Esping-Andersen G (1999) Social foundations of postindustrial economies. Oxford University Press, Oxford

Eurofound (2017) Sixth European working conditions survey – overview report (2017 update). Publications Office of the European Union, Luxembourg

Fletcher JM, Sindelar JL, Yamaguchi S (2011) Cumulative effects of job characteristics on health. Health Econ 20:553–570. https://doi.org/10.1002/hec.1616

Frøyland K, Schafft A, Spjelkavik Ø (2019) Tackling increasing marginalization: can support-side approaches contribute to work inclusion? In: Hvid H, Falkum E (eds) Work and wellbeing in the Nordic countries. Critical perspectives on the world's best working lives. Routledge, Oxon, pp 194–216

Fuchs M (2014) Quota systems for disabled persons: parameters, aspects, effectivity. European Centre for Social Welfare Policy and Research, Vienna

Geiger BB (2017) Benefits conditionality for disabled people: stylised facts from a review of international evidence and practice. J Poverty Soc Justice 25:107–128. https://doi.org/10.1332/175982717x14939739331010

Geiger BB, van der Wel KA, Toge AG (2017) Success and failure in narrowing the disability employment gap: comparing levels and trends across Europe 2002–2014. BMC Public Health 17:928. https://doi.org/10.1186/s12889-017-4938-8

Goldgruber J, Ahrens D (2010) Effectiveness of workplace health promotion and primary prevention interventions: a review. J Public Health 18:75–88. https://doi.org/10.1007/s10389-009-0282-5

Grammenos S (2018) European comparative data on Europe 2020 & people with disabilities. Centre for European Social and Economic Policy/Academic Network of European Disability Experts (ANED), Brussels

Greenan N, Kalugina E, Walkowiak E (2007) The transformation of work? D9. 2.2 Å Trends in work organisation. CEE, France. https://www.researchgate.net/publication/265114156_The_Transformation_of_Work_Trends_in_Work_Organisation_in_Europe

Halvorsen R, Hvinden B, Bickenbach J, Ferri D, Rodriguez AMG (2017a) The contours of the emerging disability policy in Europe. Revisiting the multi-level and multi-actor framework. In: Hvinden B, Halvorsen R, Bickenbach J, Ferri D, Guillén Rodriguez A (eds) The changing disability policy system. Active citizenship and disability in Europe, vol 1. Routledge, Oxford, pp 215–234

Halvorsen R, Waldschmidt A, Hvinden B, Bøhler K (2017b) Diversity and dynamics of disability policy in Europe: an analytical framework. In: Hvinden B, Halvorsen R, Bickenbach J, Ferri D, Guillén Rodriguez A (eds) The changing disability policy system. Active citizenship and disability in Europe, vol 1. Routledge, Oxford, pp 12–33

Heggebo K (2016) Hiring, employment, and health in Scandinavia: the Danish 'flexicurity' model in comparative perspective. Eur Soc 18:460–483. https://doi.org/10.1080/14616696.2016.1207794

Holland P et al (2011) How do macro-level contexts and policies affect the employment chances of chronically ill and disabled people? Paper I: the impact of recession and de-industrialisation. Int J Health Serv 41:395

Jones MK, Latreille PL (2011) Disability and self-employment: evidence for the UK. Appl Econ 43:4161–4178. https://doi.org/10.1080/00036846.2010.489816

Joyce S, Modini M, Christensen H, Mykletun A, Bryant R, Mitchell PB, Harvey SB (2016) Workplace interventions for common mental disorders: a systematic meta-review. Psychol Med 46:683–697. https://doi.org/10.1017/S0033291715002408

Karasek R (1979) Job demands, job decision latitude, and mental strain: implications for job redesign. Adm Sci Q 24:285–308

Landsbergis PA, Grzywacz JG, LaMontagne AD (2014) Work organization, job insecurity, and occupational health disparities. Am J Ind Med 57:495–515. https://doi.org/10.1002/ajim.22126

Lindsay C, Greve B, Cabras I, Ellison N, Kellett S (2015) Assessing the evidence base on health, employability and the labour market – lessons for activation in the UK. Soc Policy Adm 49:143–160. https://doi.org/10.1111/spol.12116

MacInnes T, Tinson A, Gaffney D, Horgan G, Baumberg B (2014) Disability, long term conditions and poverty. New Policy Institute, London

Malmberg-Heimonen I, Vuori J (2005) Activation or discouragement – the effect of enforced participation on the success of job-search training Aktivointi vai lannistaminen – Työnhakuryhmään velvoittamisen vaikutukset. This article has been published in the doctoral dissertation: Malmberg-Heimonen I (2005) Public welfare policies and private responses: studies of European labour market policies in transition, Finnish Institute of Occupational Health, People and Work, research reports 68. AU – Malmberg-Heimonen, Ira Eur J Soc Work 8:451–467. https://doi.org/10.1080/13691450500314178

McAllister A, Nylen L, Backhans M, Boye K, Thielen K, Whitehead M, Burstrom B (2015) Do 'flexicurity' policies work for people with low education and health problems? A comparison of labour market policies and employment rates in Denmark, The Netherlands, Sweden, and the United Kingdom 1990-2010. Int J Health Serv 45:679–705. https://doi.org/10.1177/0020731415600408

Morris Z (2017) The Wind before the storm: aging, automation, and the disability crisis. University of California-Berkeley, Berkeley

Nøkleby H, Blaasvær N, Berg R (2017) Supported employment for arbeidssøkere med bistandsbehov: en systematisk oversikt. [Supported employment for people with disabilities: a systematic review]. Folkehelseinstituttet, Oslo

OECD (2010) Sickness, disability and work: breaking the barriers. A synthesis of findings across OECD countries. Paris. https://doi.org/10.1787/9789264088856-en

OECD (2017) Preventing ageing unequally. Paris. https://doi.org/10.1787/9789264279087-en

Oesch D (2015) Occupational structure and labor market change in Western Europe since 1990. In: Kriesi H, Kitschelt H, Beramendi P, Häusermann S (eds) The politics of advanced capitalism. Cambridge University Press, Cambridge, pp 112–132. https://doi.org/10.1017/CBO9781316163245.005

Origo F, Pagani L (2009) Flexicurity and job satisfaction in Europe: the importance of perceived and actual job stability for well-being at work. Labour Econ 16:547–555. https://doi.org/10.1016/j.labeco.2009.02.003

Owens J (2015) Exploring the critiques of the social model of disability: the transformative possibility of Arendt's notion of power. Sociol Health Illn 37:385–403. https://doi.org/10.1111/1467-9566.12199

Pagan R (2012) Transitions to part-time work at older ages: the case of people with disabilities in Europe. Disabil Soc 27:95–115. https://doi.org/10.1080/09687599.2012.631800

Reeves A, Karanikolos M, Mackenbach J, Mckee M, Stuckler D (2014) Do employment protection policies reduce the relative disadvantage in the labour market experienced by unhealthy people? A natural experiment created by the great recession in Europe. Soc Sci Med 121:98–108. https://doi.org/10.1016/j.socscimed.2014.09.034

Roulstone A (2012) Disabled people, work and employment: a global perspective. In: Watson N, Roulstone A, Thomas C (eds) Routledge handbook of disability studies. Routledge, London, pp 222–235

Sainsbury R, Coleman-Fountain E, Trezzini B (2017) How to enhance active citizenship for persons with disabilities in Europe through labour market participation. European and national perspectives. In: Hvinden B, Halvorsen R, Bickenbach J, Ferri D, Guillén Rodriguez A (eds) The changing disability policy system. Active citizenship and disability in Europe, vol 1. Routledge, Oxford, pp 90–107

Siegrist J, Wahrendorf M (eds) (2016) Work stress and health in a globalized economy: the model of effort-reward imbalance. Springer, Cham

Sjoberg O (2017) Positive welfare state dynamics? Sickness benefits and sickness absence in Europe 1997–2011. Soc Sci Med 177:158–168. https://doi.org/10.1016/j.socscimed.2017.01.042

Standing G (2011) The precariat: the new dangerous class. Bloomsbury Academic, London

Stansfeld S, Candy B (2006) Psychosocial work environment and mental health–a meta-analytic review. Scand J Work Environ Health 32:443–462

Taylor-Gooby P (2004) New risks, new welfare: the transformation of the European welfare state. Oxford University Press, Oxford

Thomas C (2010) Medical sociology and disability theory. In: Scambler G, Scambler S (eds) New directions in the sociology of chronic and disabling conditions: assaults on the Lifeworld. Palgrave Macmillan, London/New York

van der Wel KA, Dahl E, Birkelund GE (2010) Employment inequalities through busts and booms the changing roles of health and education in Norway 1980–2005. Acta Sociol 53:355–370. https://doi.org/10.1177/0001699310380063

van der Wel KA, Bambra C, Dragano N, Eikemo TA, Lunau T (2015) Risk and resilience: health inequalities, working conditions and sickness benefit arrangements: an analysis of the 2010 European Working Conditions survey. Sociol Health Illn 37:1157–1172. https://doi.org/10.1111/1467-9566.12293

Van Kersbergen K, Hemerijck A (2012) Two decades of change in Europe: the emergence of the social investment state. J Soc Policy 41:475–492. https://doi.org/10.1017/S0047279412000050

van Oostrom S, Boot C (2013) Workplace interventions. In: Loisel P, Anema JR (eds) Handbook of work disability prevention and management. Springer, New York, NY, pp 335–371

Vooijs M, Leensen MCJ, Hoving JL, Wind H, Frings-Dresen MHW (2015) Interventions to enhance work participation of workers with a chronic disease: a systematic review of reviews. Occup Environ Med 72:820–826. https://doi.org/10.1136/oemed-2015-103062

Vornholt K et al (2018) Disability and employment – overview and highlights. Eur J Work Organ Psy 27:40–55. https://doi.org/10.1080/1359432x.2017.1387536

Waddel G, Burton K (2006) Is work good for your health and wellbeing? The Stationary Office, London

Waddington L, Lawson A (2009) Disability and non-discrimination law in the European Union. An analysis of disability law within and beyond the employment field. Publications Office of the European Union, Luxembourg

Burden of Injury Due to Occupational Exposures

7

Jukka Takala

Contents

Introduction	106
History and Background	106
Materials and Methods	107
Sources of Data on the Burden of Injuries and Illnesses at Work	107
Estimation Method	113
Identification of Fatal Occupational Injuries in the ILO Estimates 2017	113
Non-fatal Occupational Injuries	114
Results and Trends from Statistical Sources	114
Non-fatal Injury Surveys	118
The Relationship Between Serious and Less Serious Outcomes for Occupational Injuries	119
Occupational Injury Burden Is Unequally Shared by Various Groups of Workers	120
Cost Estimates of Injuries and Illnesses at Work	121
Policies and Practices to Prevent Injuries Include a Range of Traditional and New Measures	121
Conclusions	124
Cross-References	125
References	125

Abstract

Occupational injuries, also called occupational accidents, have existed as long as the humankind. Such injuries have often been considered to "go with the business." Injuries are, however, not caused by a law of nature. They are preventable as has been demonstrated by best practices elsewhere. This chapter provides an overview of important global trends of occupational injuries, with data sources coming mostly from developed countries. Moreover, good policy and practice solutions are emphasized.

J. Takala (✉)
International Commission on Occupational Health, ICOH, Rome, Italy
e-mail: jstakala@gmail.com

The best available data and numbers of injuries have been estimated by the International Labour Organisation (ILO), based on thorough investigation. These findings indicate that, globally, the annual number of *fatal* occupational injuries is 380,000. This is composed mainly of an Asian burden of 250,000 deaths and 65,000 deaths in Africa, with only 10,760 deaths taking place in the high-income region. Occupational injury rates vary widely within and between regions, being highest in the riskiest sectors and occupations in less-developed countries. The average annual range between countries varies from 0.5/100,000 to 27.5/100,000. The range between the safest and most hazardous jobs annually varies between 0 and 500 deaths/100,000, the most hazardous jobs being in tropical logging. The estimated global cost of poor or non-existing safety and health measures has been estimated to be around 3 trillion USD, equivalent of 3.9% of the global GDP. Globally, the number of occupational injuries is still growing, despite successful reductions in the high-income regions. The human burden and economic price of occupational injuries are very high.

Keywords

Occupational injuries · Accident prevention · Safety at work · Costs · Burden of injury · Exposures to risks

Introduction

History and Background

More organized work started when individuals were not just working for the family but as requested or ordered to work for an outsider either as an exchange of services or for a leader such as a landowner, slave master, duke, king, pharaoh, or emperor. Employment as a concept and industrial work started when individual craftsmen were needed in larger scale and when industrial revolution took place.

Over the years, high-income (WHO classification) countries have done well to reduce occupational injuries (Hämäläinen et al. 2006, 2009, 2010, 2017; Takala et al. 1997, 1999, 2014; Takala 2017; García et al. 2007), despite having an increasingly complex work environment.

As seen in many high-income countries, the health component of workplace safety and health is rapidly increasing in importance compared to the safety component. The "high-income" group of countries include the USA, EU, Japan, Australia, New Zealand, and Singapore. The relatively higher importance of health issues is caused by:

- Improvements in technology, processes, and methods
- Better leadership, management, and efforts in safety and health
- Reduction of the number of workers in hazardous industries
- Shift in economic structures

Furthermore, hazardous and labor-intensive workplaces, such as those in manufacturing and construction sectors, have decreased in most developed countries, and much of such work takes place in other locations, in particular in Asia. It is common that in developed countries, more than two thirds of all workers are already working in service occupations. The processes of mechanization, automation, and prefabrication are also foreseen to contribute to jobs less exposed to injury risks. However, most of the population is exposed to "new and emerging" work risks related to long-term health effects, such as psychosocial factors, stress, musculoskeletal disorders, and exposures to carcinogens.

Globally the population living in extreme poverty has been radically reduced to some 800 million people, and global life expectancy is today about 70 years (Rosling et al. 2018). The poorest group needs to be taken care of by eliminating extreme poverty. The rest or some seven billion of the global population have already been elevated from extreme poverty, and prevention of occupational injuries and work-related diseases has a major role in further avoiding also their hardship and in improving the well-being of workers and their families. The workforce including the household workers – some 3.5 billion workers – is the sole productive component of the society upon which children and students, retired and older population groups, and the disabled will have to rely on getting their livelihood. An occupational injury, fatal or non-fatal, and disabling disease or disorder immediately affect the well-being of the depending populations. The breadwinner becomes dependent on others as well.

This chapter reviews latest global and country numbers of occupational injuries within the framework related to not only work-related injuries but also related illnesses and presents data of selected countries and regions. It is a summary of the evolution, present state of art, and possible future trends in the global burden of injury and measures to reduce and eliminate such burden.

Materials and Methods

Sources of Data on the Burden of Injuries and Illnesses at Work

Employment figures, mortality rates, occupational burden of injuries, selected diseases, and reported accidents were reviewed for this chapter. These were complemented by surveys on self-reported occupational injuries, economic cost estimates of work-related injuries, and the most recent information on the problems from published papers, documents, and electronic data sources of international and regional organizations, in particular ILO, WHO, EU and ASEAN, safety and health institutions, agencies, and public websites (Driscoll et al. 2005; 't Mannetje and Pearce 2005; García et al. 2007; Hämäläinen et al. 2006, 2010; Takala 2005, 1997, 1999).

While it is difficult to compare national data related to occupational injuries due to differences in legal and compensation criteria, the comparison between the number of *fatal* injuries (accidents) is easier, and, although not completely, it is reasonably

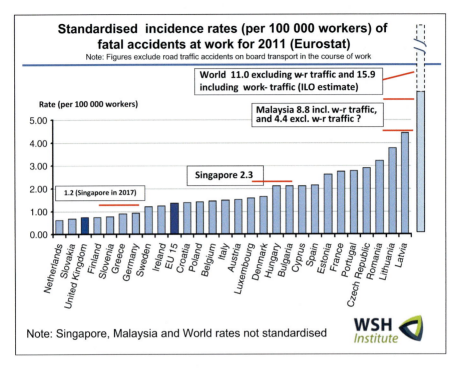

Fig. 1 Standardized incidence rates (per 100,000 workers) of fatal accidents at work for 2011 (Eurostat 2009; HSE 2014 includes latest EU data); Singapore rates not standardized

comparable when the recording criteria, denominators, and economic structures are well documented. Usually fatal injuries are expressed per 100,000 employed persons in national statistics or per 1 million working hours which may be converted to 100,000 full-time employed.

Some international and regional organizations collect such data, notably the International Labour Organisation (ILO), the World Health Organization (WHO), and the European Union (EU). In addition, other research mechanisms and institutions and published scientific papers complement these sources. Data collection systems for these still vary, so their comparability has limitations. Using a combination of these sources, a selection of such data is presented in Figs. 1 and 2. For example, Singapore had 2.3 fatal injuries per 100,000 employed in 2010 which has since gone down to 1.2 fatal injuries per 100,000 workers in 2017. These numbers exclude fatal commuting injuries between home and workplace. Sometimes, those work injuries that took place in work-related traffic on public roads and in other public traffic were also excluded, for instance, in the in the UK's Health and Safety Executive reports (HSE 2014) based on EU's Eurostat numbers. The removal of fatalities arising from work-related traffic injuries enables more accurate comparison. The best countries included major countries

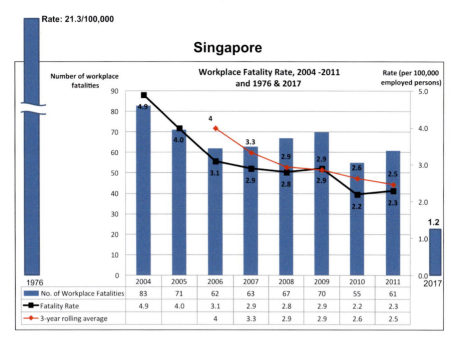

Fig. 2 Singapore fatal injury rate performance from Singapore as a typical model in high-income countries. (Source: Takala et al. 2017, updates by author)

such as the UK with 0.74 fatal injuries per 100,000 employed and Germany 0.9 per 100,000. Comparative global outcomes are based further on ILO estimates (ILO 2017; Hämäläinen et al. 2017) as sources for global data. Data including work-related traffic included in the estimates have significantly increased the rates including those in the EU28 up to double of those presented in Fig. 1.

The standardized numbers in Fig. 1 included adjustments based on average industry structures in the EU. Countries that have a relatively high level of activity in high-risk industries, such as construction work, would otherwise show much higher rates as compared to those with a high service industry component even though within each economic sector, their safety levels and rates would be equal to those in another country. While Eurostat rates have been standardized, the added non-EU country rates have not been adjusted due to lack of comparable data. Fatal injury rates in industrialized countries are gradually going down, partly due to a shift in the countries' economic structure from dangerous sectors to less risky ones, such as the service sector (Fig. 1).

Data from Singapore illustrates the trend in many industrialized countries where fatal occupational injuries are gradually becoming a smaller problem as compared to health issues (Fig. 2). However, this is not the case for most populous countries in the world where the injury rates are high and the rates are increasing in many areas.

Furthermore, while several work-related diseases are the main killers, such as occupational cancer and work-related cardiovascular diseases, injuries take place for much younger worker groups. Long latency diseases and disorders are often linked to ageing. As a result, the fatal injuries form a much bigger share of the disability-adjusted life years, DALYs, as compared to those of deaths due to work-related diseases (GBD 2016).

The ILO statistics complemented with published data provide a reasonably reliable picture of a limited number of countries. Singapore data from the Ministry of Manpower provide a typical picture of the declining trend in high-income countries (Fig. 2). The fatal injury trend has gone down from 21.3 to 1.2 in 40 years. In small countries the random fluctuation of relatively small numbers can be compensated by calculating a rolling average of 3–10 years. The number of workers covered and gradual increase are better covered when rates/100,000 workers are used at the country level. In enterprises and workplaces, Lost Time Injury rates are often used where the denominator is the number of hours – or million hours – worked in the location concerned. One million working hours are roughly equivalent of 500 workers in a year if a worker performs 2,000 h a year.

Underreporting is common in both fatal and, in particular, non-fatal cases. Another major problem in comparing data from different countries is what is really required by the authorities. In some highly developed countries, work-related traffic accidents are not covered by reporting requirements and consequently do not appear in statistics. These could be injuries of bus, truck, and taxi drivers, pizza delivery workers, salespeople, and many others present in road, rail, sea, and air traffic and logistics. They may be well compensated but not counted in statistics. Usually travels in traffic from home to work and back are covered separately but not in direct occupational injury statistics.

There are often major further omissions of coverage. Some sectors and groups of workers are not covered, such as uniform workers, military, police, government in general, housemaids working in other peoples' homes, agricultural workers, self-employed farmers, and other self-employed. In an Australian study, comparing all sources of information of injury numbers including compensation bodies, labor inspectorates, coronary reports, hospital records, deaths certificates, and media reports, none of the sources were complete and at best covered some 50–60% of the cases. The burden to find out such details makes it simpler to use fatal cases as a baseline when comparing the outcomes in different countries. The pyramid method in Fig. 8 can be useful for such estimates.

The same trend of gradually improving injury records in high-income countries is shown in Fig. 3 on Norway and Finland when using absolute numbers and considering that the population and workforce in Finland are about 10% higher than that of Norway. The rates are somewhat different due to economic structures and their development in time. In Norway the rate came down from 12/100,000 workers in 1970 to 1.5 in 2015. In Finland the numbers have come down from an annual average of 370 in the period 1961–1965 (injuries only) to 24 (wage earners, no

7 Burden of Injury Due to Occupational Exposures

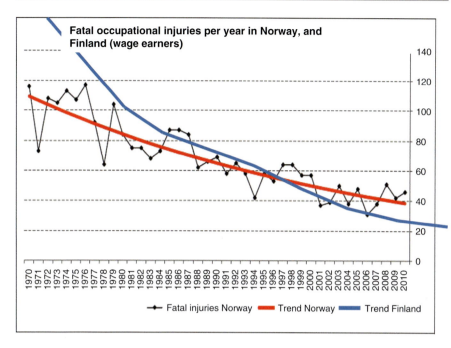

Fig. 3 Fatal injury trends in Norway and Finland. (Sources: country statistics)

traffic) or from 9.7/100,000 in 1976 to 1.1/100,000 in 2017 (wage earners, no traffic). The covered numbers may exclude work-related traffic, no self-employed are included, and other exclusions may affect the obtained numbers and rates.

The fatal injury rates per 100,000 employed in various countries vary widely as seen in the following examples (Table 1) (ILOSTAT 2018):

The overall fatality rates in the whole economy vary considerably depending on the national practices and definitions of injury categories and coverage of legal requirements. As a result and to avoid over- or underestimates based on these statistics, a generally accepted method has been to use fatal injury rates of specific industrial sectors, in particular the three main sectors that have a wide difference of the risk level between them. The ILO practice has used this method in covering the three main economic sectors.

Selection of data for these sectors and using proxy countries was based on the reliability and credibility of such data based on national reporting and documentation and representativeness for the region concerned. The rates where then applied to the country concerned and the summing up of the sectoral estimates for the country. The description of the estimation method is presented below and covers all countries and regions in the world (Hämäläinen et al. 2017).

Table 1 Fatal injury rates per 100,000 employed worldwide

Sub-Saharan Africa		
Burkina Faso	8.96/100,000	5-year average
Gabon	26.4/100,000	5-year average
Kenya	126/100,000	1 year
Niger	147.2/100,000	10-year average
South Africa	27.8/100,000	5-year average
Togo	16.6/100,000	10-year average
Zimbabwe	7.7/100,000	5-year average
India	103.9/100,000	5-year average
Indonesia	58.7/100,000	3-year average
Malaysia[a]	11.6/100,000	5-year average
China[b]	13.4/100,000	2-year average
Hong Kong	6.8/100,000	5-year average[c]
Taiwan	7.32/100,000	5-year average
EURO area		
Ukraine	8.58/100,000	5-year average
Russia	6.6/100,000	5-year average
Kazakhstan	16.44/100,000	5-year average
Belarus	5.76/100,000	5-year average
High-income areas		
USA	3.94/100,000	5-year average
EU28	1.54/100,000	in 2014
EMRO Eastern Mediterranean		
Occupied Arab Territories	38/100,000	1 year
Algeria	21.7/100,000	5-year average
Jordan	14.9/100,000	3-year average
AMRO		
Argentina	4.8/100,000	5-year average
Chile	5.3/100,000	5-year average
Colombia	18/100,000	1 year
Costa Rica	8.2/100,000	5-year average
Cuba	24.0/100,000	2-year average
El Salvador	40.1/100,000	5-year average
Venezuela	57.1/100,000	5-year average

[a]Confirmed by national statistics
[b]Source: Chinese Statistical Communique, 69,434 and 68,061 deaths in 2013 and 2014 "Work accidents in industrial mining and commercial enterprises," non-covered self-employed farmers form some 30% of workforce), ILO estimate 2014 was 99,197 including farm workers and service sector
[c]Practically no agriculture

Estimation Method

Identification of Fatal Occupational Injuries in the ILO Estimates 2017

The number of fatal occupational accidents was estimated from the ILOSTAT 2014 frequency rates of fatal accidents (fatalities per 100,000 workers) from selected ILO member States that reported their accident data in three economic sectors:

- Agriculture including farming, fishing and forestry
- Industry including mining, manufacturing, energy production, and construction
- Services

For countries where fatal data was not available, the substitute data from closely related countries of the corresponding WHO Economic Divisions were used. WHO places countries of similar income and health structures to seven WHO divisions groups of seven divisions (Fig. 4):

- High-income countries (HIGH)
- Low- and middle-income countries of the African Region (AFRO)
- Low- and middle-income countries of the Americas (AMRO)
- Low- and middle-income countries of the Eastern Mediterranean Region (EMRO)
- Low- and middle-income countries of the European Region (EURO)
- Low- and middle-income countries of the Southeast Asia Region (SEARO)
- Low- and middle-income countries of the Western Pacific Region (WPRO)

For each division, the available fatality rates of the three economic sectors are shown in Table 3.

The previous rates of fatal occupational injuries were used for HIGH, AFRO, and EMRO division because of lack of data. The percentage of labor force for each

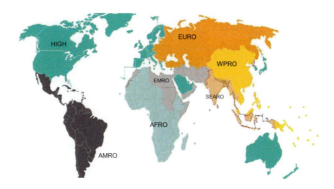

Fig. 4 Geographical Coverage of WHO economic divisions used in calculations and presentation

economic sector in each country was retrieved from *The World Factbook* of the Central Intelligence Agency (CIA). These percentages can also be obtained from ILOSTAT Database, but they are percentages of the employed instead of the labor force. Together with the labor force, total employment (comprising both paid employment and self-employment), and respective divisions' fatality rates in 2014, the number of fatalities of each country was then computed.

Non-fatal Occupational Injuries

As non-fatal (causing at least 4 days of absence) occupational accidents are not usually well reported by most countries, they are estimated by using lower and upper limit estimates. The lower limit of 0.14% was obtained by averaging the proportion of fatal and non-fatal injuries of the European Union (EU) 15 countries except Greece. The upper limit of 0.08% was obtained similarly from Finland, France, and Germany. The lower and upper limits used for 2010 were 0.13% and 0.10%, respectively. The lower and upper limit estimates of the number of non-fatal injuries of each country in 2014 are then calculated as follows:

$$\text{Estimated number of non} - \text{fatal injuries (Lower Limit)} = \frac{\text{No. of fatalities} \times 100\%}{0.14}$$

$$\text{Estimated number of non} - \text{fatal injuries (Upper Limit)} = \frac{\text{No. of fatalities} \times 100\%}{0.08}$$

The estimated non-fatal injury is then finally obtained by taking the mean of the two limits.

Results and Trends from Statistical Sources

The latest estimates show that globally, the major causes of work-related deaths are circulatory diseases and occupational cancer followed by respiratory diseases and occupational injuries. The term "work-related diseases" is different from "occupational diseases." Occupational diseases and occupational injuries are usually recorded, reported, and compensated, while the compensation criteria are widely different in countries and depend on the national laws and practice. One could say that:

Cancer is a disease – occupational cancer is an administrative decision.

The same reservation applies to *occupational injuries*. It is easier to see the occupational causes for injuries but the coverage equally varies widely. For example, in many Asian and African countries, the legal coverage, the enforcement coverage, coverage of compensation systems, recording and reporting systems, and coverage of prevention services, such as occupational health services, are in the range of 0–10% of the workforce. Almost no country has a full 100% coverage of these systems.

Work-relatedness is usually based on epidemiological and scientific studies and based on the latest data. These may be based on risk ratios obtained through case-control studies and measured by related population-attributable fractions of various diseases. Work-relatedness of injuries – even though injuries are not recorded and compensated – is estimated through best practices of reporting and/or through household surveys. At best these two methods provide reasonably close results. This depends, however, on the knowledge, awareness, and cultures of different economies.

The latest global estimates have been made by a coalition of several of institutions – ILO/ICOH/Ministries and Institutes of Singapore and Finland/EU – under the umbrella of the International Labour Organisation (Fig. 5).

There was an estimated 2.78 million fatalities – injuries and diseases at work – in the latest survey results of 2017, based on data from 2015, compared to 2.33 million estimated in 2011.

There were 380,500 deaths by occupational injuries, an increase of 8% in 2014 compared to 2010. Some 7,500 people die every day: 1,000 from occupational injuries and 6,500 from work-related illnesses. The rate of fatal occupational injuries decreased from 1998 (see Table 2). The number of non-fatal occupational injuries

Table 2 Estimation method

Estimates of work-related deaths	Methods/data sources

Total number of deaths due to occupational injuries (occupational accidents)	Number of fatal injuries reported to the ILO and EU28 based on member States reporting systems (ILOSTAT and Eurostat)
	  Included fatal injuries, injury rates in three major economic sectors separately, in particular, in agriculture, forestry, mining, and other basic (primary) industries. These rates included work-related traffic fatalities and suicides but excluded fatalities via commuting to work and back
	  As ILO data includes data from a limited number of countries, those countries where no information was available were grouped in specific regions, in particular WHO regions and subregions, and fatal injury rates per 100,000 employed of one or several countries of comparable production and economic systems that had produced injury rates were used as proxy values
	  To increase the accuracy, separate injury rates were used for (1) agriculture and fishing, mining, and other primary economic sectors, (2) industry sectors including construction, and (3) service (tertiary) sector. This balances some of the potential differences between reporting proxy countries and non-reporting countries

Table 3 Identified fatal occupational injury rates per 100,000 employees

	Fatality rates of each economic sector					
	Agriculture		Industry		Service	
Division	2010	2014	2010	2014	2010	2014
HIGH	7.8	No change	3.8	No change	1.5	No change
AFRO	18.9	No change	21.1	No change	17.7	No change
AMRO	9.3	8.7↓	9.5	11.2↑	6.0	5.7↓
EMRO	13.0	No change	14.9	No change	12.3	No change
EURO	15.7	17.0↑	10.3	13.4↑	5.5	3.5↓
SEARO	24.0	27.5↑	9.7	9.9↑	5.1	4.4↓
WPRO	24.0	27.5↑	9.7	9.9↑	5.1	4.4↓

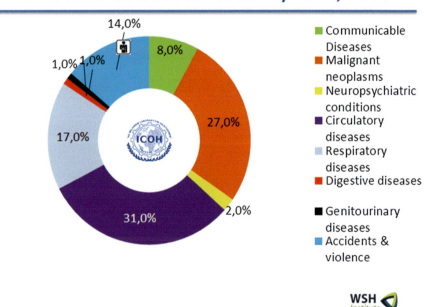

Fig. 5 Global division of deaths caused by occupational injuries and work-related diseases

was estimated to be 374 million, increasing significantly from 2010. The main reason was that a higher underreporting estimate was used compared to the previous estimates (Table 4).

As a comparison to the global picture, in the European Union, EU28, cardiovascular and circulatory diseases account for 28% and cancers at 53%. They were the top illnesses responsible for 4/5 of deaths from work-related diseases in EU28. Occupational injuries (2.4%) and infectious diseases (2.5%) together amount

7 Burden of Injury Due to Occupational Exposures

Table 4 Global trend of occupational accidents and fatal work-related diseases (1998–2015)

Year	Fatal occupational accidents Number	Rate[a]	Non-fatal occupational accidents at least 4 days absence Number	Rate[a]	Fatal work-related disease
1998	345,436	16.4	263,621,966	12,534	
2000					2,028,003
2001	351,203	15.2	268,023,272	12,218	
2002					1,945,115
2003	357,948	13.8	336,532,471	12,966	
2008	320,580	10.7	317,421,473	10,612	2,022,570
2010	352,769	11.0	313,206,348	9,786	
2011					1,976,021
2014	380,500	11.3	373,986,418	11,096	
2015					2,403,965

[a]Number of occupational accidents per 100,000 persons in the labor force. (Source: Hämäläinen et al. 2017)

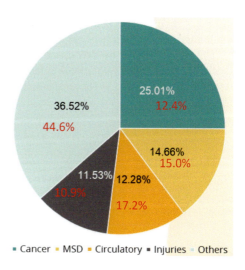

Fig. 6 Share of DALY's, mortality and morbidity, in EU28, in addition the Central and South America estimates are given in red numbers

accounts for less than 5%. On the other hand, in the non-high-income countries and regions, the share of occupational injuries is much higher; e.g., in Western Pacific Region dominated by China, it was 17% of all fatal injuries and diseases (Hämäläinen et al. 2017).

As indicated earlier the disability-adjusted life years are providing a more comprehensive picture. The percentage of total DALYs in EU28 is given in Fig. 6 (black and white % characters).

Comparative values for Central and South America, AMRO are given in the pie chart as red % characters (Fig. 7).

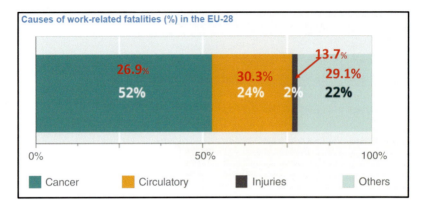

Fig. 7 Share of mortality or deaths in EU28, and in Central and South America in red characters

Long-term disabilities caused by musculoskeletal and psychosocial (mental) disorders are expected to affect the female population (GBD 2017) more seriously, while injuries are a much larger problem for males.

The picture of the burden at work becomes more gender balanced if not just deaths are counted but rather work-related years of lost life, YLL_{work}, and years lived with disability, YLD_{work}. These two indicators together form the disability-adjusted life years, $DALY_{work's}$, as follows:

$$YLL + YLD = DALY$$

The method and results for EU28 are explained on the website of the European Agency for Safety and Health at Work (Elsler et al. 2018). The baseline for the cost estimates is the number of DALYs in a country in relation to DALYs in an ideal situation where no occupational accidents or work-related disorders take place.

Non-fatal Injury Surveys

A common additional method to identify non-fatal injuries is to use an additional statistical module as a part of labor force surveys carried out regularly in many countries and regions. Based on such surveys where data is obtained through interview surveys or self-reporting, households can be also used to estimate the level of underreporting of official statistics. Countries where the reported rate of non-fatal injuries is high have usually much more minor injuries reported. The results from such surveys on non-fatal injuries and illnesses at work can be summarized as follows (Table 5):

7 Burden of Injury Due to Occupational Exposures

Table 5 Injuries by occupational accidents in selected countries including 1 *day* or longer absence Eurostat Statistics in focus 63/2009 (Eurostat 2009)

Finland	6.3% of the workforce
Sweden	5.1%
Denmark	4.9%
France	5.4%
EU average	3.2%
Hungary	1.0%
Singapore	5.4% (data from WSH Institute, Ministry of Manpower)
Work-related ill health	
Finland	24.5% of the workforce
Sweden	14.3%
Denmark	12.9%
EU average	8.6%
Hungary	5.8%
Singapore	10.0% (data from WSH Institute, Ministry of Manpower)

It appears that minor injuries are more frequent in Germany and the Nordic countries, in fact only the *reporting* of minor injuries appears to be better. The rates may also be obtained for just compensable injuries, which in many countries include accidents that cause an absence of work for 4 *days* or more.

The Relationship Between Serious and Less Serious Outcomes for Occupational Injuries

Drawing a combined picture of both lives lost and burden of disabilities needs an accurate picture of the severity distribution of the injury and illness burden. Figure 8 shows the pyramid of severity of occupational injuries. If the injury recording and reporting systems are accurate, this survey-based data collection can be used to verify and validate the official records. Unfortunately, this is not often the case. As a result, the countries that have most non-fatal injury cases in EU and possibly in the world are Germany and Finland. This result indicates that reporting of non-fatal accidents is poor in most parts of the world. The economic structure has an impact on the country pyramid of shape; countries with a large number of construction workers or other high-risk occupations tend to have a relatively higher number of fatal cases as compared to non-fatal injuries and a narrower pyramid (see also the Eurostat adjustment system in Fig. 1). Country reporting appears to be better when reporting is linked to compensation through the employers. This means that the employer will have to cover all expenses if not reported. Nevertheless, if no control systems exist, small injuries are not well reported.

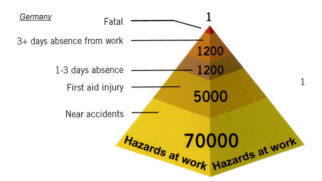

Singapore 2011- 2014
1 fatal
  42 -   93 accidents, 30 days+
284 - 623 accidents, 4 days+
516 - 1087 accidents w.sick leave
685 - 2111 accidents, all

EU 28 average 2011
1 fatal
362 accidents, 30 days+
880 accidents, 4 days+
1208 accidents with sick leave
1646 accidents , all

Fig. 8 Division of fatal and non-fatal injuries in relation to one fatal case in Singapore and selected reference populations

Occupational Injury Burden Is Unequally Shared by Various Groups of Workers

As in many social setups, the burden of injuries concentrates very unfairly on specific groups. Dirty, dangerous, and demanding jobs are poorly paid and very risky. There are major differences between:

- Workers in high-risk sectors in any country may have radically different risks; construction workers may have a 50 times higher risk of fatal and other accidents than in office or banking jobs.
- Some occupations and jobs are particularly dangerous anywhere, such as logging with traditional methods in tropical forests, small vessel fishermen, coal and other miners, small plane pilots, farmers, pizza delivery drivers in traffic, street sweepers, carpenters, etc.
- Injuries concentrate on male workers due to the selection of jobs and occupations, while even in exactly similar jobs such as female taxi drivers, they have less injuries; however female workers have more other types of occupational risks.
- Small-scale industry workers have much higher injury risk than large enterprises.
- Young workers and child laborers are, in particular, in a vulnerable position due to non-existing experience and training.

Some of the injury risks concentrate when work is carried out by young workers or even by children, often without any training, work in high-risk sectors, and jobs in small enterprises in some low-income countries. Such work may be carried out for bigger enterprises as contractors or subcontractors. This sort of unethical treatment of vulnerable workers that have no choice to select a better job must be eliminated.

Table 6 provides a summary of rates and exact numbers of occupational injuries in selected countries (Takala et al. 2017; Government of China 2014 and 2015).

Cost Estimates of Injuries and Illnesses at Work

Various cost estimates have been carried out by Australia, the USA, Finland, Norway, EU, and others. The ILO and EU jointly updated their cost estimates in 2017. Usually such cost estimates cover direct and production losses only and not the intangible costs, such as the cost of the virtual statistical life, which could multiply the costs by a factor of 3–4. However, the share of occupational injuries is about 11% of this 3 trillion or 323 billion USD ($323 * 10^9$ USD), roughly equal to that of occupational cancer globally 12.4% of all costs. These rates vary considerably, for example, the highest share is for the EURO Eastern European Region: 16.2% of the region's total costs.

The costs estimates are presented in Fig. 9. They cover direct costs and indirect loss of productivity costs. The estimates have been made by the ILO/ICOH/Finland/Singapore/EU Coalition Project. It neither includes any estimates of the intangible costs nor estimates of costs of pain and suffering to victims and family members. Including such costs will multiply the total costs by a factor of 3–4, for example, in Finland it has been estimated to be four times higher when including the intangibles. The global cost ended up in a loss or rather opportunity to gain equal to 3.94% global GDP (see earlier also the presentation in Fig. 6 for EU28) (Elsler et al. 2018). DALY estimate for different diseases and injuries corresponds to the costs.

Policies and Practices to Prevent Injuries Include a Range of Traditional and New Measures

Considering the risks involved and the fact that both traditional and new and emerging risks need to be studied, new innovations and solutions need to be identified. Singapore, based on models in the USA and elsewhere, has decided to concentrate on two aspects:

1. Establishing a Research Agenda setting priorities for the continuous search for evidence for policy and practice (Takala et al. 2014)
2. Building a Risk Observatory or *Observatory for Workplace Landscape* (OWL)

Often perceptions drive action more than real evidence, and it is important to highlight the difference between media interest, public attention, and real evidence for policy and practice. Media, including social media, are vital for communication, for reaching large numbers of stakeholders, workers, small and medium-sized enterprises (SMEs), the informal sector, migrant workers, and vulnerable groups,

Table 6 Rates and numbers of occupational injuries in selected countries

Fatal injuries at work (occupational accidents) including and excluding those related to traffic in selected countries and regions, absolute numbers (N*) and fatal injury rate (N*/100,000)

Year & Type/Area	Singapore[a]	Finland[b]	Germany[b]	Spain[b]	U.K.[b]	EU15[b]	EU28[b]	EU28/ILOad[d]	China, Gvt2013[d]	China, IHME/GBD 2013	China. ILO 2010[d]	ILO/World[d]	GBD/IHME[e]
Rate, 2011–2013, excl. traffic@ work	2.3	0.75	0.94	2.16	0.74	1.39	2.0	2.15				11.0[i]	5.0[i]
N*, 2011 excl. traffic@work	61	26[f]			194								
N*, 2010–2011, incl. traffic@work	80[g]	28	507	365	~650[h]	2,910	4,103	4,692	69,434	31,715	99,197	352,800[i]	159,000[i]

[a]Singapore WSH Statistics, WSH Institute
[b]EUROSTAT numbers referred by the Health and Safety Executive, U.K. web page: http://www.hse.gov.uk/statistics/pdf/fatalinjuries.pdf (accessed 11.9.2014), work-related traffic injuries excluded, rate for Finland in year 2013 including work-related traffic was 0.8/100,000 workers, in Singapore 1.8/100,00 in 2014
[c]EUROSTAT Fatal Accidents at Work by Economic Activity 18 July 2014, includes road traffic at work, web page http://epp.eurostat.ec.europa.eu/statistics_explained/index.php/Health_and_safety_at_work statistics (accessed 11.9.2014)
[d]See end note references referring to ILO Global Estimates 2014 (Takala et al. 2014; Nenonen et al. 2014), adjusted: includes all employed and road traffic at work, and Government of China (Government of China 2014) see http://www.stats.gov.cn/english/PressRelease/201402/t20140224_515103.html
[e]Institute of Health Metrics, GBD Cause Patterns, Occupational Risks, Rate, Both sexes, Global, webpage: http://vizhub.healthdata.org/gbd-cause-patterns/ (accessed 18.09.2015)
[f]Statistics Finland, Official Statistics of Finland (OSF): Occupational accident statistics (e-publication).ISSN=1797-9544. 2011. Helsinki: Statistics Finland (referred: 11.9.2014).Access method: http://www.stat.fi/til/ttap/2011/ttap_2011_2013-11-27_tie_001_en.html and http://www.stat.fi/til/ttap/2011/ttap_2011_2013-11-27_tau_001_fi.html
[g]Work-related traffic fatalities included, seamen and other assigned workers' fatalities excluded, all injuries compensated was 115
[h]The Royal Society for the Prevention of Accidents: "Around one third of fatal and serious road crashes involve someone who was at work." In 2012: 1754 road fatalities altogether, of which 1/3 is more than 500, web page: http://www.rospa.com/faqs/detail.aspx?faq=296 (accessed 11.9.2014)
[i]For the Global Burden of illness and injuries the denominator is calculated for total population and converted to cover labour force in 2011 (3,200,509,548 million)

7 Burden of Injury Due to Occupational Exposures

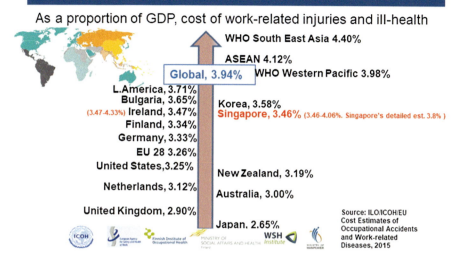

Fig. 9 Cost comparison of selected countries and regions. Injury costs globally are 11% of the total globally but different in each region, this about 323 billion USD

and to foster a safety culture at places of work. However, misperceptions in assessing risks exist. Statistical risks are not easy to assess and understand correctly. Further, common everyday risks are underestimated, and complicated technological risks that are not easily controlled by individuals are overrated.

Leadership, management, and systems thinking at all levels and related worker engagement have been identified as key for efforts to ensure workplace safety and health. Recent experiences from mega-projects such as the London Olympics construction effort were successful exactly because of emphasis on and continuous follow-up of these factors. The numbers presented in Tables 2 and 3 are alarmingly high and often poorly understood, and their importance has been underestimated. One should also keep in mind that the targets or "goal posts" are gradually moving due to changes in work, workplace, and work force. A systems approach is necessary at all levels. An enterprise management system is the strategic component for an organization, but an action program for risk assessment and priority setting for risk management are also needed. Collaboration between management and workers at the organizational (enterprise) level must be followed by a national-level mechanism, such as a tripartite advisory council, that looks after wider issues like new legal measures and better strategic enforcement.

Contrary to some perceptions – according to USA/OSHA (government) view – enforcement supports employers in reducing injuries and injury claims, and saving compensation costs, on average 26% or USD355,000, as a result of inspection of the company, and saving employers US$6 billion nationwide in the USA. This counts neither the costs of lost production of the injured workers nor the pain and suffering.

Several key processes have been gaining momentum, such as design for safety, and control banding based on the new Globally Harmonized System for Classification and Labelling of Chemicals (GHS) labelling requirements. One groundbreaking and new longer-term concept, or philosophy, is *Vision Zero*. The idea is to change the values and mindset of all stakeholders from business as usual and ensure zero accidents, zero illnesses, zero exposures, zero violence, zero harassment, and simply *zero harm* during an entire working life as the objective. So far it has been launched for selected special needs already, such as the Swedish traffic vision. It is not a key performance objective but a new mindset.

Conclusions

Globally, occupational injuries are still going up, while they have been successfully and continuously reduced in the high-income countries and regions. However, much of the progress has been achieved in "exporting" these injuries with the global production to locations where manufacturing – and construction – takes place, such as Asia. In the rapidly industrializing countries and regions, the injury numbers have gone up and may go down gradually only later, while the evidence is very limited.

This transfer of technologies has been incomplete. Machinery and production methods are easy to move from a continent to another, but the "software" or safety as a value, zero harm thinking, and concrete management goals as well as the measuring of progress through relevant indicators will need to be taken seriously.

While the negative outcomes, death, and permanent or temporary disability caused by occupational injuries are easy to detect, these are globally poorly recognized and reported. All injuries are avoidable; we do have all measures to prevent them everywhere in the world. This requires a paradigm change in thinking at workplaces around the world.

Key action programs should concentrate on finding solutions, reducing exposures to various injury risks, and on including illnesses that have a long latency period. For each injury and illness, there are many factors with influence on the negative outcomes. Cultures that start from committed and capable leadership in the organization need to be developed, and presently known best practices as well as new innovations at an organization and country level need to be identified and used. In addition to laws, enforcement, and health and safety services, media including social media should be better used for promotion of safety, health, and well-being at work.

Occupational injuries and work-related diseases and disorders are a bigger problem than estimated earlier. Longer-term risks are gradually increasing in importance at workplaces. A toolbox comprising (i) legal measures; (ii) enforcement; (iii) knowledge and solutions; (iv) incentives; (v) awareness raising and campaigns; (vi) services available to enterprises and organizations, such as occupational health services; and (vii) networking for best exchange of good practice is vital for any successful strategy for safety, health, and well-being at work.

A comprehensive toolbox model is the ILO Convention no. 187 on the Promotional Framework for Occupational Safety and Health. Furthermore, ILO Code of Practice on Recording and Notification of Occupational Accidents and Diseases provide further guidance in a compact form.

Safe work is about *decent work*, good work, for life. In the words of the former Secretary General of the United Nations, Mr. Kofi Annan: "Health and safety at work is not just sound economic policy – it is a basic human right."

Cross-References

▸ Policies of Reducing the Burden of Occupational Hazards and Disability Pensions
▸ Surveillance, Monitoring, and Evaluation
▸ Trends in Work and Employment in Rapidly Developing Countries

References

't Mannetje A, Pearce N (2005) Quantitative estimates of work-related deaths, diseases and injury in New Zealand. Scand J Work Environ Health 31(4):266–276. https://doi.org/10.5271/sjweh.882

Driscoll T, Takala J, Steenland K, Corvalan C, Fingerhut M (2005) Review of estimates of the global burden of injury and illness due to occupational exposures. Am J Ind Med 48:491–502

Elsler D, Takala J, Remes J (2018) An international comparison of the cost or work-related accidents and illnesses. European Agency for Safety and Health at Work. Bilbao, Spain, Oct 2017. https://osha.europa.eu/en/tools-and-publications/publications/international-comparison-cost-work-related-accidents-and. Accessed 10 Mar 2018

Eurostat (2009) Statistics in focus 63, 2009. European Commission, Luxembourg 2009. https://osha.europa.eu/en/safety-health-in-figures/eurostat-labour-force-survey-2007. Accessed 16 Nov 2016

García AM, Merino RG, Martínez VL (2007) Estimación de la mortalidad atribuible a enfermedades laborales en España, 2004. Rev Esp Salud Pública 81(3):261–270

GBD 2016 Causes of Death Collaborators (2017) Global, regional, and national age-sex specific mortality for 264 causes of death, 1980–2016: a systematic analysis for the Global Burden of Disease Study 2016. Lancet 390:1151–1210. https://doi.org/10.1016/S0140-6736(17)32152-9

Government of China (2014 and 2015) Statistical Communiqué of the People's Republic of China on the 2013 National Economic and Social Development, item XII. Resources, Environment and Work Safety. National Bureau of Statistics of China. http://www.stats.gov.cn/english/PressRelease/201402/t20140224_515103.html. Accessed 29 Dec 2018

Hämäläinen P (2010) Global estimates of occupational accidents and fatal work-related diseases. Doctoral dissertation, Publication 917, Tampere University of Technology, Finland. https://tutcris.tut.fi/portal/files/1314205/hamalainen.pdf. Accessed 30 Jan 2019

Hämäläinen P, Takala J, Saarela KL (2006) Global estimates of occupational accidents. Saf Sci 44:137–156. https://doi.org/10.1016/j.ssci.2005.08.017

Hämäläinen P, Takala J, Tan BK (2017) Global estimates of occupational accidents and work-related illnesses 2017. WSH Institute, Ministry of Manpower, ICOH et al. https://goo.gl/2hxF8x. Accessed 28 Dec 2018

HSE (2014) Health and safety executive, U.K. Based on EUROSTAT numbers referred by the HSE web page. http://www.hse.gov.uk/statistics/pdf/fatalinjuries.pdf. Includes also latest data, see further http://www.hse.gov.uk/statistics/. Accessed 28 Dec 2018

ILO (2017) Director-general guy ryder opening address at XXI World Congress on Safety and Health. World Congress on Safety and Health at Work, Singapore, 3–6 Sept 2017. https://www.ilo.org/global/about-the-ilo/how-the-ilo-works/ilo-director-general/statements-and-speeches/WCMS_639102/lang%2D%2Den/index.htm. Accessed 29 Dec 2018

ILOSTAT (2018) Dataset on safety and health at work. International Labour Statistics, International Labour Organisation, Geneva. https://www.ilo.org/ilostat/. Accessed 28 Dec 2018

Nenonen N, Saarela KL, Takala J, Kheng LG, Yong E, Ling LS, Manickam K, Hämäläinen P (2014) Global Estimates of Occupational Accidents and Work-related Illnesses 2014. Singapore: WSH Institute. 25

Rosling H, Rosling O, Rosling Rönnlund A (2018) Factfulness. Flatiron Books, New York, pp 89–114. (Finnish version: Faktojen maailma, Otava, Finland, 2018. ISBN 978-951-1-30371-8)

Takala J (1997) Occupational and major accidents. In: Brune D, Gerhardsson G, Crockford GW, D'Auria D (eds) The workplace, vol. 1: Part 4.2, Oslo, CIS/ILO. Scandinavian Science Publisher, Geneva, pp 228–243

Takala J (1999) Global Estimates of Fatal Occupational Accidents. Epidemiology, 10, 640–646. https://doi.org/10.1097/00001648-199909000-00034

Takala J (2005) ILO introductory report: decent work – safework. ILO introductory report, XVII World Congress on Safety and Health at Work, Orlando. ISBN 92-2-117750-5. http://ohsa.org.mt/Portals/0/docs/intrep_05.pdf. Accessed 15 Dec 2018

Takala J, Hämäläinen P, Saarela KL, Loke YY, Manickam K, Tan WJ, Heng P, Tjong C, Lim GK, Lim S, Gan SL (2014) Global estimates of the burden of injury and illness at work in 2012. J Occup Environ Hyg 11:326–337. https://doi.org/10.1080/15459624.2013.863131

Takala J, Hämäläinen P, Nenonen N, Takahashi K, Chimed-Ochir O, Rantanen J (2017) Comparative analysis of the burden of injury and illness at work in selected countries and regions. Cen Eur J Occup Environ Med 23(1–2):7–31. http://www.efbww.org/pdfs/CEJOEM%20Comparative%20analysis.pdf

Occupational Causes of Cancer

Jack Siemiatycki and Mengting Xu

Contents

Introduction	128
Early Discoveries	128
Sources of Evidence on Risk to Humans due to Chemicals	129
Epidemiology	130
Animal Experimentation	131
Short-Term Tests and Understanding of Mechanisms	132
Listing of Occupational Carcinogens	132
IARC Monographs	133
Occupational Agents or Exposure Circumstances Evaluated as Carcinogenic or Probably Carcinogenic	135
Interpreting the Lists	140
Illustrative Examples and Controversies	141
Polycyclic Aromatic Hydrocarbons (PAHs)	141
Diesel and Gasoline Engine Emissions	142
Asbestos	143
Cadmium and Cadmium Compounds	144
Styrene	144
Vinyl Chloride	145
Occupational Cancer Risk Factors Among Women	146
Fraction of Cancer Attributable to Occupation	147
Additional Considerations	148
Prevention and Compensation	149
Cross-References	149
References	150

J. Siemiatycki (✉) · M. Xu
École de santé publique, Université de Montréal, Montreal, QC, Canada

Université de Montréal Hospital Research Centre, (CRCHUM), Montreal, QC, Canada
e-mail: j.siemiatycki@umontreal.ca

Abstract

Many recognized human carcinogens are chemicals or physical agents found in the occupational environment. The present chapter is intended to summarize current information on occupational carcinogens. Most discoveries have been based on epidemiologic research; however, animal experimentation and basic science research have also contributed to this body of knowledge. Establishing a list of occupational carcinogens is not straightforward; since many occupational agents are also found in consumer products and the general environment, it requires judgment as to what should be considered an occupational agent. It is important to synthesize this information for both scientific and public health purposes. The International Agency for Research on Cancer (IARC) publishes lists of human carcinogens based on evaluations conducted by expert panels. Based largely on the evaluations published by IARC, and supplemented by our knowledge of the occupations and industries in which they are found, and their target organs, we list 50 definite occupational carcinogens and 51 probable occupational carcinogens. The evidence base for some of these is described. In various countries it has been estimated that between 4% and 14% of all cancer deaths among males are attributable to occupational exposures, and the corresponding range is from 1% to 3% of cancer deaths among females.

Keywords

Occupation · Cancer · Etiology · Epidemiology · IARC Monographs

Introduction

Occupational carcinogens occupy a special place among the different classes of modifiable risk factors for cancer. The occupational environment has been a most fruitful one for investigating the etiology of human cancer. Indeed, nearly half of all recognized human carcinogens are occupational carcinogens. Although it is important to discover occupational carcinogens for the sake of preventing occupational cancer, the potential benefit of such discoveries goes beyond the factory walls since most occupational exposures find their way into the general environment, sometimes at higher concentrations than in the workplace, and, for some agents, with more people exposed in the general environment than in the workplace.

Early Discoveries

From the late eighteenth century to the early twentieth century, there were some reports of clusters of various types of cancer (scrotum, lung, bladder) among workers in certain occupations (chimney sweeps, coal tar and shale oil workers, metal miners, dyestuff production). These discoveries were usually sparked by a clinician observing a cluster of cases in his clinical practice and following it up with some documentation of a case series which made a persuasive case for a causal association, particularly because the background incidence of cancer was very low at the time.

Rigorous scientific investigation of cancer etiology began in the early twentieth century with experimental animal research. It was found that skin tumors could be induced in rabbits by applying coal tar, and it was found that the active carcinogenic components were in the family of polycyclic aromatic hydrocarbons (PAHs). These compounds may have been responsible for many of the excess risks of scrotal cancer in various groups exposed to soot and oils. Several other PAHs were subsequently shown to be carcinogenic to laboratory animals, but so were substances of many other chemical families. For instance, 2-naphthylamine, an aromatic amine, was shown to cause bladder tumors in dogs, and this was thought to explain the bladder cancers seen earlier among dyestuff workers.

The era of modern cancer epidemiology began around 1950 with several studies of smoking and lung cancer, and with the conduct of some important studies of occupational cohorts such as nickel refinery workers, coal carbonization workers, chromate workers, asbestos products manufacture, and workers producing dyestuffs in the chemical industry (Siemiatycki 2014). The findings of these early studies highlighted some significant workplace hazards. Indeed, until the 1970s, virtually the only proven causes of human cancer were smoking and various occupational exposures.

In the 1960s and 1970s, there was a sharp increase in the amount of research aimed at investigating links between the environment and cancer. Particular attention was paid to the occupational environment for several reasons. Most of the historic observations of environmental cancer risks were discovered in occupationally exposed populations. As difficult as it is to characterize and study groups of workers, it is much harder to study groups of people who share other characteristics, such as diet or general environmental pollution. Not only are working populations easier to delineate, but, often, company personnel and industrial hygiene records permit some, albeit crude, forms of quantification of individual workers' exposure to workplace substances. Also, the pressure of organized labor was an important force in attracting attention to the workplace. Finally, the workplace is a setting where people have been exposed to high levels of many substances which could potentially be harmful.

Sources of Evidence on Risk to Humans due to Chemicals

Direct evidence concerning human carcinogenicity of a substance comes from epidemiologic studies. Experimental studies of animals (usually rodents) provide evidence of carcinogenicity, but the interspecies differences preclude automatic inferences regarding human carcinogenicity. Complementary evidence comes from the results of studies of mutagenicity, genotoxicity, and other studies of biological mechanisms.

Epidemiology

Epidemiologic research provides the most relevant data for identifying occupational carcinogens and characterizing their effects in humans. Such research requires the juxtaposition of information on illness or death due to cancer among workers and information on their past occupations, industries, and/or occupational exposures. A third, optional data set which would improve the validity of inferences drawn from that juxtaposition is the set of concomitant risk factors which may confound the association between occupation and disease. Confounding is a well-known potential problem in all nonexperimental empirical research, including in epidemiology. It refers to the possible distortion of the relationship between a factor and a disease by another factor. For instance, in estimating the relationship between an occupational chemical and lung cancer, it is important to consider whether the people exposed to the occupational chemical are more often smokers than the people unexposed to the chemical. That would distort the true relationship between the chemical under investigation and lung cancer.

Each human experiences, over his or her lifetime, an idiosyncratic and bewildering pattern of exposures. Not only is it impossible to completely and accurately characterize the lifetime exposure profile of an individual, but even if we could it is a daunting statistical task to tease out the effects of a myriad of specific substances. The possibility of mutual confounding among different occupational chemicals is sometimes particularly challenging in occupational epidemiology because of some highly correlated chemical co-exposures in the occupational environment. Blue-collar workers tend to be exposed to many different chemicals, not just one. Because of long induction periods for most cancers, it is necessary to ascertain exposure information about workers many years before cancer onset. The statistical power of a study to detect hazards depends among other things on the number of people in the study, and this is often limited by the size of a workforce in a given company or plant. Despite all of these challenges, epidemiology has made significant contributions to our knowledge of occupational carcinogens.

Epidemiologic investigation of occupation-cancer associations has usually been conducted by one of the following research designs: retrospective cohort study of a group of workers in a certain company or workplace or a case-control study in the population. Each of these designs has pros and cons in regard to ability to ascertain exposure histories, relevant confounder information, valid cancer incidence data, and statistical power.

An occupational retrospective cohort study is one in which the investigator obtains a list of workers from a company or union who worked in the company at some point in the past. Using the worker's employment history, the investigator reconstructs an employment history and, if there are historic industrial hygiene records, a history of exposure to agents in that company's workplace. With the worker's identification, the investigator could trace the worker through national mortality or cancer incidence registers to determine if the worker had a cancer diagnosis since starting to work there. This can be used to estimate risks of different types of cancer in relation to the exposure circumstances of the worker. One weakness of this design is that it usually does not involve communication with workers, and thus the investigator rarely has access to information about nonoccupational potential confounding variables like smoking.

A case-control study is one where the investigator starts with a series of cancer cases, typically identified through a cancer registry or a hospital, and a series of controls who do not have cancer, chosen from the general population or from among hospital patients with other conditions, and the investigator contacts each person to obtain information about the work they have done and about potential confounding variables. When carried out properly, the results from a case-control study should be of equivalent validity to those of a well-conducted cohort study.

Recently there have been increasing numbers of prospective cohort studies in the general population that collect occupational information and information on potential confounders, from initially cancer-free study subjects, and follow them over time to ascertain the incidence of cancer among study participants. This type of cohort study is potentially very valid, but it might take decades of follow-up time and huge investments of resources to conduct such studies. Few such studies have thus far produced useful results on occupational carcinogens.

Since the revolution in genomics research, there has been considerable effort and investment to integrate genetic markers in occupational cancer studies to estimate so-called gene-environment interactions. While this is an interesting and worthwhile pursuit, it has not yet led to a significant increase in knowledge of new carcinogens.

Animal Experimentation

Partly in consequence of the difficulty of generating adequate data among humans and partly because of the benefits of the experimental approach, great efforts have been devoted to studying the effects of substances in controlled animal experiments. Results generated by animal studies do bear on carcinogenicity among humans. Certain fundamental genetic and cellular characteristics are similar among all mammalian species. Most recognized human carcinogens have been reported to be carcinogenic in one or more animal species; and there is some correlation between species in the target organs affected and in the carcinogenic potency.

Still, there are several reasons for caution in extrapolating from animal evidence to humans. The animal experiment is not designed to emulate the human experience but rather to maximize the sensitivity of the test to detect animal carcinogens. Doses administered are usually orders of magnitude higher than levels to which humans are exposed. The route of exposure is sometimes unrealistic (e.g., injection or implantation), and the controlled and limited pattern of co-exposures is unlike the human situation. The "lifestyle" of the experimental animal is not only different from that of humans, but it is unlike that of its species in the wild. Animals used are typically from pure genetic strains, and susceptibility to carcinogens may be higher in such populations than in genetically heterogeneous human populations. Metabolism, immunology, DNA repair systems, life spans, and other physiologic characteristics differ between species. Tumors seen in animals often occur at sites that do not have a counterpart among humans or that are much more rarely affected among humans. Some experimental carcinogens operate via mechanisms which may not be relevant to humans. While there remain disagreements about the predictive value of animal experimentation (Cohen 1995; Gold et al. 1998), it remains an important arm in the effort to identify human carcinogens.

Short-Term Tests and Understanding of Mechanisms

A number of rapid in vitro tests have been developed to detect presumed correlates of or predictors of carcinogenicity (Ashby and Tennant 1988). However, neither alone nor in combination have these approaches proven to be consistently predictive of animal carcinogenicity, much less human carcinogenicity (Huff et al. 1996; Kim and Margolin 1999).

Deeper understanding of mechanisms of carcinogenesis has provided insight into the plausibility of a specified chemical having a carcinogenic effect on particular sites of cancer, and this can be useful in complementing the results on carcinogenicity that come from epidemiology or animal experimentation (International Agency for Research on Cancer 2006).

Listing of Occupational Carcinogens

This chapter includes a tabular listing of known occupational carcinogens, the occupations and industries in which they are found, and their target organs. Although seemingly simple, drawing up an unambiguous list of occupational carcinogens is challenging. The first challenge is define what is meant by an "occupational carcinogen." Exposures to most occupational carcinogens also occur in the general environment and/or in the course of using consumer products, and reciprocally, most environmental exposures and those associated with using certain consumer products, including medications, foods, and others, also occur in some occupational context. For instance, whereas exposures to tobacco smoke, sunlight, and immunosuppressive medications are generally not identified as occupational exposures, there are people whose occupation results in them being in contact with these agents to a degree that would not otherwise occur. Also, whereas asbestos, benzene, diesel engine emissions, and radon gas are considered to be occupational carcinogens, exposure to these agents is also experienced by the general population, and indeed many more people are probably exposed to these substances in the course of day-to-day life than are exposed at work. Given the definitional ambiguity, we adopt the following operational rule: a carcinogen is considered to be "occupational"

8 Occupational Causes of Cancer

if there is significant human exposure to the agent in the workplace, as measured in terms of prevalence of exposure or level of exposure, or if the main epidemiological studies that led to the identification of an elevated risk of cancer were undertaken among workers. Even this operational definition requires judgment in its implementation.

The strength of the evidence for an association can vary. For some associations the evidence of excess risk seems incontrovertible (e.g., liver angiosarcoma and vinyl chloride monomer (IARC 2012b); bladder cancer and benzidine (IARC 2012b)). For some associations the evidence is suggestive (e.g., breast cancer and shift work (Hansen and Stevens 2012); bladder cancer and employment as a painter (IARC 2012b)). Among the many substances in the industrial environment for which there are no human data concerning carcinogenicity, there are hundreds that have been shown to be carcinogenic in some animal species and thousands that have been shown to have some effect in assays of mutagenicity or genotoxicity. These considerations complicate the attempt to devise a list of occupational carcinogens.

IARC Monographs

One of the key sources of information for listing of occupational carcinogens is the monograph program of the International Agency for Research on Cancer (IARC) – Evaluation of the Carcinogenic Risk of Chemicals to Humans. The objective of the IARC program, which has been operating since 1971, is to publish critical reviews of epidemiological and experimental data on carcinogenicity for chemicals, groups of chemicals, industrial processes, other complex mixtures, physical agents, and biological agents to which humans are known to be exposed and to evaluate the data in terms of human risk.

Once it is decided to evaluate a given agent or set of related agents, an international working group of experts, usually numbering between 15 and 25, is convened by IARC, and all relevant data on the topic is assembled. The meetings may evaluate only one agent, such as silica, they may address a set of related agents, or they may even address exposure circumstances such as an occupation or an industry. The working group is comprised of experts covering the following domains: (i) exposure and occurrence of the substances being evaluated, (ii) human evidence of cancer risk (i.e., epidemiology), (iii) animal carcinogenesis, and (iv) other data relevant to the evaluation of carcinogenicity and its mechanisms. They determine whether the epidemiological evidence supports the hypothesis that the substance causes cancer and, separately, whether the animal evidence supports the hypothesis that the substance causes cancer. The judgments are not simply dichotomous (yes/no), but rather they allow the working group to express a range of opinions on each of the dimensions evaluated. (In the IARC jargon, these are labeled sufficient evidence of carcinogenicity; limited evidence of carcinogenicity; inadequate evidence of carcinogenicity; evidence indicating lack of carcinogenicity.)

The overall evaluation of human carcinogenicity is based on the epidemiological and animal evidence of carcinogenicity, plus any other relevant evidence on genotoxicity, mutagenicity, metabolism, mechanisms, or others. Epidemiological evidence, where it exists, is given greatest weight. Direct animal evidence of carcinogenicity is next in importance, with increasing attention paid to mechanistic evidence that can inform the relevance of the animal evidence for human risk assessment.

Table 1 shows the categories for the overall evaluation and how they are derived from humans, animals, and other evidence. In the end, each substance is classified into one of the following classes (which IARC refers to as "groups": carcinogenic (Group 1), probably carcinogenic (Group 2A), possibly carcinogenic (Group 2B), not classifiable (Group 3), probably not carcinogenic (Group 4)). However, the

Table 1 Classifications and guidelines used by IARC working groups in evaluating human carcinogenicity based on the synthesis of epidemiological, animal, and other evidence[a]

Group	Definition of group	Combinations which fit in this group		
		Epidemiological evidence	Animal evidence	Other evidence
1	The agent, mixture, or exposure circumstance is carcinogenic to humans	Sufficient	Any	Any
		Less than sufficient	Sufficient	Strongly supportive
2A	The agent, mixture, or exposure circumstance is probably carcinogenic to humans	Limited	Sufficient	Less than strongly supportive
		Inadequate or not available	Sufficient	Strongly supportive
2B	The agent, mixture, or exposure circumstance is possibly carcinogenic to humans	Limited	Less than sufficient	Any
		Inadequate or not available	Sufficient	Less than strongly supportive
		Inadequate or not available	Limited	Strongly supportive
3	The agent, mixture, or exposure circumstance is not classifiable as to its carcinogenicity to humans	Inadequate or not available	Limited	Less than strongly supportive
		Not elsewhere classified		
4	The agent, mixture, or exposure circumstance is probably not carcinogenic to humans	Suggesting lack of carcinogenicity	Suggesting lack of carcinogenicity	Any
		Inadequate or not available	Suggesting lack of carcinogenicity	Strongly nonsupportive

[a]This table shows our interpretation of the IARC guidelines used by the working groups to derive the overall evaluation from the combined epidemiological, animal, and other evidence. However, the working group can, under exceptional circumstances, depart from these guidelines in deriving the overall evaluation. For example, the overall evaluation can be downgraded if there is less than sufficient evidence in humans and strong evidence that the mechanism operating in animals is not relevant to humans. For details of the guidelines, refer to the Preamble of the IARC Monographs (International Agency for Research on Cancer 2006)

algorithm implied by Table 1 is only indicative, and the working group may derive an overall evaluation that departs from the strict interpretation of the algorithm. For example, neutrons have been classified as human carcinogens (Group 1) despite the absence of epidemiological data, because of overwhelming experimental evidence and mechanistic considerations (IARC 2000). The IARC process relies on consensus, and this is usually achieved, but sometimes, differing opinions among experts lead to split decisions. The published evaluations reflect the views of at least a majority of participating experts. The results of IARC evaluations are published in readily available and user-friendly volumes, and summaries are published on a web site (IARC 2013).

As of 2018, over 120 meetings have been held and almost 1100 agents have been evaluated, many of which are occupational. IARC evaluations are respected worldwide and are widely used by government regulatory agencies.

Occupational Agents or Exposure Circumstances Evaluated as Carcinogenic or Probably Carcinogenic

We used the IARC Monographs as the basis for listing of occupational carcinogens. There are some limitations to bear in mind. First, IARC does not provide any explicit indication as to whether the substance evaluated should be considered as an "occupational" exposure. We have made these judgments. Second, the evaluations are anchored in the time that the working group met and reviewed the evidence; it is possible that evidence that appeared after the IARC review could change the evaluation. Third, the evaluation is a qualitative hazard evaluation; it is not a quantitative risk assessment. This means that IARC does not quantify the potency of the carcinogen or indicate what the risks may be at different levels of exposure.

Table 2 lists 50 occupational agents, occupations, and industries that have been classified as Group 1, carcinogenic to humans. The table explicitly distinguishes 38 chemical or physical agents from 12 occupations and industries that involve an increased risk of cancer but for which the responsible agent has not yet been identified.

Some of the carcinogens listed occur naturally, such as wood dust or solar radiation, whereas some are man-made, such as 1,3-butadiene or vinyl chloride. Some are single chemical compounds, such as benzene or trichloroethylene; others are families of compounds that include some carcinogens, and still others are mixtures of varying chemical composition, of which diesel engine emissions and mineral oils are examples. Most known human carcinogens have been shown to induce only one or a few different types of cancer.

Among the high-risk occupations and industries shown in Table 2 for which the agents responsible for the excess cancer risk have not yet been identified, most are industries in which the number of workers is quite small, at least in developed countries. But one occupational group – painters – stands out as an occupation that is very prevalent. Aromatic amines may be responsible for some of the excess bladder cancer risk among painters, and some of the dusts in the construction

Table 2 Occupational exposures, occupations, industries, and occupational circumstances classified as definite carcinogenic exposures (Group 1) by the *IARC Monographs*, Volumes 1–123

Agent, occupation, or industry	Target organ	Main industry or use
Chemical or physical agent		
Acid mists, strong inorganic	Larynx, lung	Pickling operations; steel and petrochemical industries; phosphate fertilizer manufacturing
4-Aminobiphenyl	Bladder	Rubber
Arsenic and inorganic arsenic compounds	Lung, skin, bladder	Glass, metals, pesticides
Asbestos (all forms)	Larynx, lung, mesothelioma, ovary	Insulation, construction, renovation
Benzene	Leukemia (acute nonlymphocytic), leukemia (acute myeloid)	Starter and intermediate in chemical production, solvent
Benzidine	Bladder	Pigments
Benzo[a]pyrene	Uncertain	Coal liquefaction and gasification, coke production, coke ovens, coal-tar distillation, roofing, paving, aluminum production, and others
Beryllium and beryllium compounds	Lung	Aerospace, metals
Bis(chloromethyl) ether; chloromethyl methyl ether	Lung	Production of BCME; manufacturing of plastics, resins, and polymers
1,3-Butadiene	Leukemia and/or lymphoma	Plastics, rubber
Cadmium and cadmium compounds	Lung	Pigments, batteries
Chromium (VI) compounds	Lung	Metal plating, pigments
Coal-tar pitch	Lung, skin	Construction, electrodes
1,2-Dichloropropane	Biliary tract	Production of chlorinated chemicals
Diesel engine exhaust	Lung	Transportation, mining
Ethylene oxide	Uncertain	Many, including chemical, sterilizing agent
Formaldehyde	Nasopharynx, leukemia	Formaldehyde production; plastics, textiles
Ionizing radiation (including radon-222 progeny)	Thyroid, leukemia, salivary gland, lung, bone, esophagus, stomach, colon, rectum, skin, breast, kidney, bladder, brain	Radiology, nuclear industry, underground mining

(continued)

8 Occupational Causes of Cancer

Table 2 (continued)

Agent, occupation, or industry	Target organ	Main industry or use
Leather dust	Nasal cavity	Shoe manufacture and repair
Lindane	Non-Hodgkin's lymphoma	Pesticide
4,4'-Methylenebis(2-chloroaniline) (MOCA)	Uncertain	Rubber
Mineral oils, untreated or mildly treated	Skin	Lubricant
2-Naphthylamine	Bladder	Pigments
Nickel compounds	Nasal cavity, lung, paranasal sinus	Metal alloy
Outdoor air pollution	Lung	Outdoor workers
Pentachlorophenols	Non-Hodgkin's lymphoma	Pesticide
Pentachlorobiphenyl (PCBs)	Melanoma of skin	Transformer manufacturing, electric power workers
Shale oils	Skin	Lubricant, fuel
Silica dust, crystalline, in the form of quartz or cristobalite	Lung	Construction, mining
Solar radiation	Skin, melanoma	Outdoor work
Soot	Lung, skin	Chimney sweeps, masons, firefighters
Tobacco smoke, second-hand	Lung	Bars, restaurants, offices
Ortho-Toluidine	Bladder	Pigments
Trichloroethylene	Kidney	Solvent, dry cleaning
Ultraviolet radiation from welding	Melanoma of eye	Welding
Vinyl chloride	Liver	Plastics
Welding fumes	Lung	Welders, construction workers
Wood dust	Nasal cavity, nasopharynx	Wood sawing, construction, furniture
Occupation or industry, without specification of the responsible agent		
Acheson process	Lung	Production of silicon carbide fibers
Aluminum production	Lung, bladder	–
Auramine production	Bladder	–
Coal gasification	Lung	–
Coal-tar distillation	Skin	–
Coke production	Lung	–
Hematite mining (underground)	Lung	–

(continued)

Table 2 (continued)

Agent, occupation, or industry	Target organ	Main industry or use
Iron and steel founding	Lung	–
Isopropyl alcohol manufacture using strong acids	Nasal cavity	–
Magenta production	Bladder	–
Painter	Bladder, lung, mesothelioma	–
Rubber manufacture	Stomach, bladder, leukemia	–

Table 3 Occupational exposures, occupations, industries, and occupational circumstances classified as probable carcinogenic exposures (Group 2A) by the *IARC Monographs*, Volumes 1–123

Agent, occupation, or industry	Suspected target organ	Main industry or use
Chemical or physical agent		
Acrylamide	–	Plastics
Bitumens (combustion products)	Lung	Roofing
Captafol	–	Fungicide
α-Chlorinated toluenes combined with benzoyl chloride	–	Pigments, chemicals
4-Chloro-*ortho*-toluidine	Bladder	Pigments, textiles
Cobalt metal with tungsten carbide	Lung	Hard-metal production
Creosotes	Skin	Wood preserving, brick making
Diazinon	Lung, non-Hodgkin lymphoma	Insecticide
4,4′-Dichlorodiphenyltrichloroethane (DDT)	Liver, testis, non-Hodgkin lymphoma	Biocide
Dichloromethane (Methylene chloride)	–	Organic solvent
Dieldrin and aldrin metabolized to dieldrin	–	Pesticides
Diethyl sulfate	–	Production of dyes, pigments, textiles
Dimethylcarbamoyl chloride	–	Production and manufacture of pharmaceuticals, pesticides, and dyes
Dimethylformamide	–	Solvent in production of acrylic fibers, plastics, pharmaceuticals, pesticides, adhesives, synthetic leathers, and surface coatings

(continued)

8 Occupational Causes of Cancer

Table 3 (continued)

Agent, occupation, or industry	Suspected target organ	Main industry or use
1,2-Dimethylhydrazine	–	Laboratory use only – DNA methylation
Dimethyl sulfate	–	Used in methylation of phenols, amines, and thiols – plastics, pharmaceuticals, herbicides
Epichlorohydrin	–	Plastics
Ethylene dibromide	–	Fumigant
Glycidol	–	Pharmaceutical industry
Glyphosate	Non-Hodgkin's lymphoma	Herbicide, agriculture
Hydrazine	Lung	Production of gases, propellants, pharmaceuticals, pesticides, solvent
Indium phosphide	–	Semiconductors
Lead compounds, inorganic	Lung, stomach	Metals, pigments
Malathion	Prostate, non-Hodgkin lymphoma	Organophosphate insecticide
2-Mercaptobenzothiazole	–	Sulphur vulcanization of rubber
Methyl methanesulfonate	–	Methylating agent
6-Nitrochrysene	–	Transportation, vehicle mechanic
1-Nitropyrene	–	Transportation, vehicle mechanic
2-Nitrotoluene	–	Production of dyes
Non-arsenical insecticides	–	Agriculture
Polybrominated biphenyls	–	Plastics
Polychlorinated biphenyls	Non-Hodgkin lymphoma	Electrical components

Polycyclic aromatic hydrocarbons
  Cyclopenta[cd]pyrene
  Dibenz[a,h]anthracene
  Dibenz[a,j]acridine
  Dibenzo[a,l]pyrene
	–	Combustion of organic matter, coal liquefaction and gasification, coke production, coke ovens, coal-tar distillation, roofing, paving, aluminum production, foundries; steel mills; firefighters; vehicle mechanics

1-3-Propane sultone	–	Laboratory use, photographic chemicals, pharmaceuticals, insecticides, dyes, chemical industry
Silicon carbide whiskers	–	Mineral, abrasives
Styrene	–	Plastics
Styrene-7,8-oxide	–	Plastics
Tetrabromobisphenol A	–	Fire retardant
3,3′,4,4′-Tetrachloroazobenzene	–	Contaminant in the production of some commonly used herbicides
Tetrachloroethylene (perchloroethylene)	–	Solvent

(continued)

Table 3 (continued)

Agent, occupation, or industry	Suspected target organ	Main industry or use
Tetrafluoroethylene	–	Alkylating agent used in production of polymers, nonstick coatings, resistant tubing
1,2,3-Trichloropropane	–	General purpose solvent
Tris(2,3-dibromopropyl) phosphate	–	Plastics, textiles
Vinyl bromide	–	Plastics, textiles
Vinyl fluoride	–	Production of various polymers, solar panels
Occupation or industry, without specification of the responsible agent		
Art glass, glass containers, and pressed ware (manufacture of)	Lung, stomach	–
Carbon electrode manufacture	Lung	–
Hairdressers or barbers	Bladder, lung	–
Petroleum refining	–	–
Occupational circumstance, without specification of the responsible agent		
Food frying at high temperature	–	–
Shift work involving circadian disruption	Breast	Nursing, others

industry (e.g., asbestos, silica) may be responsible for some of the excess lung cancer risk.

Table 3 lists occupational agents, occupations, and industries that have been classified as Group 2A, probably carcinogenic to humans. The table explicitly distinguishes 45 chemical or physical agents from 4 occupations and industries that have been found to present a probable risk but for which a causative agent has not been identified and the two other at-risk occupational circumstances – food frying and shift work. Whereas most agents in Table 2 (definite carcinogens) have been evaluated in several epidemiologic studies, most agents in Table 3 do not have a large body of epidemiologic evidence but rather have been found to be carcinogenic in animal experiments.

Interpreting the Lists

The designation of an agent as carcinogenic is an important public health statement, as well as a scientific one.

The determination that a substance or circumstance is carcinogenic depends on the strength of evidence at a given point in time. The evidence is sometimes clear-cut, but more often it is not. The balance of evidence can change in either direction as new data emerge.

The characterization of an occupation or industry group as a "high-risk group" is strongly rooted in time and place. For instance, the fact that some groups of nickel refinery workers experienced excess risks of nasal cancer does not imply that all workers in all nickel refineries will be subject to such risks. The particular circumstances of the industrial process, raw materials, impurities, and control measures may produce risk in one nickel refinery but not in another or in one historic era but not in another. The same can be said of rubber production facilities, aluminum refineries, and other industries and occupations. Labeling a chemical substance as a carcinogen in humans is a more timeless statement than labeling an occupation or industry as a high-risk group. A determination of carcinogenicity of a specified chemical is a statement about the properties of that chemical that is invariant in time and place; conditional on the amount of exposure to the agent, it should always be considered that a carcinogenic chemical is capable of causing cancer.

Different carcinogens produce different levels of risk, and for a given carcinogen, there may be vast differences in the risks incurred by different people exposed under different circumstances. Indeed there may also be interactions with other factors, environmental or genetic, that produce no risk for some exposed workers and high risk for others.

This raises the issue of quantitative risk assessment, which is an important tool in prevention of occupational cancer. While it would be valuable to have such information, for many agents, the information base on dose-response to support such quantification is fragmentary. As much as the designation of an agent as carcinogenic should raise flags that could lead to changes in industrial processes or regulations, we must be careful to avoid needless panic in regard to the presence of carcinogens. For most carcinogens, exposure to low concentrations for brief periods of time is unlikely to measurably influence a person's risk of cancer. Many of the already recognized carcinogens are very widespread and even ubiquitous in the occupational or general environment, and this has not been shown to lead to epidemics of cancer.

Illustrative Examples and Controversies

In this section, we present a few examples to illustrate some of the difficulties inherent in research to evaluate occupational carcinogens.

Polycyclic Aromatic Hydrocarbons (PAHs)

PAHs comprise a large family of chemical compounds which are produced during incomplete combustion of organic material and in particular fossil fuels. PAHs are found in many occupations and industries, and they are found in such non-occupational settings as vehicle roadways, homes heated by burning fuel, barbequed foods, cigarette smoke, and many more.

As described above, the earliest known occupational carcinogens were coal-derived soots, oils, and fumes that caused skin cancers. Animal experiments showed that several of the chemicals found in these complex mixtures were carcinogenic. These chemicals were in the family of PAHs. When epidemiologic evidence accumulated on lung cancer risks among workers exposed to complex mixtures derived from combustion of coal, petroleum, and wood, it was widely felt that the responsible agents were likely to be PAHs. Several of the complex mixtures (coal tars and pitch, mineral oils, shale oils, soot) which are classified as IARC Group 1 carcinogens include PAHs, and several of the industries in which cancer risks have been identified (coal gasification, coke production, aluminum production, iron and steel founding) are industries in which PAHs are prevalent. Paradoxically, however, there is only one specific PAH on the Group 1 list – benzo(a)pyrene. Some others are classed in Group 2A. This is because it is virtually impossible to epidemiologically isolate the effect of one versus another of the components of these carcinogenic mixtures. Because of the non-feasibility of measuring all PAHs when they are measured for industrial hygiene purposes, benzo(a)pyrene has typically been considered a representative marker of PAHs. While this marker may be available for epidemiologic purposes, it cannot be assumed that this is the only PAH present or how its presence is correlated with those of other PAHs. It is possible that biomarker and genetic studies will provide the additional information that would permit the determination that specific PAHs are definite human carcinogens.

Diesel and Gasoline Engine Emissions

Engine emissions are common in many workplaces and are ubiquitous environmental pollutants. Engine emissions are complex and variable mixtures of chemicals, including many PAHs. There has long been suspicion that emissions from diesel-powered engines may be lung carcinogens; but, until recently, the epidemiologic evidence was considered inconclusive (Boffetta et al. 1997; Katsouyanni and Pershagen 1997; Nauss et al. 1995). The difficulty of drawing inferences was partly due to the crudeness of the use of the job titles of truck driver as a proxy for occupational exposure to diesel exhaust and partly because few studies were able to control for the potential confounding effect of cigarette smoking and of other occupational exposures. Also, many of the studies had low statistical power and/or insufficient follow-up time. Finally, the relative risk estimates in most studies ranged from 1.0 to 1.5, making it difficult to exclude the possibility of chance or bias. The number of diesel-powered vehicles is increasing in many countries. Because of the significant scientific and public policy implications, it is important to derive more definitive inferences regarding the potential human carcinogenicity of diesel emissions. Recently some studies of diesel-exposed mine workers and railroad workers have provided more definitive evidence that the associations previously observed are probably true (Attfield et al. 2012; Garshick et al. 2004; Silverman et al. 2012) and IARC classified diesel engine emissions as a human carcinogen.

By contrast, there is no evidence for a carcinogenic effect of exposure to gasoline engine emissions (IARC 2014; Xu et al. 2018).

Engine emission provides an example of a common dilemma in occupational and environmental cancer risk assessment. A chemical analysis of both gasoline and diesel exhaust shows the presence of many substances which are considered carcinogenic, notably some nitro-PAHs which are classed by IARC as 2A and 2B. Should the presence of a carcinogen within a complex mixture automatically trigger a labeling of the mixture as carcinogenic, irrespective of the epidemiologic evidence on the mixture? There is no wide consensus on this issue, but it has important consequences. For instance, it would have meant that both diesel and gasoline engine emissions would have been classified long ago as probable or definite human carcinogens.

Asbestos

Few health issues have sparked as much public concern, controversy, and expense as has asbestos-related cancer risk. Asbestos is a term describing a family of naturally occurring fibrous silicates which have varied chemical and physical compositions and which have been widely used in industrial and consumer products for over a century. The main fiber types are called chrysotile and amphibole. Exposure to asbestos fibers has occurred in many occupations, including mining and milling, manufacture of asbestos-containing products, and use of these products. Currently, in developed countries, construction and maintenance workers constitute the largest group of asbestos-exposed workers, resulting from application and removal of asbestos products and building demolition. Asbestos was one of the most ubiquitous workplace exposures in the twentieth century. Not only is asbestos found in occupational environments, but it is found, albeit at lower concentrations, in the air of urban centers and even rural areas.

Case reports linking asbestos with lung cancer started to appear in the 1930s and 1940s, but the first formal investigations were published in the 1950s and 1960s (Selikoff 1990). In the early 1960s, reports appeared linking asbestos exposure to a hitherto unrecognized tumor of the pleura and peritoneum called mesothelioma. By the mid-1960s, it was clear that the very high and virtually uncontrolled exposure conditions prevalent up to then could induce lung cancer and mesothelioma.

While asbestos production and use has declined dramatically in most industrialized countries since 1975, public concern and controversy have not (IPCS (International Programme on Chemical Safety) 1998; Upton et al. 1991). Asbestos fibers are highly persistent and widespread in the environment, partly because of its widespread industrial use in the past and partly because it is a natural geological component of outcroppings in many areas of the world. Measurements carried out in all kinds of non-occupational settings have detected asbestos fibers, and it has become clear that asbestos is a widespread environmental pollutant, albeit at much lower levels than in some workplaces. Also, because of long latency periods, we are still seeing the cancer impact of high occupational exposure levels experienced 30 to 50 years ago, and we will for some time to come. Since exposure levels are much lower than they used to be, it is of interest to determine the risk due to low levels of asbestos exposure. Risk assessment models have been developed to extrapolate from high to low exposure levels, but these models have not been validated.

Many countries have banned use of asbestos, while some others have instituted regulatory limits orders of magnitude below levels that had been known to produce harmful effects. The availability of alternative non-asbestos substitution products makes such strategies feasible. Perhaps because they are not carcinogenic, or perhaps because exposure levels to the substitution products is much lower than that experienced by asbestos-exposed workers in the past, there has been no demonstrated cancer risk related to the substitution products.

While asbestos use has declined in developed countries, its use has been increasing in some developing countries.

Cadmium and Cadmium Compounds

Cadmium has been produced and used in alloys and various compounds for several end products including batteries, pigments, electroplating, and some plastics (IARC 2012a). Exposure varies widely between industries in both types of cadmium compounds and level of exposure. Following reports in a few small cohorts of excess cases of prostate cancer among workers in battery plants, an early IARC working group concluded that there was moderately persuasive evidence of an excess risk of prostate cancer as a result of cadmium exposure (IARC 1976). They noted in passing that one of the cohorts also reported an excess of lung cancer. In the following decade, a number of additional cohort studies were undertaken in cadmium-exposed workers (IARC 1993). There was no additional evidence of an increase in prostate cancer risk. But the evidence on lung cancer, which was unremarkable in the first few studies, became much more pronounced as additional data were accumulated. By 1993, another IARC working group pronounced cadmium a Group 1 carcinogen but solely on the basis of its association with lung cancer. Still, the assessment of carcinogenicity of cadmium highlighted several methodological problems. The number of long-term, highly exposed workers was small, the historical data on exposure to cadmium was limited, and the ability to define and examine a gradient of exposure was limited to one study. Confounding by cigarette smoking in relation to lung cancer was difficult to address, as was possible confounding by other occupational chemicals.

Styrene

Styrene is one of the most important industrial chemicals. The major uses are in plastics, latex paints and coatings, synthetic rubbers, polyesters, and styrene-alkyd coatings. These products are used in construction, packaging, boats, automotive (tires and body parts), and household goods (e.g., carpet backing). Nearly 18 million tons were used worldwide in 1998, with millions of workers exposed in different industries. In addition, there is widespread low-level environmental exposure.

The first evidence of a possible cancer risk came from case reports of leukemia and lymphoma among workers in various styrene-related industries. A number of cohort studies have been carried out since then in Europe and the USA in various industries (Bond et al. 1992). The interpretation of these studies has been bedeviled by four main problems: the different types of industries in which these studies were carried out make it difficult to compare results across studies; within most industries, styrene is only one of several chemical exposures, and these tend to be highly correlated with styrene exposure; the pattern of results has been unpersuasive, though there are a couple of hints of excess risk of leukemia in some subgroups of some cohorts; and finally, the classification of hematopoietic malignancies is complicated (IARC 2002).

The substantial body of epidemiologic evidence can reasonably be interpreted as showing no cancer risk, or it can be interpreted as showing suggestions of risk of leukemia in some subgroups of some cohorts. The IARC working group leaned in the latter direction as they categorized the human evidence as "limited" rather than "inadequate." The studies already conducted have been large and there have been several of them. It is not clear that another study would resolve the issue (Boffetta et al. 2009).

Nor does the experimental evidence provide clear guidance. The animal experimental evidence is equivocal and human biomarker studies show some signs of DNA adduct formation.

Vinyl Chloride

Vinyl chloride is a large-volume industrial chemical with many practical applications. In the early 1970s, clinicians observed a cluster of cases of a rare type of liver cancer called angiosarcoma among a group of workers in a plant using vinyl chloride (Creech and Johnson 1974). Within a very short time of the initial publication, other similar clusters were reported in other plants using vinyl chloride, and the association was quickly accepted as causal. The discovery was facilitated by the rarity of the tumor, the strength of the association, and the fact that there are no other known risk factors for this tumor and thus little danger of confounding. Early cohort studies confirmed the strong effect of vinyl chloride on risk of angiosarcoma of the liver and also raised questions about a possible association with lung cancer. In fact the data were suggestive enough in the 1980s that an effect on lung cancer was considered likely (Doll 1988). However, subsequent studies have failed to demonstrate such an effect, and it is likely that the early reports were distorted by confounding or by chance (Boffetta et al. 2003). While there is growing evidence that lung cancer is not a target organ for vinyl chloride, it is becoming more plausible that exposure to vinyl chloride may cause other types of liver cancer as well as angiosarcoma (Boffetta et al. 2003). Detecting an association of low to moderate strength with a fairly rare tumor which has a long latency is difficult. Because of the drastic decrease in exposure levels that took place in the vinyl chloride industry after the discovery of its carcinogenic activity, it is unlikely that there will be new cohorts of highly exposed workers to investigate. It is conceivable that new data can be generated from further follow-up of existing cohorts; however, the maximum latent period for most cancers has likely passed, and additional cancers are increasingly likely to reflect background risk factors for liver cancer.

Occupational Cancer Risk Factors Among Women

Until quite recently, in most countries, blue-collar jobs involving significant and long-term exposure to chemicals were mainly held by men. Consequently, most research on cancer risks among workers focused on male workers. Almost all the evidence that has led to the identification of occupational cancer risk factors has been derived from studies among male workers. However, and increasingly with the shift in workplace roles of women, many women are exposed at work to agents identified as carcinogens among men. In the absence of contrary empirical evidence, it is assumed that occupational carcinogens identified among males, and listed in Tables 2 and 3, are dangerous for female workers as they are for male workers when the exposure circumstances are similar. This general assumption has not been validated, but it is reasonable to accept it as a precaution.

What is more troubling is the possibility that there may be occupational agents that are carcinogenic among women but not among men or that there are exposures experienced predominantly by women workers that have not been evaluated at all because there are few men exposed. A well-known historic example of the latter possibility is the discovery in the early 1930s that radium exposure is a risk factor for bone cancer. This was discovered because of a cluster of bone cancer among young women working as radium dial painters (Winkelstein 2002).

Although there have been few studies of cancer risks among female workers, and those that have been conducted tended to be rather small, we nevertheless enumerate here some of the findings that have hinted at cancer risks to female workers. This review is not based on a consensus process such as those conducted by IARC, and it should not be interpreted as a listing of established or probable causal associations. Some evidence of increased risk of lung cancer was observed among female workers exposed to asbestos, arsenic, chromium, nickel, and mercury or in industries including motor vehicle manufacturing, food service, or cosmetology (Zahm and Blair 2003). Some evidence of leukemia risk was observed among female workers exposed to solvents, vinyl chloride, antineoplastic drugs, radiation, and pesticides and in women who worked in food processing or textile industry (Zahm and Blair 2003). For bladder cancer, an increase in risk was observed among women who worked as painters, dry cleaners, and health-care workers, as well as women who worked in the textile and dyestuff, rubber and plastic, and leather industries (Zahm and Blair 2003). A higher risk of breast cancer was observed in female white-collar workers (Kullberg et al. 2017) and shift workers (Yuan et al. 2018). Most of the associations listed above were based on limited number of studies with small study sample, and thus further investigations are warranted to strengthen the current evidence on occupational cancer risk factors among women.

Fraction of Cancer Attributable to Occupation

Given the lengthy list of established occupational carcinogens, it is natural to wonder how much of the total number of cancers in our society could be prevented if we eliminated all occupational carcinogens. Such a fraction is referred to as an attributable fraction, and it can be estimated for any known carcinogen. By far the most important risk factor for cancer is smoking; in North America, about 85% of lung cancers and about 30% of all cancers are attributable to smoking (Jacobs et al. 2015).

To estimate the fraction of cancers attributable to occupational exposures, it is necessary to have a list of occupational carcinogens, to know what the potency of each is (as measured by relative risk), and to know the prevalence of each one in the population. Conducting such analyses is complicated and is beyond the scope of this chapter. However other investigators have conducted such analyses. We compile in Table 4 a set of estimates that have been made since 2001 in various countries. The results depend on various features of the analysis, including which chemical agents are included and which types of cancer are included in the analysis, as well as whether the focus is on incident cases or deaths. The different analyses have been based on different decisions and assumptions, but they largely coincide.

In the various analyses, it has been estimated that between 4% and 14% of all cancer deaths among males are attributable to occupational exposures, and the corresponding range is from 1% to 3% of cancer deaths among females. In many countries this would translate to thousands of deaths per year. The WHO Global Burden of Disease project estimated that in 2017, approximately 334,000 cancer deaths worldwide were due to occupational exposures (Stanaway et al. 2018). The most detailed and extensive of the national analyses was that of Rushton et al. in

Table 4 Population attributable fraction (PAF) of cancer due to occupation: selected national estimates

Lead author (year)	Country	Nbr agents[a]	Nbr types of cancer	Incidence or mortality	PAF (%) M	F
Nurminen (2001) (Nurminen and Karjalainen 2001)	Finland	>40	26	Mortality	14	2
Steenland (2003) (Steenland et al. 2003)	USA	>40	9	Mortality	4	1
Fritschi (2006) (Fritschi and Driscoll 2006)	Australia	>40	26	Incidence	11	2
Boffetta (2010) (Boffetta et al. 2010)	France	17	7	Mortality	4	1
Rushton (2012) (Rushton et al. 2012)	UK	>40	24	Mortality	8	2
Labrèche (2014) (Labrèche et al. 2014)	Canada (Quebec)	>40	28	Mortality	12	3

[a]For the most part, these agents were IARC Group 1 and Group 2A agents

Britain; there it was estimated that the occupational agents that led to the greatest numbers of attributable cancers were (in descending order) asbestos, shift/night work, mineral oils, solar radiation, silica, and diesel engine exhaust.

Additional Considerations

In the 1960s and 1970s, the field of occupational cancer research was one of the most thriving areas of epidemiological research. This was fed by the social trends which raised the profile of environmentalism and workers' health and by important discoveries of occupational carcinogens such as asbestos. Workers' organizations were active and vocal in calling for improved working conditions and for the research that would support such action. Many young investigators, influenced by the zeitgeist of the 1960s, were ideologically drawn to a research area which would dovetail with their political and social interests. Over time there has been a waning of interest and enthusiasm.

The reasons for this decline are complex but may well include the following. The political/social climate that fostered research on occupational health has greatly changed. In western countries, the economies and workforces have shifted, and there are fewer blue-collar industrial workers than there were 30 years ago. Union membership, especially in blue-collar unions, has declined, and the unions have become less militant and influential. These trends have been fostered by technology (e.g., computerization and robotization) and by globalization. Many "dirty jobs" have been eliminated or exported from western to developing countries. The bottom line is that a smaller fraction of the western workforce is involved in traditional "dirty jobs." Another factor is that most large workplaces have become much cleaner, at least in some industrialized countries. But this should not be exaggerated. There remain many industries and hundreds of thousands of workers in industrialized countries who are in jobs that involve exposure to dusts and fumes to agents that may be dangerous. This is particularly the case of small companies.

There are many thousands of chemicals in workplaces. Many of them are obscure and involve relatively few workers; but many involve exposure for thousands of workers. Of these, only a small fraction has been adequately investigated in epidemiological studies. One of the foremost problems in occupational epidemiology is to reveal as-yet-unrecognized carcinogens and carcinogenic risks.

In the past, epidemiological research of occupational risk factors has largely focused on occupational exposures associated with "dirty" industrial environments. In recent decades, however, occupational hygiene in many industries has improved, or different technologies have been adopted such that the historical circumstances no longer apply, at least in developed countries. Increasing attention is now being paid to nonchemical agents in the work environment. Physical agents such as solar radiation and electromagnetic fields have been investigated, as have behavioral and ergonomic characteristics of particular occupations, such as physical activity and shift work. For almost all these risk factors, the distinction between occupational and non-occupational exposure is becoming more blurred.

Industries and occupations are constantly evolving. Even if we knew all there was to know about the cancer risks in today's occupational environments – which we do not – continuing to monitor cancer risks in occupational settings would remain an important activity because occupational exposure circumstances change over time and novel exposures may be introduced. Recent examples of "new" exposures are nanoparticles and indium phosphide in the semiconductor industry.

As much as the occupational environment in industrialized countries remains an area of concern, the problem in developing countries is much more precarious. Occupational hygiene conditions in developing countries are generally not subject to the same levels of regulation as those in industrialized countries. Enormous numbers of people are now working in insalubrious conditions. As life expectancy in these populations rises with improved living conditions and medical care, the numbers of cancer cases and most likely the numbers of occupationally related cancers will increase.

Many chemicals in the workplace find their way into the general environment, either via industrial effluent or via their use in consumer products. Hazards identified in the workplace often have an importance that goes beyond the factory walls.

Prevention and Compensation

The listing of occupational carcinogens in Tables 2 and 3 is useful in occupational medicine, in compensation, and in prevention. Approaches to preventing workplace exposures to occupational carcinogens include eliminating the production or use of such agents or reducing exposure levels. For some agents, reduction of exposure levels is feasible and appropriate; for others, more draconian measures, like banning use, may be appropriate. Education of workers and industries and regulators is an important component of prevention.

Where a worker has been diagnosed with a cancer known to be linked to the occupation he or she exercised, it is appropriate to look into the possibility of compensation, depending on the national policies for compensation. We offer the listing of occupational carcinogens as a tool that can be used for such a purpose.

Cross-References

▶ Cancer Survivors at the Workplace
▶ Surveillance, Monitoring, and Evaluation

References

Ashby J, Tennant RW (1988) Chemical structure, Salmonella mutagenicity and extent of carcinogenicity as indicators of genotoxic carcinogenesis among 222 chemicals tested in rodents by US NCI/NTP (MYR 01277). Mutat Res 204(1):17–115

Attfield MD et al (2012) The diesel exhaust in miners study: a cohort mortality study with emphasis on lung cancer. J Natl Cancer Inst 104(11):869–883

Boffetta P, Jourenkova N, Gustavsson P (1997) Cancer risk from occupational and environmental exposure to polycyclic aromatic hydrocarbons [review]. Cancer Causes Control 8(3):444–472

Boffetta P, Matisane L, Mundt KA, Dell LD (2003) Meta-analysis of studies of occupational exposure to vinyl chloride in relation to cancer mortality. Scand J Work Environ Health 29(3):220–229

Boffetta P, Adami HO, Cole P, Trichopoulos D, Mandel JS (2009) Epidemiologic studies of styrene and cancer: a review of the literature. J Occup Environ Med 51(11):1275–1287

Boffetta P et al (2010) An estimate of cancers attributable to occupational exposures in France. J Occup Environ Med 52(4):399–406

Bond GG, Bodner KM, Olsen GW, Cook RR (1992) Mortality among workers engaged in the development or manufacture of styrene-based products – an update. Scand J Work Environ Health 18(3):145–154

Cohen SM (1995) Human relevance of animal carcinogenicity studies. Regul Toxicol Pharmacol 21(1):75–80

Creech JL Jr, Johnson MN (1974) Angiosarcoma of liver in the manufacture of polyvinyl chloride. J Occup Med 16(3):150–151

Doll R (1988) Effects of exposure to vinyl chloride. An assessment of the evidence. Scand J Work Environ Health 14(2):61–78

Fritschi L, Driscoll T (2006) Cancer due to occupation in Australia. Aust N Z J Public Health 30(3):213–219

Garshick E et al (2004) Lung cancer in railroad workers exposed to diesel exhaust. Environ Health Perspect 112(15):1539

Gold LS, Slone TH, Ames BN (1998) What do animal cancer tests tell us about human cancer risk? Overview of analyses of the carcinogenic potency database. Drug Metab Rev 30(2):359–404

Hansen J, Stevens RG (2012) Case-control study of shift-work and breast cancer risk in Danish nurses: impact of shift systems. Eur J Cancer 48(11):1722–1729

Huff J, Weisburger E, Fung VA (1996) Multicomponent criteria for predicting carcinogenicity: dataset of 30 NTP chemicals. Environ Health Perspect 104(Suppl 5):1105–1112

IARC (1976) Cadmium, nickel, some epoxides, miscellaneous industrial chemicals and general considerations on volatile anaesthetics. IARC monographs on the evaluation of the carcinogenic risk of chemicals to man, vol 11. IARC (International Agency for Research on Cancer, Lyon

IARC (1993) Beryllium, cadmium, mercury, and exposures in the glass manufacturing industry. IARC monographs on the evaluation of carcinogenic risks to humans, vol 58. IARC (International Agency for Research on Cancer, Lyon

IARC (2000) Ionizing radiation, part 1. X-radiation and g-radiation, and neutrons. IARC monographs on the evaluation of carcinogenic risks to humans, vol 75. IARC (International Agency for Research on Cancer, Lyon

IARC (2002) Some traditional herbal medicines, some mycotoxins, naphthalene and styrene. IARC monographs on the evaluation of carcinogenic risks to humans, vol 82. IARC (International Agency for Research on Cancer, Lyon

IARC (2012a) A review of human carcinogens, part C: arsenic, metals, fibres, and dusts. IARC monographs on the evaluation of carcinogenic risks to humans, vol 100. IARC (International Agency for Research on Cancer, Lyon

IARC (2012b) A review of human carcinogens, part F: chemical agents and related occupations. IARC monographs on the evaluation of carcinogenic risks to humans, vol 100. IARC (International Agency for Research on Cancer, Lyon

IARC (2013) IARC monographs on the evaluation of carcinogenic risks to humans. International Agency for Research on Cancer. http://monographs.iarc.fr/. Accessed 27 June 2013

IARC (2014) Diesel and gasoline engine exhausts and some Nitroarenes. IARC monographs on the evaluation of carcinogenic risks to humans, vol 105. IARC (International Agency for Research on Cancer, Lyon

International Agency for Research on Cancer (2006) Preamble to the IARC monographs. https://monographs.iarc.fr/wp-content/uploads/2018/06/CurrentPreamble.pdf. Accessed 7 Jan 2019

IPCS (International Programme on Chemical Safety) (1998) Chrysotile asbestos. Environmental health criteria. World Health Organization, Geneva

Jacobs EJ et al (2015) What proportion of cancer deaths in the contemporary United States is attributable to cigarette smoking? Ann Epidemiol 25(3):179–182. e1

Katsouyanni K, Pershagen G (1997) Ambient air pollution exposure and cancer [review]. Cancer Causes Control 8(3):284–291

Kim BS, Margolin BH (1999) Prediction of rodent carcinogenicity utilizing a battery of in vitro and in vivo genotoxicity tests. Environ Mol Mutagen 34(4):297–304

Kullberg C, Selander J, Albin M, Borgquist S, Manjer J, Gustavsson P (2017) Female white-collar workers remain at higher risk of breast cancer after adjustments for individual risk factors related to reproduction and lifestyle. Occup Environ Med 74(9):652–658. https://doi.org/10.1136/oemed-2016-104043

Labrèche F, Duguay P, Boucher A, Arcand R (2014) Estimating the number of cases of occupational cancer in Quebec. Institut de recherche Robert-Sauvé en santé et en sécurité du travail (IRSST), Montréal

Nauss KM et al (1995) Critical issues in assessing the carcinogenicity of diesel exhaust: a synthesis of current knowledge diesel exhaust: a critical analysis of emissions, exposure, and health effects. Health Effects Institute, Cambridge, MA, pp 11–61

Nurminen M, Karjalainen A (2001) Epidemiologic estimate of the proportion of fatalities related to occupational factors in Finland. Scand J Work Environ Health 27:161–213

Rushton L et al (2012) Occupational cancer burden in Great Britain. Br J Cancer 107(S1):S3

Selikoff IJ (1990) Historical developments and perspectives in inorganic fiber toxicity in man. Environ Health Perspect 88(Aug):269–276

Siemiatycki J (2014) Historical overview of occupational cancer research. In: Anttila S, Boffetta P (eds) Occupational cancers. Springer, London, pp 1–20

Silverman DT et al (2012) The diesel exhaust in miners study: a nested case–control study of lung cancer and diesel exhaust. J Natl Cancer Inst 104(11):855–868

Stanaway JD et al (2018) Global, regional, and national comparative risk assessment of 84 behavioural, environmental and occupational, and metabolic risks or clusters of risks for 195 countries and territories, 1990–2017: a systematic analysis for the Global Burden of Disease Study 2017. Lancet 392(10159):1923–1994

Steenland K, Burnett C, Lalich N, Ward E, Hurrell J (2003) Dying for work: the magnitude of US mortality from selected causes of death associated with occupation. Am J Ind Med 43(5):461–482

Upton ABJBM et al (1991) Asbestos in public and commercial buildings: a literature review and synthesis of current knowledge. Report to: Health Effects Institute – Asbestos Research (HEI-AR). Health Effects Institute, Cambridge, MA

Winkelstein W Jr (2002) Deadly glow: the radium dial worker tragedy. Am J Epidemiol 155(3):290–291

Xu M et al (2018) Occupational exposures to leaded and unleaded gasoline engine emissions and lung cancer risk. Occup Environ Med 75(4):303–309

Yuan X, Zhu C, Wang M, Mo F, Du W, Ma X (2018) Night shift work increases the risks of multiple primary cancers in women: a systematic review and meta-analysis of 61 articles. Cancer Epidemiol Prev Biomark 27(1):25–40

Zahm SH, Blair A (2003) Occupational cancer among women: where have we been and where are we going? Am J Ind Med 44(6):565–575

Respiratory Work Disability in Relation to Occupational Factors

9

Paul D. Blanc and Kjell Torén

Contents

Introduction	154
Asthma	156
COPD	158
Upper Airway Conditions	159
Cystic Fibrosis (CF)	161
Obstructive Sleep Apnea (OSA)	162
Pulmonary Fibrosis	162
Lung Transplantation	163
Conclusion	164
Cross-References	164
References	164

Abstract

Respiratory work disability refers to compromised work ability due to a respiratory tract condition. Respiratory work disability subsumes the adverse effects on working life of occupational (work-caused) lung disease and extends far beyond that. Whatever the etiology of a disease of the respiratory tract, it can interfere with the ability to be employed fully and productively. Respiratory work disability can be manifested in multiple ways. Although traditionally health-related work disability has been quantified by work cessation or work absences (lost workdays) due to the condition in question, a number of other measures can be used to assess respiratory work disability, for example, change of job, change

P. D. Blanc (✉)
Division of Occupational and Environmental Medicine, Department of Medicine, University of California San Francisco, San Francisco, CA, USA
e-mail: paul.blanc@ucsf.edu

K. Torén
Department of Occupational and Environmental Medicine, Sahlgrenska Academy, University of Gothenburg, Gothenburg, Sweden
e-mail: kjell.toren@amm.gu.se

in job hours, and, while still on the job, decreased work productivity. This chapter will present the findings from a range of studies that have analyzed respiratory work disability in multiple respiratory tract conditions, including asthma, chronic obstructive lung disease (COPD), rhinitis, cystic fibrosis, and obstructive sleep apnea.

Keywords

Work disability · Occupational impairment · Respiratory tract disease · Asthma · COPD · Cystic fibrosis · Obstructive sleep apnea

Introduction

Clinicians, researchers, and policy makers easily may confuse *impairment* and *disability*. These are distinct albeit interrelated constructs that should not be applied interchangeably. Impairment refers to a decrement in function below an expected norm. This is very relevant to respiratory status because functional impairment is easily and commonly quantified physiologically through lung function testing. This is typically accomplished through measuring pulmonary function using simple spirometry to measure the volumes and rate of air that the person being tested is able to blow out from the lungs. In addition to simple spirometry, other more sophisticated testing also can be carried out quantifying additional aspects of pulmonary physiology, such as how the lungs access and utilize oxygen. The key aspect of lung function testing is that there are generally accepted values of expected performance standardized to age, height, and sex, thus making it straightforward to quantify the degree of "impairment" from population-based normative values.

Disability, in contradistinction, rather than being an objective matter of quantification, can be highly subjective. Moreover, theoretical models of disablement take this to be a dynamic process. In such models, impairment affects individuals in the context of a range of life activities, one of which can be a person's working life, and only through life activities contributes to disablement (Verbrugge and Jette 1994; Katz et al. 2010). As importantly, there are many other contributors to disability from respiratory disease beyond impairments in lung physiology. Factors promoting respiratory disability but not subsumed by impairment can be related, directly or indirectly, to various aspects of the disease process itself. Examples include a propensity for acute exacerbations, the side effects of medications, or the need for frequent medical visits, all of which can interfere with work ability but also can contribute to disability more broadly through disrupting other valued life activities or more basic activities of daily living.

Working life or better-stated, vocational life (e.g., salaried or unsalaried work) is particularly relevant to respiratory disease-associated disability because this is a human activity central to economic welfare as well as to self-identity and social integration and because respiratory ill-health commonly impacts adversely vocational status. Moreover, not only respiratory conditions themselves but also the nature of the job itself may promote disability. As one key example, this can derive directly from the physical demands of a job. An individual with a respiratory condition leading to moderate lung impairment may be able to function in a sedentary job with modest physical demands but will be disabled in the performance of activities with a heavy exertional requirement. But beyond physical attributes, the structure and organization of work also may promote respiratory disability. Jobs with little scheduling flexibility, for example, may lead to disability because frequent days missed are not tolerated by the employer. In contrast, a person with very same degree of respiratory disease severity and "impairment" might be able to continue at the job under conditions that allowed self-scheduled telecommuting or more flexible work hours.

A particularly relevant aspect of respiratory work disability is that the respiratory condition itself may have been caused by the very job in which the affected individual can no longer be engaged. Examples include lung fibrosis (e.g., miners), chronic obstructive pulmonary disease (COPD) (e.g., in cotton mill workers), and occupational asthma (e.g., in urethane workers). These are distinctly different scenarios than work disability linked to other chronic conditions in which etiology is not from the occupation itself, for example, diabetes. Occupationally related disease brings into play medicolegal factors that can impact the likelihood of respiratory work disability. This can include regulatory proscription of specific work activities and various insurance compensation schemes that define work ability.

The construct of respiratory work disability is further complicated because it can be assessed using a wide range of measures. These can include disease-related complete cessation of work (withdrawal from the labor force), change in job or job duties, reduced salary, lost workdays (whole day or partial days missed), and decreased productivity or impaired "presenteeism" even while still on the job. Some of these measures can be obtained from administrative data such as employer personnel records or health insurance data, although they can also be ascertained by self-report from the person with disease. Other measures of work disability, such as changes in job duties or level of presenteeism, typically are defined by survey responses obtained from affected individuals.

For non-salaried workers, such as persons working in the home, disability assessment is wholly dependent on self-report and lacks standardly defined measures (e.g., non-salaried work cessation or absence). For that reason, non-salaried vocational impairment has typically been addressed in assessment either of activities of daily living or as alluded to above, disability in valued life activities, topics that are beyond the scope of this review. Another topic indirectly related to respiratory work disability that will not be considered further here is the work impact of childhood lung disease on adult caretakers. Work absence for dependent care, for example, has been identified as a substantial contributor in estimates to the indirect costs of childhood asthma.

In summary, respiratory work disability is an import aspect of lung disease. Physiologic impairment is one but not the only contributor to such disability. Indeed, respiratory work disability is a complex construct, with multifactorial contributors. This is all the more so true because work exposures themselves can lead to respiratory disease, and the nature of the job itself, independent of the etiology of the lung disease at hand, can help promote disability. Broadening work disability to additionally consider non-salaried vocations further expands the complexity of this topic. In the following sections, we will consider aspects of respiratory work disability in relation to a series of specific conditions: asthma, COPD, and a group of other heterogeneous respiratory conditions including upper airway disorders, cystic fibrosis, obstructive sleep apnea, hypersensitivity pneumonitis, and advanced lung disease leading to lung transplantation.

Asthma

Asthma is quite common in the working population because it is a relatively frequent respiratory condition among adults of working age. Hence, asthma-related respiratory work disability may carry large consequences for work-life participation. This can be in the form of absenteeism or restrictions in possible job duties or tasks. Asthma-related work disability occurs both among persons with work-caused asthma (i.e., asthma etiologically related to occupation) and among those having asthma where the onset is totally unrelated to occupational exposures. In support of the latter scenario, work disability defined as sickness absence or disability pension utilization was significantly more common among persons with asthma exacerbations due to different triggering exposures outside work (Karvala et al. 2018). It has also been shown that the presence of different comorbidities in persons with asthma, such as depression, diabetes, or coronary heart disease, increases the risk for asthma-related work disability (Hakola et al. 2011). Thus, different aspects of work disability, including nonoccupational factors, are important components for evaluating the consequences and risk factors among persons with asthma.

In a large prospective study (European Community Respiratory Health Survey, ECRHS) comprising a European random population sample, it was found that during 9 years of follow-up, 4.9% of the subjects with asthma reported change of work due to respiratory problems, compared to 1.1% in the random control sample (Torén et al. 2009). Further, it was found that exposure to biological dust, and gases, and fumes in the subsample of persons with asthma markedly increased the risk of changing work because of respiratory complaints compared to randomly selected population controls. Exposure to mineral dust (stone, quartz, sand, etc.) was not associated with any increased risk for respiratory-related change of work (work disability). Atopy was not a modifying factor in that study. In a large Norwegian cross-sectional study, job change among women due to respiratory symptoms was more common among certain occupations such as chefs, hairdressers, and cleaners (Fell et al. 2016). Among men, job change due to respiratory symptoms was seen among gardeners, sheet metal workers, and welders. Further analyses of the occupational exposures show that both inorganic and organic dust increased the risk for respiratory-related job change. These findings support the conclusion that work-related exposures induce asthma exacerbations, thus causing persons to change jobs.

Severe asthma is a disease often refractory to therapy, and it will also affect a substantial subset of those with asthma. Severe asthma is clearly associated with work disability defined as self-reported decreased work ability (Hiles et al. 2018). Occupational exposures have severe impact as found in a US study of subjects with severe asthma (Eisner et al. 2006). Among 465 ever-employed adults with clinically ascertained asthma, 14% reported asthma-related complete work disability, and among those without current employment, 25% attributed their unemployment to previous occupational exposures.

In terms of sickness absence, the number of workdays lost by workers with asthma has been found to be related both to severity of asthma (Gonzalez Barcala et al. 2011) and also to current exposure to vapor, gas, dust, and fumes, where such exposures seem to double the risk for respiratory sickness absence among subjects with asthma or respiratory symptoms (wheeze or breathlessness) (Kim et al. 2013a). A similar observation was made among healthcare workers, where cleaners had increased prevalence of respiratory symptoms and significantly higher sickness absence than other working groups (Kim et al. 2013b). There are a number of studies indicating that employed asthmatics have a reduced productivity (impaired presenteesim) because of their disease (Balder et al. 1998; Blanc et al. 2001).

The exacerbation of asthma is a scenario that has particular relevance to respiratory work disability. There are multiple studies indicating that occupational exposure to vapor, gas, dust, and fumes increases the prevalence of symptoms among asthmatics, hence increasing the risk for respiratory disability, a relationship affirmed in an American Thoracic Society Task Force report (Henneberger et al. 2011). Three studies are of particular relevance to this question. In a Finnish general-population-based case-control study, workplace exposure to gas, dust, and fume (i.e., nonspecific exposures) and work in abnormal temperatures both increased the occurrence of asthma symptoms (Saarinen et al. 2003). In the previously cited ECRHS study, unplanned care for asthma was linked to high exposure to dust and fumes (Henneberger et al. 2010). Finally, in a Swedish general population study, exposure to gas, dust, and fumes and to cold work also was associated with exacerbations of asthma (Kim et al. 2016).

Among workers with occupational asthma (work-caused asthma, as opposed to asthma unrelated in its etiology to workplace factors), longitudinal studies have consistently showed that occupational asthma is associated with a high risk of work disability, defined either as complete work cessation or reduced income levels (Vandenplas et al. 2003). The magnitude of the effect appears to differ among countries, with the lowest asthma-related work-loss rate observed in a Finnish population study (Piirilä et al. 2005).

In summary, both cross-sectional and longitudinal studies clearly have shown that subjects with asthma are at increased risk for work loss, work absence, and job change due to the disease. Workplace exposure and disease severity appear to interact with each other in causing the disability.

COPD

"Work capacity," in a purely physiologic sense, has long been a topic of study in chronic obstructive pulmonary disease (COPD) (Carter et al. 1994). Nonetheless, until recent years COPD-association respiratory work disability in the social sense of labor force participation was not given extensive consideration. A key explanatory factor in failing to consider COPD and employment may be because this disease process manifests its predominant adverse effects among persons already beyond standard retirement age. When the question of COPD and respiratory work disability began to be explored in greater depth, however, it became clear that among persons with COPD, work disability is a frequent occurrence. The evolving recognition that approximately 15% of COPD may be at least partially attributable to work itself has also contributed to greater interest in the question of respiratory work disability from COPD. Finally, temporal trends (e.g., delayed age of retirement) mean that persons increasingly are still in the labor force at an age range at which COPD prevalence rapidly increases (e.g., age 60–70).

In an early investigation of this subject, it was shown among a population-based sample of 3805 California adults that compared to adults with no chronic health conditions and taking covariates into account, adults with COPD had 60% reduced odds of having current employment (OR = 0.41; 95% CI = 0.24, 0.71) (Eisner et al. 2002). In another early study from the same group of investigators using a different cohort, among the 234 subjects analyzed, 1 in 4 reported that they had left work altogether due to their lung disease, the definition in that study of respiratory-related work disability (Blanc et al. 2004).

The association between COPD defined by airflow obstruction has been studied using large, national data sets that include measurement of lung function by spirometry. An analysis of the US National Health and Nutrition Examination Survey (NHANES), based on more than 12,436 participants involved in NHANES III, found that increasing mild, moderate, and severe severity of COPD was associated with a 3.4%, 3.9%, and 14.4% reduction in the labor force participation (Sin et al. 2002). Subsequently, a national study from Korea using its own NHANES analyzed data for nearly 10,000 adults aged 40 to 60 who had spirometry data defining obstruction (present in 8%). They observed a falloff in labor force participation with increasing severity of airflow obstruction (with a nadir of 72% in the most severely obstructed) and more than threefold odds of ill-health attributed work cessation (OR 3.38; 95% CI 1.03,11.02). They also explored a novel measure of work disability, "precarious employment," that was defined as part-time or hourly as opposed to regularly salaried work. Those with severe obstruction still working nonetheless had more than fourfold odds of being in precarious jobs (OR 4.71; 95% CI 1.70,13.06) (Shin et al. 2018).

Using a different national US data set, the Health and Retirement Study, investigators showed that among persons 51 years and older, COPD was associated with decreased odds of labor force participation (OR 0.58; 95% CI 0.50,0.67). Relative to other chronic conditions, this was comparable to the impact of heart disease, cancer, hypertension, and diabetes. This analysis also found that the increased likelihood of receipt US Social Security Disability Insurance payment associated with COPD (OR 2.52; 95% CI 2.00,3.17) was even greater than for those other conditions (Thornton Snider et al. 2012).

The UK-based Birmingham COPD cohort study of nearly 2000 adults of working age has provided insights into the relationship between various cofactors and employment in the presence of disease. In a cross-sectional analysis in that study, taking COPD severity into account, past occupational exposures to the highest level of vapors, gases, dust, or fumes (VGDF, reported by approximately one in four) and the lowest level of educational attainment (a similar proportion) were each associated with decreased odds of being employed (ORs 0.32 and 0.43, respectively) (Rai et al. 2017a).

Beyond national-specific studies, the observation that COPD is associated with substantially increased likelihood of employment loss has been replicated around the world in two major multinational studies of COPD: the PLATINO study from South America and the global BOLD study (Montes de Oca et al. 2011; Grønseth et al. 2017). Short of complete cessation of employment, COPD has been strongly associated with respiratory work disability by other measures as well. Studies from Scandinavia have documented that work absences among persons with COPD still employed are higher than among persons without disease (Jansson et al. 2013; Erdal et al. 2014).

A further analysis of a subset of 338 persons from the Birmingham cohort studied both absenteeism (self-reported work absence) and presenteeism using a standard measure (the Stanford Presenteeism Scale). Absenteeism was common, with 17.0% reported COPD-related work absences in the previous year. Further, 77 of the sample were categorized as having little to no presenteeism. In a multivariate analysis, severity of shortness of breath was significantly associated with both absenteeism and presenteeism, while work-related VGDF severity was significantly associated only with presenteeism (p-values for trend <0.01 for each relationship). Additionally, increasing history of occupational exposure to vapors, gases, dusts, or fumes was independently associated with presenteeism (p for trend<0.01) (Rai et al. 2017b).

Despite the increasing attention that is being given to respiratory work disability in COPD, a recent comprehensive review of COPD-related work disability underscores the relatively limited nature of published data directly pertinent to this topic (Rai et al. 2018). Despite such data limitations, it is abundantly clear that COPD is linked to decreased labor force participation among working age adults.

Upper Airway Conditions

Rhinitis is often omitted from consideration of respiratory work disability both because the upper respiratory tract manifests patterns of disease quite distinct from the lower respiratory tract and also because the morbidity of rhinitis is far less than that most major lung conditions, for example, asthma and COPD as previously addressed. Failing to consider rhinitis as a factor in respiratory work disability is ill-advised, however, on multiple grounds. Rhinitis is a very common condition, such that even a small proportion of more severe disease overall still affects a relatively large number of persons. Further, as with asthma but unlike COPD, rhinitis impacts young adults at the age of peak labor force participation. Like asthma as well, a subset of rhinitis arises etiologically from work itself, making it likely that continued employment in job that caused the disease will not be tolerated. Finally, although complete work cessation is unlikely to be linked to rhinitis, lost workdays from episodic exacerbations of disease and symptoms not severe enough to prevent work but rather sufficient to impair productivity while on-the-job would be entirely consistent with the clinical nature of this condition.

One of the earliest studies of this question assessed work disability among adults with rhinitis as compared to persons with asthma, already cited previously in regard to asthma. Current adult labor force participation was not reduced among those with rhinitis (97%) although it was reduced significantly in asthma (88%) ($p < 0.05$). Among those still actively employed, however, self-assessed diminished job effectiveness was more frequent in rhinitis (36%) than in asthma (19%) ($p < 0.05$). Condition-attributed lost work time was common in both conditions: more than 20% with asthma or rhinitis reported one or more complete or partial workdays lost in the 4 weeks previous to interview (Blanc et al. 2001). Allergic rhinitis also has a greater than might be anticipated impact on working life than manifested by various other chronic conditions. Among more than 600 patients in a multicenter cross-sectional observational study, for example, absenteeism was similar for allergic rhinitis (4.6 ± 1.1%), diabetes mellitus (4.2 ± 1.7%) and hypertension patients (2.1 ± 1.5%). But global loss of productivity was substantively higher in in allergic rhinitis (26.6 ± 1.8%) compared to diabetes (16.7 ± 2.8%) or hypertension (8.8 ± 2.5%) (de la Hoz et al. 2012).

The most thorough review of the work impact of allergic rhinitis, covering publications appearing from 2005 to 2015, identified 19 observational surveys and 9 interventional studies. Pooled analysis estimated the proportion of missed work time to be 3.6% (95% CI 2.4; 4.8%) In contrast to this measure of morbidity, the prevalence of impaired productivity (decreased presenteeism) was substantial: 35.9% (95% CI, 29.7; 42.1%) (Vandenplas et al. 2018). In summary, the most important manifestation of respiratory work disability associated with rhinitis appears to be decreased productivity while on the job (impaired presenteeism), rather than lost workdays or cessation of work altogether.

Vocal cord dysfunction, also termed paradoxical vocal fold motion disorder, is another upper airway condition that affects adults of working age. This syndrome is marked by dysfunction of the larynx characterized by inappropriate vocal fold closure with breathing, manifested by shortness of breath, change in voice, cough, and other symptoms, and it is frequently misdiagnosed as asthma (Dunn et al. 2015). Clinically, it is well recognized that this functional syndrome can be associated with substantial interference in daily activities. Although respiratory work disability is likely to occur in vocal cord dysfunction, its extent and frequency have not been characterized quantitatively or qualitatively. A qualitative open-ended interview study of a different vocal cord condition related to nerve damage, unilateral vocal fold paralysis (UVFP), noted that, "Many patients found that UVFP limited their work performance. One participant mentioned, 'If I needed to make a call about something, business-wise, I couldn't, because people couldn't hear me at the other end'" (Francis et al. 2018: 436).

Cystic Fibrosis (CF)

The survival of persons with cystic fibrosis (CF) has increased to the extent that, currently, adult working life participation is a reality for most individuals with this condition. A substantial proportion of the persons with CF is employed, and there have been multiple observational studies of work disability in patients with this disease. These studies have shown that despite high rates of labor force participation, persons with CF frequently report that their disease has hampered the job career.

In an early British study of 866 subjects with CF, 54% were in paid employment compared to 69% in the general population, with nonmanual occupations more frequent in the CF (Walters et al. 1993). A study from the USA found that 27% of persons with CF were currently employed and almost 50% attributed job change or work cessation due to the disease (Gillen et al. 1995). The majority (84%) had nonmanual occupations. Notably, nearly 100% reaching adulthood did have some degree of labor force participation. In multiple regression modeling in that study, work disability was associated with adult onset of CF, female gender, and living alone.

As the care of patients with CF improved, later studies found a higher prevalence of work life participation. In a study from Australia, 72% were currently employed, and 40% worked more than 30 h/week (Hogg et al. 2007). Still, over 50% attributed job changes or ceased work to the CF. In regression modeling, disease severity was associated with work disability, but there were no factors studied that reflected the workplace itself. Further studies support the impression that the labor force participation among adults with CF continues to increase. In a French study from 2012, 70% of those with CF were employed, while 94% reported a job in the past (Laborde-Castérot et al. 2012). The majority had nonmanual works; only 4% were classified as blue-collar workers. Half of those studied had been counseled to avoid certain jobs such as healthcare work, physical work, or dusty work. In multiple regression modeling, severity of CF and educational level was significantly associated with employment status. An even more recent study reported that 65% of persons with CF were employed or students, and 80% had worked at some time (20% had blue-collar jobs). Nonetheless, 40% reported that CF had negatively affected their work. In regression modeling, disease severity, male gender, quality of life, and educational level were associated with employment status (Targett et al. 2014).

Working life participation is now a reality for most subjects with CF, but there is still knowledge gap regarding the importance of workplace exposures, including psychosocial factors, even if it seems plausible that dusty and heavy work are not beneficial for the CF group.

Obstructive Sleep Apnea (OSA)

Obstructive sleep apnea (OSA) is a common albeit underdiagnosed breathing disorder characterized by recurrent episodes of airflow limitation during sleep caused by recurrent upper airway obstruction (Hirsch Allen et al. 2015; Gugliemi et al. 2015). The prevalence in a working population is high, estimated to range from 5% among women to 15% among men (Hirsch Allen et al. 2015). A prevalence as high as 24% has been reported in middle-aged men giving reason to believe that this condition is overlooked in a working population (Young et al. 1993).

Due to the fragmented sleep and hypoxemia, OSA is associated with a number of health problems affecting many of the body's function. The most important effects are neurocognitive impairments and cardiovascular diseases. These conditions affect alertness and ability to concentrate. Consistent with this, OSA is also a risk factor for car accidents and workplace accidents (Young et al. 2002; Lindberg et al. 2001). Hence, it is reasonable to assume that OSA would be a risk factor for work disability. There are also several studies and two reviews, showing that individuals with OSA have an increased frequency of sickness absence and disability pension (Sjösten et al. 2009a, b; Gugliemi et al. 2015; Hirsch Allen et al. 2015). Excessive daytime sleepiness is the component of OSA that seems to be most associated with work disability (Omachi et al. 2009).

Even if a person with OSA is at work, the performance (productivity, also characterized as presenteeism) is affected by the disease. It has been shown in several studies that individuals with OSA have impaired on-the-job performance (Grunstein et al. 1995; Ulfberg et al. 1999; Gugliemi et al. 2015). The first-line treatment of OSA is continuous positive airway pressure (CPAP). It has been shown that CPAP treatment improves job performance, but there is a need for either randomized controlled studies or prospective observational studies (Ulfberg et al. 1999; Hirsch Allen et al. 2015).

Pulmonary Fibrosis

Lung fibrosis without an identifiable cause, known as idiopathic pulmonary fibrosis (IPF), is a severe, potentially life-threatening disease. Because of its severity, it would be anticipated that IPF leads to profound respiratory work disability. Although considerable attention has been given to health-related quality of life in IPF, however, direct data are sparse on its impact specifically on working life. A qualitative study based on 20 in-depth interviews developed 12 domains of concern to IPF patients, 1 of which was "employment and finances." The patients fell into three categories: those that retired prior to the IPF diagnosis, those who had lost their job or career due to IPF, and remarkably those who felt that they could not retire because their medical costs were so great. The study noted, "Some of the patients who were still working felt the need to conceal their chronic illness from business colleagues, because the patients believed it made them 'appear weak'" (Swigris et al. 2005: 5).

Lung fibrosis caused by occupation itself falls under the rubric of *pneumoconioses*, for example, silicosis or coal worker's pneumoconiosis. Much of the epidemiologic research on these conditions has focused on the dust inhalation in relation to limitations in lung function rather than the quantification of disability. Nonetheless, it is clear from descriptive data that among persons with pneumoconiosis, the adverse impact on working life is profound. For example, in a cohort of 157 relatively young Turkish workers with exposure to silica through sandblasting denim jeans, not a single person studied remained employed in that industry, although the frequency of complete loss of any kind of job was not reported (Akgun et al. 2008). In another silicosis outbreak, in this case from artificial stone work, among cohort of 25 workers with advanced disease all but 6 were on supplemental oxygen, making any employment dubious (even though respiratory work disability was not directly quantified) (Kramer et al. 2012). There is also a phenomenon of job loss simply from receiving a diagnosis of pneumoconiosis. As a recent commentary on the US resurgence of coal workers' pneumoconiosis in the *Journal of the American Medical Association* noted, "The chance that he might file a worker's compensation claim if occupational lung disease was diagnosed was enough for the miner to lose his job" (Voelker 2019: 17).

Extrinsic allergic alveolitis (EAA, also known as hypersensitivity pneumonitis) is a lung condition leading to fibrosis that, by definition, is caused by factors in the environment, including specific workplace settings. In farming and other sectors where organic material is handled, EAA is particularly important. A study from Finland described the clinical course of 86 farmers with EAA and found that after 5-year follow-up, 57 (66%) continued as farmers despite presumed continued exposure (Mönkäre and Haahtela 1987). Two farmers changed occupation, and the remaining 29 gave up their work. Those who gave up their work had more severe disease. Cooling fluid in metalworking is another important source of EAA. In 1 metalworking shop series, 35 workers were diagnosed as having EAA (Bracker et al. 2003). After 2 years, only just over half had returned to work, presumably with better control of exposure; no information was provided on predictors of return to work.

Lung Transplantation

A substantial proportion of patients with advanced lung disease undergo lung transplantation, including persons with CF, COPD, and lung fibrosis. This intervention is increasing and leading to larger numbers of subjects that are participating in the labor force after transplantation. Indeed, return to work has become increasingly important as part of the rehabilitation process among such patients. In an early study of this question, among 99 patients from Canada and the USA, 60% were assessed to have work ability posttransplantation, but only 37% were indeed employed. Positive factors for work life participation were pretransplantation employment, self-report of work ability, and good lung function and physical capacity after the transplantation (Paris et al. 1998). A study of 281 patients having undergone various organ transplantations, those who had undergone lung transplantation, had significantly lower rate of return to work compared to the kidney transplant. Positive factors for return to work were employment before the transplantation, high self-assessed work ability, being married, and male gender (de Baere et al. 2010). It has been argued that heart-lung transplant patients have an inferior return to work compared to other transplant patients (Paris and White-Williams 2005).

For lung diseases with an occupational or environmental etiology, there is also the question of posttransplantation resumption of exposure. For example, in a case series of lung transplant for EAA, two patients developed recurrent disease with renewed environmental exposure (Kern et al. 2015). The observation that exposure to higher levels of air pollution is linked to increased risk of chronic lung allograft dysfunction (CLAD) following lung transplantation raises further concern regarding the potential adverse effects of return to work were this to include exposure to vapors, gases dust, or fumes (Ruttens et al. 2017). Thus, in post-lung transplantation, there may be conflicting impetuses encouraging return to work and work avoidance. Lung transplantation, however, is a field currently marked by a scarcity of data on work outcomes in either direction. Probably, as in the case of CF, we can expect that with extended post-lung transplantation survival, greater attention will be given to questions of respiratory work disability.

Conclusion

Respiratory work disability is common across a wide range of respiratory tract conditions but is manifested with a heterogeneous pattern of outcomes. Because these impairments have been studied inconsistently across disease groups, it is challenging to draw firm conclusions as to the relative importance of different domains of respiratory work disability. It is clear that assessing multiple manifestations of respiratory work disability, using both quantitative and qualitative approaches, is critical if we are to gauge accurately the full extent of this problem.

Cross-References

▶ Concepts and Social Variations of Disability in Working-Age Populations
▶ Reducing Inequalities in Employment of People with Disabilities

References

Akgun M, Araz O, Akkurt I, Eroglu A, Alper F, Saglam L, Mirici A, Gorguner M, Nemery B (2008) An epidemic of silicosis among former denim sandblasters. Eur Respir J 32:1295–1303
Balder B, Lindholm NB, Löwhagen O, Palmqvist M, Plaschke P, Tunsäter A, Torén K (1998) Predictors of self-assessed work ability among subjects with recent onset asthma. Respir Med 92:729–734
Blanc PD, Trupin L, Eisner M, Earnest G, Katz PP, Israel L (2001) The work impact of asthma and rhinitis: findings from a population-based survey. J Clin Epidemiol 54:610–618

Blanc PD, Eisner MD, Trupin L, Yelin EH, Katz PP, Balmes JR (2004) The association between occupational factors and adverse health outcomes in chronic obstructive pulmonary disease. Occup Environ Med 61:661–667

Bracker A, Storey E, Yang C, Hodgson MJ (2003) An outbreak of hypersensitivity pneumonitis at a metalworking plant: a longitudinal assessment of intervention effectiveness. Appl Occup Environ Hyg 18:96–108

Carter R, Nicotra B, Huber G (1994) Differing effects of airway obstruction on physical work capacity and ventilation in men and women with COPD. Chest 106:1730–1739

De Baere C, Delva D, Kloeck A, Remans K, Vanrenterghem Y, Verleden G, Vanhaecke J et al (2010) Return to work and social participation: does type of organ transplantation matter? Transplantation 89:1009–1015

de la Hoz CB, Rodríguez M, Fraj J, Cerecedo I, Antolín-Amérigo D, Colás C (2012) Allergic rhinitis and its impact on work productivity in primary care practice and a comparison with other common diseases: the cross-sectional study to evaluate work productivity in allergic rhinitis compared with other common diseases (CAPRI) study. Am J Rhinol Allergy 26:390–394

Dunn NM, Katial RK, Hoyte FCL (2015) Vocal cord dysfunction: a review. Asthma Res Pract 22(1):9

Eisner MD, Yelin EH, Trupin L, Blanc PD (2002) The influence of chronic respiratory conditions on health status and work disability. Am J Public Health 92:1506–1513

Eisner MD, Yelin EH, Katz PP, Lactao G, Iribarren C, Blanc PD (2006) Risk factors for work disability in severe adult asthma. Am J Med 119:884–891

Erdal M, Johannessen A, Askildsen JE, Eagan T, Gulsvik A, Grønseth R (2014) Productivity losses in chronic obstructive pulmonary disease: a population-based survey. BMJ Open Respir Res 1: e000049

Fell AKM, Abrahamsen R, Henneberger PK, Svendsen MV, Andersson E, Torén K, Kongerud J (2016) Breath-taking jobs: a case-control study of respiratory work disability by occupation in Norway. Occup Environ Med 73:600–606

Francis DO, Sherman AE, Hovis KL, Bonnet K, Schlundt D, Garrett CG, Davies L (2018) Life experience of patients with unilateral vocal fold paralysis. JAMA Otolaryngol Head Neck Surg 144:433–439

Gillen M, Lallas D, Brown C, Yelin E, Blanc PD (1995) Work disability in adults with cystic fibrosis. Am J Respir Crit Care Med 152:153–156

Gonzalez Barcala FJ, La Fuente-Cid RD, Alvaraez-Gil R, Tafalla M, Nuevo J, Caamaño-Isorna F (2011) Factors associated with a higher prevalence of work disability among asthmatic patients. J Asthma 48:194–199

Grønseth R, Erdal M, Tan WC, Obaseki DO, Amaral AFS, Gislason T, Juvekar SK, Koul PA, Studnicka M, Salvi S, Burney P, Buist AS, Vollmer WM, Johannessen A (2017) Unemployment in chronic airflow obstruction around the world: results from the BOLD study. Eur Respir J 50(3). pii: 1700499 (online)

Grunstein RR, Stenlöf K, Hedner JA, Sjöström L (1995) Impact of self-reported sleep-breathing disturbances on psychosocial performance in the Swedish Obese Subjects (SOS) study. Sleep 18:635–643

Gugliemi O, Jurado-Gámez B, Gude F, Buela-Casal G (2015) Occupational health of patients with obstructive sleep apnea syndrome: a systematic review. Sleep Breath 19:35–44

Hakola R, Kauppi P, Leino T, Ojajärvi A, Pentti J, Oksanen T, Haahtela T, Kivimäki M, Vahtera J (2011) Persistent asthma, comorbid conditions and the risk of work disability: a prospective cohort study. Allergy 66:1598–1603

Henneberger PK, Mirabelli MC, Kogevinas M, Plana E, Dahlman-Höglund A, Jarvis DL, Olivieri M, Torén K, Urrutia I, Villani S, Zock JP (2010) The occupational contribution to severe exacerbation of asthma. Eur Respir J 36:743–750

Henneberger PK, Redlich C, Callahan DB, Harber P, Lemiere C, Martin J, Tarlo SM, Vandenplas O, Torén K (2011) American thoracic society statement: work-exacerbated asthma. Am J Respir Crit Care Med 184:368–378

Hiles SA, Harvey ES, McDonald VM, Peters M, Bardin P, Revnolds PN, Upham JW, Baraket M, Bhikoo Z, Bowden J et al (2018) Working while unwell: workplace impairment in people with severe asthma. Clin Exp Allergy 48:650–662

Hirsch Allen AJM, Bansback N, Ayas NT (2015) The effect of OSA on work disability and work related injuries. Chest 147:1422–1428

Hogg M, Barithwaite M, Baiuley M, Kotsimbos T, Wilson JW (2007) Work disability in adults with cystic fibrosis and its relation to quality of life. J Cyst Fibros 6:223–227

Jansson SA, Backman H, Stenling A, Lindberg A, Rönmark E, Lundbäck B (2013) Health economic costs of COPD in Sweden by disease severity – has it changed during a ten years period? Respir Med 107:1931–1938

Karvala K, Uitti J, Taponen S, Luukkonen R, Lehtimäki L (2018) Asthma trigger perceptions are associated with work disability. Respir Med 139:19–26

Katz PP, Gregorich S, Eisner M, Julian L, Chen H, Yelin E, Blanc PD (2010) Disability in valued life activities among individuals with COPD and other respiratory conditions. J Cardiopulm Rehabil Prev 20:126–136

Kern RM, Singer JP, Koth L, Mooney J, Golden J, Hays S, Greenland J, Wolters P, Ghio E, Jones KD, Leard L, Kukreja J, Blanc PD (2015) Lung transplantation for hypersensitivity pneumonitis. Chest 147:1558–1565

Kim JL, Blanc PD, Zock JP, Kogevinas M, Radon K, Kromhout H, Antó JM, Torén K (2013a) Predictors for respiratory-related sickness absence in subjects with asthma, wheeze, breathlessness or chronic bronchitis. Am J Ind Med 56:541–549

Kim JL, Torén K, Lohman S, Lötvall J, Lundbäck B, Andersson E (2013b) Respiratory symptoms and respiratory-related absence from work among health care workers in Sweden. J Asthma 50:174–179

Kim JL, Henneberger PK, Lohman S, Olin AC, Dahlman-Höglund A, Andersson E, Torén K, Holm M (2016) Impact of occupational exposures on exacerbation of asthma: a population-based cohort study. BMC Pulm Med 16:148

Kramer MR, Blanc PD, Fireman E, Amital A, Guber A, Rhahman NA, Shitrit D (2012) Artificial stone silicosis: disease resurgence among artificial stone workers. Chest 142:419–424

Laborde-Castérot H, Donnay C, Chapron J, Burgel PR, Kanaan R, Honoré D, Dusser D et al (2012) Employment and work disability in adults with cystic fibrosis. J Cyst Fibros 11:137–143

Lindberg E, Carter N, Gislason T, Janson C (2001) Role of snoring and daytime sleepiness in occupational accidents. Am J Respir Crit Care Med 164:2031–2035

Mönkäre S, Haahtela T (1987) Farmer's lung- a 5-year follow-up of eighty-six patients. Clin Allergy 17:143–151

Montes de Oca M, Halbert RJ, Talamo C, Perez-Padilla R, Lopez MV, Muiño A, Jardim JR, Valdivia G, Pertuzé J, Moreno D, Menezes AM (2011) Paid employment in subjects with and without chronic obstructive pulmonary disease in five Latin American cities: the PLATINO study. Int J Tuberc Lung Dis 15:1259–1264

Omachi TA, Claman DM, Blanc PD, Eisner MD (2009) Obstructive sleep apnea: a risk factor for work disability. Sleep 32:791–798

Paris W, White-Williams C (2005) Social adaptation after cardiothoracic transplantation. J Cardiovasc Nurs 20:567–573

Paris W, Diercks M, Bright J, Zamora M, Kesten S, Scavuzzo M, Paradis I (1998) Return to work after lung transplantation. J Heart Lung Transplant 17:430–436

Piirilä PL, Keskinen HM, Luukkonen R, Salo SP, Tuppurainen M, Nordman H (2005) Work, unemployment and life satisfaction among patients with diisocyanate induced asthma – a prospective study. J Occup Health 47:112–118

Rai KK, Jordan RE, Siebert WS, Sadhra SS, Fitzmaurice DA, Sitch AJ, Ayres JG, Adab P (2017a) Birmingham COPD cohort: a cross-sectional analysis of the factors associated with the likelihood of being in paid employment among people with COPD. Int J Chron Obstruct Pulmon Dis 12:233–242

Rai KK, Adab P, Ayres JG, Siebert WS, Sadhra SS, Sitch AJ, Fitzmaurice DA, Jordan RE (2017b) Factors associated with work productivity among people with COPD: Birmingham COPD cohort. Occup Environ Med 74:859–867

Rai KK, Adab P, Ayres JG, Jordan RE (2018) Systematic review: chronic obstructive pulmonary disease and work-related outcomes. Occup Med (Lond) 68:99–108

Ruttens D, Verleden SE, Bijnens EM, Winckelmans E, Gottlieb J, Warnecke G et al (2017) An association of particulate air pollution and traffic exposure with mortality after lung transplantation in Europe. Eur Respir J 49:1600484

Saarinen K, Karjalainen A, Martikainen R, Uitti J, Tammilehto L, Klaukka T, Kurppa K (2003) Prevalence of work-aggravated symptoms in clinically established asthma. Eur Respir J 22:305–309

Shin SH, Park J, Cho J, Sin DD, Lee H, Park HY (2018) Severity of airflow obstruction and work loss in a nationwide population of working age. Sci Rep 8(1):9674

Sin DD, Stafinski T, Ng YC, Bell NR, Jacobs P (2002) The impact of chronic obstructive pulmonary disease on work loss in the United States. Am J Respir Crit Care Med 165:704–707

Sjösten N, Kivimäki M, Oksanen T, Salo P, Saaresranta T, Virtanen M, Pentti J, Vahtera J (2009a) Obstructive sleep apnea syndrome as a predictor of work disability. Respir Med 103:1047–1055

Sjösten N, Vahtera J, Oksanen T, Salo P, Saaresranta T, Virtanen M, Pentti J, Kivimäki M (2009b) Increased risk of lost workdays prior to the diagnosis of sleep apnea. Chest 136:130–136

Swigris JJ, Stewart AL, Gould MK, Wilson SR (2005) Patients' perspectives on how idiopathic pulmonary fibrosis affects the quality of their lives. Health Qual Life Outcomes 3:61

Targett K, Bourke S, Nash E, Murphy E, Ayres J, Devereux G (2014) Employment in adults with cystic fibrosis. Occup Med 64:87–94

Thornton Snider J, Romley JA, Wong KS, Zhang J, Eber M, Goldman DP (2012) The disability burden of COPD. COPD 9:513–521

Torén K, Kogevinas M, Zock J-P, Sunyer J, Kromhout H, Jarvis D, Payo F, Antó JM, Blanc PD (2009) A prospective longitudinal general population study of respiratory work-disability among adults. Thorax 64:339–344

Ulfberg J, Jonsson R, Edling C (1999) Improvement of subjective work performance among obstructive sleep apnea patients after treatment with continuous positive airway pressure. Psychiatry Clin Neurosci 53:677–679

Vandenplas O, Torén K, Blanc PD (2003) Health and socio-economic impacts of work-related asthma. Eur Respir J 22:689–697

Vandenplas O, Vinnikov D, Blanc PD, Agache I, Bachert C, Bewick M, Cardell LO, Cullinan P, Demoly P, Descatha A, Fonseca J, Haahtela T, Hellings PW, Jamart J, Jantunen J, Kalayci Ö, Price D, Samolinski B, Sastre J, Tian L, Valero AL, Zhang X, Bousquet J (2018) Impact of rhinitis on work productivity: a systematic review. J Allergy Clin Immunol Pract 6:1274–1286

Verbrugge LM, Jette AM (1994) The disablement process. Soc Sci Med 38:1–14

Voelker R (2019) Black lung resurgence raises new challenges for coal country physicians. JAMA 321:17–19

Walters S, Britton J, Hodson ME (1993) Demographic and social characteristics of adults with cystic fibrosis in the United Kingdom. Br Med J 306:549–552

Young T, Palta M, Dempsey J, Skatrud J, Weber S, Badr S (1993) The occurrence of sleep-disordered breathing among middle-aged adults. N Engl J Med 328:1230–1235

Young T, Peppard PE, Gottlieb DJ (2002) Epidemiology of obstructive sleep apnea: a population health perspective. Am J Respir Crit Care Med 165:1217–1239

Occupational Determinants of Musculoskeletal Disorders

10

Alexis Descatha, Bradley A. Evanoff, Annette Leclerc, and Yves Roquelaure

Contents

Introduction	171
General Consideration on Determinants of Musculoskeletal Disorders	172
Nonoccupational Factors	173
Occupational Factors	173
Combination of Determinants	174
Main Disorders and Their Occupational Determinants	176
Shoulder Disorders	176
Elbow Disorders	178
Hand Disorders	178
Cervical Spine Disorders	180

A. Descatha (✉)
INSERM, U1085, IRSET (Institute de recherché en santé, environnement et travail), ESTER Team, University of Angers, Angers, France

University of Versailles Saint-Quentin-en-Yvelines, Versailles, France

INSERM, UMS 011 UMR1168, Villejuif, France

AP-HP, Occupational Health Unit, Raymond Poincaré University Hospital, Garches, France

Inserm U1085-Unité de santé professionnelle AP-HP UVSQ, Garches, France
e-mail: alexis.descatha@inserm.fr

B. A. Evanoff
Division of General Medical Sciences, School of Medicine, Washington University in St. Louis, St. Louis, MI, USA
e-mail: bevanoff@wustl.edu

A. Leclerc
INSERM, UMS 011 UMR1168, Villejuif, France
e-mail: annette.leclerc@inserm.fr

Y. Roquelaure
INSERM, U1085, IRSET (Institute de recherché en santé, environnement et travail), ESTER Team, University of Angers, Angers, France
e-mail: yvroquelaure@chu-angers.fr

© Springer Nature Switzerland AG 2020
U. Bültmann, J. Siegrist (eds.), *Handbook of Disability, Work and Health*, Handbook Series in Occupational Health Sciences, https://doi.org/10.1007/978-3-030-24334-0_8

Lumbar Spine Disorders	181
Specific Radicular Disorders in the Lumbar Spine	181
Non-specific Back Pain	181
Other Trunk Disorders	182
Lower Limb Disorders	182
Osteoarthritis of the Hip	183
Osteoarthritis of the Knee	183
Other Disorders of the Lower Limbs	183
Conclusion	183
Cross-References	184
References	184

Abstract

Musculoskeletal disorders (MSDs) related to working conditions are the leading cause of work disability. MSD related to work is due to non-traumatic injury of soft tissue structures such as the muscles, tendons, ligaments, and nerves that are caused and/or exacerbated by a person's interactions with the work environment. Diagnostic criteria for MSD differ for different disorders, ranging from clinical diagnoses based on symptoms and signs for some to diagnoses based on structural and functional criteria for others. MSDs are multifactorial disorders, where both nonoccupational factors and occupational factors interact in both etiology and recovery. Biomechanical exposures increase risk for MSD based on their intensity (or level), frequency, and duration. Exposures can be estimated through expert judgments, systematic observations, and direct measurements or through use of a job exposure matrix. Psychosocial factors may play an important role in recovery and disability from MSD, and in non-specific pain disorders, and can be defined on many scales based on validated questionnaires.

In addition to the general considerations above, specific causal associations exist between disorders and working conditions, mainly between disorders and biomechanical factors. There is good evidence for associations between biomechanical factors such as hand-arm elevation and shoulder load in the etiology of rotator cuff tendinopathies, the most common shoulder disorder. There is also a positive association between epicondylitis and nerve entrapment at the elbow and combined biomechanical exposures (strength, repetition, and/or awkward posture) involving the wrist and/or the elbow. For carpal tunnel syndrome, associations are consistently found with forceful and repetitive hand exposures, particularly when combined, with strong evidence of a dose-response relationship. Hand-arm vibration syndrome is seen in specific populations exposed to vibrating tools. There is an association between neck pain and biomechanical factors such as static work with maintained awkward postures. Whole-body vibration and vehicle driving, carrying or pulling heavy loads, awkward postures, and psychological demands including lack of support from the social environment are consistently associated with non-specific back pain. Occupational determinants of hip and knee osteoarthritis have been found in several studies in jobs

10 Occupational Determinants of Musculoskeletal Disorders

with high biomechanical exposures from carrying loads and from kneeling/squatting (for knee osteoarthritis).

There are many determinants of musculoskeletal disorders, which vary according to nature and location of the disorder. A better global approach toward prevention of these disorders requires a life course perspective and consideration of all relevant risk factors, both those common to many MSD and those specific to particular MSD.

Keywords

Musculoskeletal · Occupational · Diagnosis · Pain · Syndrome · Biomechanical · Psychosocial organizational · Global approach · Lifetime perspective

Introduction

Musculoskeletal disorders (MSDs) related to repetitive and physically demanding working conditions continue to represent one of the largest work-related problems in industrialized countries. Through pain, difficulty performing work-related tasks, long periods of absence from work, and disability, these disorders engender high social and economic costs. They are usually considered as the leading cause of work disability, sickness absence from work, "presenteeism," and loss of productivity in industrialized countries. In the European Union states, it has been estimated that the total cost of lost productivity attributable to MSDs among people of working age could be as high as 2% of gross domestic product (Bevan 2015). According to the ESENER survey carried out in 2014 by the European Agency for Safety and Health at Work, MSDs are the second most pressing occupational health concern for European companies after work-related accidents, and almost 80% of companies believe that MSDs represent a major challenge (EU OSHA 2014). In the United States, the Bureau of Labor Statistics reported 365,580 WMSDs in private industry and an annual incidence rate of 333.8 per 10,000 workers. Estimated annual workers' compensation costs were estimated at $14 billion in direct costs accounting for 23% of the overall national burden (Liberty Mutual 2017). They contribute to high levels of social inequality in health and are partially avoidable, because a substantial proportion of them could be prevented by workplace interventions (Madan and Grime 2015).

Work-related MSD has been known since the early 1700s, when Bernardino Ramazzini noted the harmful effects of unnatural postures and repetitive movements, such as numbness in the upper extremity among scribes due to "incessant movement of the hand and always in the same direction," or sciatica among potters due to continual turning of the potter's wheel with their feet (Ramazzini 1700; Dembe 1996). In the late 1990s, major collaborative works clarified classifications and determinants of such disorders (Hagberg et al. 1995; Bernard 1997;

Table 1 Example of lesions and locations

Types of disorders	Locations
1. Tendinopathies	Shoulder rotator cuff
	Lateral/medial epicondylian tendon
	Flexors and extensors of the hands/fingers
2. Entrapment neuropathies or radiculopathies	Median (carpal tunnel)
	Ulnar at elbow
	Radial at elbow (radial tunnel)
	Shoulder: Suprascapular, serratus anterior, musculocutaneous, circumflex nerves
	Cervicothoracic (thoracic outlet syndrome)
	Lumbar roots
3. Hygromas	Elbow
	Knee
4. Osteoarthritis	Hip
	Knee
5. Vascular syndromes	Angioneurotic disorders
6. Meniscus lesions	Knee
7. Non-specific disorders	All regions

Yassi 1997; Buckle and Devereux 1999; Inserm 2000; Palmer et al. 2000; Sluiter et al. 2001).

MSD related to work is due to non-traumatic injury of soft tissue structures such as the muscles, tendons, ligaments, joint bones, and nerves that are caused and/or exacerbated by a person's interactions with the work environment (Table 1). Diagnostic criteria for MSD differ for different disorders, ranging from clinical diagnoses based on symptoms and signs for some to diagnoses based on structural and functional criteria for others. We note that "disorder" is a broader category than "disease" and better captures the range of phenomena being considered. Later on, we will consider specific disorders where the diagnosis is based on clear clinical diagnosis and in some cases requiring imaging, nerve conduction studies, and non-specific disorders where symptoms are present but more vague (Sluiter et al. 2001). We will detail first some general considerations on determinants of MSDs and then address main anatomic areas (shoulder, elbow, hand/wrist, cervical spine, back, hip, and knee), differentiating determinants of major specific disorders and non-specific disorders. Acute traumatic injuries are not addressed here.

General Consideration on Determinants of Musculoskeletal Disorders

The World Health Organization (WHO) defined work-related disorders as multifactorial to indicate the inclusion of physical, organizational, psychosocial, and sociological risk factors. A disorder is work related when work procedures, equipment, or environment contribute significantly to the cause of the disorder. Using this description of MSD, there is a broad consensus on their multifactorial nature, where both nonoccupational factors and occupational factors interact in etiology and prognosis.

Nonoccupational Factors

It is well established that certain personal characteristics are factors of individual susceptibility, such as genetic background, pregnancy, female sex, obesity, and some comorbid medical conditions. Age is an important personal factor that also integrates work trajectory and cumulative exposures. Furthermore, some personal factors such as obesity and tobacco use are related to some working conditions and social factors.

Some medical conditions are considered as risk factors of onset of MSDs: history of inflammatory or endocrine disease (especially diabetes) may be factors in some specific disorders (for instance, neuropathies, tendinopathies). A previous history of MSD is a major factor of recurrence and onset of another disorder. Personal psychological factors with anxiety and mood symptoms, personality traits, sleep disturbances, and fear of pain due to movement can be barriers to favorable recovery.

Finally, musculoskeletal overuse due to sports and leisure activities has been described, but its association with onset of MSD among manual workers should not be overestimated. Indeed, though some leisure activities can be a source of musculoskeletal overuse, the intensity, frequency, and duration are typically much lower than musculoskeletal demands at work among manual workers. Moderately intense physical activity and physical fitness also represent a source of activation and maintenance of the musculoskeletal tissues and have been described as protective for work-related MSD.

Occupational Factors

Occupational factors involved in MSD are biomechanical, psychosocial, and organizational factors.

The evaluation of biomechanical exposures can be done in different ways, depending on the objectives and means available. It should be expressed around three principal dimensions, intensity (or level), duration, and frequency (van der Beek and Frings-Dresen 1998). The exposure assessment can be obtained by estimations on the basis of subjective judgments (self-reports, expert judgments), systematic observations (observations at the workplace, video recording), and direct measurements (at the workplace or in laboratory). In particular for the intensity of exposure to postures, movements, and exerted forces, the direct methods of measurement yield higher precision than other methods, such as data from systematic observations. In terms of cost and effort, however, exposures are most easily obtained by subjective judgments, are accurate for some exposure evaluations compared to other methods, and more accurately include the global evaluation of the exposure, particularly for variable jobs (Stock et al. 2005). There has been rapid improvement in the availability and technology of sensors used in direct measurements in the last decade: both size and price are diminishing. Future studies will make increasing use of directly measured exposures as this technology improves. However, other types of approaches, such as job exposure matrices, are useful, especially if assessment of past exposure is needed.

A job exposure matrix is a common method used in occupational epidemiology research to estimate workers' exposures to chemical and other physical risk factors based on job titles, industry information, and population exposure data. The use of job exposure matrix has recently increased for the assessment of physical exposures such as posture, repetition, and force in the study of work-related MSD. While these exposure estimates represent global and average levels for workers in a given job, these measures are inexpensive and useful for general population studies (Descatha et al. 2018).

The main biomechanical risk factors for MSD are high repetition of gestures (frequency, velocity), high force (strength exertion, carrying or moving loads, overall physical demands of work), prolonged maintenance of an awkward posture (arms above the shoulders, flexion/extension of the elbow and wrist, flexion of the trunk, kneeling, and squatting), large ranges of motion, and vibration exposure, either whole body or hand-transmitted vibrations. A combination of biomechanical factors increases the risk for many disorders. While exposures over weeks or months are most relevant to the etiology of some disorders (such as tendinitis), for other disorders (such as osteoarthritis), cumulative lifetime exposures are most relevant to associations between work and disease. In order to assess the potential benefits of specific preventive interventions, the knowledge on temporal dimensions – short-term effect versus long-term or cumulative effect – is important.

Psychosocial factors include psychological job demand, decision latitude, social support, effort reward imbalance, and social injustice. Consistent among common models for workplace psychosocial factors is that worker well-being is lowest in the context of high psychological job demands, low control over work, and low social support. These factors are assessed by worker-completed questionnaires.

Organizational factors have been linked to MSD. Relevant factors include work under time pressure, short cycle times, lack of recovery time, rigidity of procedures and controls, lack of individual or collective autonomy, lack of time or capacity to do quality work, monotony of tasks, and gender discrimination. Other factors include the availability of alternative work or job modifications and the safety culture and safety climate of the workplace. These determinants are increasingly being shown to influence the occurrence and prognosis of work-related MSDs and can be measured by self-evaluation, objective evaluation, and economic indicators or other data from employers.

Combination of Determinants

There are now more and more models for understanding risk factors for the onset and chronicity of MSDs, as well as work disability related to MSD. Whatever model is used, it is important to note the combination of different factors at different levels, with both occupational and nonoccupational determinants, during the whole working life. Overall, most societal and work organization factors can be considered as distal factors and determinants of personal, biomechanical, and also psychosocial factors.

Several risk models for MSDs have been proposed in the literature focusing on the biomechanical, psychosocial, and organizational dimensions (Roquelaure 2016). The classical biomechanical model is based on the imbalance between soft tissue recovery and physical demands, determined by exposure to high forces, awkward postures and repetitive movements, and the worker's functional capacities. The biopsychosocial and organizational risk models of work-related MSDs are more pertinent than the classical biomechanical model for preventive purposes, because they take into account the complexity of multiple determinants. According to these models, the multifactorial nature of MSDs justifies a multidimensional approach based on a global and systemic approach in assessment of the work situation in order to identify the various risk factors and their determinants with reference to a complex model of MSDs as shown in Fig. 1. This kind of model illustrates the complexity of the interactions between different types of determinants, first at an individual level. For example, psychosocial factors can have a direct effect through muscle activation; they can also have indirect effects by an increasing of biomechanical exposure. In addition, such an integrated multidimensional and multilevel conceptual model of MSDs takes into account not only biomechanical and psychosocial factors at the level of the individual worker but also factors related to overall workplace organization and management practices at the company level. These factors largely determine the biomechanical and psychosocial conditions of individual workers.

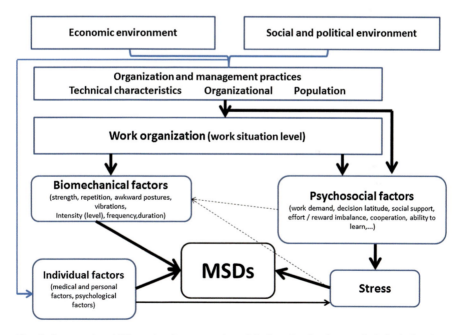

Fig. 1 Integrated multidimensional conceptual model of work-related musculoskeletal disorders (MSDs) (Roquelaure 2016)

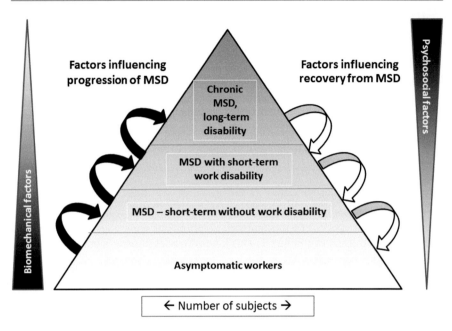

Fig. 2 Diagram presenting a conceptual model of the "pyramid of disability" (Evanoff et al. 2014)

Finally, more general "macro ergonomic" risk factors related to the economic, social, and political environment at market and society levels should be evaluated. Such an integrated multidimensional and multilevel conceptual model suggests enlarging the scope of the assessment of risk factors (Fig. 1): (1) biomechanical factors at the job station level; (2) psychosocial and stress factors at the job levels; (3) organizational factors at work situation and company levels; and (4) socioeconomic factors at the society level.

Biomechanical workplace exposures play a strong role in the incidence of specific MSD, including those which are consequences of psychosocial or organizational exposures. Psychological and psychosocial factors such as job satisfaction and social support seem to play an important role in subsequent disability and chronicity of disease (Fig. 2) (Evanoff et al. 2014). A global approach is needed to prevent new MSD and to limit work disability following an MSD in a lifetime perspective.

In addition to these general considerations, major work-related disorders and their determinants will be described separately below.

Main Disorders and Their Occupational Determinants

Shoulder Disorders

Shoulder diseases are the leading causes of consultation for upper extremity musculoskeletal problems: shoulder pain affects more than 20% of the adult population and nearly 30% in working populations (Carton et al. 2013, 2016).

Rotator Cuff Tendinopathy

The main specific disorder of the shoulder is the rotator cuff tendinopathy (or syndrome, also called impingement syndrome) (Linaker and Walker-Bone 2015). Though diagnosis is mainly clinical, imaging (ultrasound, magnetic resonance imaging, arthro-CT scan) may be also helpful. This condition affects 6.6% of men and 8.5% of women (clinically diagnosed), incidence of first time surgery of 11 per 10,000 people by year (Bodin et al. 2012; Dalbøge et al. 2014).

There is abundant literature on the risk factors for these disorders, for which there is evidence for biomechanical factors such as hand-arm elevation and shoulder load (Bernard 1997; Sluiter et al. 2001; van Rijn et al. 2010; van der Molen et al. 2017). Hand force exertion and hand-arm-transmitted vibrations seem to have weaker evidence, as do some psychosocial factors (job demand, work with temporary workers (van der Molen et al. 2017). In order to give global dose quantification, a previous systematic review studied significant levels of exposure (van Rijn et al. 2010). A force requirement greater than 10% of the maximum voluntary contraction, lifting more than 20 kilos more than 10 times per day, and a high level of hand force (greater than one hour per day) have been associated with the onset of rotator cuff tendinopathies. Repetitive movements of the shoulder, repetitive motion of the hand or wrist greater than 2 h per day, hand-arm vibration, working with hands above shoulder level, upper arm flexion greater or equal to 45° more than 15% of time, duty cycle of forceful exertions more than 9% time, or forceful pinch at any time, were also risk factors.

With regard to duration, the incidence of rotator cuff tendinopathies increases with the cumulative duration of exposure over time (Dalbøge et al. 2018). While this study found levels of safe exposure for repetition (median angular velocity lower than 45°/s), it also found increased risks after 10 years at low intensities for force (exertion greater or equal to 10% of maximal voluntary activity) and for upper arm elevation (greater than 90° more than 2 min/day).

Other Specific Disorders of the Shoulder

There have been too few studies to determine whether work-related exposures are related to the occurrence of other specific shoulder disorders including acromioclavicular arthropathies, retractile capsulitis, macrocalcifications in shoulder tendons, or scapula-humeral osteoarthritis.

Non-specific Disorders of the Shoulder

Some studies have examined risk factors for shoulder pain, finding that both physical risk factors and psychosocial factors contributed (Bodin et al. 2018). Such studies of non-specific disorders of the shoulder likely encompass a spectrum of disorders, including early stages of rotator cuff syndrome, joint disorders, advanced staged with major disability without specific sign or lesion anymore, muscle or tendon pain with functional hypersollicitation, and multisite pain syndrome. Notably, the same biomechanical and psychosocial factors are associated with specific and non-specific disorders, and workers who do not meet an epidemiological case definition may nonetheless have work disability related to pain and activity limitation. For shoulder disorders and other MSD, organizational, psychosocial, and biomechanical factors must all be considered for effective prevention of disability related to musculoskeletal symptoms.

Elbow Disorders

Lateral and Medial Epicondylitis

Lateral and medial epicondylitis are tendinopathies of the lateral and medial epicondylar insertions (Shiri and Viikari-Juntura 2011). Diagnosis is clinically based. These are common disorders, affecting, respectively, 1% (lateral epicondylitis) and 0.5% (medial epicondylitis) of working people (Shiri et al. 2006). The prevalence can be much higher depending on sectors and professional activities (van Rijn et al. 2009a). Overall, there is a positive association between lateral epicondylitis incidence and combined biomechanical exposure (strength, repetition, and/or awkward posture) involving the wrist and/or the elbow with a meta-odds ratio of 2.6 [1.9–3.5] (Descatha et al. 2016). In detail, handling tools heavier than 1 kg, handling loads over 20 kg at least 10 times per day, and repetitive movements more than 2 h per day have found to be associated with lateral epicondylitis (van Rijn et al. 2009a). Handling loads more than 5 kg at least two times per minute for 2 or more hours per day, handling loads more than 20 kg at least ten times per day, high handgrip forces for more than 1 h per day, repetitive movements for more than 2 h per day, and working with vibrating tools more than 2 h per day have found to be associated with medial epicondylitis. The psychosocial factors of low job control and social support have also been associated with the incidence of lateral epicondylitis.

Other Elbow Disorders

Ulnar nerve entrapment at the elbow, diagnosed by clinical criteria and nerve conduction studies, is often associated with medial epicondylitis or carpal tunnel syndrome. Ulnar nerve entrapment at the elbow is associated with forceful hand and arm exposures and sustained or frequent non-neutral postures at the elbow (van Rijn et al. 2009a; Svendsen et al. 2012). Radial nerve syndrome at the elbow is rare and difficult to diagnose and often confused with lateral epicondylitis. Diagnosis requires imaging and/or nerve conduction study. This disorder has been associated with handling loads more than 1 kg, static work of the hand during the majority of the work cycle time, and frequent full extension of the elbow. Elbow hygroma might be related to specific pressure on the joint, and osteoarthritis of the elbow joint (with osteophytes) was associated with repeated high intensity microtrauma and vibration from percussive tools but with a low quality of evidence (Palmer and Bovenzi 2015). Similar to shoulder disorders, non-specific disorders of the elbow likely encompass a wide variety of conditions with different causes.

Hand Disorders

Occupational hand diseases mainly include carpal tunnel syndrome, tendinitis or tenosynovitis of the hands and fingers, hand-arm vibration syndrome, Dupuytren's disease, and non-specific disorders. Carpal tunnel syndrome, defined by examination and nerve conduction study, is the major hand disorder with an incidence of 1 per 1000 persons/years in the general population (higher among populations with intensive hand work) and prevalence of 1–19% depending on the diagnostic criteria used and the population studied (Newington et al. 2015). The prevalence of other diseases is less than 5% in the general population at work but may increase with exposure (Roquelaure et al. 2006; Dale et al. 2013).

Carpal Tunnel Syndrome (CTS)
There is strong evidence for an association between the incidence of carpal tunnel syndrome and forceful and repetitive hand exposures, particularly when combined, with strong evidence of a dose-response relationship. In detail, hand force requirement of more than 4 kg, repetitiveness at work with a cycle time lower than 10 s, or more than 50% of cycle time performing the same movements, and a daily 8-h energy-equivalent frequency-weighted acceleration of 3.9 m/s^2 were related to carpal tunnel syndrome (van Rijn et al. 2009b). Recent studies found that low-force repetition alone was not a significant risk factor for CTS but that peak hand force and the duration or frequency of forceful hand exertion ($\geq$9 N pinch force or $\geq$45 N of power grip) were strongly associated with the incidence of CTS (Harris-Adamson et al. 2015). Large cohort studies in the United States and in Italy found that incident CTS was strongly associated with exposure values that combine peak hand force with the level of hand activity (Kapellusch et al. 2014; Violante et al. 2016).

With regard to psychosocial factors, some statistically significant but weak associations have been found between psychosocial factors and carpal tunnel syndrome independent of biomechanical factors (Harris-Adamson et al. 2016). In addition, organizational factors including fast work pace and piece work have been identified as risk factors for CTS in different studies (Petit et al. 2015). Contrary to common belief, computer work by itself is not a risk factor for carpal tunnel syndrome (Andersen et al. 2011; Mediouni et al. 2014).

Tendonitis and Tenosynovitis of the Hand and Fingers
The prevalence of tendonitis and tenosynovitis of the hand/fingers is as high as 5% in existing studies, though population estimates are lacking. These disorders, clinically diagnosed, have been little studied except in particular occupational groups (Palmer et al. 2007). Diagnosis is based on physical examination (Sluiter et al. 2001). The determinants found in the literature are primarily from cross-sectional studies, though it is well accepted clinically that repeated forceful movements or unaccustomed postures can lead to the development of these disorders. Biomechanical factors that have been highlighted for de Quervain's disease were work pace dependent on technical organization, repeated or sustained wrist bending in extreme posture, and repeated movements associated with the twisting or screwing (Petit Le Manac'h et al. 2011). Tendinitis and tenosynovitis have mainly been studied in hand-intensive industries (Palmer et al. 2007).

Hand-Arm Vibration Syndrome

Disorders secondary to vibration exposure, also known as hand-arm vibration syndromes or Raynaud's syndromes or vibration-induced white finger, are found in specific populations exposed to vibration (Palmer and Bovenzi 2015). These conditions have vascular and neurologic components. Diagnosis is usually clinically based though functional testing or photographs during vasospastic episodes (Poole et al. 2018). Measurement of exposure is complex, as it involves both frequencies of vibration and amplitudes. European standards exist for limiting exposure to vibrating tools: daily 8-h energy-equivalent frequency-weighted acceleration at 2.5 m/s^2 for an exposure action value and 5 m/s^2 for exposure limit value (Palmer and Bovenzi 2015).

Dupuytren's Disease and Non-specific Disorders of the Hand, Wrist, and Fingers

For Dupuytren's disease, the diagnosis is also clinically based, with well-identified genetic determinants (Eaton et al. 2011). Vibration exposures and, to a lesser degree, forceful work have been identified as etiological or aggravating factors (Descatha et al. 2011). Necrosis of the hand bones (lunate, scaphoid) has been described in relation to high-energy microtrauma (from percussive tool use more than vibrating tool use) in similar fashion to elbow osteoarthritis, with a low quality of evidence (Palmer and Bovenzi 2015). Finger and hand osteoarthritis have been associated with high pinch grip forces, without sufficient evidence to show a clear causal relationship (Hammer et al. 2014). Non-specific disorders of the hand, wrist, and fingers have no particular determinants compared to other non-specific disorders.

Cervical Spine Disorders

Disorders of the cervical spine include neck pain, non-specific disorders of muscular origin, and cervical radiculopathy related to a disc lesion or osteoarthritis. These conditions are diagnosed clinically and might be confirmed by imaging (magnetic resonance imaging) and nerve conduction study in some cases (Sluiter et al. 2001).

Specific Cervical Disorders: Cervical Radiculopathy

There are very few specific data on work-related causes of cervical radiculopathy (Cote et al. 2008). Association with whole-body vibrations exposure was not consistently found. The only work-related factor for radiculopathy was direct bearing on the head and neck of very heavy loads that has been described with a biological plausibility (Linaker and Walker-Bone 2015).

Non-specific Disorders: Neck Pain

Non-specific neck pain is a common disorder in the general population and in the working population, with variable prevalence depending on the definition and the working sector studied. The prevalence is between 10% and 20% but can range from 70% to 80% in sectors of activity with certain risk factors (Carroll et al. 2008).

Unlike specific neck radiculopathy, there are consistent and sufficient elements in the literature to recognize an association with certain factors in combination with personal factors (McLean et al. 2010): static work with maintained awkward postures was a significant factor related to non-specific neck pain, especially for women who regularly work with their arms above the shoulders and in men with fast work pace (Petit et al. 2018). There are also many physiological studies confirming these relationships (Aptel 2007).

Psychosocial factors including psychological demand and job strain are found consistently in the literature (McLean et al. 2010). Interactions between these factors and personal factors are important, with relatively complex causal conceptual models (Chouaniere et al. 2011).

Lumbar Spine Disorders

As for cervical spinal disorders, back pain can be classified as non-specific back pain or pain with radicular symptoms (sciatica or cruralgia). Imaging (magnetic resonance imaging, CT scan) and nerve conduction might be used for treatment of specific radicular disorders. In both specific and non-specific disorders, there is an association between these disorders and work exposure in the literature.

Specific Radicular Disorders in the Lumbar Spine

The prevalence rates of radicular disorders in the lumbar spine vary from 1% to 43% according to the exposure, gender, but also the surveillance system used, and the definition used (symptoms, symptoms and radiological abnormalities, surgery for herniated discs) (Konstantinou and Dunn 2008; Fouquet et al. 2018). The biomechanical factors found were exposure to whole-body vibrations (drive for more than 2 h more than once by week), manual work (more than 2 h by day), and awkward posture (twisting of the trunk, working with the trunk forward). However, these results are found in few studies compared to non-specific back pain, and the level of evidence is low, and some are disputed (such as active walking) (Roquelaure and Petit 2014; Cook et al. 2014; Parreira et al. 2018). Indeed, the common lack of consistency between pain and abnormal imaging partly explains that most studies focus on pain.

Non-specific Back Pain

Given the human and social cost of non-specific low back pain, there are many studies and reviews in this area. Depending on the definition used, the prevalence varies on chronic low back pain between 25% and 30%, with a period prevalence within 6 months, between 40% and 50% (Roquelaure and Petit 2014; Schaafsma et al. 2015). This represents 8–10% of sick leave in industrialized countries and the main cause of job loss for health reasons (Burton et al. 2005).

The occupational factors found in the literature are biomechanical, mostly whole-body vibration and vehicle driving (for more than 2 h by day), lifting frequently, heavy lifting or pulling loads (greater than 25 kg), and awkward postures like prolonged flexion to more than 60° or for more than 5% of the time (Palmer and Bovenzi 2015; Parreira et al. 2018). Prolonged sitting, a postural factor also found during driving, has also been described as a risk for low back pain. Several studies indicate that exposure to biomechanical strains has long-lasting effects, with a specific role for duration of exposure (Plouvier et al. 2008; Lallukka et al. 2017).

In addition to biomechanical factors, psychosocial factors, including psychological demands and lack of support from the social environment, are also found consistently, and to a lesser extent lack of decision latitude and job strain, with interactions between these factors and personal and social factors (Chouaniere et al. 2011; Ramond et al. 2011).

Other Trunk Disorders

There is very little data on determinants of thoracic spine disorders, although a prevalence between 5% and 10% of thoracic pain has been found in the literature. Spine postural factors and vehicle driving have been identified in men and a significant perceived burden of work in women and often associated with personal factors (Roquelaure et al. 2014). Nevertheless, further studies are necessary to better define risks for this relatively understudied yet relatively common symptom.

Although inguinal and femoral hernias are considered to be primarily traumatic disorders, recent studies have found a significant excess of risk in different studies from cumulative prolonged standing and other postural exposure, in association with personal risk factors such as obesity (Svendsen et al. 2013).

Lower Limb Disorders

Osteoarthritis of the hip and knee will be mostly discussed here, since these are the most frequent work-related MSDs that are not related to an acute trauma. The non-traumatic meniscopathies come from degenerative origin and are included with knee osteoarthritis. The prevalence of hip and knee disorders is high, affecting about 20% of the population in their 50s (all disorders included) (Fransen et al. 2011). The diagnosis requires imaging (plain radiographs, most commonly, CT scan and/or magnetic resonance imaging in some cases).

Osteoarthritis of the Hip

The prevalence of confirmed symptomatic hip osteoarthritis is estimated at less than 1% of the population (all ages), more common in women than in men and increasing with age (Vignon et al. 2006; Fransen et al. 2011; Harris and Coggon 2015). Occupational determinant is found consistently in several studies on activity sectors with very high biomechanical exposure such as farming or construction (Richmond et al. 2013). In these sectors, carrying loads of more than 10 kg for more than 10 years increases the risk with a dose-response relationship. Other exposures such as walking and climbing ladders or stairs were not consistent, and no association with psychosocial factors was found (Fouquet et al. 2016).

Osteoarthritis of the Knee

The prevalence of knee osteoarthritis has been estimated at 3.8% (Dulay et al. 2015). There is convergent data among men on the combination of carrying heavy loads and kneeling/squatting for many years, particularly in mining, farming, or construction sectors (Jensen 2008; McWilliams et al. 2011). Carrying loads independent of kneeling/squatting work have more limited evidence, as does climbing stairs (Verbeek et al. 2017). These associations are weaker among women (Fouquet et al. 2016). No association with psychosocial factors was found for etiology.

Other Disorders of the Lower Limbs

Knee hygromas, like elbow ones, may be associated with forced or prolonged pressure on the joint. Tendinopathies, and foot disorders such as plantar fasciitis, have been described following particular biomechanical exposure circumstances, but overall this literature is sparse, and additional studies are needed (Descatha et al. 2009; Waclawski et al. 2015).

Conclusion

There are many determinants of musculoskeletal disorders, which vary according to their nature and location. A better application of causal models with combination of all relevant risk factors, using a life course perspective and more knowledge on temporal links between exposure and MSD, would allow a better global approach toward prevention of these disorders. There is a need for better exposure assessment methods and the use of common and precise diagnoses or case definitions. Despite the economic importance of MSDs, there has been relatively little study of the risk factors for prolonged disability following most MSDs, in particular how workplace physical and psychosocial factors influence prognosis and return to work.

Cross-References

▸ Policies of Reducing the Burden of Occupational Hazards and Disability Pensions
▸ Reducing Inequalities in Employment of People with Disabilities
▸ Work-Related Burden of Absenteeism, Presenteeism, and Disability: An Epidemiologic and Economic Perspective
▸ Work-Related Interventions to Reduce Work Disability Related to Musculoskeletal Disorders

References

Andersen JH, Fallentin N, Thomsen JF, Mikkelsen S (2011) Risk factors for neck and upper extremity disorders among computers users and the effect of interventions: an overview of systematic reviews. PLoS One 6:e19691. https://doi.org/10.1371/journal.pone.0019691

Aptel M (2007) De l'épidémiologie à la physiopathologie des TMS: le modèle de Bruxelles un référentiel intégrateur. In: Neuropathies et pathologies professionnelles. Masson, Paris, pp 51–62

Bernard BP (1997) Musculoskeletal disorders and workplace factors: a critical review of epidemiologic evidence for work-related musculoskeletal disorders of the neck, the upper-limb, and low back. Cincinnati, Department of Health and Human Services, National Institute for Occupational Safety and Health

Bevan S (2015) Economic impact of musculoskeletal disorders (MSDs) on work in Europe. Best Pract Res Clin Rheumatol 29:356–373. https://doi.org/10.1016/j.berh.2015.08.002

Bodin J, Ha C, Chastang J-F et al (2012) Comparison of risk factors for shoulder pain and rotator cuff syndrome in the working population. Am J Ind Med 55:605–615. https://doi.org/10.1002/ajim.22002

Bodin J, Garlantézec R, Costet N et al (2018) Risk factors for shoulder pain in a cohort of French workers: a structural equation model. Am J Epidemiol 187:206–213. https://doi.org/10.1093/aje/kwx218

Buckle P, Devereux JJ (1999) Work-related neck and upper limb musculoskeletal disorders. European Agency for Safety and Health at Work, Bilbao

Burton AK, Balagué F, Cardon G et al (2005) How to prevent low back pain. Best Pract Res Clin Rheumatol 19:541–555. https://doi.org/10.1016/j.berh.2005.03.001

Carroll LJ, Hogg-Johnson S, Cote P et al (2008) Course and prognostic factors for neck pain in workers: results of the bone and joint decade 2000–2010 task force on neck pain and its associated disorders. Spine Phila Pa 1976 33:S93–S100

Carton M, Leclerc A, Plouvier S et al (2013) Description of musculoskeletal disorders and occupational exposure from a field pilot study of large population-based cohort (CONSTANCES). J Occup Environ Med 55:859–861. https://doi.org/10.1097/JOM.0b013e31825fa545

Carton M, Santin G, Leclerc A et al (2016) Prevalence of musculoskeletal disorders and occupational biomechanical factors: preliminary estimates from the French CONSTANCES cohort. Bull Épidémiol Hebd 2016(35–36):630–639. http://invs.santepubliquefrance.fr/beh/2016/35-36/2016_35-36_4.html

Chouaniere D, Cohidon C et al (2011) Expositions psychosociales et santé: état des connaissances épidémiologiques – [Psychosocial exposure and health. Epidemiological state of the art]. http://www.inrs.fr/media.html?refINRS=TP%2013. Accessed 26 Oct 2018

Cook CE, Taylor J, Wright A et al (2014) Risk factors for first time incidence sciatica: a systematic review. Physiother Res Int 19:65–78. https://doi.org/10.1002/pri.1572

Cote P, van der Velde G, Cassidy JD et al (2008) The burden and determinants of neck pain in workers: results of the bone and joint decade 2000–2010 task force on neck pain and its associated disorders. Spine Phila Pa 1976 33:S60–S74

Dalbøge A, Frost P, Andersen JH, Svendsen SW (2014) Cumulative occupational shoulder exposures and surgery for subacromial impingement syndrome: a nationwide Danish cohort study. Occup Environ Med 71:750–756. https://doi.org/10.1136/oemed-2014-102161

Dalbøge A, Frost P, Andersen JH, Svendsen SW (2018) Surgery for subacromial impingement syndrome in relation to intensities of occupational mechanical exposures across 10-year exposure time windows. Occup Environ Med 75:176–182. https://doi.org/10.1136/oemed-2017-104511

Dale AM, Harris-Adamson C, Rempel D et al (2013) Prevalence and incidence of carpal tunnel syndrome in US working populations: pooled analysis of six prospective studies. Scand J Work Environ Health 39:495–505. https://doi.org/10.5271/sjweh.3351

Dembe A (1996) Occupation and disease: how social factors affect the conception of work-related disorders. Yale University Press, Yale, 358p

Descatha A, Plenet A, Leclerc A, Roquelaure Y (2009) Atteintes du pied au cours de la pratique professionnelle (revue de la litterature épidémiologique) [Knee pain in occupational setting: a systematic review of epidemiological literature]. In: Le pied dans la pratique professionnelle. Masson, Paris

Descatha A, Jauffret P, Chastang J-F et al (2011) Should we consider Dupuytren's contracture as work-related? A review and meta-analysis of an old debate. BMC Musculoskelet Disord 12:96. https://doi.org/10.1186/1471-2474-12-96

Descatha A, Albo F, Leclerc A et al (2016) Lateral epicondylitis and physical exposure at work? A review of prospective studies and meta-analysis. Arthritis Care Res 68:1681–1687. https://doi.org/10.1002/acr.22874

Descatha A, Despréaux T, Petit A et al (2018) Développement d'une matrice emplois-expositions française ("MADE") pour l'évaluation des contraintes biomécaniques. Sante Publique 30:333–337. https://doi.org/10.3917/spub.183.0333

Dulay GS, Cooper C, Dennison EM (2015) Knee pain, knee injury, knee osteoarthritis & work. Best Pract Res Clin Rheumatol 29:454–461. https://doi.org/10.1016/j.berh.2015.05.005

Eaton C et al (2011) Dupuytren's disease and related hyperproliferative disorders – principles, research, and clinical perspectives. Springer, Berlin/New York, p339

EU OSHA (2014) ESENER study. https://osha.europa.eu/en/surveys-and-statistics-osh/esener/2014

Evanoff B, Dale AM, Descatha A (2014) A conceptual model of musculoskeletal disorders for occupational health practitioners. Int J Occup Med Environ Health 27:145. https://doi.org/10.2478/s13382-014-0232-5

Fouquet B, Descatha A, Roulet A, Hérisson C (2016) Arthrose et activités professionnelles. Sauramps Médical, Montpellier

Fouquet N, Bodin J, Chazelle E et al (2018) Use of multiple data sources for surveillance of work-related chronic low-back pain and disc-related sciatica in a French region. Ann Work Expo Health 62:530–546. https://doi.org/10.1093/annweh/wxy023

Fransen M, Agaliotis M, Bridgett L, Mackey MG (2011) Hip and knee pain: role of occupational factors. Best Pract Res Clin Rheumatol 25:81–101. https://doi.org/10.1016/j.berh.2011.01.012

Hagberg M, Silverstein BA, Wells R et al (1995) Work related musculoskeletal disorders (WMSDs). A reference book for prevention. Taylor and Francis, Bristol

Hammer PEC, Shiri R, Kryger AI et al (2014) Associations of work activities requiring pinch or hand grip or exposure to hand-arm vibration with finger and wrist osteoarthritis: a meta-analysis. Scand J Work Environ Health 40:133–145. https://doi.org/10.5271/sjweh.3409

Harris EC, Coggon D (2015) HIP osteoarthritis and work. Best Pract Res Clin Rheumatol 29:462–482. https://doi.org/10.1016/j.berh.2015.04.015

Harris-Adamson C, Eisen EA, Kapellusch J et al (2015) Biomechanical risk factors for carpal tunnel syndrome: a pooled study of 2474 workers. Occup Environ Med 72:33–41. https://doi.org/10.1136/oemed-2014-102378

Harris-Adamson C, Eisen EA, Neophytou A et al (2016) Biomechanical and psychosocial exposures are independent risk factors for carpal tunnel syndrome: assessment of confounding using causal diagrams. Occup Environ Med 73:727–734. https://doi.org/10.1136/oemed-2016-103634

Inserm, collective work (2000) Back pain at work. Risk factors and prevention? [Lombalgies en milieu professionnel: Quels facteurs de risque et quelle prévention? expertise collective] Les éditions Inserm. http://www.ipubli.inserm.fr/handle/10608/36

Jensen LK (2008) Knee osteoarthritis: influence of work involving heavy lifting, kneeling, climbing stairs or ladders, or kneeling/squatting combined with heavy lifting. Occup Environ Med 65:72–89

Kapellusch JM, Gerr FE, Malloy EJ et al (2014) Exposure-response relationships for the ACGIH threshold limit value for hand-activity level: results from a pooled data study of carpal tunnel syndrome. Scand J Work Environ Health 40:610–620. https://doi.org/10.5271/sjweh.3456

Konstantinou K, Dunn KM (2008) Sciatica: review of epidemiological studies and prevalence estimates. Spine 33:2464–2472. https://doi.org/10.1097/BRS.0b013e318183a4a2

Lallukka T, Viikari-Juntura E, Viikari J et al (2017) Early work-related physical exposures and low back pain in midlife: the Cardiovascular Risk in Young Finns Study. Occup Environ Med 74:163–168. https://doi.org/10.1136/oemed-2016-103727

Liberty Mutual (2017) 2017 Liberty Mutual Workplace Safety Index. https://www.libertymutualgroup.com/about-liberty-mutual-site/news-site/Pages/2017-Liberty-Mutual-Workplace-Safety-Index.aspx. Accessed 24 Oct 2018

Linaker CH, Walker-Bone K (2015) Shoulder disorders and occupation. Best Pract Res Clin Rheumatol 29:405–423. https://doi.org/10.1016/j.berh.2015.04.001

Madan I, Grime PR (2015) The management of musculoskeletal disorders in the workplace. Best Pract Res Clin Rheumatol 29:345–355. https://doi.org/10.1016/j.berh.2015.03.002

McLean SM, May S, Klaber-Moffett J et al (2010) Risk factors for the onset of non-specific neck pain: a systematic review. J Epidemiol Community Health 64:565–572. https://doi.org/10.1136/jech.2009.090720

McWilliams DF, Leeb BF, Muthuri SG et al (2011) Occupational risk factors for osteoarthritis of the knee: a meta-analysis. Osteoarthritis Cartilage 19:829–839. https://doi.org/10.1016/j.joca.2011.02.016

Mediouni Z, de Roquemaurel A, Dumontier C et al (2014) Is carpal tunnel syndrome related to computer exposure at work? A review and meta-analysis. J Occup Environ Med 56:204. https://doi.org/10.1097/JOM.0000000000000080

Newington L, Harris EC, Walker-Bone K (2015) Carpal tunnel syndrome and work. Best Pract Res Clin Rheumatol 29:440–453. https://doi.org/10.1016/j.berh.2015.04.026

Palmer KT, Bovenzi M (2015) Rheumatic effects of vibration at work. Best Pract Res Clin Rheumatol 29:424–439. https://doi.org/10.1016/j.berh.2015.05.001

Palmer K, Walker-Bone K, Linaker C et al (2000) The Southampton examination schedule for the diagnosis of musculoskeletal disorders of the upper limb. Ann Rheum Dis 59:5–11

Palmer KT, Harris EC, Coggon D (2007) Compensating occupationally related tenosynovitis and epicondylitis: a literature review. Occup Med Lond 57:67–74

Parreira P, Maher CG, Steffens D et al (2018) Risk factors for low back pain and sciatica: an umbrella review. Spine J 18:1715. https://doi.org/10.1016/j.spinee.2018.05.018

Petit Le Manac'h A, Roquelaure Y, Ha C et al (2011) Risk factors for de Quervain's disease in a French working population. Scand J Work Environ Health 37:394–401. https://doi.org/10.5271/sjweh.3160

Petit A, Ha C, Bodin J et al (2015) Risk factors for carpal tunnel syndrome related to the work organization: a prospective surveillance study in a large working population. Appl Ergon 47:1–10. https://doi.org/10.1016/j.apergo.2014.08.007

Petit A, Bodin J, Delarue A et al (2018) Risk factors for episodic neck pain in workers: a 5-year prospective study of a general working population. Int Arch Occup Environ Health 91:251–261. https://doi.org/10.1007/s00420-017-1272-5

Plouvier S, Renahy E, Chastang JF et al (2008) Biomechanical strains and low back disorders: quantifying the effects of the number of years of exposure on various types of pain. Occup Environ Med 65:268–274. https://doi.org/10.1136/oem.2007.036095

Poole CJM, Bovenzi M, Nilsson T et al (2018) International consensus criteria for diagnosing and staging hand-arm vibration syndrome. Int Arch Occup Environ Health 92:117. https://doi.org/10.1007/s00420-018-1359-7

Ramazzini B (1700) De morbis artificum diatriba [Diseases of workers]. Modena. Mutinae, Episcopal publisher

Ramond A, Bouton C, Richard I et al (2011) Psychosocial risk factors for chronic low back pain in primary care–a systematic review. Fam Pract 28:12–21. https://doi.org/10.1093/fampra/cmq072

Richmond SA, Fukuchi RK, Ezzat A et al (2013) Are joint injury, sport activity, physical activity, obesity, or occupational activities predictors for osteoarthritis? A systematic review. J Orthop Sports Phys Ther 43:515–B19. https://doi.org/10.2519/jospt.2013.4796

Roquelaure Y (2016) Promoting a shared representation of workers' activities to improve integrated prevention of work-related musculoskeletal disorders. Saf Health Work 7:171–174. https://doi.org/10.1016/j.shaw.2016.02.001

Roquelaure Y, Petit A (2014) Surveillance médico-professionnelle du risque lombaire pour les travailleurs exposés à des manipulations de charges. Recommandations de Bonne Pratique. Arch Mal Prof Environ 75(1):6–33

Roquelaure Y, Ha C, Leclerc A et al (2006) Epidemiologic surveillance of upper-extremity musculoskeletal disorders in the working population. Arthritis Care Res 55:765–778

Roquelaure Y, Bodin J, Ha C et al (2014) Incidence and risk factors for thoracic spine pain in the working population: the French pays de la loire study. Arthritis Care Res 66:1695–1702. https://doi.org/10.1002/acr.22323

Schaafsma FG, Anema JR, van der Beek AJ (2015) Back pain: prevention and management in the workplace. Best Pract Res Clin Rheumatol 29:483–494. https://doi.org/10.1016/j.berh.2015.04.028

Shiri R, Viikari-Juntura E (2011) Lateral and medial epicondylitis: role of occupational factors. Best Pract Res Clin Rheumatol 25:43–57. https://doi.org/10.1016/j.berh.2011.01.013

Shiri R, Viikari-Juntura E, Varonen H, Heliövaara M (2006) Prevalence and determinants of lateral and medial epicondylitis: a population study. Am J Epidemiol 164:1065–1074. https://doi.org/10.1093/aje/kwj325

Sluiter BJ, Rest KM, Frings-Dresen MH (2001) Criteria document for evaluating the work-relatedness of upper-extremity musculoskeletal disorders. Scand J Work Environ Health 27(Suppl 1):1–102

Stock SR, Fernandes R, Delisle A, Vezina N (2005) Reproducibility and validity of workers' self-reports of physical work demands. Scand J Work Environ Health 31:409–437

Svendsen SW, Johnsen B, Fuglsang-Frederiksen A, Frost P (2012) Ulnar neuropathy and ulnar neuropathy-like symptoms in relation to biomechanical exposures assessed by a job exposure matrix: a triple case-referent study. Occup Environ Med 69:773–780. https://doi.org/10.1136/oemed-2011-100499

Svendsen SW, Frost P, Vad MV, Andersen JH (2013) Risk and prognosis of inguinal hernia in relation to occupational mechanical exposures–a systematic review of the epidemiologic evidence. Scand J Work Environ Health 39:5–26. https://doi.org/10.5271/sjweh.3305

van der Beek AJ, Frings-Dresen MH (1998) Assessment of mechanical exposure in ergonomic epidemiology. Occup Environ Med 55:291–299

van der Molen HF, Foresti C, Daams JG et al (2017) Work-related risk factors for specific shoulder disorders: a systematic review and meta-analysis. Occup Environ Med 74:745–755. https://doi.org/10.1136/oemed-2017-104339

van Rijn RM, Huisstede BM, Koes BW, Burdorf A (2009a) Associations between work-related factors and specific disorders at the elbow: a systematic literature review. Rheumatology (Oxford) 48:528–536 van Rijn RM, Huisstede BM, Koes BW, Burdorf A (2009b) Associations between work-related factors and the carpal tunnel syndrome–a systematic review. Scand J Work Environ Health 35:19–36

van Rijn RM, Huisstede BM, Koes BW, Burdorf A (2010) Associations between work-related factors and specific disorders of the shoulder–a systematic review of the literature. Scand J Work Environ Health 36:189–201

Verbeek J, Mischke C, Robinson R et al (2017) Occupational exposure to knee loading and the risk of osteoarthritis of the knee: a systematic review and a dose-response meta-analysis. Saf Health Work 8:130–142. https://doi.org/10.1016/j.shaw.2017.02.001

Vignon E, Valat JP, Rossignol M et al (2006) Osteoarthritis of the knee and hip and activity: a systematic international review and synthesis (OASIS). Joint Bone Spine 73:442–455

Violante FS, Farioli A, Graziosi F et al (2016) Carpal tunnel syndrome and manual work: the OCTOPUS cohort, results of a ten-year longitudinal study. Scand J Work Environ Health 42:280–290. https://doi.org/10.5271/sjweh.3566

Waclawski ER, Beach J, Milne A et al (2015) Systematic review: plantar fasciitis and prolonged weight bearing. Occup Med Oxf Engl 65:97–106. https://doi.org/10.1093/occmed/kqu177

Yassi A (1997) Repetitive strain injuries. Lancet 349:943–947

Occupational Determinants of Cardiovascular Disorders Including Stroke

11

Töres Theorell

Contents

Introduction	190
Obtaining Scientific Evidence	191
What Can we Make out of this?	197
Societal Relevance	202
Cross-References	203
References	203

Abstract

This review builds firstly on summaries of high-quality studies between 1985 and 2018 of the relationship between organizational and psychosocial exposures on one hand and ischemic heart disease (IHD) and stroke on the other hand. Secondly, a similar review was made of scientific studies of the relationship between exposure to chemicals at work on one hand and IHD and stroke on the other hand.

There was moderately strong to limited evidence for a significant relationship between job strain, small decision latitude, iso-strain, effort-reward imbalance, low support, lack of justice, lack of skill discretion, insecure employment, night work, long working week, and noise on one hand and increased IHD risk on the other hand. For chemicals, it was shown that job exposure to quartz dust, motor exhaust smoke, welding, benzo-a-pyrene, plumb, dynamite, carbon disulfide, carbon monoxide, liquids for cutting metal, phenoxy acids, asbestos, and tobacco smoking increases IHD risk. Stroke has not been examined to the same extent as IHD, so the evidence is still less convincing although for some exposures the same findings were made as for IHD.

T. Theorell (✉)
Stress Research Institute, Stockholm University, Stockholm, Sweden
e-mail: tores.theorell@su.se

Conclusion: Many types of job exposure may accelerate the onset of cardiovascular disease. For some factors the scientific evidence is on level three on a four-graded scale. There is need for more studies of combined effects of psychosocial and chemical risk factors on cardiovascular risk. There is also need for evaluations of interventions in the psychosocial field. In the chemical and physical exposure field, decreased exposure constitutes the intervention!

Keywords

Ischemic heart disease · Stroke · Psychosocial work conditions · Chemical job exposure

Introduction

Cardiovascular disease is one of the major reasons for death and disability in the developed countries – despite the fact that in most of these countries cardiovascular mortality has decreased since the 1980s. In my own country, Sweden, which has ten million inhabitants, the cardiovascular mortality for men decreased from 352 to 113 in 100,000 between 1987 and 2012. The corresponding numbers for women were 128 to 49. The incidence of cardiovascular disease is much higher, however, since "only" one fourth of patients with myocardial infarction die. Presently 60,000 persons receive hospital care for cardiovascular disease (including both myocardial infarction and angina pectoris and related ischemic heart disease conditions) every year out of whom 26,000 have a myocardial infarction. High age is a strong risk factor – only 1400 women and 4600 of these 26,000 are below age 65 (Nationella kvalitetsregister). Correspondingly 25,000 subjects receive care every year for stroke, but 80% of them are 65 years old or older. Our statistics from Sweden are approximately representative for developed countries (Feigin et al. 2014). Both cardiovascular disease and stroke cause considerable disability and loss of quality of life. For those who develop these illnesses while still in working age, work ability could be a major problem which causes individual suffering and societal costs.

The risk of developing ischemic heart disease or stroke is determined to a great extent outside work by genetic factors and by lifestyle, for instance, smoking habits, physical exercise, and diet, but today there is agreement among cardiologists that psychosocial stress at work is contributing to cardiovascular risk (see Piepoli et al. 2016). Some of the psychosocial risk factors that are discussed in the European guidelines are behavioral individual factors, such as hostility and depression. In this contribution I will focus on environmental working conditions, and both psychosocial and chemical exposure will be considered on the basis of our present level of knowledge. The review will focus on epidemiological evidence rather than on mechanisms.

In the scientific literature on the role of working conditions in the pathogenesis of IHD, stress and psychosocial factors have been in focus since the 1980s. Epidemiological studies in the field have become more and more sophisticated. Although there were theoretical models available for the study of psychosocial factors already in the 1960s to 1970s, these were not widely used in epidemiological studies. This changed when the demand control model was introduced by Karasek in the international scientific literature in 1979 (Karasek 1979). The demand control model with the addition of social support at work (Johnson and Hall 1988; Karasek and Theorell 1990) has been extensively used in this research since 35 years. During later years other theoretical models have been competing with the demand control support model, first of all the effort-reward imbalance model (Siegrist 1996) and second the demand resource model (Demerouti et al. 2001). In cardiovascular epidemiology the demand control support and effort-reward models have been dominating during later years. Descriptions of the theoretical foundations of these models will be found in other chapters of this book. However, as will be obvious in this review, other factors related to job organization have also been studied in relation to risk of cardiovascular disease development, such as long working hours, shift work and night work, noise, injustice at work, job insecurity, and lack of skill discretion (boring jobs). In this review all of these risk factors are included.

Obtaining Scientific Evidence

Several reviews of prospective studies of psychosocial factors at work in relation to cardiovascular disease have been published, for instance, Kristensen et al. (1998), Belkic et al. (2004), and Eller et al. (2009). There are consistent findings indicating that perceived adverse psychosocial factors in the workplace are likely to be related to an elevated risk of subsequent elevated cardiovascular disease risk. The field has recently taken an important step with the establishment of the IPD Work study. This is a network of epidemiologists who have collaborated in combining cohort studies. Measures both of exposures and outcomes have been "homogenized" which means that the comparability of assessments between cohorts has been optimized. This also means that very large cohorts can be studied.

Illness risks associated with exposure to physical (such as irradiation and heat) as well as chemical toxic substances have been studied for a long period in occupational medicine. For instance, carbon disulfide exposure at work was documented in a prospective study to be associated with increased risk of developing cardiovascular disease already in 1976 (Hernberg et al. 1976).

The system for grading evidence (GRADE) that we used has four levels of evidence, ranging from high (4) to insufficient (1).

Only studies with a prospective design or comparable case-control design were included. In addition, a valid and reliable assessment of working conditions preceding illness should have been used. The main focus of the study should have been the relationship between working conditions and development of IHD and stroke among working subjects. We conducted these systematic reviews within the framework for the Swedish Agency for Health and Technology Assessment and Assessment of Social Services, using the PRISMA framework (Moher et al. 2009). Since it is of potential interest to readers to see how the different levels of scientific evidence assessments are made, I shall go into some detail describing the process.

The inclusion criteria for studies were:

1. The study should have examined the work environment (psychosocial, organizational, physical, and other ergonomic job factors as well as chemical) in relation to heart disease and stroke. It should have been published during the period 1985 to 2014. Work environments studied in the whole world were included. In the review of chemical exposure, the time interval 1970–2016 was used in the literature search because methods for assessment of chemical exposure have been available for a longer period and since the chemical review was finished later than the psychosocial one.
2. IHD should have been defined according to accepted criteria. The outcome should have been certified through diagnostic investigation and with established methods including type of illness onset, enzyme elevation, and ECG changes.
3. Prospective or comparable case-control design. Prospective cohort studies with at least 1000 persons (500 persons in the chemical review since risks are more easily established for some chemical exposures than for most psychosocial ones) and case-control studies with at least 50 cases (with design equivalent to prospective) were accepted. In this case, case-control studies are studies with strict definition of cases recruited in a representative way in the same population as the control subjects and with exposure data as well as IHD data from the period before disease onset. The study design should have considered age and gender, e.g., by adjustment or stratification.

Multiple publications investigating the same population were systematically identified, and only the most relevant publication in a doublet was included in the graded result.

Experts used relevance and quality criteria. Concordance in judgments of relevance and quality was trained. After the training session, the group was divided in pairs, and the articles were distributed randomly to the pairs. Each member of the pair did the (the same) assessments separately, and then discordances were discussed within the pair. In the final grading process, only studies with medium high and high quality were accepted.

As in all studies using the GRADE methodology, five general aspects of quality were assessed, namely, *representativeness* of the study sample (including attrition in different steps); *confounding* such as age, gender, and life habits; *data collection* and statistics; *validation of methods*; and *possibility of graded exposure* (for instance, several longitudinal assessments of exposure).

Even between studies of specific work environment factors, there were differences with regard to operationalization of exposure. Examples are job strain (combination of high psychological demands and low decision latitude) and effort-reward imbalance (combination of high effort and poor reward).

An important aspect of the systematic review process was to systematically and transparently assess the scientific evidence. According to the GRADE instructions, explicit consideration should be given to each of the GRADE criteria for assessing the quality of evidence (risk of bias/study limitations, directness, consistency of results, precision, publication bias, magnitude of the effect, dose-response gradient, influence of residual plausible confounding, and bias "antagonistic bias") although different terminology may be used. For level 4 (=High), randomized trials are required, and there were no such published relevant studies in our search. For observational studies of the kind included in the present review, the highest possible grade is Moderate = 3.

We allowed for upgrading the scientific evidence when there was strong coherence of results between studies. Accordingly, when there were many published observational studies of medium or high quality with homogenous results (almost all pointing in the same direction although all findings may not have been statistically significant), the evidence was graded on level 3.

Forest plots were constructed for visual interpretation – associations calculated by different methods (e.g., hazard ratios, odds ratios, and relative risk) were included in the same graph. To assist in illustrating the results and as a contribution to the overall assessment, these forest plots (meta-analyses) were conducted when in at least two studies the same risk factor was analyzed using the *Comprehensive Meta-Analysis* software package (www.meta-analysis.com/index.php).

Informal homogeneity tests were performed in order to compare results from studies using general population studies versus specific occupational cohorts, men versus women, case-control studies versus prospective studies, and early versus late publications and geographical origin (North America versus Nordic and other European countries). In these tests, we conducted sub-analyses of the presented findings and compared results between the subcategories, e.g., if the association between job exposure and IHD differed according to study design.

In the literature search, we accepted a wide range of heart diseases, e.g., ischemic heart disease, arrhythmia, and cardiomyopathy. To provide an idea of the quantity of articles perused, in the psychosocial and physical exposure search for the years 1984 to 2014, there were 11,766 records identified in the database search (with the outcome cardiovascular disease). After the exclusion of articles which turned out not to fill inclusion criteria, articles that lacked relevance and finally articles with low scientific quality, 96 studies of ischemic heart disease remained.

Most studies were based on population samples although studies of samples from companies and occupational groups were also present. Few studies that were judged to be relevant were based upon objective assessments of exposure; these studies were mainly focused on physical exposure (e.g., noise) or time aspects (e.g., night work). Subjective assessments based upon standardized and validated questionnaires (for instance, demand/control/support, effort/reward, procedural justice, and bullying) were used in most studies.

Two exposures, low decision latitude and the combination of high psychological demands and low decision latitude, were judged to have moderate evidence (grade 3), while ten exposures (the combination of job strain and poor support at work = iso-strain, "pressing job," effort-reward imbalance, low support at work, low workplace justice, poor skill discretion, insecure employment, night work, long working week, and noise) were judged to have limited (grade 2) evidence in relation to IHD. Thirteen exposures (psychological demands, active work, passive work, poor social climate, bullying, conflicts, shift work, physically strenuous work, physically inactive in sitting position, heavy lifting, electromagnetic fields, ionizing irradiation (gamma and other kinds), and radon exposure) were judged to have insufficient evidence (grade 1).

The number of studies with sufficient quality varied considerably for the different exposures. Low decision latitude had been studied in relation to IHD in 25 studies and job strain (the combination of high demand and low decision latitude) in 16 studies. Low support had been studied in 11, noise in 9, long working hours in 7, "pressing job" in 7, effort-reward imbalance in 5, and poor skill discretion in 5 studies, respectively. The numbers of study participants were just above 1,000,000 for each of one the exposures "pressing work," long working hours, and low skill discretion. In the studies of low decision latitude, there were 800,000, in the studies of noise, almost 600,000, and, in the studies of job strain, more than 200,000 participants.

Figure 1 shows the forest plot for job strain that was judged with evidence grade 3 to be related to incidence of IHD. For this exposure there was data from 18 studies. In addition one study showed data separately for blue-collar and white-collar workers. These data are also presented separately in the diagram. Accordingly, the diagram includes 23 estimates with 95% confidence limits. All estimates except one are above 1. Twelve of the lower confidence limits are above 1. This was judged as a homogenous finding across the studies that motivated an upgrading from evidence level 2 to level 3 (Fig. 2).

Homogeneity tests were performed for all exposures for which we could conclude that there was an association to ischemic heart disease. The tests showed that results were comparable for men and women, for general population versus specific occupation cohorts, and for prospective studies versus case-control studies. For job strain, the homogeneity test showed that the findings were similar for participants with low and high socioeconomic status. For low decision latitude, however, when socioeconomic group was taken into account, the association had a lower magnitude for white-collar workers than for blue-collar workers. For both exposures, adjustment for lifestyle factors such as smoking and physical activity during leisure time had small effects on the associations with IHD. The homogeneity tests also showed that the association between job strain and IHD was stronger during recent years than previously.

In order to explore the possibility that we had had a positive bias in our quality assessments, we produced "funnel plots" for some of the associations. This pertained, for instance, to 22 studies of job strain. The figure showed that in these medium high to high-quality studies, those with "positive findings" that had a large standard error and a disproportionately large odds ratio had not been favored in the assessment process.

With regard to chemical job exposure, a large number of exposures were reviewed (SBU 2017), and grades 2 to 3 evidence for chemical job exposure and heart disease risk was found for arsenic, asbestos, benzo-a-pyrene, plumb,

11 Occupational Determinants of Cardiovascular Disorders Including Stroke

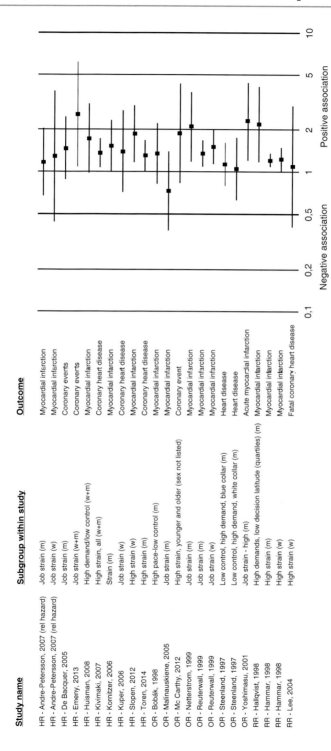

Fig. 1 Association (mostly gender specific) between job strain and development of ischemic heart disease. The graph is based on age-standardized data in studies expressing the strength of the association either as hazard ratios (HR), odds ratios (OR), or relative risk (RR). (From Theorell et al. 2016)

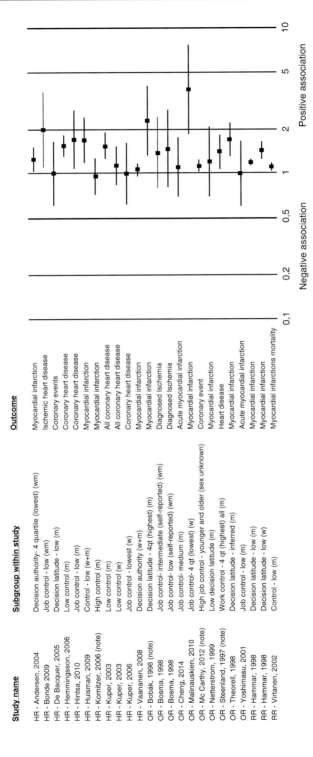

Fig. 2 Association between low decision latitude and development of ischemic heart disease. (From Theorell et al. 2016)

electrolytic aluminum production, phenoxy acids with TCDD (pesticides), carbon disulfide, carbon monoxide, quartz dust, motor exhaust, nitroglycerine, metalworking fluids, welding, and tobacco smoke. Among those the strongest evidence (grade 3) was found for asbestos, phenoxy acids with TCDD, quartz dust, and motor exhaust. It should be pointed out that for quartz dust, there was evidence only for cor pulmonale (lung-related disease in the right side of the heart) and not for ischemic heart disease. The excess risks associated with chemical job exposure were broadly speaking of the same magnitude as those for psychosocial and organizational factors. Many more factors were reviewed, and for most of those, there were few studies of sufficient quality. Hence it was not possible to draw any conclusions regarding associations for those factors.

There are not so many published medium- to high-quality studies of chemical job exposure in relation to stroke risk. However grade 2 evidence was found for exposure to plumb, electrolytic aluminum production, phenoxy acids, and carbon disulfide.

What Can we Make out of this?

For some of the chemical exposures, a direct chemical biological effect is likely. The toxicity could be expressed in many different ways. Breakdown of a toxic agent may require large amounts of an enzyme needed for regulation of normal functions. In this way a competition may arise in which natural regulatory functions will be weakened. One example, the breakdown of some toxic agents containing alcohol molecules, requires alcohol dehydrogenase. This enzyme is needed also for the breakdown of some steroids, for instance, cortisol. This means that these kinds of toxic agents could prolong the effects of cortisol which is one of the key agents in long-term stress reactions. Another example, during later years immunological mechanisms have been discussed, and these seem to be particularly relevant for quartz dust, tobacco smoke, and motor exhaust. These kinds of chemical exposures activate the same immunological mechanisms that are relevant for psychosocial factors – exposure to inhaled dust, tobacco smoke, and motor exhaust gives rise to endothelial dysfunction activating proinflammatory cytokines which start inflammatory reactions in the vessel walls which are exactly the mechanism we discuss in relation to cardiovascular long-term effects of psychosocial stress. Regenerative functions related among other things to the parasympathetic system may in such situations protect the artery wall from long-term adverse effects. Long-term stress may inhibit such protective mechanisms. Hence when there is adverse exposure, the same injuring and protecting biological mechanisms are operating for psychosocial and organizational factors as for adverse chemical exposure (see Theorell et al. 2015 for a more detailed discussion).

There is considerable accumulating evidence showing that psychosocial factors with relevance to work organization are related to risk of developing premature ischemic heart disease and stroke. The most established theoretical model, the demand control model, has been subjected to many observational high to medium high-quality studies. The number of such studies including the effort-reward imbalance model has increased since 2014 (for instance, Dragano et al. 2017). It is reasonable to say that there is now evidence on the third GRADE level (moderate) for a relationship between those two models and development of ischemic heart disease. Even for those models, the number of published controlled intervention studies is still too small for an upgrading to level 4, so there is a strong need for more controlled intervention studies. A new development in the literature is that the risk of experiencing recurring events of ischemic heart disease with exposure to job strain and effort-reward imbalance has been studied more systematically (Li et al. 2015). The results from four published studies of high quality indicate that the relative excess risk associated with job strain or effort-reward imbalance may be greater than the relative excess risk for a first event among persons without previous heart disease. Furthermore, in the review by Kivimäki and Steptoe (2018), it was concluded that job stress may be an even more important target in populations with accepted risk factors (such as smoking, adverse lipoprotein patterns, obesity, or high blood pressure) than in populations without such risk factors.

Several theoretical problems are however still being discussed regarding the two dominating job stress models.

Firstly, it has been argued that there is no empirical solid basis for the hypothesis that there is an interaction between high psychological demands and low decision latitude (Karasek 1979) in generating cardiovascular risk. This is true of both models. It is very hard to prove the existence of multiplicative interaction since such interaction tests require very large samples. However, with regard to the demand control model, many researchers have reasoned that this may not be crucial since there is additive interaction – the effects are added to one another. The joint use of the demand and decision latitude scales mostly improves predictions (see Kivimäki et al. 2015b, Peter et al. 2002, and Bosma et al. 1998). Additive effects are also important because such effects imply that subjects who have both high demands and low decision latitude tend to have a higher risk than those with either high demands or low decision latitude. These kinds of problems have been discussed extensively for the demand control model but so far less extensively for the effort-reward imbalance model.

Secondly the operational definitions of job strain and effort-reward imbalance vary in different studies. The most common definition of job strain is based upon median split. This means that subjects who report psychological demands above and decision latitude below the median of the respective distributions are operationally defined as having job strain. Since we are dealing with normal distributions, there will be a large number of participants centered around the means. In some samples the majority in this group are not really exposed to job strain since they are located in the middle and will not differ very much from other subjects who are also in the middle but happened to place themselves on the other side of the median. Definitions in which the middle group is excluded – with comparisons made between groups with more contrast – should be preferred. The net result of the median split operation is underestimation of the true association between job strain and cardiovascular risk. It has been pointed out, however, that it is important to use an agreed-upon definition since otherwise the temptation to "fishing for significance" increases (Kivimäki et al. 2015b). To publish operational definitions in advance and then stick rigidly to them during the analysis of epidemiological data has been a hallmark of the IPD Work study.

Thirdly there are several versions of the demand control and effort-reward questionnaires. It has been pointed out that the use of questionnaires with imprecise assessments may increase the risk of underestimation of true associations (Choi et al. 2013). Another risk arises if the questionnaires do not conform with the original theory. Psychological demands and effort are theoretically different, and the questionnaires tapping those two should be different. It has happened in the past that psychological demands and effort have been assessed with the same questionnaire. Sometimes social support has been used as a proxy for reward. Such measurements make it impossible to disentangle the effects of the two models. However, when adequate assessments are made, it has been shown that the two models add to one another in cardiovascular prediction.

There was evidence for several other work conditions being linked to IHD among the employees. Limited evidence (grade 2) was found for the combination of job strain and poor support at work = iso-strain as well as for low support at work per se, low work place justice, poor skill discretion, insecure employment, night work, long working week, and noise.

Few studies have used both ischemic heart disease and stroke as outcomes in the same study. One exception was the study by Torén et al. (2014) which showed that among men (no women in the study) there was a significant relationship between job strain and IHD risk even after adjustment for other risk factors with a hazard ratio of 1.31. But in the same study, there was no relationship between job strain and stroke risk. A large study based upon the IPD Work collaboration examining the relationship between long working hours and incidence of coronary heart disease was published in August 2015. This study was based upon 5 published and 17 hitherto unpublished prospective studies of the relationship between long working hours and coronary heart disease. The general conclusion was that there is a weak relationship between long working hours and cardiovascular disease but that this may be mediated or confounded by other risk factors (Kivimäki et al. 2017). On the other hand, in the same study, long working hours showed a robust progressive relationship to stroke risk even after adjustment for other risk factors. 55 working hours per week or more were associated with a relative risk of stroke development of 1.33 (1.11–1.61) compared to regular working hours.

That there is moderately strong evidence from observation studies that job strain is associated with increased cardiovascular disease risk is consistent with the large IPD Work study (Kivimäki et al. 2012) with its standardization of exposure and outcome data in a number of European cohort studies. The findings showed a clear relationship that was consistent across gender, geographical region, socioeconomic status, publication status (published/unpublished), and lifestyle. It was possible in the IPD cohort study to examine delayed onset of myocardial infarction – 3 years or more after the work environment description. This showed that the findings in the delayed version were very similar to the findings for more near-future events –

illustrating that symptoms heralding heart disease did not influence the work descriptions (something that could possibly have inflated the association).

Results published after 2014 do not change these conclusions regarding the demand control model. Based upon the results from our review, we concluded that case-control studies with hard endpoint cardiovascular outcome (mostly myocardial infarction) show findings that are very similar to the prospective studies. Our conclusions are also consistent with the conclusions made by Kivimäki and Kawachi (2015) in their recent review. In all the reviews, the authors have concluded that there is convincing evidence for an association between job strain and cardiovascular risk although intervention studies are lacking which makes it impossible to use grade 4 for the evidence. For job strain the conclusion was even *that more observational studies are not needed*. Kivimäki and Kawachi recommended intervention studies examining the cardiovascular preventive potential of working with these work risk factors.

We note that low decision latitude in itself is a risk factor with the same evidence grade as job strain – albeit with lower odds ratios. Low decision latitude at work is correlated with social class, and accordingly adjustment for social class reduces the magnitude of the association. Subjects who grow up in poor socioeconomic conditions, particularly those maintaining poor conditions as adults, are more likely to be exposed to adverse working conditions than other people. However, adjusting for social class means that the adverse effects of these conditions may be "controlled away." Such adverse conditions partly explain why socioeconomic status is related to higher illness risk. There is no ideal solution to this theoretical problem – we need information about associations both adjusted and non-adjusted for social class.

Job insecurity is less established than job strain and poor decision latitude (grade 2). However, since job insecurity is an important potential risk factor in the modern working world with more and more jobs becoming redundant, more studies are recommended in the future. The same statement relates to low support, unfavorable social climate, lack of procedural and relational justice, conflicts with superiors and colleagues, and limited skill discretion.

It should be pointed out that some of the adverse conditions discussed in this review show some overlap but are also partly unrelated to one another. The implication of this is important since it means that the total effect of adverse working conditions is much greater than each one of the relatively small odds ratios indicate. The population attributable risk for job strain in relation to acute IHD is in the order of 5%. This is if we assume a relative risk of 1.3 and a prevalence of job strain of 22%. If the risks related to insecure employment, long working hours, effort-reward imbalance, noise, night work, poor social climate, lack of social support, conflicts, and lack of procedural and relational justice are added to one another, the effects on a societal level are substantial despite the fact that each one of the excess risks is moderate or small. There is also increasing evidence showing that a similar set of adverse working conditions is associated with increased incidence of stroke (Torén et al. 2014) and with the onset of diabetes 2 (Nyberg et al. 2014).

Among the exposures included in this review, there are some that are more objectively assessed, such as number of working hours and noise, whereas the assessments of others are more subjectively flavored. Conflicts, lack of justice, and social support are examples of psychosocial dimensions that are difficult to assess by means of objective assessments. Decision latitude is interesting from this point of view since it has been shown that self-reported decision latitude correlates highly with expert ratings and job exposure matrix measures of decision latitude (Theorell and Hasselhorn 2005). Psychological demands could be divided into several kinds of demands such as quantitative, cognitive, and emotional (Kristensen et al. 2004). In the demand control model, the five questions about psychological demands mainly reflect quantitative demands. Correlations with expert ratings and job exposure matrix assessments are lower for psychological demands than for decision latitude.

Decision latitude has two components (Karasek 1979), namely, decision authority (which corresponds to everyday workplace democracy) and skill discretion (which corresponds to possibility to develop skills which are needed for decision latitude). In most studies the two components are added to one another, but in some studies (for instance, in the British Whitehall II studies of British state employees), decision latitude only includes decision authority. This does not seem to have any importance for the job strain findings. There is some evidence (grade 2) however that low skill discretion when treated separately is associated with elevated IHD incidence.

During later years research studies of the association between work environment factors and illness outcomes have become increasingly sophisticated. For instance, Shields (2006), Stansfeld et al. (2012), and De Lange et al. (2002) have examined possible effects of exposure at least twice, or even three times, in the follow-up survey waves to job strain. Their findings indicate that accumulated or increasing job strain has a stronger adverse statistical effect on risk of experiencing increased ratings of depressive symptoms during follow-up than decreasing job strain. As might be expected, these studies show that two or more assessments of the job situation provide more precise information regarding risk than only one measurement. Similar observations have been made on the relationship between psychosocial working conditions and coronary heart disease. This has been shown, for instance, in the Whitehall II study (Chandola et al. 2008). Accordingly stronger evidence regarding the influence of working conditions on poor health may be expected in future research with a growing body of studies with such methodology.

Finally it should be pointed out that that chemical and psychosocial job exposure might also interact. Carreon et al. (2014) showed that subjects who had been exposed to both shift work and carbon disulfide had almost three times higher risk of developing cardiovascular disease than those exposed to neither of those factors, whereas subjects who either worked shift work or were exposed to carbon disulfide did not have a significantly elevated IHD risk. There may be many such interactions although they have not yet been studied. In addition, interaction between psychosocial and chemical job conditions could take place on a less sophisticated level. When workers have psychosocial working conditions (i.e., with job strain and lack of social support), they may be less likely to use protection equipment because they lack control or because they have insufficient time to apply the equipment (Torp et al. 2005).

Our results showed that similar work conditions were related to a similar increase in incidence of IHD among men and women. However, although there is no gender difference in excess risk associated with adverse work conditions, studies have shown that women actually have higher levels of job strain than men (Theorell and Hasselhorn 2005). This is despite the fact that working women have a lower incidence of IHD than working men.

A limitation of our review could be that we may have underestimated the importance of work environment factors that have not been subjected to many empirical studies. This illustrates the need for more detailed studies of different aspects of working conditions.

Societal Relevance

It could be argued that individual psychological treatments may be sufficient to handle psychosocial problems related to cardiovascular risk and that accordingly work organization and working condition for the subject could be disregarded. A recent Cochrane review (Richards et al. 2017) concluded that individual psychological treatments directly tailored to patients with heart disease did reduce the risk of cardiac deaths and also reduced participant-reported symptoms of depression, anxiety, and stress. Psychological interventions did not reduce mortality related to other causes, however. Nor did they reduce the risk associated with cardiac surgery or having another heart attack. In the Cochrane review, the age range of the patients was 59 to 67 (median 59.6). This means that job conditions were important for a majority of them. The duration of the beneficial effects of psychological treatments in secondary prevention is likely to improve if the intervention involves a thorough job discussion and an adaptation of them to the psychosocial needs of the patient and his/her colleagues.

Another argument has been that the odds ratios associated with specific work environment factors are relatively small. Richards et al. make the point (2017) that the relative excess risk of developing IHD among subjects with job strain is lower than the corresponding risk associated with unemployment and that most of the accepted biological risk factors are associated with higher levels of excess risk. While this is not the topic of the present chapter, it has been shown that specified work environment problems are associated not only with increased IHD and stroke risk. Job strain, for instance, is also associated with increased risk of developing depression, diabetes, and low back pain. This means that an improved work environment is important also for other health outcomes. Accordingly, there are strong arguments for decreased job strain if we widen the perspective to other health outcomes. It should also be pointed out that similar conclusions are made, for instance, with regard to other identified work environment problems such as exposure to carbon disulfide, tobacco smoke at work, noise, effort-reward imbalance, night work, extremely long work weeks, and lack of social support. Some individuals may concomitantly have several of these psychosocial adverse job conditions as well as IHD-relevant chemical exposure at work. If we take into account all the exposures and all possible health outcomes at once, it becomes obvious that working conditions constitute a major public health concern.

As has been argued by several authors (see, for instance, Theorell 2012), improvement of working conditions is not only about eliminating and reducing adverse factors but also about stimulation of regenerative and protective biological processes. In psychosocial terms I am referring to improved social support and leadership as well as improved decision latitude for employees.

The work environment factors for which we found scientific evidence for an association to IHD development are possible to influence by means of work organization changes and reduced exposure to chemical agents. It should be pointed out that certain psychosocial work conditions can make it difficult for employees to protect themselves against adverse physical (for instance, noise) and chemical exposures. Accordingly, the psychosocial factors are intertwined with the chemical and physical exposures.

It has been shown that decision latitude for employees can be improved by analysis of the work organization with subsequent goal-directed organization intervention (Michie and Williams 2003) or by a year-long education of managers about psychosocial factors (Theorell et al. 2001; Romanowska et al. 2011). Reviews of natural experiments designed to reduce psychosocial risks in the work environment have shown that such interventions may result in reduced biological stress and improved health in that group (Jauregui and Schnall 2009; Hasson et al. 2012; Montano et al. 2014). The present results also suggest that in assessment and treatment plans for patients with already manifest IHD, work environment should be taken into account since the work environment seems to be even more important in secondary prevention than it is in primary prevention.

Cross-References

- ▶ Coronary Heart Disease and Return to Work
- ▶ Occupational Determinants of Affective Disorders
- ▶ Return to Work After Stroke
- ▶ Work-Related Burden of Absenteeism, Presenteeism, and Disability: An Epidemiologic and Economic Perspective

References

Belkic KL, Landsbergis PA, Schnall PL, Baker D (2004) Is job strain a major source of cardiovascular disease risk? Scand J Work Environ Health 30:85–128

Bosma H, Peter R, Siegrist J, Marmot M (1998) Two alternative job stress models and the risk of coronary heart disease. Am J Public Health 88:68–74

Carreon T, Hein MJ, Hanley KW, Viet SM, Ruder AM (2014) Coronary artery disease and cancer mortality in a cohort of workers exposed to vinyl chloride, carbon disulfide, rotating shift work, and o-toluidine at a chemical manufacturing plant. Am J Ind Med 57:398–411

Chandola T, Britton A, Brunner E, Hemingway H, Malik M, Kumari M, Badrick E, Kivimaki M, Marmot M (2008) Work stress and coronary heart disease: what are the mechanisms? Eur Heart J 29:640–648

Choi B, Dobson M, Landsbergis PA, Ko S, Yang H, Schnall P, Baker DRE (2013) Need for more individual-level meta-analyses in social epidemiology: example of job strain and coronary heart disease. Am J Epidemiol 178:1007–1008

de Lange AH, Taris TW, Kompier MA, Houtman IL, Bongers PM (2002) Effects of stable and changing demand-control histories on worker health. Scand J Work Environ Health 28:94–108

Demerouti E, Bakker AB, Nachreiner F, Schaufeli WB (2001) The job demands-resources model of burnout. J Appl Psychol 86:499–512

Dragano N, Siegrist J, Nyberg ST, Lunau T, Fransson EI, Alfredsson L, Bjorner JB, Borritz M, Burr H, Erbel R, Fahlén G, Goldberg M, Hamer M, Heikkilä K, Jöckel KH, Knutsson A, Madsen IEH, Nielsen ML, Nordin M, Oksanen T, Pejtersen JH, Pentti J, Rugulies R, Salo P, Schupp J, Singh-Manoux A, Steptoe A, Theorell T, Vahtera J, Westerholm PJM, Westerlund H, Virtanen M, Zins M, Batty GD, Kivimäki M, IPD-Work consortium (2017) Effort-reward imbalance at work and incident coronary heart disease: a Multicohort Study of 90,164 individuals. Epidemiology 28:619–626. https://doi.org/10.1097/EDE.0000000000000666

Eller NH, Netterstrøm B, Gyntelberg F, Kristensen TS, Nielsen F, Steptoe A, Theorell T (2009) Work-related psychosocial factors and the development of ischemic heart disease: a systematic review. Cardiol Rev 17:83–97

Feigin VL, Forouzanfar MH, Krishnamurthi R, Mensah GA, Connor M, Bennett DA, Moran AE, Sacco RL, Anderson L, Truelsen T, O'Donnell M, Venketasubramanian N, Barker-Collo S, Lawes CM, Wang W, Shinohara Y, Witt E, Ezzati M, Naghavi M, Murray C (2014) Global burden of diseases, injuries, and risk factors study 2010 (GBD 2010) and the GBD Stroke Experts Group. Global and regional burden of stroke during 1990–2010: findings from the Global Burden of Disease Study 2010. Lancet 383(9913):245–254

Hasson H, Gilbert-Ouimet M, Baril-Gingras G, Brisson C, Vézina M, Bourbonnais R, Montreuil S (2012) Implementation of an organizational-level intervention on the psychosocial environment of work: comparison of managers' and employees' views. J Occup Environ Med 54:85–91

Hernberg S, Tolonen M, Nurminen M (1976) Eight-year follow-up of viscose rayon workers exposed to carbon disulphide. Scand J Work Env Health 2:27–30

Jauregui M, Schnall PL (2009) Work, psychosocial stressors and the bottom line. In: Schnall PL, Dobson M, Rosskam E (eds) Unhealthy work. Baywood Publishing, Amityville

Johnson JV, Hall EM (1988) Job strain, work place social support, and cardiovascular disease: a cross-sectional study of a random sample of the Swedish working population. Am J Public Health 78:1336–1342

Karasek R (1979) Job demands, job decision latitude and mental strain: implications for job redesign. Adm Sci Q 24:285–307

Karasek RA, Theorell T (1990) Healthy work. Basic Books, New York

Kivimäki M, Kawachi I (2015) Work stress as a risk factor for cardiovascular disease. Curr Cardiol Rep 17:74

Kivimäki M, Steptoe A (2018) Effects of stress on the development and progression of cardiovascular disease. Nat Rev Cardiol 15:215–229. https://doi.org/10.1038/nrcardio.2017.189. Epub 2017 Dec 7

Kivimäki M, Nyberg ST, Batty GD, Fransson EI, Heikkilä K, Alfredsson L, Bjorner JB, Borritz M, Burr H, Casini A, Clays E, De Bacquer D, Dragano N, Ferrie JE, Geuskens GA, Goldberg M, Hamer M, Hooftman WE, Houtman IL, Joensuu M, Jokela M, Kittel F, Knutsson A, Koskenvuo M, Koskinen A, Kouvonen A, Kumari M, Madsen IE, Marmot MG, Nielsen ML, Nordin M, Oksanen T, Pentti J, Rugulies R, Salo P, Siegrist J, Singh-Manoux A, Suominen SB, Väänänen A, Vahtera J, Virtanen M, Westerholm PJ, Westerlund H, Zins M, Steptoe A, Theorell T, IPD-Work Consortium (2012) Job strain as a risk factor for coronary heart disease: a collaborative meta-analysis of individual participant data. Lancet 380:1491–1497

Kivimäki M, Jokela M, Nyberg ST, Singh-Manoux A, Fransson EI, Alfredsson L, Bjorner JB, Borritz M, Burr H, Casini A, Clays E, De Bacquer D, Dragano N, Erbel R, Geuskens GA, Hamer M, Hooftman WE, Houtman IL, Jöckel KH, Kittel F, Knutsson A, Koskenvuo M, Lunau T, Madsen IE, Nielsen ML, Nordin M, Oksanen T, Pejtersen JH, Pentti J, Rugulies R, Salo P, Shipley MJ, Siegrist J, Steptoe A, Suominen SB, Theorell T, Vahtera J, Westerholm PJ, Westerlund H, O'Reilly D, Kumari M, Batty GD, Ferrie JE, Virtanen M, IPD-Work Consortium (2015a) Long working hours and risk of coronary heart disease and stroke: a systematic review and meta-analysis of published and unpublished data for 603 838 individuals. Lancet 386:1739–1746

Kivimäki M, Nyberg ST, Kawachi I (2015b) Authors' reply: calculation of population attributable risk should to be based on robust estimates. Scand J Work Environ Health 41:506–507

Kivimäki M, Nyberg ST, Batty GD, Kawachi I, Jokela M, Alfredsson L, Bjorner JB, Borritz M, Burr H, Dragano N, Fransson EI, Heikkilä K, Knutsson A, Koskenvuo M, Kumari M, Madsen IEH, Nielsen ML, Nordin M, Oksanen T, Pejtersen JH, Pentti J, Rugulies R, Salo P, Shipley MJ, Suominen S, Theorell T, Vahtera J, Westerholm P, Westerlund H, Steptoe A, Singh-Manoux A, Hamer M, Ferrie JE, Virtanen M, Tabak AG, IPD-Work consortium (2017) Long working hours as a risk factor for atrial fibrillation: a multi-cohort study. Eur Heart J 38:2621–2628

Kristensen TS, Kornitzer M, Alfredsson L (1998) Social factors, work, stress and cardiovascular disease prevention. The European Heart Network, Brussels

Kristensen TS, Bjorner JB, Christensen KB, Borg V (2004) The distinction between work pace and working hours in the measurement of quantitative demands at work. Work Stress 18:305. https://doi.org/10.1080/02678370412331314005

Li J, Zhang M, Loerbroks A, Angerer P, Siegrist J (2015) Work stress and the risk of recurrent coronary heart disease events: a systematic review and meta-analysis. Int J Occup Med Environ Health 28:8–19

Michie S, Williams S (2003) Reducing work related psychological ill health and sickness absence: a systematic literature review. Occup Environ Med 60.3–9

Moher D, Liberati A, Tetzlaff J, Altman DG (2009) Preferred reporting items for systematic reviews and meta-analyses: the PRISMA statement. Ann Internal Med 151:264–269

Montano D, Hoven H, Siegrist J (2014) Effects of organisational-level interventions at work on employees' health: a systematic review. BMC Public Health 14:135

Nationella Kvalitetsregister. Nationellt register för hjärtintensivvård, kranskärlsröntgen, PCI, hjärtkirurgi och sekundärprevention – SWEDE-HEART (National register for acute coronary care, coronary artery X-ray, PCI, heart surgery and secondary prevention – SWEDE-HEART, Jernberg, T. http://www.kvalitetsregister.se/hittaregister/registerarkiv/hjartkarlsjukdom.187.htmal

Nyberg ST, Fransson EI, Heikkilä K, Ahola K, Alfredsson L, Bjorner JB, Borritz M, Burr H, Dragano N, Goldberg M, Hamer M, Jokela M, Knutsson A, Koskenvuo M, Koskinen A, Kouvonen A, Leineweber C, Madsen IE, Magnusson Hanson LL, Marmot MG, Nielsen ML, Nordin M, Oksanen T, Pejtersen JH, Pentti J, Rugulies R, Salo P, Siegrist J, Steptoe A, Suominen S, Theorell T, Väänänen A, Vahtera J, Virtanen M, Westerholm PJ, Westerlund H, Zins M, Batty GD, Brunner EJ, Ferrie JE, Singh-Manoux A, Kivimäki M, IPD-Work Consortium (2014) Job strain as a risk factor for type 2 diabetes: a pooled analysis of 124,808 men and women. Diabetes Care 37:2268–2275

Peter R, Siegrist J, Hallqvist J, Reuterwall C, Theorell T, SHEEP Study Group (2002) Psychosocial work environment and myocardial infarction: improving risk estimation by combining two complementary job stress models in the SHEEP Study. J Epidemiol Comm Health 56:294–300

Piepoli MF, Agewall S, Albus C, Brotons C, Catapano AL, Cooney M-T, Corra U, Cosyns B, Deaton C, Graham I, Hall MS, Hobbs FDR, Löchen M-L, Löllge HL, Marques-Vidal P, Perk J, Prescott E, Redon J, Richter DJ, Sattar N, Smulders Y, Tiberi M, van der Worp HB, van Dis I, Verschuren WMM (2016) 2016 European guidelines on cardiovascular disease prevention in clinical practice: the sixth joint task force of the European Society of Cardiology and Other

Societies on Cardiovascular Disease Prevention in Clinical Practice. Eur Heart J 37:2315–2381. https://doi.org/10.1093/eurheartj/ehw106

Richards SH, Anderson L, Jenkinson CE, Whalley B, Rees K, Davies P, Bennett P, Liu Z, West R, Thompson DR, Taylor RS (2017) Psychological interventions for coronary heart disease: cochrane systematic review and meta-analysis. Cochrane Library

Romanowska J, Larsson G, Eriksson M, Wikström BM, Westerlund H, Theorell T (2011) Health effects on leaders and co-workers of an art-based leadership development program. Psychother Psychosom 80:78–87

SBU (2017) Arbetsmiljöns betydelse för hjärtkärlsjukdom – exponering för kemiska ämnen. (The significance of the work environment to heart disease – exposure to chemical agents. Albin M, Hall C, Hogstedt C, Sjögren B, Theorell T) Stockholm: Statens beredning för medicinsk och social utvärdering (SBU); SBU-rapport nr 261/2017

Shields M (2006) Stress and depression in the employed population. Health Rep 17:11–29

Siegrist J (1996) Adverse health effects of high-effort/low-reward conditions. J Occup Health Psychol 1:27–41

Stansfeld SA, Shipley MJ, Head J, Fuhrer R (2012) Repeated job strain and the risk of depression: longitudinal analyses from the Whitehall II study. Am J Public Health 102:2360–2366

Theorell T (2012) Stress reduction programmes for the workplace. In: Gatchel RJ, Schultz IZ (eds) Handbook of occupational health and wellness. Springer, Boston, pp 383–403

Theorell T, Hasselhorn HM (2005) On cross-sectional questionnaire studies of relationships between psychosocial conditions at work and health – are they reliable? Int Arch Occup Environ Health 78:517–522

Theorell T, Emdad R, Arnetz B, Weingarten AM (2001) Employee effects of an educational program for managers at an insurance company. Psychosom Med 63:724–733

Theorell T, Brisson C, Vezina M, Milot A, Gilbert-Ouimet M (2015) Psychosocial factors in the prevention of cardiovascular disease. Chapter 18. In: Gielen S, de Backer G, Piepoli MF, Wood D (eds) The ESC textbook of preventive cardiology. Oxford University Press, London

Theorell T, Jood K, Slunga Järvholm L, Vingård E, Perk J, Östergren P-O, Hall C (2016) A systematic review of studies in the contribution of the work environment to ischemic heart disease development. BMC Public Health 26:470–477

Torén K, Schiöler L, Giang WK, Novak M, Söderberg M, Rosengren A (2014) A longitudinal general population-based study of job strain and risk for coronary heart disease and stroke in Swedish men. BMJ Open 4(3):e004355. https://doi.org/10.1136/bmjopen-2013-004355

Torp S, Grøgaard JB, Moen BE, Bråtveit M (2005) The impact of social and organizational factors on workers' use of personal protective equipment: a multilevel approach. J Occup Environ Med 47:829–837

Occupational Determinants of Affective Disorders

12

Reiner Rugulies, Birgit Aust, and Ida E. H. Madsen

Contents

Introduction	208
What Are Affective Disorders?	208
Definition and Diagnosis	209
Prevalence	211
Etiology	213
Working Conditions and Risk of Depressive Disorders	217
Theoretical and Methodological Issues	217
Results from Systematic Reviews and Meta-analyses	218
Interpretation and Discussion of the Epidemiological Evidence	222
Future Research Needs	225
Summary and Conclusion	230
Cross-References	231
References	231

Abstract

Affective disorders encompass mental disorders related to excessively elated and depressed mood, referred in clinical diagnostic terms as manic episode, bipolar disorders, and depressive disorders. The etiology of affective disorders is complex and only partly understood. Regarding the role of working conditions in the etiology of affective disorders, research evidence is currently limited to depressive disorders. We present results from recent reviews and meta-analyses of prospective cohort

---

R. Rugulies (✉)
National Research Centre for the Working Environment, Copenhagen, Denmark

Department of Public Health, University of Copenhagen, Copenhagen, Denmark

Department of Psychology, University of Copenhagen, Copenhagen, Denmark
e-mail: rer@nfa.dk

B. Aust · I. E. H. Madsen
National Research Centre for the Working Environment, Copenhagen, Denmark
e-mail: bma@nfa.dk; ihm@nfa.dk

© Springer Nature Switzerland AG 2020
U. Bültmann, J. Siegrist (eds.), *Handbook of Disability, Work and Health*, Handbook Series in Occupational Health Sciences, https://doi.org/10.1007/978-3-030-24334-0_10

studies showing that the combination of high job demands and low job control (denoted as job strain), low job control in itself, the imbalance between high efforts and low rewards at work, and high job insecurity are associated with a moderately increased risk of depressive disorders. Long working hours are associated with a weak, albeit statistically significant increased risk; however the associations vary across different world regions. Exposure to workplace bullying is strongly associated with risk of depressive disorders; however, this result is based on only a few studies. We critically discuss the epidemiological evidence while considering various potential biases leading to both over- and underestimation of the reported associations. We conclude with pointing to future research needs for a better understanding of the role of working conditions in the etiology of depressive disorders, including strategies to address biases; a stronger focus on a work-life course perspective; the analyses of possible effect modification by other variables, including contextual factors; approaches for advancing theory and understanding mechanisms; and the development, implementation, and comprehensive evaluation of workplace intervention studies.

Keywords

Occupational health · Psychosocial work environment · Stress · Depression · Anxiety · Social psychiatry · Psychosocial epidemiology · Meta-analysis

Introduction

In this chapter we review and discuss the current research evidence regarding the contribution of working conditions to the development of affective disorders. We have divided the chapter into two parts. The first part addresses what affective disorders are and discusses their definition, diagnoses, prevalence, and etiology. The second part presents results from systematic reviews and meta-analyses on the association between working conditions and depressive disorders, provides an interpretation and discussion of the research evidence, and considers future research needs. The chapter closes with a summary and conclusion.

We recently published a book chapter on a specific psychosocial working condition, effort-reward imbalance, and risk of affective disorders (Rugulies et al. 2016). For the current chapter, we reused some parts of this previous chapter, in particular regarding definition, diagnoses, prevalence, and etiology of affective disorders. We also sometimes refer to this previous chapter for more detailed information and for additional references.

What Are Affective Disorders?

In this first part of the chapter, we describe and discuss the main characteristics of affective disorders, in terms of their definition and diagnosis, prevalence, and etiology.

Definition and Diagnosis

The term "affective disorders," also called "mood disorders," is a superordinate concept encompassing different types of mental disorders related to peoples' emotions and feelings. It pertains to both excessively elated and depressed mood. The concept evolved in the eighteenth century, parallel to the rise of psychiatry as a new medical discipline (Blazer 2005). A key figure in the rise of psychiatry was the German psychiatrist Emil Kraepelin (1856–1926) who developed a comprehensive nosology of mental disorders including the distinction between *dementia praecox* and *manic-depressive insanity* that correspond to the diagnoses of schizophrenia and affective disorders in contemporary psychiatry (Kendler 1986).

There are two main diagnostic tools for mental disorders. One tool is the *International Classification of Diseases and Related Health Problems* of the World Health Organization (WHO), currently in its 10th version, covering both somatic diseases and mental disorders (ICD-10, World Health Organization 2015; the ICD-11 has been released by WHO in June 2018 and will come into effect in 2022). The other tool is the *Diagnostic and Statistical Manual of Mental Disorders* of the American Psychiatric Association, currently in its 5th edition, solely covering mental disorders (DSM-5, American Psychiatric Association 2013). Whereas the ICD-10 lists manic episode, bipolar disorders, and depressive disorders under the common header "mood (affective) disorders," the DSM-5 does no longer have a common header for these disorders but uses the separate headers "depressive disorders" and "bipolar and related disorders."

The Paradigm Shift in Psychiatry in 1980

The diagnosis of mental disorders in both ICD-10 and DSM-5 are, with a few exceptions, based on the presence of specific symptoms and do not consider possible causes of the disorder. This is a consequence of a paradigm shift in the classification of mental disorders that occurred in 1980 when the American Psychiatric Association replaced the DSM-II with the DSM-III. The DSM-III revolutionized psychiatry, discarding the previous etiological concepts of mental disorders and replacing them with atheoretical and etiology-free symptom lists. With regard to depressive disorders, for example, the previous distinction between *endogenous depressive disorders*, i.e., depressive disorders primarily originating from within the individual (encompassing the diagnoses of *involutional melancholia* and *manic-depressive illness, depressive type*), and *exogenous depressive disorders*, i.e., depressive disorders as an excessive reactions to life experiences (encompassing the diagnoses of *psychotic depressive reaction* and *depressive neurosis*), was replaced with the new diagnosis of *major depressive episode* that is based on the number and severity of symptoms and level of impairment (Blazer 2005).

The DSM-III paradigm shift, also called a *neo-Kraepelinian* revolution, ended the dominance of a psychodynamic-oriented psychiatry in a Freudian tradition, at least in the United States. According to Mayes and Horwitz (2005), the paradigm shift had multiple reasons, including concerns that the government and insurance companies no longer were willing to pay for psychotherapies for the "worried well" but instead wanted to identify those with the more severe disorders. Psychiatrists were further concerned about facing increasing competition by clinical psychologists and social workers who were offering "talk therapy" at relatively inexpensive rates. There was also a general desire among psychiatrists to make psychiatry more research-focused like other branches of medicine. Mayes and Horwitz concluded that this paradigm shift "was not the result of a carefully orchestrated conspiracy, but neither was it an accident or 'chance-like-sequence' of event as some have argued." It also "did not stem from any new knowledge about the causes of mental illnesses nor their treatments." Instead, the paradigm shift was mainly the result of "efforts of research-oriented psychiatrists who wanted to standardize diagnostic criteria and focus attention on the symptoms of mental disorders, rather than on their underlying causes" (Mayes and Horwitz 2005, p. 265).

For a more detailed discussion on this paradigm shift and past and current controversies on the DSM and the ICD, in particular with regard to the diagnoses of depressive disorders, see Mayes and Horwitz (2005), Blazer (2005), Bolwig and Shorter (2007), Wakefield (2015), Rugulies et al. (2016). For a discussion of the fundamental question if mental health and mental disorders should be viewed as categorical (as DSM and ICD do) or dimensional (i.e., be on a continuous scale), see the article by Krueger et al. (2018), including the commentaries to the article.

The Diagnosis of Affective Disorders in the ICD-10

In ICD-10, mood (affective) disorders belong to *Chapter V: Mental and Behavioral Disorders* and encompass the diagnostic codes in the block F30 to F39 (World Health Organization 1992, 2015). Table 1 gives an overview of these codes. Disorders related to elated mood or the mixture of elated and depressed mood are classified under F30 (manic episode) and F31 (bipolar affective disorders). Disorders related to depressive mood without phases of elation are classified under F32 (depressive episode) and F33 (recurrent depressive disorder). Affective disorders that are persistent but less severe than the disorders classified in F30 to F33 are classified under F34 with a main distinction between cyclothymia (F34.0, related to a persistent and relatively mild bipolar disorder) and dysthymia (F34.1, related to a persistent and relatively mild depressive disorder). Other affective disorders and unspecified affective disorders are classified under F38 and F39, respectively.

The ICD-10 diagnoses of depressive episode (F32) and recurrent depressive disorders (F33) and the corresponding DSM-5 diagnosis of major depression are those with the greatest relevance for this chapter. Table 2 shows the ICD-10 diagnostic criteria for a depressive episode (DSM-5 diagnostic criteria for major depression are similar). There are three core symptoms (depressed mood, loss of interest and enjoyment, and reduced energy) and seven accompanying symptoms, and the number and combination of these symptoms yield diagnoses of a mild, moderate, or severe depressive episode (Table 2). The symptoms should be present for at least 2 weeks, although the ICD-10 allows shorter periods if "symptoms are unusually severe or of rapid onset" (World Health Organization 1992, p. 100). It is assumed that depressive episodes will be accompanied with reduced functioning in core areas of life (work, education, domestic, social), with more severe impairments in the case of a severe depressive episode.

Table 1 ICD-10 diagnoses for mood [affective] disorders (F30-F39)

F30 Manic episode

Hypomania (F30.0); mania without psychotic symptoms (F30.1); mania with psychotic symptoms (F30.2); other manic episodes (F30.8); manic episode, unspecified (F30.9)

F31 Bipolar affective disorder

Current episode hypomanic (F31.0); current episode manic without psychotic symptoms (F31.1); current episode manic with psychotic symptoms (F31.2); current episode mild or moderate depression (F31.3); current episode severe depression without psychotic symptoms (F31.4); current episode severe depression with psychotic symptoms (F31.5); current episode mixed (F31.6); currently in remission (F31.7); other bipolar affective disorders (F31.8); bipolar affective disorders, unspecified (F31.9)

F32 Depressive episode

Mild (F32.0); moderate (F32.1); severe without psychotic symptoms (F32.2); severe with psychotic symptoms (F32.3); other depressive episodes (F32.8); depressive episodes, unspecified (F32.9)

F33 Recurrent depressive disorder

Mild (F33.0); moderate (F33.1); severe without psychotic symptoms (F33.2); severe with psychotic symptoms (F33.3); in remission (F33.4); other recurrent depressive disorders (F33.8); recurrent depressive disorder, unspecified (F33.9)

F34 Persistent mood [affective] disorders

Cyclothymia (F34.0); dysthymia (F34.1); other persistent mood [affective] disorders (F34.8); persistent mood [affective] disorders, unspecified (F34.9)

F38 Other mood [affective] disorders

Other single mood [affective] disorders (F38.1); other recurrent mood [affective] disorders (F38.1); other unspecified mood [affective] disorders (F38.8)

F39 Unspecified mood [affective] disorder

Information in this table derived from (1) World Health Organization (1992). Available from: http://www.who.int/classifications/icd/en/bluebook.pdf and (2) World Health Organization (2015). International Statistical Classification of Diseases and Related Health Problems 10th Revision. ICD-10: Version 2015 (Web Page). Available from: http://apps.who.int/classifications/icd10/browse/2016/en (Accessed 5 November 2018)

Prevalence

Twelve-Month Prevalence

Affective disorders are highly prevalent, worldwide, which is mostly due to the high prevalence of depressive disorders. Figure 1 shows the results from a major review on the 12-month prevalence of selected mental disorders in Europe (Wittchen et al. 2011). The mental disorder with the highest 12-month prevalence (14.0%) was anxiety disorders, encompassing disorders such as panic disorders, phobias, and generalized anxiety disorders. Of the two affective disorders, depressive disorders (denoted as "major depression" in the study) were estimated with a 12-month prevalence of 6.9% (corresponding to 30.3 million affected individuals in Europe), whereas bipolar disorders were estimated with a 12-month prevalence of only 0.9% (corresponding to 3.0 million affected Europeans). The female-male ratio also differed substantially between the two disorders. For depressive disorders it was estimated that women were more than twice as often affected than men (ratio: 2.3),

Table 2 ICD-10 diagnostic criteria for depressive episode (F32, F33)

Core symptoms
•Depressed mood •Loss of interest and enjoyment •Reduced energy leading to increased fatigability and diminished activity
Accompanying symptoms
•Reduced concentration and attention •Reduced self-esteem and self-confidence •Ideas of guilt and unworthiness (even in a mild type of episode) •Bleak and pessimistic views of the future •Ideas or acts of self-harm or suicide •Disturbed sleep •Diminished appetite
Diagnosis
•Symptoms should be present for at least 2 weeks •Mild depressive episode: at least four symptoms including two core symptoms •Moderate depressive episode: at least five, preferable six symptoms including two core symptoms •Severe depressive episode: at least six symptoms including all three core symptoms

Information in this table derived from World Health Organization (1992). Available from: http://www.who.int/classifications/icd/en/bluebook.pdf (Accessed 5 November 2018)

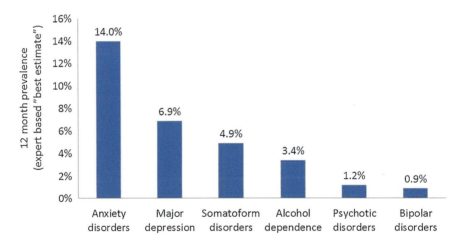

Fig. 1 Twelve-month prevalence of selected mental disorders in Europe (27 European Union member states plus Switzerland, Iceland, and Norway, expert-based "best estimate"). (Own visualization based on results from a study by Wittchen et al. (2011))

whereas for bipolar disorders, the prevalence was similar for women and men (ratio: 1.2).

Lifetime Prevalence

Lifetime prevalence of affective disorders is more difficult to estimate than 12-month prevalence as investigators usually have to rely on the ability of the participants to accurately recall depressive episodes in the past. Some researchers have argued that previously reported lifetime prevalence rates of depressive disorders in the magnitude of about 15% are underestimations, because individuals tend to forget single episodes of depressive disorders, in particular if they have recovered well (Moffitt et al. 2010). Prevalence rates may be further underestimated because studies often do not include specific groups with high prevalence of mental disorders, such as those who are homeless or imprisoned (Moffitt et al. 2010). To overcome these limitations, Moffitt et al. assessed lifetime prevalence of mental disorders in accordance with DSM-IV in the Dunedin New Zealand birth cohort at age 18, 21, 26, and 32. Retention rate at age 32 was 96%, i.e., almost all participants were kept in the cohort. Combining 12-month prevalence at the different points of measurement, the authors calculated a lifetime prevalence of depressive disorders of 41.4% at the age of 32 years (Moffitt et al. 2010). The results were received with great interest, with some researchers pointing out that such a high prevalence may indicate that the definition of depressive disorders in the DMS is flawed and pathologizes normal discomfort, sorrow, and grief (Wakefield 2015).

Etiology

The etiology of affective disorders, including manic episodes, bipolar disorders, and depressive disorders, appears to be highly complex and is to date only partly understood. Research on occupational determinants of affective disorders has almost exclusively focused on depressive disorders. This is understandable, considering that manic episodes and bipolar disorders have a much lower prevalence and seem to be less strongly determined by environmental factors than depressive disorders (Marangoni et al. 2016). Consequently, we will in the following focus on the etiology of depressive disorders only. For a recent systematic review on possible causes of disorders in the manic and bipolar spectrum, see Marangoni et al. (2016).

The Monoamine Hypothesis

As psychiatry is rooted in medicine, it is not surprising that psychiatric research traditionally has a strong focus on biological causes of depressive disorders. The most dominant theory is the *monoamine hypothesis*, postulating that a deficiency of certain neurotransmitters in the brain (serotonin, noradrenalin, dopamine) causes depressive disorders (France et al. 2007). The hypothesis emerged in the 1950s, following the discovery of chlorpromazine for treatment of psychotic disorders and the testing of iproniazid and imipramine for treatment of depressive disorders. The idea that chemical imbalances in the brain cause depression became very popular in both scientific and public debates, and antidepressant medication targeting neurotransmitters is today the primary choice for treating depressive disorders (France et al. 2007). However, research has not succeeded yet in identifying biomarkers for depressive disorders, and neither measures of neurochemicals nor neuroimaging can distinguish individuals with depressive disorders from individuals without such a disorder (France et al. 2007). Thus, there is still only limited support for the monoamine hypothesis.

Psychological and Sociological Theories

Numerous psychological and sociological theories for explaining the development of depressive disorders have been proposed during the last 100 years. Regarding psychological theories, this includes psychodynamic explanations emphasizing the key role of intrapsychic conflicts in reaction to both material and symbolic loss (Davison and Neale 1990), theories from cognitive psychology pointing to mechanisms related to dysfunctional cognitions and negative schemata (Beck 1967), and social psychological theories stressing the role of loss of control and enhanced feelings of helplessness (Seligman 1975) and of problematic interactions between individuals with a disposition for depression and their social environment (Sacco 1999). Regarding sociological theories, prevalence rates of depressive disorders have been shown to be higher in individuals of lower socioeconomic position compared to individuals of higher position (Lorant et al. 2003), and it has been argued that this is due to a higher level of adversity and a lower level of resources among individuals of lower socioeconomic position (Brown and Harris 1978). It has also been argued that the societies of the twenty-first century to a higher degree than earlier societies confront the individuals with opportunities for failure and feelings of inadequacy and insufficiency that may contribute to an increased risk for developing depressive disorders (Ehrenberg 1998). See Rugulies et al. (2016) for a more detailed discussion of these psychological and sociological theories of depressive disorders.

Most psychological and sociological research on depressive disorders considers exposure to adversity an important part in the etiological process. In childhood, the loss of a parent, neglect, and physical and sexual abuse seem to be potent risk factors for onset of depressive disorders later in life (Harris 2001). In adulthood, it seems that in particular the loss of a loved one and experiences related to humiliation and threats to self-esteem are important contributors to the risk of depressive disorders (Brown and Harris 1978; Harris 2001; Kendler et al. 2003). The key role of adversities that undermine individuals' self-esteem has also been emphasized by Brown and Harris in their seminal book *Social Origins of Depression*, where they describe "loss events as the deprivation of sources of value or reward" as the key factors leading to "an inability to hold good thoughts about ourselves, our lives, and those close to us" (Brown and Harris 1978, p. 233).

Psychophysiological Mechanisms

A major challenge for research on psychological and social determinants of both somatic diseases and mental disorders is to understand the biological mechanisms through which these determinants may affect health. With regard to cardiovascular disease (see ▶ Chap. 11, "Occupational Determinants of Cardiovascular Disorders Including Stroke") and depressive disorders, it has been discussed for some time that psychophysiological stress responses, particularly a dysregulation of the hypothalamic-pituitary-adrenal (HPA) axis, likely is a key mechanism for understanding how psychological and social factors may affect health (Horowitz and Zunszain 2015; Kivimäki and Steptoe 2018). Inflammatory processes are also increasingly considered as a potential link between psychological and social factors and risk of ill-health (Horowitz and Zunszain 2015; Kivimäki and Steptoe 2018). But there is still a lot of research needed in this area to fully understand how psychological and social factors elicit biological processes that may affect somatic and mental health.

Genetic Risk Factors and Gene-Environment Interaction

While psychiatry had always shown a great interest in the heritability of mental disorders, this interest increased even further with the mapping of the human genome. However, a recent review on the "genetics of major depression" concluded that genetic research on depressive disorders has not yet reached a stage where it would cast "light on known, suspected or indeed novel biological processes that explain why some people fall ill" (Flint and Kendler 2014, p. 497). Instead "genetics does not support any of the biological theories [of depression] put forward to date (p. 498)." As a possible explanation, the authors suggest that depressive disorders may be influenced by multiple genetic loci and that each only contributes with a small effect. Numerous studies are currently conducted aiming to identify these multiple loci that may have some association with risk of depressive disorders.

It is possible that genes do not directly cause depression but that individuals with a certain genetic disposition might be more likely to develop a depressive disorder when exposed to environmental adversity than individuals without such a disposition. An apparent breakthrough for this gene-environment interaction hypothesis was a study published by Caspi et al. (2003) demonstrating that a polymorphism in the serotonin transporter gene (5-HTTLPR) modified the association of adverse life events with risk of depressive disorders. The association between adverse life events and risk of depressive disorder at age 26 was strongest among participants with two short alleles, weaker among those with one short and one long allele, and even weaker (but still clearly visible) among those with two long alleles. This spectacular result led to numerous replication studies conducted all over the world; however, these replication studies showed mixed results. Some studies found similar associations as Caspi et al. (2003), whereas others found no gene-environment interaction. Several reviews and meta-analyses have summarized these mixed results (for an overview see Rugulies et al. 2016, pp. 112–113). The most recent meta-analyses by Culverhouse et al. (2018), a collaborative study on 31 data sets with more than 38,000 participants of European ancestry, reported a clear main effect of current and lifetime adversity (including childhood maltreatment and broad stress definitions) on risk of depressive disorders (odds ratio: 2.16, 95%; CI: 1.65 to 2.82), no main effect of polymorphism of the serotonin transporter gene (odds ratio: 1.00, 95%; CI: 0.95 to 1.05), and no gene-environment interaction (odds ratio: 1.05, 95%; CI: 0.91 to 1.21).

Influence of Multiple Risk Factors over the Life Course

Considering that no single major cause of depressive disorders has been identified, it is today widely assumed that depressive disorders are caused by multiple risk factors, including biological, psychological, and social factors. Figure 2 shows a selection of risk factors of depressive disorders at different stages of life (childhood, early adolescence, late adolescence, adulthood), derived from research on a developmental model of depressive disorders by Kendler and colleagues (2002, 2006). It is assumed in the figure that risk factors may influence each other, both at the same

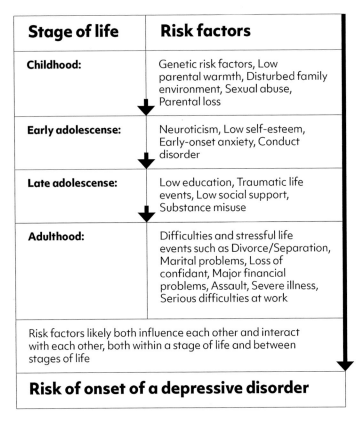

Fig. 2 Risk factors in the etiology of depressive disorders over the life course. Own visualization based on analyses on a developmental model of depressive disorders by Kendler et al. (2002), and (2006)

stage of life (e.g., that a disturbed family environment may cause parental loss in childhood) and between stages (e.g., that low self-esteem in early adolescence may cause substance misuse in late adolescence). It is further assumed that risk factors may interact with each other, again both within a stage of life (e.g., that the effect of marital problems on risk of depressive disorders in adulthood may be modified by major financial problems in adulthood) and between stages (e.g., that the effect of traumatic life events in late adolescence may be modified by low parental warmth in childhood).

Occupational determinants of depressive disorders would belong to the broad category of "difficulties and stressful life events in adulthood" in Fig. 2. Kendler et al. point here, among many other things, to "serious difficulties at work" (Kendler et al. 2002, p. 1135) but do not further specify what type of difficulties should be considered as depressogenic. In the following second part of this book chapter, we will examine what type of working conditions may be considered as risk factors in the etiology of depressive disorders.

Working Conditions and Risk of Depressive Disorders

In this second part of the chapter, we examine the relation of working conditions with risk of depressive disorders. We address theoretical and methodological issues, present results from systematic reviews and meta-analyses, and provide an interpretation and discussion of the epidemiological evidence. This part closes with considerations about future research needs for better understanding the occupational determinants of depressive disorders.

Theoretical and Methodological Issues

Psychosocial Working Conditions
Although a few studies have considered physical working conditions (e.g., exposure to pesticides) in the etiology of depressive disorders, most studies have focused on psychosocial working conditions as potential risk factors (Theorell et al. 2015). Psychosocial working conditions pertain to various factors and constellations at work, including, but not limited to, quantitative workload, work pace, emotional demands, work organization, rewards, conflicts, and the social interactions of workers with their supervisors, colleagues, clients, and customers (Clausen et al. 2019; Rugulies 2019).

Several theoretical models have described specific constellations at work that are thought to be particularly health hazardous. The most widely used models in psychosocial occupational epidemiology are the *job strain model*, positing that health hazardous work is characterized by a combination of high job demands and low job control (Karasek and Theorell 1990), and the *effort-reward imbalance model*, positing an increased risk of ill-health due to the mismatch of spending high efforts at work while receiving low rewards, in terms of salary, respect, appreciation, promotion prospects, and job security (Siegrist 2016). Both models have been tested mostly with regard to risk of cardiovascular disorders (see ▶ Chap. 11, "Occupational Determinants of Cardiovascular Disorders Including Stroke") but since the late 1990s have also increasingly been used in studies on other health outcomes, including mental health.

Study Design Considerations
For ethical and practical reasons, it is not feasible to conduct randomized controlled trials (RCTs), in which a treatment group is first deliberately exposed to adversity at the workplace (e.g., workplace bullying) and then is monitored for rates of onset of depressive disorders compared to a nonexposed control group. Cross-sectional studies and case-control studies measuring working conditions in participants who already have developed a depressive disorder are of only limited value, as depressive disorders can cause a negative perception of the environment (Harmer et al. 2009), making it impossible to determine whether the working condition caused the depressive disorder or the depressive disorder caused the reporting of adverse working conditions.

Therefore, the best available research design for studying adverse working conditions and depressive disorders is a prospective cohort study. In such studies, researchers assess working conditions in individuals who are free of depressive disorders at baseline and then follow the participants for some time. If workers who are exposed to adverse working conditions at baseline have a higher risk of onset of depressive disorders during follow-up compared to workers not exposed at baseline, if these differences remain after adjustment for potential confounders, and if unmeasured confounding and other biases are unlikely, then it may be concluded that adverse working conditions contribute to the risk of depressive disorder.

Measuring Depressive Disorders in Epidemiological Studies

The gold standard method for measuring depressive disorders in epidemiological studies is a Clinical Interview (usually either Structured Clinical Interview or Clinical Diagnostic Interview), conducted by a trained interviewer, allowing diagnoses in accordance with ICD or DSM (Drill et al. 2015). However, as a Clinical Interview is laborious and expensive, it is not an attractive choice for large-scale epidemiological studies. Self-administered questionnaires assessing the occurrence of symptoms typical of depressive disorders offer an alternative measurement. These questionnaires usually provide a score indicating the presence or absence of a depressive disorder. A questionnaire that previously has been tested against a Clinical Interview and showed good validity may be considered as a low-cost alternative in epidemiological studies. However, questionnaires do not provide sensual clues (e.g., subdued behavior of the respondent) and do not allow clarifying questions.

It is a major limitation of both Clinical Interviews and questionnaires that they ascertain depressive disorders only at a particular point of time during follow-up. Consequently, individuals who developed a depressive disorder early during follow-up but are in remission at the time when a Clinical Interview or a questionnaire is administered may be falsely classified as non-cases. Such a misclassification can be avoided when study participants are continuously monitored in national health registers that provide the exact date when an individual, for example, purchases an antidepressant, is admitted to a hospital, or is granted a disability pension due to a depressive disorder. Disadvantages of national health registers are that they are available for research purposes in a few countries only and that they can only identify those cases of depressive disorders where the individual contacted the healthcare system and was diagnosed. This is an important restriction because many individuals with depressive disorders do not seek help from the healthcare system and are never diagnosed (Hämäläinen et al. 2009).

Results from Systematic Reviews and Meta-analyses

Epidemiological research on working conditions and mental health, including depressive disorders, emerged on a larger scale first in the late 1990s. A pioneering study was conducted by Stansfeld and colleagues in a cohort of British civil servants in the Whitehall II study, showing that job strain, low workplace social support, and effort-reward imbalance were associated with an increased risk of psychiatric disorders (Stansfeld et al. 1999).

In 2015, Theorell and colleagues published the most comprehensive systematic review and meta-analysis on work environment and depressive disorders to date, identifying 59 cohort studies of moderate or high quality (Theorell et al. 2015). The level of scientific evidence was assessed in accordance with the GRADE (*G*rading of *R*ecommendations *A*ssessment, *D*evelopment and *E*valuation) procedure (GRADE Working Group 2018). In GRADE, results from observational epidemiological studies are in principle considered of only "limited evidence," because these studies are more vulnerable to bias due to selection and unmeasured confounding than RCTs. However, GRADE allows upgrading the evidence from observational studies under certain conditions to "moderate evidence" or even "high evidence."

Table 3 shows the main results of the review. Three working conditions were upgraded to "moderate evidence," job strain and low job control because of

Table 3 Results of a systematic review by Theorell et al. (2015) on the scientific evidence for the associations between 31 working conditions and risk of depressive disorders

Scientific evidence level	Work factor (number of studies in the review)
Moderate scientific evidence (3 factors)	Job strain (14)
	Job control (19)
	Workplace bullying (4)
Limited scientific evidence (18 factors)	Psychological job demands (10)
	Combination of low job demands with low decision latitude (2)
	High-pressure job (5)
	Effort-reward imbalance (3)
	Low support at the workplace (17)
	Low supervisor support (8)
	Low co-worker support (6)
	Poor social climate at the workplace (2)
	Poor social capital at the workplace (2)
	Low workplace justice (5)
	Procedural injustice (5)
	Relational injustice (3)
	Workplace conflicts (3)
	Conflicts with superiors (3)
	Conflicts with co-workers (2)
	Low job development (4)
	Job insecurity (7)
	Long working week (6)
Insufficient scientific evidence (10 factors)	Several different types of demands
	Emotional demands
	Distributive justice
	Threats
	Violence
	Irregular work hours
	Physical demanding work
	Pesticides
	Solvents
	Heavy metals
	(Number of studies not reported at this evidence level)

Table 4 Association between selected psychosocial working conditions and risk of depressive disorders from eight meta-analyses (from five systematic reviews), published in 2015 or later

Reference	Working condition	Measurement of depressive disorders (number of studies)	Pooled estimate (95% CI)
Theorell et al. (2015)	Job strain	C-Int. SAQ, SRDD ($n = 14$)	1.74 (1.53–1.96)
Madsen et al. (2017)	Job strain	C-Int. ($n = 7$)	1.77 (1.47–2.13)
Madsen et al. (2017)	Job strain	HT ($n = 14$)	1.27 (1.04–1.55)[a]
Theorell et al. (2015)	Low job control	C-Int., SAQ, SRDD ($n = 19$)	1.37 (1.30–1.47)[b]
Rugulies et al. (2017)	Effort-reward imbalance	C-Int., SAQ, SRDD, AD, DP ($n = 8$)	1.49 (1.23–1.80)
Kim and Knesebeck (2016)	Job insecurity	SAQ ($n = 6$)	1.29 (1.06–1.57)
Virtanen et al. (2018)	Long working hours	C-Int., SAQ ($n = 28$)	1.14 (1.03–1.25)[c,d]
Theorell et al. (2015)	Workplace bullying	SAQ, SRDD ($n = 4$)	2.82 (2.21–3.59)

Abbreviations: *C-Int.* Clinical Interview, *SAQ* self-administered questionnaire, *SRDD* self-reported doctor-diagnosed depressive disorders, *HT* hospital treatment for depressive disorders, *AD* treatment with antidepressants, *DP* disability pension due to depressive disorders
[a] Based on individual participant data from previously unpublished cohort studies
[b] Theorell et al. (2015) reported pooled estimates for the association between high job control and depressive disorders that was 0.73 (95% CI: 0.68–0.77). We converted the estimate and the CI, so the pooled estimate shows the association between low job control and depressive disorders
[c] The 28 studies combined 10 published studies and 18 individual participant data from previously unpublished cohort studies
[d] The meta-analysis also included some studies that measured psychological distress instead of depressive disorders

the large number of studies with consistent results and workplace bullying because of a large effect size. In addition, 18 other working conditions were graded with "limited evidence," indicating that these conditions might be related to risk of depressive disorders but that uncertainty about the results was considerable. For ten further working conditions, the evidence was graded as "insufficient."

After the publication of the comprehensive review by Theorell et al., several new reviews focusing on specific psychosocial working conditions were published with updated literature searches. Table 4 gives an overview of the pooled estimates and the 95% confidence intervals (CI) from eight meta-analyses, including three meta-analyses from Theorell et al. and five meta-analyses from four newer reviews. The examined working conditions were job strain, low job control, effort-reward imbalance, job insecurity, long working hours, and workplace bullying.

Job Strain and Low Job Control

Job strain was examined in three of the eight meta-analyses. Theorell et al. (2015) reported that individuals exposed to job strain had a 1.74 higher risk of depressive disorders compared to nonexposed individuals, when depressive disorders were measured with a wide range of methods, including Clinical Interviews, questionnaires, and self-reported doctor-diagnosed depressive disorders. Madsen et al. (2017) conducted two meta-analyses on job strain with strictly clinical measures of depressive disorders. When they examined job strain and risk of depressive disorders measured with Clinical Interviews in the published literature, they found a pooled estimate of 1.77, almost identical to the estimate reported by Theorell and colleagues. Madsen et al. further examined job strain and risk of depressive disorders in unpublished data from 14 cohort studies with registered hospital treatment of depressive disorders as the outcome that yielded a weaker, albeit still statistically significant, pooled estimate of 1.27. Hospital treatment of depressive disorders is a relatively rare event and may be an indicator for particular severe forms of depressive disorders. The fact that job strain showed a weaker association with hospital-treated depressive disorders than with depressive disorders assessed by other methods in previous studies could indicate that job strain is a more important contributor to risk of light and moderate depressive disorders than severe depressive disorders. However, other explanations are also possible, such as an overestimation of the association in the meta-analyses of the previous studies due to publication bias (as these meta-analyses were based on published studies, whereas the meta-analysis on hospital-treated depression was based on unpublished data) or underestimation of the association in the meta-analysis on hospital-treated depressive disorders because of confounding from unknown third variables (e.g., socioeconomic variables) that were related to hospital referral.

Theorell et al. also calculated the pooled estimate for job control, a component of the job strain model. Based on 19 studies, they found that low control predicted risk of depressive disorders with a pooled estimate of 1.37 that was statistically significant.

Effort-Reward Imbalance and Job Insecurity

Effort-reward imbalance was only measured in three studies in the review by Theorell et al. and was graded with limited evidence, and no pooled estimate was reported. In a more recent review, Rugulies et al. (2017) identified eight studies on effort-reward imbalance with a pooled estimate of 1.49. Job insecurity, a component of effort-reward imbalance, contributed with seven studies to the review by Theorell et al. and was graded with limited evidence (no pooled estimate). A year later, Kim and Knesebeck (2016), using slightly different inclusion criteria, identified six studies, only partly overlapping with the studies identified by Theorell et al., and reported a pooled estimate of 1.29.

Long Working Hours

Long working hours showed a small, but statistically significant, pooled estimate of 1.14 in a review by Virtanen et al. (2018). Two things should be noted: first, the meta-analysis included not only studies on depressive disorders but also some studies on psychological distress. Second, when results were stratified by geographical regions, the pooled estimate for the association between long working hours and risk of the outcome was strongest for studies from Asia (pooled hazard ratio (HR): 1.50, 95%; CI: 1.13–2.01, seven studies), weaker for studies from Europe (pooled HR: 1.11, 95%; CI: 1.10–1.22, 17 studies), and not existent for studies from North America (pooled HR: 0.97, 95%; CI: 0.70–1.34, six studies) and a single study from Australia (HR: 0.95, 95%; CI: 0.70–1.29). This indicates that the association between psychosocial work environment and risk of depressive disorders (and psychological distress) might be modified by country-specific characteristics.

Workplace Bullying

The by far strongest association between psychosocial working conditions and risk of depressive disorders was found for workplace bullying that had a pooled estimate of 2.82 in the review by Theorell et al. (2015). Note that the lower boundary of the 95% CI for workplace bullying was 2.21 and was therefore higher than the upper boundaries of the 95% CIs of all other psychosocial working conditions shown in Table 4.

Interpretation and Discussion of the Epidemiological Evidence

All estimates shown in Table 4 are based on prospective cohort studies with individuals free of depressive disorders at baseline and followed-up for several years. In the absence of RCTs, this is the strongest epidemiological design studying effects of working conditions on risk of depressive disorders. However, several methodological issues that might have caused over- or underestimation of the associations need to be considered. These issues pertain to (i) publication bias, (ii) magnitude of the estimates, (iii) self-report of psychosocial working conditions, (iv) selection into certain job groups, and (v) repeated exposure measurements.

Publication Bias

Publication bias refers to the well-documented phenomena that studies showing an association between a risk factor and a health outcome are more likely to be published than studies not finding an association (Ekmekci 2017). Some, but not all, of the meta-analyses presented in Table 4 examined publication bias, and it cannot be ruled out that publication bias inflated estimates to some extent.

Magnitude of the Estimates

The pooled estimates regarding job strain, low job control, effort-reward imbalance, job insecurity, and long working hours were all less than twofold; thus the associations with depressive disorders were moderate (in case of long working hours:

weak) and are therefore vulnerable to residual confounding. In contrast, the pooled estimate for workplace bullying was 2.82 indicating a strong association that is less vulnerable to residual confounding. However, the bullying estimate was based on only four studies, and none of these studies used a Clinical Interview or clinical register data as an outcome measure. Thus, even though the association of workplace bullying and risk of depressive disorders was remarkably strong, it remains to be seen if this association can be replicated when studies ascertain depressive disorders with clinical measurements.

Self-Report of Working Conditions
The vast majority of studies measured working conditions with self-report, i.e., workers responded to questionnaire items assessing specific aspects of the psychosocial work environment. This raises concern about reporting bias, because it is possible that individuals with undetected subclinical depressive symptoms overreport the adversity of their work environment. Such overreporting could be due to that either the subclinical depressive symptoms had elicited a biased, more gloomy perception of the environment or that subclinical depressive symptoms had led to reduced workability and subsequent problems at the workplace (e.g., increasing workload due to inability of workers with subclinical depressive symptoms to complete work tasks in time or conflicts with supervisors due to underperformance). As subclinical depressive symptoms strongly predict onset of a depressive disorder (Cuijpers and Smit 2004), this could mean that subclinical depressive symptoms at baseline generated spurious associations between self-reported working conditions and risk of onset of a depressive disorder (see Fig. 3, part a, confounding).

A solution to this problem would be to adjust for baseline subclinical depressive symptoms. However, if the association of subclinical depressive symptoms and self-reported adverse working conditions at baseline is not caused by an effect of the subclinical depressive symptoms on the reporting of the adverse working conditions but, conversely, is caused by an effect of the adverse working conditions on the onset of the subclinical depressive symptoms, which then over time progressed into clinically significant depressive disorder, subclinical depressive symptoms would not be a confounder but a mediator linking the working conditions to depressive disorders, and adjustment would be inappropriate (see Fig. 3, part b, mediation). In a supplementary analysis to the meta-analysis on job strain and risk of hospital treatment of depressive disorders, Madsen et al. (2017) reported that job strain predicted subclinical depressive symptoms but subclinical depressive symptoms also predicted job strain, suggesting that subclinical depressive symptoms are both a confounder and a mediator in the association of job strain with risk of depressive disorders. Consequently, neither adjustment nor refusal of adjustment for subclinical depressive symptoms might be able to show the true association between working conditions and risk of depressive disorders as the association may be underestimated by adjusting and overestimated by not adjusting.

To reduce possible reporting bias, some studies have averaged self-reported working conditions either at the job group level (job exposure matrix, e.g., Wieclaw et al. 2008) or the work unit level (e.g., Rugulies et al. 2018). Other studies

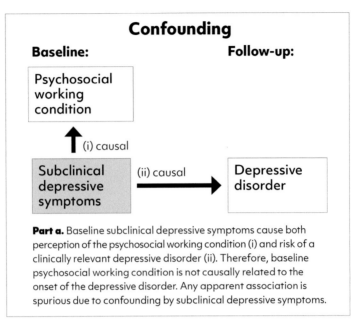

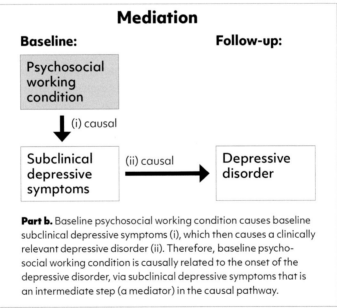

Fig. 3 The association between psychosocial working conditions and risk of onset of depressive disorders: confounding and mediation by subclinical depressive symptoms

have measured working conditions without relying on self-report, for example, by using trained workplace observers for directly assessing working conditions (e.g., Jakobsen et al. 2015) or by using information from registers to approximate working conditions (e.g., Virtanen et al. 2008). These alternative methods have shown mixed results, and all have their own strength and weaknesses, i.e., none of them provide the perfect solution for obtaining unbiased estimates. But combining these different methods, with their different risks for over- and underestimation, might currently be the best strategy for getting more insight into the possible range and magnitude of the true association between psychosocial working conditions and risk of depressive disorders.

Selection into Specific Job Groups

Stansfeld et al. (2008) showed in the British Birth Cohort Study that childhood and early adulthood psychological problems predicted mid adulthood job strain levels, probably through selection of individuals with early life psychological problems into disadvantaged jobs. The analyses, however, also showed that the association of job strain with risk of onset of depressive disorders remained, even after adjustment for earlier psychological problems. This suggests that selection into specific jobs may explain some, but not all, of the association between psychosocial working conditions and risk of depressive disorders. To examine this further, more life course cohort studies are needed that follow individuals from early life, over entry to the labor market until onset of depressive disorders.

Repeated Exposure Measurements

In the vast majority of studies, working conditions were measured at baseline only. As characteristics of jobs change over time and some individuals move from one job to another job during follow-up, measuring working conditions only once will result into exposure misclassification likely causing an underestimation of the association of working conditions and risk of depressive disorders. For example, Madsen et al. (2017) reported that individuals exposed to job strain at one point in time had a hazard ratio for depressive disorders of 1.23, whereas individuals exposed at two points in time had a hazard ratio of 1.56.

Future Research Needs

Future studies on working conditions and risk of depressive disorders should address the biases for over- and underestimation of the associations that were discussed above. Particularly, reporting bias should be addressed, for example, by aggregating self-reported exposure measures to the work unit level or the job group level, where appropriate, or measuring psychosocial working conditions with other methods than self-report, while being aware of that these alternative strategies for data analysis and exposures measurement also have their limitations. Future research may also consider a (work) life course perspective, where individuals are included into the study before entering the workforce and where exposure to adverse working conditions is assessed repeatedly throughout the study.

In addition to these challenges evolving from the above-discussed methodological issues in the current literature, we see three additional research needs. This pertains to (i) analyses of effect modification and the role of context, (ii) advancing psychosocial work environment theories and understanding psychological and biological mechanisms, and (iii) conducting workplace intervention studies.

Effect Modification and the Role of Context
So far, little is known whether the effects of working conditions on risk of depressive disorders differ depending on exposure to other factors or on contextual conditions. As delineated above (Section "Genetic Risk Factors and Gene-Environment Interaction"), there is a great interest in gene-environment interaction in the risk of depressive disorders. So far, results are inconsistent and controversially discussed (Culverhouse et al. 2018). In most of the interaction studies, environmental factors were measured by either childhood adversity or adulthood adverse life events, whereas studies on adverse working conditions are lacking. From a scientific perspective, it would be interesting to examine the possible interaction of genes and working conditions in the etiology of depressive disorders. From a societal perspective, however, such interaction research is problematic, because if an interaction between genetic disposition and working conditions was found, it might motivate genetic screenings at the workplace to avoid hiring or to remove workers who are suspected as genetically vulnerable.

The effect of working conditions on risk of depressive disorders may also be modified by social factors. Some research suggests that the association between working conditions and risk of ill health is stronger in individuals of lower socioeconomic position than in individuals of higher socioeconomic position (Hoven and Siegrist 2013). Individuals of low socioeconomic position are generally exposed to more adversity in life (e.g., due to financial constraints or limited access to resources), and adding adversity at work to the already existing adversity may exceed coping capacities. However, so far, studies have shown inconsistent results, and more research in this area is needed (Hoven and Siegrist 2013).

The adversity of working conditions may also be experienced differently depending on the context at the workplace. Figure 4 depicts the result of the interaction of individual-level reported managerial quality and workplace-mean managerial quality on risk of depressive disorders in a cohort study among about 5,000 Danish eldercare workers from 274 workplaces (Rugulies et al. 2018). Low individual-level experienced managerial quality strongly predicted risk of depressive disorders at workplaces with a high mean score of managerial quality (odds ratio: 3.10) but not at workplaces with a low mean score of managerial quality (odds ratio: 1.07). This statistically significant interaction suggests that experiencing low managerial quality is particularly health hazardous when this experience is not

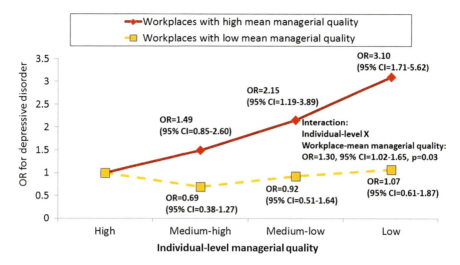

Fig. 4 Prospective association of individual-level managerial quality with risk of onset of a depressive disorder after 20 months of follow-up stratified by high and low workplace-mean managerial quality. (Source: Rugulies et al. 2018 (https://journals.lww.com/joem/), with permission from Wolters Kluwer Health, Inc. (Copyright ©2017). All rights reserved)

shared by the colleagues of the individual. It is possible that low managerial quality is more tolerable at a workplace where most of the other workers are also experiencing low managerial quality and that this congruent experience may even strengthen the bonds between the workers and result in collective actions to handle the situation. Conversely, experiencing low managerial quality at a workplace where most of the other workers are experiencing high managerial quality may be particular hurtful and may lead to isolation and decreased self-esteem. However, as this was a first explorative approach to investigate the interaction of individual level with workplace-mean levels of managerial quality, interpretations should be made with caution.

The association between working conditions and depressive disorders may also be modified by context at the macro-level. Some studies suggest that the association between adverse psychosocial working conditions and depressive disorders might be weaker in countries with more comprehensive welfare regimes and with a high level of protective labor and social policies (e.g., high active labor market policies, high unemployment benefits, low income inequality) than in countries with less comprehensive welfare regimes and less protective labor and social policies (e.g., Dragano et al. 2011). It is possible that in societies with a comprehensive welfare regime and a high level of protective policies, adverse working conditions may be less prevalent and may less often cross a health hazardous threshold or that social welfare and protective policies may buffer the hazardous effect of adverse working conditions on mental health.

Advancing Theories and Understanding Mechanisms

High-quality epidemiological research on psychosocial working conditions and depressive disorders has so far been limited by examining only a few working conditions, mostly job strain, including the component low job control, effort-reward imbalance, including the component job insecurity, long working hours, and workplace bullying (Table 4). Both job strain and effort-reward imbalance are elaborated psychosocial work environment theories; however, neither of them was originally meant to explain the potential impact of working conditions on the risk of depressive disorders, and it is not specified in the theories why the working conditions they describe should be regarded as depressogenic. Post hoc, though, some arguments can be made. For example, lack of control over job demands (i.e., job strain) might elicit a state of learned helplessness that has been considered as a mechanism in the etiology of depressive disorders (Seligman 1975). Further, workers who recognize that their level of influence over work tasks is much lower compared to other workers or who experience that their efforts are not matched by their rewards may feel humiliated by these situations and their self-esteem may be threatened, two mechanisms that are likely involved in the etiology of depressive disorders (Brown and Harris 1978; Harris 2001; Kendler et al. 2003) (see section "Psychological and Sociological Theories").

Workplace bullying has been examined in only few cohort studies; however, in these few studies, estimates for workplace bullying and risk of depressive disorders were remarkably strong. As workplace bullying likely will cause feelings of humiliation and threatened self-esteem, these results are congruent with the assumption that humiliation and threatened self-esteem might be important psychological mechanisms linking adverse working conditions to risk of depressive disorders. Further, workplace bullying may cause high levels of anxiety, which is a known precursor of depressive disorders (Wittchen et al. 2000). It seems reasonable to examine also the role of other potentially humiliating, self-esteem threatening, and anxiety-provoking experiences at work, for example, workplace violence, sexual harassment, or discrimination. Some studies exist on these exposures (Theorell et al. 2015), but more studies are needed to provide an evidence base on which conclusions can be drawn.

One theoretical framework that explicitly addresses self-esteem-threatening experiences at work is the stress-as-offense-to-self (SOS) theory (Semmer et al. 2015), which is built on the notion that having to perform unreasonable or unnecessary (illegitimate) tasks at work increases risk of reduced self-esteem and poor mental health. However, with few exceptions (e.g., Madsen et al. 2014), the theory has rarely been tested in large-scale epidemiological studies yet.

Elucidating psychophysiological mechanisms that link psychosocial working conditions to risk of depressive disorders is even more challenging than elucidating psychological mechanisms. As discussed above (Section "Psychophysiological Mechanisms"), possible psychophysiological mechanisms through which psychosocial factors may increase risk of depressive disorders are HPA axis dysregulation and inflammatory processes (Horowitz and Zunszain 2015; Kivimäki and Steptoe 2018). If research studies would consistently and convincingly show that psychosocial working conditions cause HPA axis dysregulation and inflammatory processes, then this would be a major step forward in understanding the link between working conditions and risk of depressive disorders.

Intervention Studies

The assumption that adverse psychosocial working conditions are causally related to risk of depressive disorders would be substantially strengthened if intervention studies could show that removal of these working conditions led to a decreased risk of depressive disorders. However, such studies are very difficult to conduct. If one assumes that the 1-year incidence rate of depressive disorders is 3% and that an intervention would be able to reduce this incidence rate by 50% (assuming a strong impact of the intervention), then one would need more than 3,000 participants in an individual-level randomized trial to show a significant effect. A cluster-randomized trial in which workplaces and not individuals are randomized would require even more participants.

Considering these enormous logistic and financial efforts, it is not surprising that workplace intervention studies have not focused on the prevention of depressive disorders but on reducing symptoms of mental health problems including depressive symptoms (Grawitch et al. 2015; LaMontagne et al. 2014). A recent meta-review on workplace interventions for common mental disorders identified 20 reviews of moderate or high quality that included a total of 481 primary studies (Joyce et al. 2016). The review concluded that there was moderate evidence for that workplace interventions focusing on increasing worker control over their working conditions led to a reduction of symptoms of mental ill health.

The moderate evidence for a beneficial effect of interventions focusing on increasing worker control is, however, the exception from the rule that little is known whether or not workplace interventions can improve worker mental health. Results from workplace intervention studies are inconsistent, partly due to the low methodological quality of many studies and partly due to the high degree of heterogeneity of the studies, for example, regarding interventions designs and study populations, which make it difficult to systematically review the results (Montano et al. 2014).

A major weakness of most workplace intervention studies is the lack of a comprehensive process evaluation. As pointed out by Kompier and Aust (2016, p. 355), it is not sufficient "to know 'what works', but also 'when, how, and why' this may be the case." If a workplace intervention does not show any effects, it is important to understand if this was due to a lack of efficacy of the intervention or due to that the intervention was not properly implemented. In the first case, the theory behind the intervention has failed, and the intervention should not be recommended to other workplaces. In the second case, however, not the theory behind the intervention but the implementation of the intervention has failed, and it would still be possible, although not certain, that the intervention can show the desired effect under conditions that would allow its implementation (Kompier and Aust 2016). To distinguish between theory failure and implementation failure and to understand why an intervention has succeeded or failed, a process evaluation that comprehensively examines each step in a workplace intervention and also the context in which the intervention is conducted is crucial. With more studies conducting comprehensive evaluations, including process evaluation, it might be possible in the future to compare well-implemented intervention studies and thereby identify the types of interventions that are effective and the conditions under which they are effective.

Summary and Conclusion

Depressive disorders are highly prevalent and have a complex etiology likely influenced by multiple biological, psychological, and social risk factors that act across the life course. Research on the possible contribution of psychosocial working conditions to risk of depressive disorders started only in the late 1990s and is thus a rather new endeavor, compared to research that has examined the contribution of, for example, genetics, cognitive styles, or life events. As psychosocial working conditions are – in principal – modifiable, identifying depressogenic working conditions could help to reduce the burden of depressive disorders in the population. Current reviews and meta-analyses of prospective cohort studies show that some psychosocial working conditions, namely, job strain, low job control, effort-reward imbalance, and job insecurity, are associated with a moderately increased risk of depressive disorders. Further, there is a weak association of long working hours with risk of depressive disorders; however, this association may vary between different countries. Exposure to workplace bullying is strongly and consistently associated with risk of depressive disorders; however, this conclusion is based on very few studies. When interpreting these results, several potential biases for both over- and underestimation of the associations need to be considered. Addressing these potential biases in new studies with improved designs is an important task for future research on psychosocial work environment and risk of depressive disorders.

Future studies also need to examine if and to what extent the strength of the association between psychosocial working conditions and risk of depressive disorders may be modified by other factors or by the larger context. It is further important to better understand the psychological and biological mechanisms through which specific psychosocial working conditions get under the skin and subsequently may affect the mental health of the employees. Finally, the case that psychosocial working conditions contribute to the etiology of depressive disorders would be strengthened if it could be shown that improvements in working conditions prevent the onset of depressive disorders or at least reduce the level of depressive symptoms. Developing, implementing, and comprehensively evaluating such interventions are very difficult. However, we suggest that this should not stop researchers from continuing to strive for such interventions, because if successful, they could have major impact, both on our understanding of the etiology of depressive disorders and on reducing the burden of depressive disorders in the population.

Cross-References

▶ Occupational Determinants of Cardiovascular Disorders Including Stroke

References

American Psychiatric Association (2013) Diagnostic and Statistical Manual of Mental Health Disorders, fifth edition (DSM-5). American Psychiatric Association, Arlington. https://doi.org/10.1176/appi.books.9780890425596

Beck AT (1967) Depression: clinical, experimental and theoretical aspects. Harper and Row, New York

Blazer DG (2005) The age of melancholy. "Major depression" and its social origins. Routledge, New York

Bolwig TG, Shorter E (eds) (2007) Melancholia: beyond DSM, beyond neurotransmitters. Proceedings of a conference, May 2006, Copenhagen, Denmark. Acta Psychiatr Scand 115:4–183. https://doi.org/10.1111/j.1600-0447.2007.00956.x

Brown GW, Harris T (1978) Social origins of depression. A study of psychiatric disorder in women. Tavistock, London

Caspi A et al (2003) Influence of life stress on depression: moderation by a polymorphism in the 5-HTT gene. Science 301:386–389. https://doi.org/10.1126/science.1083968

Clausen T et al (2019) The Danish Psychosocial Work Environment Questionnaire (DPQ): development, content, reliability and validity. Scand J Work Environ Health 45:356-369. https://doi.org/10.5271/sjweh.3793

Cuijpers P, Smit F (2004) Subthreshold depression as a risk indicator for major depressive disorder: a systematic review of prospective studies. Acta Psychiatr Scand 109:325–331. https://doi.org/10.1111/j.1600-0447.2004.00301.x

Culverhouse RC et al (2018) Collaborative meta-analysis finds no evidence of a strong interaction between stress and 5-HTTLPR genotype contributing to the development of depression. Mol Psychiatry 23:133–142. https://doi.org/10.1038/mp.2017.44

Davison GC, Neale JM (1990) Abnormal psychology, 6th edn. Wiley, New York

Dragano N, Siegrist J, Wahrendorf M (2011) Welfare regimes, labour policies and unhealthy psychosocial working conditions: a comparative study with 9917 older employees from 12 European countries. J Epidemiol Community Health 65:793–799. https://doi.org/10.1136/jech.2009.098541

Drill R, Nakash O, DeFife JA, Westen D (2015) Assessment of clinical information: comparison of the validity of a Structured Clinical Interview (the SCID) and the Clinical Diagnostic Interview. J Nerv Ment Dis 203:459–462. https://doi.org/10.1097/NMD.0000000000000300

Ehrenberg A (1998) La fatigue d'être soi – dépression et société. Odile Jacob, Paris

Ekmekci PE (2017) An increasing problem in publication ethics: publication bias and editors' role in avoiding it. Med Health Care Philos 20:171–178. https://doi.org/10.1007/s11019-017-9767-0

Flint J, Kendler KS (2014) The genetics of major depression. Neuron 81:484–503. https://doi.org/10.1016/j.neuron.2014.01.027

France CM, Lysaker PH, Robinson RP (2007) The "chemical imbalance" explanation for depression: origins, lay endorsement, and clinical implications. Prof Psychol Res Pract 38:411–420. https://doi.org/10.1037/0735-7028.38.4.411

GRADE Working Group (2018) GRADE. http://www.gradeworkinggroup.org/. Accessed 20 Aug 2018

Grawitch MJ, Ballard DW, Erb KR (2015) To be or not to be (stressed): the critical role of a psychologically healthy workplace in effective stress management. Stress Health 31:264–273. https://doi.org/10.1002/smi.2619

Hämäläinen J, Isometsä E, Sihvo S, Kiviruusu O, Pirkola S, Lönnqvist J (2009) Treatment of major depressive disorder in the Finnish general population. Depress Anxiety 26:1049–1059. https://doi.org/10.1002/da.20524

Harmer CJ et al (2009) Effect of acute antidepressant administration on negative affective bias in depressed patients. Am J Psychiatry 166:1178–1184. https://doi.org/10.1176/appi.ajp.2009.09020149

Harris T (2001) Recent developments in understanding the psychosocial aspects of depression. Br Med Bull 57:17–32

Horowitz MA, Zunszain PA (2015) Neuroimmune and neuroendocrine abnormalities in depression: two sides of the same coin. Ann N Y Acad Sci 1351:68–79. https://doi.org/10.1111/nyas.12781

Hoven H, Siegrist J (2013) Work characteristics, socioeconomic position and health: a systematic review of mediation and moderation effects in prospective studies. Occup Environ Med 70:663–669. https://doi.org/10.1136/oemed-2012-101331

Jakobsen LM, Jorgensen AFB, Thomsen BL, Greiner BA, Rugulies R (2015) A multilevel study on the association of observer-assessed working conditions with depressive symptoms among female eldercare workers from 56 work units in 10 care homes in Denmark. BMJ Open 5: e008713. https://doi.org/10.1136/bmjopen-2015-008713

Joyce S, Modini M, Christensen H, Mykletun A, Bryant R, Mitchell PB, Harvey SB (2016) Workplace interventions for common mental disorders: a systematic meta-review. Psychol Med 46:683–697. https://doi.org/10.1017/S0033291715002408

Karasek R, Theorell T (1990) Healthy work: stress, productivity, and the reconstruction of working life. Basic Books, New York

Kendler KS (1986) Kraepelin and the differential diagnosis of dementia praecox and manic-depressive insanity. Compr Psychiatry 27:549–558

Kendler KS, Gardner CO, Prescott CA (2002) Toward a comprehensive developmental model for major depression in women. Am J Psychiatry 159:1133–1145. https://doi.org/10.1176/appi.ajp.159.7.1133

Kendler KS, Hettema JM, Butera F, Gardner CO, Prescott CA (2003) Life event dimensions of loss, humiliation, entrapment, and danger in the prediction of onsets of major depression and generalized anxiety. Arch Gen Psychiatry 60:789–796. https://doi.org/10.1001/archpsyc.60.8.789

Kendler KS, Gardner CO, Prescott CA (2006) Toward a comprehensive developmental model for major depression in men. Am J Psychiatry 163:115–124. https://doi.org/10.1176/appi.ajp.163.1.115

Kim TJ, Knesebeck O (2016) Perceived job insecurity, unemployment and depressive symptoms: a systematic review and meta-analysis of prospective observational studies. Int Arch Occup Environ Health 89:561–573. https://doi.org/10.1007/s00420-015-1107-1

Kivimäki M, Steptoe A (2018) Effects of stress on the development and progression of cardiovascular disease. Nat Rev Cardiol 15:215–229. https://doi.org/10.1038/nrcardio.2017.189

Kompier M, Aust B (2016) Organizational stress management interventions: is it the singer not the song? Scand J Work Environ Health 42:355–358. https://doi.org/10.5271/sjweh.3578

Krueger RF et al (2018) Progress in achieving quantitative classification of psychopathology. World Psychiatry 17:282–293. (commentaries 241–242 and 294–305). https://doi.org/10.1002/wps.20566

LaMontagne AD et al (2014) Workplace mental health: developing an integrated intervention approach. BMC Psychiatry 14:131. https://doi.org/10.1186/1471-244X-14-131

Lorant V, Deliege D, Eaton W, Robert A, Philippot P, Ansseau M (2003) Socioeconomic inequalities in depression: a meta-analysis. Am J Epidemiol 157:98–112

Madsen IEH, Tripathi M, Borritz M, Rugulies R (2014) Unnecessary work tasks and mental health: a prospective analysis of Danish human service workers. Scand J Work Environ Health 40:631–638. https://doi.org/10.5271/sjweh.3453

Madsen IEH et al (2017) Job strain as a risk factor for clinical depression: systematic review and meta-analysis with additional individual participant data. Psychol Med 47:1342–1356. https://doi.org/10.1017/S003329171600355X

Marangoni C, Hernandez M, Faedda GL (2016) The role of environmental exposures as risk factors for bipolar disorder: a systematic review of longitudinal studies. J Affect Disord 193:165–174. https://doi.org/10.1016/j.jad.2015.12.055

Mayes R, Horwitz AV (2005) DSM-III and the revolution in the classification of mental illness. J Hist Behav Sci 41:249–267. https://doi.org/10.1002/jhbs.20103

Moffitt TE, Caspi A, Taylor A, Kokaua J, Milne BJ, Polanczyk G, Poulton R (2010) How common are common mental disorders? Evidence that lifetime prevalence rates are doubled by prospective versus retrospective ascertainment. Psychol Med 40:899–909. https://doi.org/10.1017/S0033291709991036

Montano D, Hoven H, Siegrist J (2014) Effects of organisational-level interventions at work on employees' health: a systematic review. BMC Public Health 14:Art 135. https://doi.org/10.1186/1471-2458-14-135

Rugulies R (2019) What is a psychosocial work environment? Scand J Work Environ Health 45:1–6. https://doi.org/10.5271/sjweh.3792

Rugulies R, Aust B, Madsen IEH (2016) Effort-reward imbalance and affective disorders. In: Siegrist J, Wahrendorf M (eds) Work stress and health in a globalized economy – the model of effort-reward imbalance. Springer International Publishing, Cham, pp 103–143. https://doi.org/10.1007/978-3-319-32937-6

Rugulies R, Aust B, Madsen IEH (2017) Effort-reward imbalance at work and risk of depressive disorders. A systematic review and meta-analysis of prospective cohort studies. Scand J Work Environ Health 43:294–306. https://doi.org/10.5271/sjweh.3632

Rugulies R, Jakobsen LM, Madsen IEH, Borg V, Carneiro IG, Aust B (2018) Managerial quality and risk of depressive disorders among Danish eldercare workers: a multilevel cohort study. J Occup Environ Med 60:120–125. https://doi.org/10.1097/JOM.0000000000001195

Sacco WP (1999) A social-cognitive model of interpersonal processes in depression. In: Joiner T, Coyne JC (eds) Advances in interpersonal approaches: the interactional nature of depression. American Psychological Association, Washington, DC, pp 329–362

Seligman M (1975) Helplessness: on depression, development, and death. Freeman, San Francisco

Semmer NK, Jacobshagen N, Meier LL, Elfering A, Beehr TA, Kalin W, Tschan F (2015) Illegitimate tasks as a source of work stress. Work Stress 29:32–56. https://doi.org/10.1080/02678373.2014.1003996

Siegrist J (2016) A theoretical model in the context of economic globalization. In: Siegrist J, Wahrendorf M (eds) Work stress and health in a globalized economy – the model of effort-reward imbalance. Springer International Publishing, Cham, pp 3–19. https://doi.org/10.1007/978-3-319-32937-6

Stansfeld SA, Fuhrer R, Shipley MJ, Marmot MG (1999) Work characteristics predict psychiatric disorder: prospective results from the Whitehall II Study. Occup Environ Med 56:302–307

Stansfeld SA, Clark C, Caldwell T, Rodgers B, Power C (2008) Psychosocial work characteristics and anxiety and depressive disorders in midlife: the effects of prior psychological distress. Occup Environ Med 65:634–642. https://doi.org/10.1136/oem.2007.036640

Theorell T et al (2015) A systematic review including meta-analysis of work environment and depressive symptoms. BMC Public Health 15:738. https://doi.org/10.1186/s12889-015-1954-4

Virtanen M et al (2008) Overcrowding in hospital wards as a predictor of antidepressant treatment among hospital staff. Am J Psychiatry 165:1482–1486. https://doi.org/10.1176/appi.ajp.2008.07121929

Virtanen M et al (2018) Long working hours and depressive symptoms: systematic review and meta-analysis of published studies and unpublished individual participant data. Scand J Work Environ Health 44:239–250. https://doi.org/10.5271/sjweh.3712

Wakefield JC (2015) DSM-5, psychiatric epidemiology and the false positives problem. Epidemiol Psychiatr Sci 24:188–196. https://doi.org/10.1017/S2045796015000116

Wieclaw J, Agerbo E, Mortensen PB, Burr H, Tüchsen F, Bonde JP (2008) Psychosocial working conditions and the risk of depression and anxiety disorders in the Danish workforce. BMC Public Health 8:280. https://doi.org/10.1186/1471-2458-8-280

Wittchen HU, Kessler RC, Pfister H, Lieb M (2000) Why do people with anxiety disorders become depressed? A prospective-longitudinal community study. Acta Psychiatr Scand 102:14–23

Wittchen HU et al (2011) The size and burden of mental disorders and other disorders of the brain in Europe 2010. Eur Neuropsychopharmacol 21:655–679. https://doi.org/10.1016/j.euroneuro.2011.07.018

World Health Organization (1992) The ICD-10 classification of mental and behavioural disorders: clinical descriptions and diagnostic guidelines. World Health Organization, Geneva

World Health Organization (2015) International classification of diseases (ICD). http://www.who.int/classifications/icd/en/. http://apps.who.int/classifications/icd10/browse/2016/en. Accessed 19 Nov 2018

Occupational Determinants of Cognitive Decline and Dementia

13

Claudine Berr and Noémie Letellier

Contents

Cognitive Reserve Hypothesis, How Does Occupational Life Contribute?	238
Psychosocial Factors at Work	240
Occupational Chemical Exposures, an Effect on Brain Functioning Long After Exposure: Focus on Solvents	242
Results from the GAZEL Cohort: An Effect on Brain Functioning Long After Solvent Exposures	243
Cognitive Aging and Retirement	246
Perspectives for the Future	246
Cross-References	247
References	247

Abstract

Cognitive decline and dementia are major burden for our aging society. The pathological processes implicated in dementia seem to be active many years before the first clinical signs. The life-course approach aims to integrate the different biological, social, clinical, psychological, and environmental components that interact all along the lifetime of a person, factors which are major determinants of our cognitive aging. Some studies illustrate how occupation and occupational exposures affect later in life cognitive functioning or dementia occurrence. Higher occupational status, complex occupational roles, or jobs that

C. Berr (✉)
Neuropsychiatry: Epidemiological and Clinical Research, INSERM U1061, University of Montpellier, Montpellier, France

Centre Mémoire Ressources et Recherche, Hôpital Gui de Chauliac, Montpellier, France
e-mail: claudine.berr@inserm.fr

N. Letellier
Neuropsychiatry: Epidemiological and Clinical Research, INSERM U1061, University of Montpellier, Montpellier, France
e-mail: noemie.letellier@inserm.fr

© Springer Nature Switzerland AG 2020
U. Bültmann, J. Siegrist (eds.), *Handbook of Disability, Work and Health*, Handbook Series in Occupational Health Sciences, https://doi.org/10.1007/978-3-030-24334-0_11

are challenging seem to have a protective effect on cognitive functioning and dementia occurrence, even when controlling for education. Conversely, high-strain work and passive jobs that lack both self-direction and complexity are associated with cognitive impairment after retirement.

More specifically, regarding exposures, most studies have focused on the place of occupational toxicant exposures, mostly chemicals suspected to have long-term neurotoxic effects. Studies show a deleterious effect of chronic occupational exposures to solvents during active life. They also evidence that these effects on cognitive functioning remain important even after retirement, particularly for subjects with low education or high level of exposures. This has implications for physicians working with formerly solvent-exposed patients as well as for policies limiting exposure in the workplace.

To what extent occupational exposures contribute to social health inequalities in older age, taking into account the influence of non-occupational factors associated with socioeconomic position (measured by education, income, or household wealth), remains to be explored.

Keywords

Dementia · Cognition · Solvent · Job strain · Lifespan exposures · Retirement · Long-term effect

Cognitive decline and dementia are major burden for our aging society (Mura et al. 2010). Alzheimer's disease (AD) is the most common cause of dementia in the elderly, accounting for around 70% of the cases. An estimated 50 million people worldwide are living with dementia in 2018, one new case every 3 s, making it a leading cause of dependency and disability. Dementia incidence is strongly associated with age in all populations. Because of a rapid aging of populations, the number of people living with dementia is projected to triple in the next 30 years (i.e., 150 million cases in 2050), and the socioeconomic burden of dementia will increase accordingly (https://www.alz.co.uk/research/world-report-2018). Projections of the burden of dementia could be mitigated if improvements in life conditions and health care over the last decades have had beneficial effects on dementia risk.

Over the past two decades, a steadily growing body of evidence has indicated that aging is accompanied by a systematic decline in performance of a wide variety of cognitive tasks, observed both in the laboratory setting and in everyday life (Adam et al. 2013). For instance, it is widely accepted that age influences several cognitive factors, such as processing speed, inhibition, and working memory, which in turn affect other cognitive functions, such as episodic memory and language. Moreover, this age-related cognitive decline is associated with structural changes in the brain. Even early in the aging process, global changes, such as cerebral atrophy, ventricular enlargement, and hippocampal atrophy, can be evident in some but not all individuals. Significant cognitive deficits may be detectable long before the typical cognitive, behavioral, and social criteria of dementia are met. The pathological processes

13 Occupational Determinants of Cognitive Decline and Dementia

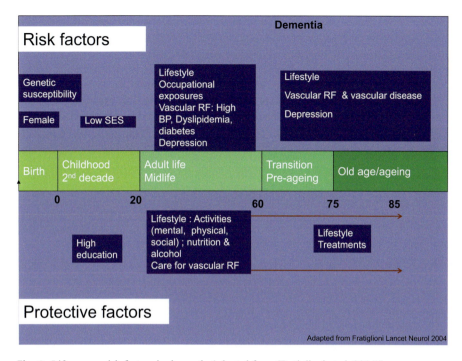

Fig. 1 Life-course risk factors in dementia (adapted from (Fratiglioni et al. 2004))

implicated in dementia (Jack et al. 2013) seem to be active many years before the first clinical signs. Medical and scientifically communities now generally accept that dementia and cognitive impairment are the result of a pathophysiological process that begins many years or decades before symptom onset (Amieva et al. 2008).

Unfortunately, even if several hypotheses are currently being explored to explain the decline in performances and dementia processes (see Fig. 1), most studies are conducted in elderly populations (Daviglus et al. 2011). Vascular risk factors – e.g., diabetes, hypertension, obesity, and physical inactivity – may occur during the midlife period, under the influence of environmental, behavioral, and lifestyle factors, in combination with genetic susceptibility and lead to disease processes in the brain that generally start to develop later in life. The life-course approach (Berr et al. 2012) aims to integrate the different biological, social, clinical, psychological, and environmental components that interact all along the lifetime of a person, including early life experiences, in order to promote healthy aging and delay the emergence of frailty and chronic diseases (Britton et al. 2008). In the Lancet Commission tribute (Livingston et al. 2017), low level of education accounts as an early life potentially modifiable factor, while only three factors are presented as midlife modifiable risk factors (hypertension, obesity, and hearing loss). No mention is made of occupational activity or exposures in this review. Only four studies on occupational level (Alvarado et al. 2002; Potter et al. 2006; Virtanen et al. 2009; Yu et al. 2009) are included in a systematic review on risk factors of cognitive decline (Plassman et al. 2010). This review considered that occupational exposures are too heterogeneous to synthetize and that there is inadequate evidence to assess associations between occupational level and cognitive decline.

Case-control studies on dementia performed mainly in the 1980s are of limited interest as they have major methodological limitations and discordant results on associations between occupation and dementia. The case-control design is vulnerable to recall bias, is mostly based on a single occupation to estimate exposure instead of full occupational histories, explores single exposures rather than combinations, and includes incomplete data on confounding factors. Thus, it remains unclear how occupational exposures during working life affect cognitive functioning later in life or dementia occurence (Smyth et al. 2004). This gap is beginning to be filled by results obtained from prospective studies.

Some (Qiu et al. 2003) but not all longitudinal studies (Helmer et al. 2001) suggest a greater risk of dementia among manual workers. In a Swedish cohort, the increased risk in lower occupation-based socioeconomic status (SES) subjects disappeared when education was entered into the model (Karp et al. 2004). This inconsistency may be due to the multifaceted nature of occupational positions, namely, as an indicator of environmental exposures, of material deprivation, and of access to medical care and attitudes to health or a surrogate marker of premorbid intelligence or cognitive abilities.

In fact, few large longitudinal studies have examined the ways in which work exposures over the life-course influence cognitive functioning in pre-aging or aging populations. Literature on aging increasingly points to the effects of long-term exposures (Richards and Deary 2005), which is difficult to document retrospectively. Most studies on aging include subjects over age 65 and did not have the opportunity to document detailed occupational exposures over the participants' working lives. Furthermore, retrospective exposure assessments are most often restricted to job titles, limiting analyses and interpretation of results.

After presenting one of the major hypotheses in cognitive aging, the cognitive reserve, we will summarize results obtained in different ways on the associations between occupational exposures/conditions and cognitive status. We will focus on two of these exposures: psychosocial stress at work and occupational exposures to solvents.

Cognitive Reserve Hypothesis, How Does Occupational Life Contribute?

The concept of cognitive reserve (Stern 2002) suggests that innate intelligence or aspects of life experience, such as educational or occupational attainment, provide a set of skills that protects individuals from cognitive decline observed in normal aging or dementia. Cognitive reserve (CR) or brain reserve capacity explains why individuals with higher IQ, education, or occupational attainment have lower risks of developing dementia, Alzheimer's disease (AD), or vascular dementia (VaD). The CR hypothesis postulates that CR reduces the prevalence and incidence of AD or

VaD. It also hypothesizes that among those who have greater cognitive reserve (in contrast to those with less reserve), the clinical symptoms of disease appear later for similar brain pathologies. CR can take two forms:

1. Neural reserve in which existing brain networks are more efficient or have greater capacity or may be less susceptible to disruption
2. Neural compensation in which alternative networks may compensate for the pathological disruption of preexisting networks (Stern 2006)

More broadly, mental and physical stimulation both early and throughout the life-course is thought to increase CR allowing cognitive function to be maintained in old age and to both protect against and delay the onset of dementia and AD. Studies on CR are based on different proxies. A large number have examined the place of education (Meng and D'Arcy 2012), whereas fewer have considered occupation (Valenzuela and Sachdev 2006). In this review, higher occupational status and educational achievement have been linked to a reduced risk of dementia (Valenzuela and Sachdev 2006). The same has been shown for a better cognitive performance in late life (Potter et al. 2008; Singh-Manoux et al. 2011). From a lifespan perspective, some studies began to examine which components of occupational activity act, in addition to the effects of education, as proxies of life-course cognitive reserve.

Occupational complexity may be important for cognition in addition to the effects of education. A recent paper exploring life-course cognitive reserve included two adult life (35–55 years) occupational-related factors (Wang et al. 2017):

1. Complexity of work with data and people for the longest held occupation in adult life based on a work complexity matrix
2. Job demands (use of skills to perform job tasks) and decision latitude derived from a job-exposure matrix

They showed that high scores on engagement in adult reserve-enhancing activities such as complex occupational roles were associated with a decreased risk of dementia.

Furthermore, jobs that are challenging (i.e., supervisory or managerial demands), or involve novelty, engagement with others, are likely to have a protective effect on cognition. Cognitive reserve could be the result of accumulated experiences throughout the life course that are influenced by childhood conditions (familial factors), prolonged periods of cognitively stimulating activities either in or out of the workplace including leisure and social activity, but also by other exogenous factors such as contextual factors as illustrated in Fig. 2. Living environment characteristics influence cognitive performance and the risk of dementia, and performing a job exposed to particular working conditions (i.e., shift work) (Marquie et al. 2015) could lead to negative effects on cognitive performance. These findings show the importance of studying the impact of occupational exposures on health with a larger overview of its complexity.

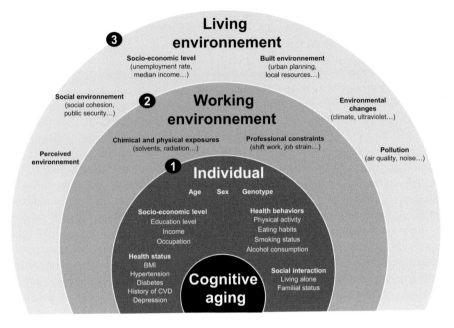

Fig. 2 Individual and contextual determinants of cognitive aging

Psychosocial Factors at Work

The potential importance of occupational status through the CR hypothesis does not preclude other approaches. A growing body of evidence from prospective studies suggests that psychosocial factors at work are significant determinants of health (Kivimaki et al. 2002). The two prominent models in this domain are the job strain model (Karasek 1979; Karasek and Theorell 1990) and the effort-reward imbalance (ERI) model (Siegrist and Marmot 2004). The job strain model assesses dimensions of psychological demands, decision latitude, and social support. It proposes that the combination of low job control and high job demands, called high job strain, increases risks for health. The ERI model postulates that a combination of high effort, low reward, and over-commitment leads to adverse health effects. The accumulated effects of psychosocial exposures are also likely to persist beyond retirement age. This pathway makes sense given the shared vascular risk factors for CVD and cognitive health and established associations between exposures such as intellectual engagement and cognitive function (cognitive reserve).

A small body of research has examined associations between job strain and cognitive function (Then et al. 2014). Most studies focused either on high-demand, low-control conditions ("high-strain" work) or on low job control more generally as the primary risk factors for disease. These studies have generally found a positive association between high-strain work – and low job control overall – and cognitive difficulties in later life. Finally, most studies of job strain and health have focused on high-strain jobs. However, from a neuropsychological perspective, passive (low-demand, low-control) jobs may be risk factors for future cognitive impairment as well; the latter portion of the demand-control matrix is not well studied in relation to cognitive function in later life.

To complete these approaches, E. Sabbath and our team (Sabbath et al. 2016) propose to study the separate and combined relationship between job demands and job control with multiple domains of cognitive function after retirement. We gave attention more specifically to passive jobs that lack both self-direction and complexity, potentially to the detriment of future brain function. We hypothesized that exposure to high-demand, low-control (high-strain) jobs, indicating high work stress, as well as low-demand, low-control (passive) jobs, indicating lack of engagement at work, would be associated with worse performance in various cognitive domains. We used data from French GAZEL cohort members who had undergone post-retirement cognitive testing ($n = 2149$). Psychosocial job characteristics were measured on average 4 years before retirement using Karasek's Job Content Questionnaire (job demands, job control, and demand-control combinations). Both high-demand, low-control (high-strain) and low-demand, low-control (passive) work are significant predictors of moderate and severe cognitive impairment in certain domains after retirement, particularly domains measuring executive function and visual-motor/psycho-motor speed.

These findings corroborate results obtained in the Kungsholmen project (Wang et al. 2012); a cohort of 931 community dwellers aged 75+ years where lifelong work-related psychosocial stress, characterized by low job control and high job strain, was associated with increased risk of AD and dementia. Passive jobs are not stimulating; an example of a passive job is a parking lot attendant. Although the majority of literature has concentrated on high-strain jobs as risk factors for cardiovascular disease, our study demonstrates that passive jobs may be a risk factor for cognitive difficulties. The plausibility of this association is suggested by the occupational complexity literature, which points to evidence that cognitive stimulation at work promotes intellectual flexibility and stability.

Thus, improving the complexity or variety in passive jobs – many of which are held by lower-wage workers who are already at increased risk of cognitive difficulties due to low education/low cognitive reserve – may reduce subsequent disparities in cognitive function at older ages. A final notable finding was marked attenuation of associations between high-strain and passive work and most cognitive tests upon adjustment for socioeconomic status. The observed attenuation may have occurred because of covariation of low job control with low SES markers. In addition, occupation-based SES may partially reflect physical and chemical occupational hazards also associated with cognitive function. These chemical exposures will be discussed in the third part of this chapter.

Occupational Chemical Exposures, an Effect on Brain Functioning Long After Exposure: Focus on Solvents

Occupational exposure to chemicals can induce a number of diseases. Besides acute toxic effects, research demonstrated long-term effects of chemical exposures for various chronic diseases such as cancers and pulmonary diseases. Evidence linking chemical exposures to cancers is strong. Many recognized human carcinogens are occupational carcinogens (Siemiatycki et al. 2004). In industrialized countries, the fraction of all cancers attributable to occupational exposure is at least 5%, contributing to social inequalities in health.

The place of environmental or occupational toxicant exposures in the development of neurodegenerative disorders including dementia, Alzheimer's disease, and Parkinson's disease is supported by a growing body of evidence. Occupational exposure to chemicals shows long-term neurotoxic effects. The list of studied exposures is long, and level of confidence in results is not so high for dementia and cognitive disorders (Genuis and Kelln 2015). Metals such as lead and aluminum, and to a lesser extent mercury, are under consideration due to their neurotoxic potentiality and some controversial epidemiological findings. Various chemical and physical factors have been implicated in neurodegenerative disorders due to their neurotoxicity at high doses (Hakansson et al. 2003). Pesticides including insecticides, herbicides, and fungicides are suspected to be involved in Parkinson's disease, with a 60% increased risk of Parkinson's disease. In a population-based study of exposed male farmers (Moisan et al. 2015), high-intensive exposure to fungicides and insecticides was associated with Parkinson's disease, even when disease onset occurred more than 20 years after exposure. It should be noted that mechanistic plausibility is difficult to establish given the large number of molecules identified in the different classes of pesticides and that assessment of pesticide exposure appears to be a crucial limitation in most studies. Long-term neurobehavioral effects of pesticides are also very controversial.

Similar questions are raised for different occupational chemical exposures, and we will now focus on a particular group, occupational solvent exposures for which we have recently published results using prospective data.

Solvents (White and Proctor 1997) are ubiquitous in industrial societies in a wide range of processes. The term "solvents" encompasses organic chemicals that differ widely in structure. All types of organic solvents are volatile liquids at room temperature and are lipophilic. Solvents are used as degreasers, adjuvants, thinners, cleaners, and purifiers. Industries in which workers are often exposed to organic solvents include automotive manufacturing and repair, paint and varnish manufacturing, the electronic industry, industrial cleaning, metal-part degreasing, dry-cleaning, the building, and furnishing sectors. They represent common occupational exposures with an increased use in new technologies. Millions of workers are exposed to organic solvents in a wide range of processes; in industrialized countries, exposure prevalence is around 8%.

The symptoms experienced after contact with these agents are generally related to the functioning of the central or peripheral nervous system. They resolve after cessation of exposure except for high-dose acute exposures, which can produce long-lasting effects characterized by cognitive and behavioral changes. Acute, low-dose exposures may be associated with specific changes in test performance that resolve after withdrawal from or a decrease in dose of exposure (White and Proctor 1997). Acute toxic encephalopathy, a rare event, can induce confusion, coma, and seizures related to cerebral edema, central nervous system capillary damage, or hypoxia.

Since the 1970s, beginning with several reports from Scandinavia, various studies have suggested that chronic low level occupational exposure to organic solvents may have a negative impact on cognitive and psychological functioning (Mikkelsen 1997; White and Proctor 1997). Indeed, a cluster of clinical symptoms, alternatively named "chronic painter's syndrome," "solvent syndrome," or "chronic toxic encephalopathy," have been reported among exposed workers. This cluster included headache, fatigue, irritability, depression, personality changes, and neurobehavioral difficulties. Typically, these neurobehavioral changes in adults have been described in earlier studies as limited to specific domains including attentional capacity, executive function, visuospatial skills, and short-term memory. Some patients have complaints and symptoms that fit diagnostic criteria for chronic fatigue syndrome. This led to the development of neuropsychological test batteries for the clinical assessment of patients exposed to potential neurotoxicants.

However, most studies were performed during active life using a cross-sectional design. They were mostly based on men, small selected samples and comparisons often lacked suitable control groups. Exposure assessment was retrospective, and potential confounders were not fully taken into account. Furthermore, as neuropsychological tests vary between studies and measures of solvent exposure differ, comparisons of results are difficult (Gamble 2000). Neuropsychological changes associated with exposure to organic solvents have been documented mainly during active occupational life (Hakansson et al. 2003). Some findings are consistent with residual central nervous system dysfunction from long-term exposure to organic solvents, persisting years after the end of exposure (Daniell et al. 1999). Whatever these limits, solvents may impact working memory, attention, and processing speed primarily due to their lipophilic and hydrophilic properties and subsequent ability to be absorbed by fatty tissue and cellular membranes (van Valen et al. 2009).

Results from the GAZEL Cohort: An Effect on Brain Functioning Long After Solvent Exposures

Our results from the GAZEL cohort on solvents exposures and cognitive impairment (Berr et al. 2010; Sabbath et al. 2012, 2014) shed new light on the long-term effects of solvent exposures in a large occupational cohort. GAZEL is a socioeconomically diverse cohort of 20,625 French civil servants employed at the national utility company, "Electricite de France-Gaz de France (EDF-GDF)," set up in 1989. Details on cohort recruitment and data collection are available elsewhere (Goldberg et al. 2007). Data on the history of professional positions are available from the company files. In 2002 and 2010, GAZEL investigators launched two campaigns to conduct cognitive examinations of participants in testing centers throughout France. Investigators documented a large numbers of covariates known to be associated with cognitive impairment in this cohort, which were considered in the analyses as potential confounding factors.

In the GAZEL cohort, lifetime exposure trajectories can be calculated because full job histories are available through company records. Chemical exposure was assessed through a job-exposure matrix called MATEX specific to EDF-GDF (Imbernon et al. 1991). The MATEX JEM has been validated, and widely used. Overall, there were a large number of male subjects exposed at least once during their career to each of the agents of the JEM; for instance, almost 40% were exposed to solvents, 26.6% to asbestos, 29.2% to PCBs, and 31.8% to herbicides-pesticides; joint exposures were common too. Linking the individual work history data with a job-exposure matrix enables lifelong exposures to be attributed to all cohort members and to allocate subject-specific cumulative exposure indices (duration and level) for each agent at yearly intervals. This allows to account for age at first exposure, latency, and different time windows of exposure. We characterize lifetime inhaled exposure to four categories of organic solvents: chlorinated solvents (tetrachloromethane, trichloroethylene, perchloroethylene, dichloromethane, trichloroethane), petroleum solvents (hydrazine, others) benzene, and non-benzene aromatic solvents (toluene diisocyanate).

In 5242 participants (aged 55–65 years) examined in 2002–2004, cognitive performance was assessed using the digit symbol substitution test (DSST), which evaluates response speed, sustained attention, visual spatial skills, associative learning, and memory. We showed a greater risk of poor cognitive performance (DSST score <25th percentile) among those with high exposure to benzene (OR = 1.58; 95% CI 1.31–1.90), chlorinated (OR = 1.39; 95% CI 1.3–2.3), aromatic (OR = 1.76; 95% CI 1.08–2.87), and petroleum solvents (OR = 1.50; 95% CI 1.23–1.81). These results suggest that occupational exposures to solvents may be associated later in life with cognitive impairment, even after taking into account the effects of education, employment grade, and numerous health factors, as well as retirement status.

The second paper on the same population (Sabbath et al. 2012) explores whether childhood educational attainment modifies the effect of career-long occupational solvent exposure on cognitive function after age 55. We hypothesized that cognitive reserve would protect those with greater education against the neurotoxic effects of occupational solvent exposure. We indeed found differential effects of solvent exposure on cognition by educational attainment. Solvent exposure rates were higher among less-educated participants. Within this group, there was a dose-response relationship between lifetime exposure to each solvent type and relative risk (RR) for poor cognition (e.g., for high exposure to benzene, RR = 1.24, 95% CI 1.09–1.41), with significant linear trends in three out of four solvent types. As solvent exposure is associated with poor cognition only among less-educated participants, we suggest that higher cognitive reserve in the more-educated group may explain this finding. This study, if confirmed, postulates that social disadvantage early in life may be exacerbated by greater vulnerability to occupational exposures, in turn leading to disparities in cognitive function in early old age. Testing whether this relationship also exists for other occupational neurotoxic exposures such as lead or pesticides would improve our understanding of the mechanism at play.

We took advantage of the second wave of neuropsychological exams in 2010 to review and detail these relationships between solvents and cognition in 2143 men who were at the time almost all retired (average age 66 years, 10 years after retirement) (Sabbath et al. 2014). These subjects benefited from a more complete neuropsychological battery exploring general cognitive functioning, verbal memory, verbal fluency, visual motor speed, executive functioning, and concentration. Individuals were first dichotomized as ever/never exposed to a given solvent type. The exposed were then dichotomized into moderate exposure (total lifetime dose below sample median) and high exposure (lifetime dose at or above median). Exposed individuals were also dichotomized by date of last exposure to a given solvent type: either 1960–1979 ("distal") or 1980–1998 ("proximal"). We thus tested whether lifetime occupational exposure to solvents was associated with cognitive deficits in retired workers by examining the role of lifetime dose, exposure timing, and a combined dose-timing metric. We hypothesized that those with high, recent exposure would be at greatest risk but also that the highly exposed would exhibit deficits regardless of exposure timing. In this population, 33% of participants were exposed to chlorinated solvents, 26% to benzene, and 25% to petroleum solvents. High exposure to solvents was significantly associated with poor cognition for almost all tests. Retirees at greatest risk for deficits had both high lifetime exposure to solvents and were last exposed 12–30 years prior to testing. Risk was also elevated among those with high lifetime exposure who were last exposed 31–50 years prior to testing. Those with high, recent exposure exhibited impairment in almost all domains, including those not typically previously associated with solvent exposure.

Several hundred million tons of organic solvents are still used worldwide each year, although regulatory pressure and concerns for the environment are gradually leading to a reduction in use. Occupational exposures are clearly modifiable factors. The solvents examined in our works have been extensively linked to cancer, with the fraction of all cancers attributable to occupational exposure being at least 5% (Boffetta et al. 1997; Harvard Report on Cancer Prevention. 1996). Their importance with regard to cognitive aging and risk of dementia needs to be more fully evaluated in future studies.

But while the risk of cognitive impairment among moderately exposed workers may attenuate with time, this may not be fully true for those with higher exposure. This has implications for physicians working with formerly solvent-exposed patients as well as for policies limiting exposure in the workplace. Furthermore, these findings strengthen evidence of detrimental effects of occupational solvents on workers' cognitive health and provide a more complete picture of long-term effects of solvent exposure on multiple domains of cognitive function in retirement.

Cognitive Aging and Retirement

Another consequence of not considering the life period preceding age 65 is the risk of missing a major life event: professional retirement. Retirement involves dealing with important changes in the social, psychological, or cognitive demands of the environment. Retirement can be expected to increase the risk of accelerated cognitive decline due to a decrease in mentally challenging tasks following the exit from the labor market. This explanation is suggested by the cognitive reserve hypothesis, but the potential negative effects of retirement may differ according to the level of the mental demand or stimulation of the job. Other phenomena linked to retirement may be involved. Impairment of cognitive functioning or various health problems associated with increased risk of cognitive impairment may prevent individuals from working and be associated with earlier retirement. Retirement status can also affect social environment and support, while social isolation is a known risk factor of cognitive dysfunction.

Very few studies have directly investigated the impact of retirement on cognition. Data issued from the European SHARE cohort study suggest that, accounting for age, sex, and education, all types of occupational activities clearly have a positive effect on cognitive functioning (Adam et al. 2013). In this study, the cognitive functioning of two individuals, one still professionally active and the other retired, will differ significantly in favor of the former, all other things being equal. In the American HRS (Health and Retirement Study) cohort (Bonsang et al. 2012), the negative impact of retirement on cognitive functioning remained significant when controlling for individual heterogeneity and the endogeneity of the retirement decision. This negative effect close to 10% is not immediate but appears with a lag.

Many questions remain unsolved in this field. Results of a meta-analysis of seven longitudinal studies (Meng et al. 2017) show only weak and contradicting evidence for an association between retirement and cognitive decline but indicate that the association is affected by the characteristics of the job the person is retiring from.

Perspectives for the Future

Occupational exposures appear to be socially stratified. To what extent they contribute to social health inequalities in older age, taking into account the influence of non-occupational factors associated with socioeconomic position (measured by education, income, or household wealth) remains to be further explored. We need to ensure that the work exposures are not simply proxies of material factors, social networks, and engagement or health behaviors.

The CONSTANCES cohort setup in 2012 (http://www.constances.fr/index_EN. php) opens exciting perspectives as it now allows us to study the impact of occupational exposures on cognitive aging in a very large sample of men and women aged 45–70 years, recruited from the general population, in most cases a long time before onset of clinical symptoms of neurodegenerative diseases. Two sources of information are available in the CONSTANCES cohort to study occupational exposures:

1. A lifetime occupational exposure questionnaire at cohort entry that includes specific questions on organic solvents
2. A professional calendar that, coupled with the use of a job and environmental exposure matrix, will allow a more detailed evaluation of exposures based on the complete history of the jobs performed

The CONSTANCES cohort will make it possible to study occupational exposures from a global perspective taking into account individual characteristics (sociodemographic factors, lifestyle factors, and health status), lifetime working conditions, and characteristics of the living environment.

Cross-References

▶ Concepts and Social Variations of Disability in Working-Age Populations
▶ Promoting Workplace Mental Wellbeing
▶ Reducing Inequalities in Employment of People with Disabilities

References

Adam S, Bonsang E, Grotz C, Perelman S (2013) Occupational activity and cognitive reserve: implications in terms of prevention of cognitive aging and Alzheimer's disease. Clin Interv Aging 8:377–390. https://doi.org/10.2147/CIA.S39921

Alvarado BE, Zunzunegui MV, Del Ser T, Beland F (2002) Cognitive decline is related to education and occupation in a Spanish elderly cohort. Aging Clin Exp Res 14:132–142

Amieva H et al (2008) Prodromal Alzheimer's disease: successive emergence of the clinical symptoms. Ann Neurol 64:492–498. https://doi.org/10.1002/ana.21509

Berr C, Vercambre MN, Bonenfant S, Manoux AS, Zins M, Goldberg M (2010) Occupational exposure to solvents and cognitive performance in the GAZEL cohort: preliminary results. Dement Geriatr Cogn Disord 30:12–19. https://doi.org/10.1159/000315498

Berr C, Balard F, Blain H, Robine JM (2012) How to define old age: successful aging and/or longevity. Med Sci (Paris) 28:281–287. https://doi.org/10.1051/medsci/2012283016

Boffetta P, Jourenkova N, Gustavsson P (1997) Cancer risk from occupational and environmental exposure to polycyclic aromatic hydrocarbons. Cancer Causes Control 8:444–472

Bonsang E, Adam S, Perelman S (2012) Does retirement affect cognitive functioning? J Health Econ 31(3):490–501. https://doi.org/10.1016/j.jhealeco.2012.03.005

Britton A, Shipley M, Singh-Manoux A, Marmot MG (2008) Successful aging: the contribution of early-life and midlife risk factors. J Am Geriatr Soc 56:1098–1105. https://doi.org/10.1111/j.1532-5415.2008.01740.x

Daniell WE, Claypoole KH, Checkoway H, Smith-Weller T, Dager SR, Townes BD, Rosenstock L (1999) Neuropsychological function in retired workers with previous long-term occupational exposure to solvents. Occup Environ Med 56:93

Daviglus ML et al (2011) Risk factors and preventive interventions for Alzheimer disease: state of the science. Arch Neurol 68:1185–1190. https://doi.org/10.1001/archneurol.2011.100

Fratiglioni L, Paillard-Borg S, Winblad B (2004) An active and socially integrated lifestyle in late life might protect against dementia. Lancet Neurol 3:343–353. https://doi.org/10.1097/01.EDE.0000078446.76859.c9

Gamble JF (2000) Low-level hydrocarbon solvent exposure and neurobehavioural effects. Occup Med (Lond) 50:81–102

Genuis SJ, Kelln KL (2015) Toxicant exposure and bioaccumulation: a common and potentially reversible cause of cognitive dysfunction and dementia. Behav Neurol 2015:1. https://doi.org/10.1155/2015/620143

Goldberg M, Leclerc A, Bonenfant S, Chastang JF, Schmaus A, Kaniewski N, Zins M (2007) Cohort profile: the GAZEL Cohort Study. Int J Epidemiol 36:32–39. https://doi.org/10.1093/ije/dyl247

Hakansson N, Gustavsson P, Johansen C, Floderus B (2003) Neurodegenerative diseases in welders and other workers exposed to high levels of magnetic fields. Epidemiology 14:420–426; discussion 427–428. https://doi.org/10.1097/01.EDE.0000078446.76859.c9

Harvard Report on Cancer Prevention (1996) Volume 1: causes of human cancer. Cancer Causes Control 7(Suppl 1):S3–S59

Helmer C et al (2001) Occupation during life and risk of dementia in French elderly community residents. J Neurol Neurosurg Psychiatry 71:303–309

Imbernon E et al (1991) Matex: une matrice emplois-expositions destin, e ... la surveillance, pid, miologique des travailleurs d'une grande entreprise (EDF-GDF). Arch Malprof 52:559

Jack CR Jr et al (2013) Tracking pathophysiological processes in Alzheimer's disease: an updated hypothetical model of dynamic biomarkers. Lancet Neurol 12:207–216. https://doi.org/10.1016/S1474-4422(12)70291-0

Karasek RA (1979) Job demands, job decision latitude, and mental strain: implications for job redesign. Adm Sci Q 24:285

Karasek RA, Theorell T (1990) Healthy work. Stress, productivity and the reconstruction of working life. Basic Book, New York

Karp A, Kareholt I, Qiu C, Bellander T, Winblad B, Fratiglioni L (2004) Relation of education and occupation-based socioeconomic status to incident Alzheimer's disease. Am J Epidemiol 159:175–183

Kivimaki M, Leino-Arjas P, Luukkonen R, Riihimaki H, Vahtera J, Kirjonen J (2002) Work stress and risk of cardiovascular mortality: prospective cohort study of industrial employees. BMJ 325:857

Livingston G et al (2017) Dementia prevention, intervention, and care. Lancet 390:2673. https://doi.org/10.1016/S0140-6736(17)31363-6

Marquie JC, Tucker P, Folkard S, Gentil C, Ansiau D (2015) Chronic effects of shift work on cognition: findings from the VISAT longitudinal study. Occup Environ Med 72:258–264. https://doi.org/10.1136/oemed-2013-101993

Meng X, D'Arcy C (2012) Education and dementia in the context of the cognitive reserve hypothesis: a systematic review with meta-analyses and qualitative analyses. PLoS One 7: e38268. https://doi.org/10.1371/journal.pone.0038268. PONE-D-12-04086 [pii]

Meng A, Nexo MA, Borg V (2017) The impact of retirement on age related cognitive decline - a systematic review. BMC Geriatr 17(1):160. https://doi.org/10.1186/s12877-017-0556-7

Mikkelsen S (1997) Epidemiological update on solvent neurotoxicity. Environ Res 73:101–112

Moisan F et al (2015) Association of Parkinson's disease and its subtypes with agricultural pesticide exposures in men: a case-control study in France. Environ Health Perspect 123:1123–1129. https://doi.org/10.1289/ehp.1307970

Mura T, Dartigues JF, Berr C (2010) How many dementia cases in France and Europe? Alternative projections and scenarios 2010–2050. Eur J Neurol 17:252–259. https://doi.org/10.1111/j.1468-1331.2009.02783.x. ENE2783 [pii]

Plassman BL, Williams JW Jr, Burke JR, Holsinger T, Benjamin S (2010) Systematic review: factors associated with risk for and possible prevention of cognitive decline in later life. Ann Intern Med 153:182–193. https://doi.org/10.7326/0003-4819-153-3-201008030-00258

Potter GG, Plassman BL, Helms MJ, Foster SM, Edwards NW (2006) Occupational characteristics and cognitive performance among elderly male twins. Neurology 67:1377–1382. https://doi.org/10.1212/01.wnl.0000240061.51215.ed

Potter GG, Helms MJ, Plassman BL (2008) Associations of job demands and intelligence with cognitive performance among men in late life. Neurology 70:1803–1808. https://doi.org/10.1212/01.wnl.0000295506.58497.7e

Qiu C, Karp A, von Strauss E, Winblad B, Fratiglioni L, Bellander T (2003) Lifetime principal occupation and risk of Alzheimer's disease in the Kungsholmen project. Am J Ind Med 43:204–211. https://doi.org/10.1002/ajim.10159

Richards M, Deary IJ (2005) A life course approach to cognitive reserve: a model for cognitive aging and development? Ann Neurol 58:617–622. https://doi.org/10.1002/ana.20637

Sabbath EL, Glymour MM, Berr C, Singh-Manoux A, Zins M, Goldberg M, Berkman LF (2012) Occupational solvent exposure and cognition: does the association vary by level of education? Neurology 78:1754–1760. https://doi.org/10.1212/WNL.0b013e3182583098

Sabbath EL et al (2014) Time may not fully attenuate solvent-associated cognitive deficits in highly exposed workers. Neurology 82:1716–1723. https://doi.org/10.1212/WNL.0000000000000413

Sabbath EL, Andel R, Zins M, Goldberg M, Berr C (2016) Domains of cognitive function in early old age: which ones are predicted by pre-retirement psychosocial work characteristics? Occup Environ Med 73:640–647. https://doi.org/10.1136/oemed-2015-103352

Siegrist J, Marmot M (2004) Health inequalities and the psychosocial environment-two scientific challenges. Soc Sci Med 58:1463–1473. https://doi.org/10.1016/S0277-9536(03)00349-6

Siemiatycki J et al (2004) Listing occupational carcinogens. Environ Health Perspect 112:1447–1459. https://doi.org/10.1289/ehp.7047

Singh-Manoux A, Marmot MG, Glymour M, Sabia S, Kivimaki M, Dugravot A (2011) Does cognitive reserve shape cognitive decline? Ann Neurol 70:296–304. https://doi.org/10.1002/ana.22391

Smyth KA, Fritsch T, Cook TB, McClendon MJ, Santillan CE, Friedland RP (2004) Worker functions and traits associated with occupations and the development of AD. Neurology 63:498–503

Stern Y (2002) What is cognitive reserve? Theory and research application of the reserve concept. J Int Neuropsychol Soc 8:448–460

Stern Y (2006) Cognitive reserve and Alzheimer disease. Alzheimer Dis Assoc Disord 20:S69–S74. 00002093-200607001-00010 [pii]

Then FS et al (2014) Systematic review of the effect of the psychosocial working environment on cognition and dementia. Occup Environ Med 71:358–365

Valenzuela MJ, Sachdev P (2006) Brain reserve and dementia: a systematic review. Psychol Med 36:441–454. https://doi.org/10.1017/S0033291705006264

van Valen E, Wekking E, van der Laan G, Sprangers M, van Dijk F (2009) The course of chronic solvent induced encephalopathy: a systematic review. Neurotoxicology 30:1172–1186. https://doi.org/10.1016/j.neuro.2009.06.002

Virtanen M et al (2009) Long working hours and cognitive function: the Whitehall II Study. Am J Epidemiol 169:596–605. https://doi.org/10.1093/aje/kwn382

Wang HX, Wahlberg M, Karp A, Winblad B, Fratiglioni L (2012) Psychosocial stress at work is associated with increased dementia risk in late life. Alzheimers Dement 8:114–120. https://doi.org/10.1016/j.jalz.2011.03.001

Wang HX, MacDonald SW, Dekhtyar S, Fratiglioni L (2017) Association of lifelong exposure to cognitive reserve-enhancing factors with dementia risk: a community-based cohort study. PLoS Med 14:e1002251. https://doi.org/10.1371/journal.pmed.1002251

White RF, Proctor SP (1997) Solvents and neurotoxicity. Lancet 349:1239–1243

Yu F, Ryan LH, Schaie KW, Willis SL, Kolanowski A (2009) Factors associated with cognition in adults: the Seattle Longitudinal Study. Res Nurs Health 32:540–550. https://doi.org/10.1002/nur.20340

Work-Related Burden of Absenteeism, Presenteeism, and Disability: An Epidemiologic and Economic Perspective

14

Marnie Dobson, Peter Schnall, Ellen Rosskam, and Paul Landsbergis

Contents

Introduction	252
The Role of Working Conditions in Disability, Absenteeism, and Presenteeism	253
Psychosocial Work Stressors, Musculoskeletal Disorders, and Occupational Injuries	254
Psychosocial Work Stressors and Chronic Mental and Physical Illness	254
Psychosocial Work Stressors and Population Attributable Risk (PAR) Percent	255
Psychosocial Stressors, Disability, and Workers' Compensation	256
Psychosocial Stressors and Absenteeism	259
Psychosocial Stressors and "Presenteeism"	260
Economic Burden of Psychosocial Work Stressors	261
Cost to Workers	261
Costs to Organizations	262
Cost to Societies	264
Conclusion	266
Barriers to Prevention of Work Stress in the USA	267
Cross-References	268
References	268

Abstract

As noncommunicable chronic diseases rise in prevalence globally, so are the years individuals are living with disability, particularly disability resulting from mental health disorders such as depression, musculoskeletal disorders, and cardiovascular disease (CVD). The psychosocial work environment including

M. Dobson (✉) · P. Schnall (✉)
Center for Occupational and Environmental Health, University of California, Irvine, CA, USA
e-mail: mdobson@uci.edu; pschnall@workhealth.org

E. Rosskam
Center for Social Epidemiology, Los Angeles, CA, USA

P. Landsbergis
SUNY Downstate School of Public Health, Brooklyn, NY, USA
e-mail: Paul.Landsbergis@downstate.edu

© Springer Nature Switzerland AG 2020
U. Bültmann, J. Siegrist (eds.), *Handbook of Disability, Work and Health*, Handbook Series in Occupational Health Sciences, https://doi.org/10.1007/978-3-030-24334-0_13

work-related psychosocial stressors, such as high demands, low job control (job strain), effort-reward imbalance, low social support, work-life conflict, bullying, and harassment, are significant contributors to these disorders, as well as to disability pensions, sickness absence, and presenteeism. These outcomes represent a substantial financial burden to workers, organizations, and societies. While many high-income countries provide social protection programs, including universal health care and state disability pensions that help to mitigate the burden of chronic disease on the worker, the USA has a very limited social safety net. Additionally, the USA is one of the few remaining high-income countries that do not officially recognize work-related psychosocial risks, which would require employers to identify and reduce psychosocial hazards to the same extent as other occupational hazards. Recognition by employers as well as by health policy-makers in the USA, that psychosocial risks pose a significant health and financial burden, is necessary.

Keywords

Psychosocial work stressors · Chronic illness · Disability · Absenteeism · Presenteeism · Costs · Productivity · Sick leave · Workers' compensation

Introduction

Disability adjusted life years (DALYs) is a measure of both years of life lost due to disability and years lived with disability. Globally, ischemic heart disease was the leading cause of DALYs in 2010 (Murray et al. 2012). While mortality rates are decreasing, particularly in high-income countries mostly due to aggressive treatments for cardiovascular disease and high blood pressure, the years lived with disability (YLDs) are increasing (Global Burden of Disease Study 2013 2015). Additionally, most cases of cardiovascular disease occur after people leave work, impacting their well-being and shortening their lifespan but not adding much to years lived with disability. Globally there have been substantial increases between 1990 and 2013 in the prevalence of and YLDs due to noncommunicable chronic diseases (NCDs) (ibidem). The leading causes of YLDs are musculoskeletal disorders (with low back pain at the top of that category) and mental and substance abuse disorders (predominantly major depressive disorders and anxiety) (ibidem). Musculoskeletal disorders (MSDs) accounted for over 20% of YLDs globally in 2010, partly a product of aging populations, but also driven by rising obesity rates and physically demanding work, as well as physical inactivity in many jobs, which are a crucial component of health-care costs in high- and middle-income countries. Mental health disorders, particularly major depressive disorder and substance abuse disorders, accounted for over 21% of YLDs (Murray et al. 2012).

There is a significant body of evidence documenting that working conditions, in particular psychosocial work stressors arising from the nature of modern work, are significant contributors to mental health disorders (Theorell and Aronsson 2015), musculoskeletal disorders (Hauke et al. 2011), hypertension, diabetes, obesity, and cardiovascular disease (Schnall et al. 2016). The contribution of the psychosocial work environment to these chronic illnesses and to the resulting disability outcomes as well as to increases in absenteeism (i.e., lost work days), presenteeism (i.e., reduced productivity due to working while ill or injured), and related costs will be explored in this chapter.

The Role of Working Conditions in Disability, Absenteeism, and Presenteeism

Working conditions can contribute to the prevalence of illness and disability via two mechanisms. Injuries and illnesses specifically related to recognized occupational hazards can result in increases in workers' compensation claims and productivity losses due to short- and long-term sick leave, absenteeism, and presenteeism. In addition, there is a robust literature recognizing that stress arising from the ways in which work tasks are organized and how policies and practices are implemented by an organization constitute psychosocial hazards that can lead to ill health, disability, and death. Research demonstrates that job strain (high demands, low control) low social support, effort-reward imbalance, bullying, as well as other work organization factors (e.g., long work hours, shift work, and precarious work) are causal factors. These work-related psychosocial and other work organization factors act as "stressors" by triggering the biological "fight or flight" stress response on a chronic basis, which, over time, can lead to long-term physiological changes, including changes in blood pressure, inflammatory effects, and metabolic changes (Landsbergis et al. 2017a). Research shows that psychosocial work stressors contribute to the incidence of occupational injuries and musculoskeletal disorders (Farnacio et al. 2017; Hauke et al. 2011) as well as chronic illnesses such as depression (Theorell and Aronsson 2015), hypertension (Landsbergis et al. 2013a), cardiovascular disease risk factors (diabetes, obesity), and cardiovascular disease (Theorell et al. 2016). These are also some of the most prevalent illnesses contributing to YLDs and DALYs globally.

Recognizing that aspects of the work environment contribute to the incidence and prevalence of disability means that the workplace and the organization of work are important points of intervention to prevent illness, therefore potentially preventing a proportion of disability related to mental health disorders, musculoskeletal disorders, and cardiovascular disease risk factors (hypertension, diabetes, and obesity). Some countries require employers to pay into a workers' compensation fund to be used in the event of a work-related injury or illness. National recognition of the contribution of psychosocial hazards, however, is largely insufficient. Encouragingly, a number of high- and middle-income countries, although not the USA, have come to recognize that work-related psychosocial hazards significantly impact organizations by negatively affecting the health and well-being of working people, increasing healthcare costs, and decreasing productivity due to absenteeism and presenteeism. Consequently, work-related psychosocial hazards are regularly researched and regulated in a number of countries because they are understood as impacting health-care and disability costs and represent a substantial economic burden on state health-care and disability systems, as well as on individuals (EU-OSHA 2014). In the USA, psychosocial stressors are mostly not recognized as work-related or compensated by workers' compensation insurance, nor are they calculated into the costs of occupational injuries and illnesses. Furthermore, they are not regulated as occupational health risks, with some exceptions, such as workplace violence, fair scheduling laws, nurse staffing laws, and bans on mandatory overtime for nurses.

Psychosocial Work Stressors, Musculoskeletal Disorders, and Occupational Injuries

Given that musculoskeletal disorders and occupational injuries are among the leading causes of disability worldwide, the impact of psychosocial work stressors on MSDs and injuries has been a robust area of investigation. Jobs requiring high physical demands, such as lifting, kneeling, or standing, are related to increased risk of injuries and musculoskeletal disorders and subsequent likelihood of long-term sickness absence or disability pension (Sundstrup et al. 2017). However, after controlling for physical work factors, some studies and reviews have found moderate evidence for the role of psychological demands, emotional demands, job insecurity, work-family imbalance, hostile relationships with supervisors or coworkers, and effort-reward imbalance on musculoskeletal disorders or occupational injuries (Farnacio et al. 2017; Hauke et al. 2011). In a review and meta-analysis of 54 longitudinal studies, statistically significant, small to medium effects were found on the risk of onset of MSDs for low social support, high job demands, low job control, low decision authority, low skill discretion, low job satisfaction, and high job strain (Hauke et al. 2011). It was estimated that the onset of MSDs is elevated 15–59% among employees exposed to psychosocial work stressors and recommended that interventions to prevent MSDs focus on both physical and psychosocial risk factors.

Psychosocial Work Stressors and Chronic Mental and Physical Illness

A growing occupational epidemiology literature, including many prospective cohort studies, has investigated the role of psychosocial work stressors on mental health problems and chronic physical illnesses (e.g., CVD and CVD-related risks) in working populations. Work stressors have also been shown to affect chronic illnesses indirectly by influencing health behaviors, including leisure time physical activity, smoking, and alcohol consumption, all of which are considered risk factors for obesity, diabetes, and heart disease (Schnall et al. 2016).

The strongest and most consistent research documents the effects of job strain – work that is high in psychological demands, and low in control or "decision latitude"– on burnout (Aronsson et al. 2017), depression (Theorell and Aronsson

2015), high blood pressure (Landsbergis et al. 2013a), diabetes (Huth et al. 2014), and cardiovascular disease (Theorell et al. 2016). Effort-reward imbalance (ERI) (i.e., work that is associated with a high level of effort or "over-commitment" with a mismatch in levels of reward) has been associated in longitudinal studies with depression (Rugulies et al. 2017), high blood pressure (Gilbert-Ouimet et al. 2014), and cardiovascular disease (Schnall et al. 2016). Bullying has also been shown in recent longitudinal reviews to be strongly associated with mental health problems (Theorell and Aronsson 2015), and more recently with cardiovascular disease (Xu et al. 2018). Low social support, low organizational justice, long work hours, work-family conflict, job insecurity, and other work stressors also have been shown to have modest levels of effect on mental and physical health problems (Theorell and Aronsson 2015).

Psychosocial Work Stressors and Population Attributable Risk (PAR) Percent

Job strain is one of the work stressors with consistently strong evidence of adverse health effects and that provides elevated estimates of population attributable risk percent (PAR%) (i.e., how much of a disease could be prevented in a population if the risk was eliminated). This is important as it allows policy- and other decision-makers to interpret how much work stressors contribute to various negative health outcomes, to disability, and other productivity outcomes and are therefore preventable. PARs help policy- and other decision-makers use evidence to set priorities and allocate funds to improve population health, economic health, and overall social well-being.

Population attributable risk percent for job strain has been estimated at 14% for common mental health disorders and at 15% for depression, which means that some 14–15% of new cases of mental health disorders or depression could be prevented by eliminating job strain (LaMontagne et al. 2010). In a study of the Australian workforce, it was estimated that 5.8% (AU$730 million) of the societal cost of depression for 1 year could be attributed to job strain (LaMontagne et al. 2010). A recent review article discussed new research that shows cumulative exposure to job strain has a stronger adverse effect on the risk of depressive symptoms at follow-up and that other work stressors, not included in these calculations, also contribute to depression and other mental health problems (Theorell and Aronsson 2015), indicating that the PAR% might be even higher.

Research on job strain and cardiovascular disease has also demonstrated significant population attributable risks. The PAR% for job strain and acute ischemic heart disease (IHD) has been estimated at 5%, assuming a job strain prevalence of 22% and a risk ratio (RR) as low as 1.3 (Theorell et al. 2016). Moreover, this is just one work stressor (job strain), and many stressors have shown independent effects (Choi et al. 2015). In 2013, the International Commission on Occupational Health (ICOH) Scientific Committee on Cardiology in Occupational Health concluded that between 10% and 20% of cardiovascular mortality in working-age populations can be attributed to work (Tokyo Declaration).

Psychosocial Stressors, Disability, and Workers' Compensation

Disability is defined as a physical or mental impairment that affects one or more areas of daily life activities, including work, but is not considered work-related. The Americans with Disabilities Act protects those with disabilities from discrimination due to their disability, requiring workplaces, schools, and other institutions to accommodate individuals who have mental or physical impairments/differences. Disability insurance programs replace some of the wages lost by workers who cannot work because of a disabling injury or illness that is not work-related. If it is considered "work-related" then workers can file for workers compensation in the USA (Monaco 2015) (Box A).

> **Box A – US Disability Insurance and Workers' Compensation: A Special Case**
> Social protection programs vary by country, impacting who bears the burden of costs related to illness or disability (i.e., the state, the employer, or the worker), and to what extent people are protected. The USA, for example, has a social safety "net," not a solid protection "floor" through which no one can fall. In the event of work-related injuries or illnesses, employer or state workers' compensation funds provide some financial protection to workers. Every state has its own workers' compensation laws defining what is a "compensable" work-related injury or illness, which are contained in statutes, and vary from state to state. Under the law in most states, every business must have some form of workers' compensation insurance to cover injured employees. Workers' compensation systems are the primary mechanisms through which employers can be held financially responsible for the health and safety of employees.
>
> In practice, there are significant barriers to workers' filing compensation claims resulting in significant underreporting of occupational injuries or work-related pain, and use of sick leave or vacation time to recover from what is, in reality, a work-related injury or illness. Financial hardship is a strong disincentive for workers to file a claim for workers' compensation, especially in low-wage occupations. There is an unknown time period between filing a claim and actually receiving any benefits; there is the likelihood of having to cover unpaid medical bills if claims are denied; and even if claims are awarded, wage replacement is significantly lower than the individual's previous wage, increasingly so as absence from work continues. In the USA, because successful claims made by workers can cause an employer's workers compensation insurance premium to increase, trigger an investigation, or create a negative reputation for the company (or all of the above), employers often discourage workers from making claims through the workers' compensation system. Workers can be "pressured" or "encouraged" to use their health insurance to pay for their health-care needs, instead of filing a legitimate

(continued)

workers' compensation claim. The protections that workers can receive through workers' compensation are not necessarily equivalent to those they may receive through health insurance. An important result of this mendacious approach is that costs incurred by work-related illnesses get externalized (i.e., not counted as part of a company or organization's bottom line) and are not counted as work-related, leading to significant underestimates in official work-related illness data (Rosskam 2007).

Unlike many other high- and middle-income countries including the European Union and Canada, in the USA psychosocial work stressors and their resultant health effects are not recognized as work-related and are, therefore, not compensable by workers' compensation. If burnout, anxiety, depression, MSDs, or cardiovascular disease prevent a worker from being able to work and require them to take short-term or long-term disability leave, their employer may provide disability benefits, but employers are not required to have disability insurance in the USA (Monaco 2015). More likely in such cases, workers would request disability payments through Social Security Disability (SSDI) or Supplemental Security Income (SSI), both of which are federal government programs offering cash benefits to disabled individuals. The programs have very different financial eligibility requirements. SSDI is available to workers who have accumulated a sufficient number of work credits, while SSI disability benefits are means-tested, available to low-income individuals who have either never worked or who have not earned enough work credits to qualify for SSDI. The amount of the monthly benefit depends on one's earnings record. The cost of disability includes money in lieu of wages paid to employees because they are unable to work, the time lost at work, and the costs of administration. These costs can include those due to temporary disability, permanent partial, and permanent total.

There are many obstacles in filing for and getting approved for disability payments through these programs. For both programs, the process of filing for disability is long. Initial claims can take 4 months (or longer) to be evaluated, after which over 60% are rejected. A request for reconsideration can take several months as well, and around 85% of those are rejected as well. If one chooses to file a new claim, they face starting all over, with the resultant waiting periods, after which they may be rejected once again. If they choose to appeal their case before an administrative judge (the most commonly recommended course of action), 2 years can pass by until the case is heard.

In the USA, relying on long-term disability benefits through either SSDI or SSI can mean living at or below the federal poverty level. The costs of work-related disability are borne by the affected individuals, employers, and by society. The loss of income has a substantial financial and general negative impact on the many working people experiencing disability. The absence of federal or state laws in the USA requiring employers to prevent illness related

(continued)

> to workplace psychosocial stressors means that afflicted workers often return to or remain in the same conditions. Because of the lack of regulation and many of the costs being externalized, there are few incentives for employers to improve the organization of work.

Psychosocial work stressors contribute to workers' compensation and disability costs when they contribute to injuries and illnesses that are recognized as compensable. However, identifying and quantifying the contribution of work stressors to these costs is quite complex. Robust evidence indicates that psychosocial work stressors can play a role in illnesses such as burnout, depression, hypertension, and heart disease, but these generally are not recognized as work-related (Jauregui and Schnall 2009). Instead, these illnesses are most often seen as the result of individual behaviors or genetic history. Recognizing, addressing, and preventing the impact of work-related psychosocial stressors in producing illnesses that may result in disability is an important point of entry for the prevention of illness and disability-related costs.

Longitudinal studies have evidenced an independent relationship between disability and psychological job demands, decision latitude, or job strain (Canivet et al. 2013). In a Finnish prospective cohort study of public sector employees, those exposed to job strain were 2.6 times more likely to have a disability pension at follow-up. This relationship was replicated in aggregated work-unit level measurements of job strain and after controlling for health behaviors, prevalent diseases, psychological distress, and self-rated health (Laine et al. 2009).

Disability has been strongly associated with psychological distress, depression, and chronic work stress. One Canadian study found an interaction effect; a combination of having a psychiatric disorder and a chronic physical condition plus chronic work stress was associated with the highest odds of disability (Dewa et al. 2007). Effort-reward imbalance was associated with disability related to depression in a large Finnish cohort, and the authors also found that the combination of job strain and ERI doubled the risk of disability pension due to depression (Juvani et al. 2018).

Disability due to cardiovascular disease may be more difficult to predict compared to depression-related disability or disability from MSDs, since the etiological time frame is longer in the development of CVD, and in older persons there are frequently multiple work- and non- work-related disorders. In certain populations, however, job characteristics have been strongly associated with disability due to CVD. Occupations requiring vigilance and responsibility for others, such as air traffic controllers, airline pilots, flight attendants, professional drivers, teachers, and manual workers (machinists, carpenters etc.), have the highest rates of cardiovascular disability. In a study of autoworkers using employer administrative data, disability claims for hypertension, CVD, and psychological disorders were higher among assembly line workers and workers in a facility with 10 more overtime hours per week than other facilities (Landsbergis et al. 2013b). Understanding the factors that might contribute to disability leave in workers with CVD could be an important area for prevention. A longitudinal study of health- and work-related predictors (e.g., alcohol, smoking, obesity, physical inactivity, job strain, ERI, social support, and shift work) of disability in employees with and without cardiometabolic diseases found these predictors accounted for 24% of the excess work disability in hypertension, 28% in diabetes, and 11% in heart or cerebrovascular disease (Ervasti et al. 2016).

In addition, a meta-analysis of four prospective studies has shown that employees who have suffered a first heart attack or other coronary heart disease and return to work to a job with job strain or effort-reward imbalance are 65% more likely to have a recurrent (second) case of coronary heart disease (Li et al. 2014). Due to improved medical care and an aging workforce, more and more employees are returning to work with heart disease. The clear implication of this research is that to reduce disability and to increase healthy and productive aging at work, sources of work stress need to be reduced.

Psychosocial Stressors and Absenteeism

Absenteeism is generally defined by employers as "a habitual pattern of absence from work obligations without good reason" and is generally considered as an employee performance problem. Some absences are protected by law (e.g., US Family Medical Leave Act) or by organizational policies (e.g., sick leave or vacation time). In the USA, however, there are no federal laws requiring employers to provide paid sick leave, and many workers, especially those in low-wage, part-time, or precarious jobs, do not receive any sick leave or vacation time from their employers. Therefore, workers without sick leave who are ill or have sick family members or other pressing obligations often have little choice but to take an "unexcused" absence without pay or to come to work sick (i.e., "presenteeism"). For women, and those with chronic health problems, absences due to sickness or to family responsibilities are generally higher than for men. Providing adequate paid sick leave for all workers would result in some progress toward addressing both "absenteeism" and "presenteeism" and address gender and class inequalities. However, sick leave is costly and is also a predictor of disability pensions and of higher morbidity and mortality (Westerlund et al. 2004), therefore preventing illness by reducing psychosocial stressors is essential.

Psychosocial work stressors have been shown in many studies, including now many prospective studies, to be strongly associated with sickness absence (Mather et al. 2015). In particular, low decision latitude has repeatedly been related to increased sickness absences, while high skill discretion and supervisor support have been associated with lower sickness absences (Rugulies et al. 2007). These studies have shown that specific psychosocial work stressors affect short-term and long-term sickness absence differently and differ by gender. Other studies addressing the demand-control-support model (job strain), effort-reward imbalance, and exposure to violence at work also have been shown to be related to increased sickness absences (Ndjaboue et al. 2014). A systematic review and meta-analysis of 17 prospective studies on workplace bullying and sickness absence showed that exposure to bullying increased the risk of sickness absence by an odds ratio of 1.58 (95% CI 1.39–1.79) (Nielsen et al. 2016).

Some research also has estimated the proportion of sickness absences due to the psychosocial work environment. In a follow-up study of 52 Danish workplaces using employer sickness absence data, etiologic fractions were estimated and showed that psychosocial factors explained 29% of all sick-leave days (in particular, decision authority, social support from supervisors, psychological demands, and predictability) (Nielsen et al. 2006). And in a 3-year follow-up study of human service workers, the authors estimated that improving the psychosocial work environment and eliminating violence and threats would reduce 32% of sickness absences in that population (Rugulies et al. 2007).

Workers exposed to psychosocial work stressors are more likely to experience chronic illnesses such as burnout, depression, and hypertension, and those with these illnesses are more likely to take sick leave, thus increasing sickness absence in an organization. There is ample evidence, therefore, that organizations could reduce absenteeism and sick leave utilization by improving the quality of work, reducing psychosocial hazards, and improving workers' health.

Psychosocial Stressors and "Presenteeism"

Presenteeism is widely referred to as working despite being physically sick, mentally ill, injured, or exhausted, resulting in reduced productivity or reduced performance. Many people go to work feeling at less than optimal because they have a commitment to the job or to clients, while others cannot afford to take sick days off or to go on disability. Many have no entitlement to paid sick days. Others are afraid to lose their jobs by not being ever-present at work. Sometimes presenteeism occurs for a combination of these reasons. While the reduction in an employee's performance is an indirect but relevant factor influencing productivity, it is not easy to estimate the prevalence of presenteeism in a workplace or to quantify the costs of lost productivity.

Presenteeism has been identified in studies of specific illnesses in the workplace, including migraines, burnout, and depression, as well as studies of work-life balance (Biron et al. 2006). Presenteeism has been shown to be a response to job stressors, overwork, and company policies and demonstrated to have substantial longitudinal relationships with excessive job demands and burnout (i.e., exhaustion and depersonalization) (Demerouti et al. 2009). Workers mobilize compensation strategies when they experience exhaustion, which can ultimately increase their exhaustion. The reciprocal nature of exhaustion and presenteeism is of considerable importance to address proactively.

The 2011 Québec Survey on Working and Employment Conditions and Occupational Health and Safety found that presenteeism affects more than half of Québec's workforce (Vézina et al. 2011). The study revealed a high prevalence of long-term presenteeism associated with a number of organizational and physical work demands, in particular low decision latitude, lack of job rewards or recognition, low social support at work, exposure to psychological harassment in the workplace, and frequent exposure to certain physical work demands. It further found women and individuals living in low-income households to be disproportionately affected by poor working conditions and more prone to long-term presenteeism.

To improve the well-being, performance, and productivity of their workforce, employers should make concerted efforts to prevent presenteeism by improving working conditions, reducing work stressors, and preventing burnout. Removing stigmas surrounding mental health problems may help more workers feel safe to report their problems and *not* go to work when they are sick. From a policy perspective, all working people deserve social protection that includes adequate paid vacation (18% of the US workforce has none), paid sick leave, and mechanisms for longer-term disability leave that protects their employment and does not sink them into poverty. While we need a better understanding of the links between presenteeism, workload intensity, and effort-reward imbalance, it is not necessary to wait for improved understanding to introduce interventions.

Economic Burden of Psychosocial Work Stressors

The economic burden of psychosocial work stressors affects workers, organizations, and society, particularly in the USA, through increased illnesses, health care costs, as well as lost time from work. We will also review some of the data showing that work stressors create increased costs to organizations through increased disability, workers' compensation, as well as the costs of absenteeism and presenteeism (EU-OSHA 2014).

Cost to Workers

Workers incur personal, health, social, and financial costs from psychosocial work stressors. Workers exposed to psychosocial work stress are at a higher risk of developing mental health disorders, chronic physical illnesses, and increased mortality (Goh et al. 2015). Psychosocial work stress and resulting illnesses can also lower quality of life and affect family relationships. The financial costs to workers are higher in societies that do not provide social protection such as guaranteed paid sick leave, state disability systems, workers' compensation, or universal health care, or in systems that do not recognize psychosocial stress and resulting illness to be work-related. In the USA, work-related psychosocial risks are not recognized through legislation or regulations, and employers are not responsible since the ill health outcomes are not commonly compensable by workers' compensation. Workers must rely on health insurance – if they have it – to cover health-care costs related to illness from psychosocial work stressors. Health insurance, however, does not provide wage reimbursement. Sometimes health-care services and treatment needed to address mental health disorders, for example, are not adequately covered by insurance. The result is that many workers with work stress-related health problems pay out of pocket for the health services they may need, go without health services, are absent from work and may lose wages/income, or go to work and function at lower levels of productivity (presenteeism) primarily because they fear losing their jobs if they are absent.

Costs to Organizations

If employers are aware of psychosocial risks in the workplace, there are often assumptions that addressing these risks are more difficult and costly than addressing physical occupational risks. As previously stated, in the USA employers are not legally required to address psychosocial risks. However, evidence suggests that failure to address these risks can also be costly for employers, workers, and societies (EU-OSHA 2014). Unfortunately, estimating the costs to employers and organizations of psychosocial work stressors is not easy as there are very few methods for determining them, and as a consequence, there is little data on financial costs by business or sector of the economy. While some guidelines have been developed to help employers estimate the costs of psychosocial work stressors related to health care, disability, absenteeism, presenteeism, etc., simpler methods are needed (EU-OSHA 2014).

Organizational Health Care Costs Due to Work Stressors

Given that health problems associated with psychosocial stressors are not recognized as work-related in the USA, these costs are not readily measured and can only be estimated. Costs of work-related stress are borne mostly by workers, employers, and society especially through increased use of health care, and increased health insurance premiums and Medicare costs. A recent US study conservatively estimated the effects of multiple workplace exposures (unemployment, lack of health insurance, shift work, long working hours, job insecurity, work-family conflict, low job control, high job demands, low social support at work, and low organizational justice) on health and health care spending using the Medical Panel Expenditure Survey and concluded that approximately 5–8% of health-care costs in the USA could be attributed to workplace stressors (Goh et al. 2015). Goh et al. (2015) suggested that "more attention should be paid to management practices as important contributors to health outcomes and costs in the United States." Some of that 5–8% of health-care costs impacts employers' bottom line, as businesses with 50 or more employees in the USA are responsible for providing employees with group health-care plans, whereas in other countries with some form of universal health care or insurance, these costs are borne by governments and taxpayers.

Organizational Costs of Disability from Work Stressors

The costs of disability to employers differ by country. In countries where disability is part of a social welfare system, employers may be less impacted by the cost of disability insurance premiums. Sometimes workers' compensation – both medical and indemnity – are included in disability costs. There are additional "hidden costs" of disability which are harder to calculate but involve lost productivity from replacing a worker (with salary and benefits) who is on disability leave. Lost work days from long-term disability leave is estimated in the billions of dollars (EU-OSHA 2014). In an EU-wide study, it was estimated that work-related depression cost the European Union €617 billion annually, and €39 billion (6%) was from the social welfare costs of disability benefit payments. In a Dutch study, it was estimated that job strain cost the country €1.7 billion in just disability payments (EU-OSHA 2014). However, for many countries, data on disability costs at the organizational level is often folded into the cost of absenteeism in general since the state bears the cost of disability pensions, whereas the loss of labor affects organizational costs.

In the USA, employers are not required to offer short or long-term disability benefits, and there are only five states that have state-mandated disability insurance requirements: California, Hawaii, New Jersey, New York, and Rhode Island. Some medium and larger companies do offer disability benefits, with 39% of private industry workers taking part in short-term disability insurance and 33% in long-term disability insurance. The cost of providing short- and long-term disability insurance in the USA is on average $624/year per full-time employee or 1% of total compensation (Monaco 2015). For an organization to be able to calculate what proportion of their disability costs could be due to work stress, they would have to calculate the proportion of disability due to work stress, which is not readily available in the USA.

Organizational Costs of Absenteeism Due to Work Stressors
Absenteeism is usually measured by measuring the days lost and calculating the lost wages. Another method, called the friction-cost method, also assesses costs such as replacement and retraining costs for the absent worker (EU-OSHA 2014). There is some evidence that job strain and other elements of the psychosocial work environment (decision latitude, skill discretion, bullying) are strongly related to sickness absence (see section above). Some studies have estimated the fraction of sick leave explained by various psychosocial factors, and several studies have concluded that around 20–40% of all sickness absence can be explained by psychosocial factors (Nielsen et al. 2006).

Organizations can use these population estimates to calculate the proportion of sickness absence that is stress-related. The next step is to estimate an organization's annual cost of sickness absence per employee (the UK Chartered Institute of Personnel and Development (CIPD 2008) estimated this figure to be £666 per employee), and multiply by number of employees applying the appropriate percentage.

Organizational Costs of Presenteeism Due to Work Stressors
For employers, presenteeism is costlier than either absenteeism or short-term disability (Biron et al. 2006). Employers are mainly affected by costs related to presenteeism through reduced productivity. For example, presenteeism has been estimated to cost British employers £605 per year/per employee, representing 58.4% of the overall cost to British employers caused by stress, anxiety, and depression (EU-OSHA 2014). In Australia, the costs of presenteeism due to

work-related stress have been estimated to be AU$9.69 billion per year, and in Germany it has been estimated to be €2,399 per employee/year (EU-OSHA 2014). In a study of US workers, those with depression reported significantly more health-related "lost productive time" (LPT) than those workers without depression, with 81% of LPT costs being explained by reduced work performance. These authors also estimated that employees with depression cost employers $44 billion per year in LPT, excluding costs from short- and long-term disability (Stewart et al. 2003).

Cost to Societies

There are multiple methodologies for determining the societal costs related to work stressors and/or to work-related illnesses (e.g., work-related depression) (EU-OSHA 2014). One way is to determine the total cost of illness, then estimate the percentage of work-related cases which gives you the total cost of work-related illness. Another methodology is to sum the different types of costs involved with work-related stress/illness (health care, disability benefits, absenteeism, presenteeism, loss of productivity due to retirement/premature death), to come up with the total cost of work-related stress. Some studies have calculated "attributable fractions" (i.e., the proportion of an illness or financial cost of that illness that can be attributed to psychosocial work stressors) (LaMontagne et al. 2010).

In 2002 the European Commission estimated the cost of work-related stress in the EU-15 at €20 billion a year, based on a total cost of work-related illness of between €189 and 289 billion/year and an estimate that 10% of work-related illness is stress-related (EU-OSHA 2014). The European Agency for Safety and Health at Work report (EU-OSHA 2014) on the costs of work-related stress included studies from multiple countries, all with different methodologies and including different elements (direct costs such as health care, indirect costs such as sick leave/absenteeism, presenteeism, turnover, lost productivity, etc.). Some studies calculated costs based on national data on job strain, others based on "work-related stress" (see Table 1). However, these data are likely to underestimate the financial costs of work stressors, when the contribution of psychosocial work stressors to several major chronic diseases (depression, hypertension, cardiovascular disease, musculoskeletal disorders, and diabetes) is also taken into consideration.

The societal cost of depression for 28 European countries was estimated in 2004 for 1 year, at €118 billion, in the USA at $83 billion, and in Australia at AU$12.6 billion (EU-OSHA 2014). The PAR% for job strain and depression was calculated at around 15%, therefore, just in Australia and for one job stressor, the cost of work stress related to depression is AU$750 million annually (LaMontagne et al. 2010). Similarly, the link between work-related stressors such as job strain and cardiovascular disease is strong (Theorell et al. 2016). The costs of CVD, the leading cause of death globally, in the EU was estimated at €196 billion in 2009 (EU-OSHA 2014). In the United States, the cost of CVD is more than US$317 billion annually (2011–2012) and is responsible for $1 of every $6 dollars spent on health care in the USA (National Center for Chronic Disease Prevention and Health 2016). According to a consensus of scientific

Table 1 Summary of societal costs of work-related stressors from a selection of countries[a,b]

Country	Type of stress	Costs considered	Estimated societal cost/year	References
EU-15	Work-related stress	Work-related illness	€20 billion	European Commission 2002
Denmark	Job strain	Health admissions, insurance benefits, sick leave, early retirement, death	DKK 2.3–14.7 billion	Juel et al. 2006
France	Job strain	Medical/health care costs, sick leave/absenteeism, loss of productivity due to premature death relative to retirement age, years of life lost relative to life expectancy	€1.9–3 billion	Bejean and Sultan-Taieb 2005
Germany	Job strain	Direct costs – prevention, rehabilitation, maintenance treatment, and administration; Indirect costs – lost working years through incapacity, disability, and premature death	€29.2 billion	Bodeker and Friedrichs 2011
Netherlands	Psychosocial load	Absenteeism, disability benefits, work-related accidents, risk prevention, safety enforcement, medical costs	€4–6 billion	Blatter et al. 2005; Koningsveld et al. 2003
Sweden	Job strain	Health care, sickness absence, loss of productivity due to early death and retirement	ECU 450 million	Levi and Lunde-Jensen 1996
United Kingdom	Stress, depression and anxiety	Work-related illness and accidents	£7-10 billion	Chandola 2010
Australia	Work-related mental stress	Work-related mental stress claims, disruption of production, medical costs	AU$5.3 billion	SafeWork Australia 2012
Canada	Work-related stress and stress-related illness	Mental health care, social services, and other costs	CA$2.9–11 billion	Shain 2008

(continued)

Table 1 (continued)

Country	Type of stress	Costs considered	Estimated societal cost/year	References
United States	Work-related stress	Stress-related absenteeism, additional overstaffing, counterproductive work performance/poor performance, and staff turnover	US$200–300 billion	Matteson and Ivancevich 1987; Rosch 2001; Jauregui and Schnall 2009

[a]European Agency for Safety and Health at Work (EU-OSHA) Report "Calculating the cost of work-related stress and psychosocial risks" (2014)
[b]This table does not include estimates made in studies from some countries regarding work-related stress costs for specific illnesses including work-related depression, work-related CVD, work-related musculoskeletal disorders, or for work stressors such as workplace violence, bullying or "mobbing," or harassment

researchers, 10–20% of all causes of CVD deaths among working-age populations can be attributed to work (Tokyo Declaration 2013).

Conclusion

Given the significant rise in the number of people worldwide that are spending years living with disability due to mental health disorders or are losing years of life due to chronic diseases such as ischemic heart disease (Global Burden of Disease Study 2015), it is imperative that we investigate effective ways of preventing these illnesses. Most major international agencies acknowledge that chronic diseases and disability are patterned by global and social inequalities that result in some of the poorest countries being burdened with some of the highest rates of disability and that even in high-income countries, the most vulnerable in terms of socioeconomic indicators suffer from the most illness and disability. However, there is also a significant research literature providing evidence that aspects of the psychosocial work environment are contributing significantly to the chronic disease burden and health inequality, as well as subsequent disability, absenteeism, and presenteeism, as explored in this chapter. As well, there is a growing worldwide literature showing that these consequences are costing businesses and society a substantial amount.

Work stress prevention strategies could reduce a significant portion (PAR%) of mental health outcomes such as burnout, anxiety, and depression, as well as chronic illnesses including hypertension and heart disease, and thus prevent or reduce disability and the resulting costs associated with disability, absenteeism, and presenteeism. Worksite-based programs and policies (LaMontagne et al. 2007), legislation, regulation (Leigh et al. 2015), and collective bargaining (Landsbergis et al. 2017b) can all be effective strategies to reduce work stressors causing disability.

Barriers to Prevention of Work Stress in the USA

Unfortunately, in the USA, two serious obstacles exist to preventing work stress or promoting healthy work and reducing the costs of disability; one is ideological, and the second is financial. First, the medical professions' limited understanding of the role of working conditions in promoting ill health and disease and second, the workers' compensation system which discourages recognizing how the organization of work is contributing to illness at the workplace because compensable diseases represent a potential economic burden to business.

Currently, in the USA, the medical profession *does* recognize that stress plays a role in disease and that working people are often beset by stress-related conditions. However, it is conceptualized as a problem of individuals (i.e., some people are less resistant to stress) like other behavioral risk factors (e.g., smoking, obesity (due to eating behaviors), lack of exercise, etc.) that are considered to be the primary factors in causing chronic illnesses such as CVD and hypertension. Occupational and environmental exposures present a challenge to the biomedical model, informing the growing public health movement in the twentieth and twenty-first centuries as more evidence demonstrated that chemical and other agents in the environment gave rise to disease. This led to an eventual understanding by some that "upstream" factors (i.e., social determinants) must be taken into consideration in addressing health, disease, and well-being. In the late twentieth century, research in Europe led to the recognition that stress at work is primarily the result of the way work is organized. Yet US national medical organizations, such as the American Medical Association and the American Heart Association, still resist the idea that it is the *conditions* of work, such as excessive demands, lack of control, inadequate support, long working hours, and effort-reward imbalance, that are major contributors to stress and ill health in working people.

The second obstacle results from the fact that in the USA, business organizations are financially responsible for the costs of officially compensable work-related diseases. Thus, it is not in the interests of businesses or insurance companies if policy-makers were to recognize additional illnesses such as those related to psychosocial factors (e.g., burnout, depression, hypertension, and cardiovascular disease) as work-related, in light of the scientific evidence. This can be a counterproductive strategy, since employers ultimately pay the costs of these chronic conditions through health or disability insurance, even while they avoid paying for workers' compensation. In fact, much of the costs of occupational disease are borne by taxpayers (through Medicare and Medicaid), workers, and their families (LaDou 2010).

These two obstacles – a limited biomedical model understanding of health and illness which neglects social causation and the mechanism of payment for workers' compensation – serve to reinforce each other. The medical profession's failure to recognize the role and significant contribution of working conditions to ill health and disability reinforces and supports the opposition of employers and workers' compensation insurers to recognize these illnesses as work-related. However, the lack of recognition of the role of working conditions is being challenged now by a looming crisis of increased incidences of depression, burnout, suicide, obesity, hypertension, and cardiovascular disease (Case and Deaton 2017; Weinberger et al. 2018). There is an urgent need for the medical profession to reexamine the basic assumptions of the current biomedical model, using the body of scientific evidence to incorporate the new epidemics of stress-related disorders into national policies on disease prevention.

The current situation in the USA is that both employers and the medical profession reject the work-relatedness of disabling MSDs, depression, burnout, hypertension, and cardiovascular disease and other health problems influenced by a poor psychosocial work environment. Stressful working conditions may continue to increase in a business environment of increasing competitiveness, and if communication remains poor between workers and management, then assuredly the causes of poor worker health will continue to be ignored and the costs of worker health will continue to be externalized and underestimated by employers, insurance companies, individuals, the state, and society.

A significant change in policies is needed, especially in the USA, whereby social causations of illness, including working conditions, are actively incorporated into our models of disease causation. Policy changes should also provide that the costs of these work-related illnesses are borne by a national health-care program, thus externalizing the costs to the government where they belong (as in the European Union, Canada, Australia, and elsewhere) while also requiring or guiding US companies to identify and reduce work stressors at an organizational level as is already occurring in other countries (Kawakami and Tsutsumi 2016; UK Health and Safety Executive 2007).

Cross-References

▶ Concepts and Social Variations of Disability in Working-Age Populations
▶ Investing in Integrative Active Labour Market Policies
▶ Policies of Reducing the Burden of Occupational Hazards and Disability Pensions
▶ Surveillance, Monitoring, and Evaluation

References

Aronsson G et al (2017) A systematic review including meta-analysis of work environment and burnout symptoms. BMC Public Health 17:264
Australia SW (2012) Cost of work related injury and disease for Australian employers, workers and the community: 2008–09. Safe Work Australia, Canberra. http://www.safeworkaustralia.gov.au/sites/SWA/about/Publications/Documents/660/Cost%20of%20Work-related%20injury%20and%20disease.pdf
Bejean S, Sultan-Taieb H (2005) Modelling the economic burden of diseases imputable to stress at work. Eur J Health Econ 50:16–23

Biron C, Brun JP, Ivers H, Cooper C (2006) At work but ill: psychosocial work environment and well-being determinants of presenteeism propensity. J Public Mental Health 5:26–37. https://doi.org/10.1108/17465729200600029

Blatter B, Houtman I, van den Bossche S, Kraan K, van den Heuvel S (2005) Gezondheidsschade en kosten als gevolg van RSI en psychosociale arbeidsbelasting in Nederland, TNO Report. Available at: http://docs.szw.nl/pdf/129/2006/129_2006_3_8656.pdf

Bodeker W, Friedrichs M (2011) Kosten der psychischen Erkrankungen und Belastungen in Deutschland. In: Kamp L, Pickshaus K (eds) Regelungslücke psychische Belastungen schliessen. Hans Bockler Stiftung, Dusseldorf, pp 69–102

Chandola T (2010) Stress at work. The British Academy, London

Canivet C, Choi B, Karasek R, Moghaddassi M, Staland-Nyman C, Ostergren PO (2013) Can high psychological job demands, low decision latitude, and high job strain predict disability pensions? A 12-year follow-up of middle-aged Swedish workers. Int Arch Occup Environ Health 86:307–319. https://doi.org/10.1007/s00420-012-0766-4

Case A, Deaton A (2017) Mortality and morbidity in the 21(st) century Brookings papers on economic activity. Brookings Pap Econ Act 397–476. https://www.ncbi.nlm.nih.gov/pubmed/29033460

Choi B et al (2015) Recommendations for individual participant data meta-analyses on work stressors and health outcomes: comments on IPD-work consortium papers. Scand J Work Environ Health 41:299–311

CIPD (2008) Building the business case for managing stress in the workplace. Chartered Institute for Professional Development (CIPD), London. http://www.cipd.co.uk/NR/rdonlyres/F5B27EA2-1A75-4C26-9140-1C9242F7A9C6/0/4654StressmanagementWEB.pdf

Demerouti E, Le Blanc PM, Bakker AB, Schaufeli WB, Hox J (2009) Present but sick: a three-wave study on job demands, presenteeism and burnout. Career Development Int 14:50–68. https://doi.org/10.1108/13620430910933574

Dewa CS, Lin E, Kooehoorn M, Goldner E (2007) Association of chronic work stress, psychiatric disorders, and chronic physical conditions with disability among workers. Psychiatr Serv 58:652–658. https://doi.org/10.1176/ps.2007.58.5.652

Ervasti J, Kivimaki M, Pentti J, Salo P, Oksanen T, Vahtera J, Virtanen M (2016) Health- and work-related predictors of work disability among employees with a cardiometabolic disease–a cohort study. J Psychosom Res 82:41–47. https://doi.org/10.1016/j.jpsychores.2016.01.010

EU-OSHA (2014) Calculating the costs of work-related stress and psychosocial risks – a literature review. European Agency for Safety and Health at Work. https://doi.org/10.2802/20493

European Commission (2002) Guidance on work-related stress: spice of life or kiss of death. European Communities, Luxembourg. Available at: https://osha.europa.eu/data/links/guidance-on-work-related-stress

Farnacio Y, Pratt ME, Marshall EG, Graber JM (2017) Are workplace psychosocial factors associated with work-related injury in the US workforce?: National Health Interview Survey, 2010. J Occup Environ Med 59:e164–e171. https://doi.org/10.1097/jom.0000000000001143

Gilbert-Ouimet M, Trudel X, Brisson C, Milot A, Vezina M (2014) Adverse effects of psychosocial work factors on blood pressure: systematic review of studies on demand-control-support and effort-reward imbalance models. Scand J Work Environ Health 40:109–132. https://doi.org/10.5271/sjweh.3390

Global Burden of Disease Study 2013 (2015) Global, regional, and national incidence, prevalence, and years lived with disability for 301 acute and chronic diseases and injuries in 188 countries, 1990–2013: a systematic analysis for the Global Burden of Disease Study 2013 Lancet Published Online June 8, 2015

Goh J, Pfeffer J, Zenios SA (2015) The relationship between workplace stressors and mortality and health costs in the United States. Management Science March:1–12

Hauke A, Flintrop J, Brun E, Rugulies R (2011) The impact of work-related psychosocial stressors on the onset of musculoskeletal disorders in specific body regions: a review and meta-analysis of 54 longitudinal studies. Work Stress 25:243–256. https://doi.org/10.1080/02678373.2011.614069

Huth C et al (2014) Job strain as a risk factor for the onset of type 2 diabetes mellitus: findings from the MONICA/KORA Augsburg cohort study. Psychosomatic Medicine 76(7):562–568

Jauregui M, Schnall P (2009) Work, psychosocial stressors and the bottom line. In: Schnall P, Rosskam E, Dobson M, Gordon D, Landsbergis P, Baker D (eds) Unhealthy work: causes, consequences and cures. Baywood Publishing, Amityville, pp 153–167

Juel K, Sorensen J, Bronnum-Hansen H (2006) Risikofaktorer og folkesundhed i Danmark. Statens Institut for Folkesundhed, Copenhagen

Juvani A, la Oksanen T, Virtanen M, Salo P, Pentti J, Kivimaki M, Vahtera J (2018) Clustering of job strain, effort-reward imbalance, and organizational injustice and the risk of work disability: a cohort study. Scand J Work Environ Health 44:485–495. https://doi.org/10.5271/sjweh.3736

Kawakami N, Tsutsumi A (2016) The Stress Check Program: a new national policy for monitoring and screening psychosocial stress in the workplace in Japan. J Occup Health 58:1–6

Koningsveld EAP, Zwinkels W, Mossink JCM, Thie X, Abspoel M (2003) Maatschappelijke kosten van arbeidsomstandigheden van werknemers in 2001, Werkdocument 203. Ministry of Social Affairs and Employment, The Hague

LaDou J (2010) Workers' Compensation in the United States: cost shifting and inequities in a dysfunctional system. New Solut 20:291–302

Laine S et al (2009) Job strain as a predictor of disability pension: the Finnish Public Sector Study. J Epidemiol Community Health 63:24–30. https://doi.org/10.1136/jech.2007.071407

LaMontagne A, Keegel T, Louie A, Ostry A, Landsbergis P (2007) A systematic review of the job stress intervention evaluation literature: 1990–2005. Int J Occup Environ Health 13:268–280

LaMontagne AD, Sanderson K, Cocker F (2010) Estimating the economic benefits of eliminating job strain as a risk factor for depression. Victorian Heath Promotion Foundation (VicHealth), Melbourne

Landsbergis P, Dobson M, Koutsouras G, Schnall P (2013a) Job strain and ambulatory blood pressure: a meta-analysis and systematic review. Am J Public Health 103:e61–e71

Landsbergis P, Janevic T, Rothenberg L, Adamu M, Johnson S, Mirer F (2013b) Disability rates for cardiovascular and psychological disorders among autoworkers by job category, facility type, and facility overtime hours. Am J Ind Med 56:755–764

Landsbergis P, Dobson M, LaMontagne A, Choi B, Schnall P, Baker D (2017a) Occupational stress. In: Levy B, Wegman D, Baron S, Sokas R (eds) Occupational and environmental health, 7th edn. Oxford University Press, UK, pp 325–343

Landsbergis P, Zoeckler J, Rivera B, Alexander D, Bahruth A, Hord W (2017b) Organizational interventions to reduce sources of K-12 teachers' occupational stress. In: McIntyre T, McIntyre S, Francis D (eds) Stress in educators: an occupational health perspective. Springer, Switzerland, pp 369–410

Leigh J, Markis C, Losif A, Romano P (2015) California's nurse-to-patient ratio law and occupational injury. Int Arch Occup Environ Health 88:477–484

Levi L, Lunde-Jensen P (1996) A model for assessing the costs of stressors at national level. European Foundation for Living and Working Conditions, Dublin

Li J, Zhang M, Loerbroks A, Angerer P, Siegrist J (2014) Work stress and the risk of recurrent coronary heart disease events: a systematic review and meta-analysis. Int J Occup Med Environ Health. https://doi.org/10.2478/s13382-014-0303-7

Mather L, Bergström G, Blom V, Svedberg P (2015) High job demands, job strain, and iso-strain are risk factors for sick leave due to mental disorders: a prospective Swedish twin study with a 5-year follow-up. J Occup Environ Med 57:858–865. https://doi.org/10.1097/jom.0000000000000504

Matteson MT, Ivancevich JM (1987) Controlling work stress: effective human resource and management strategies. Jossey-Bass, San Francisco

Monaco K (2015) Disability insurance plans: trends in employee access and employer costs, vol 4. U.S. Bureau of Labor Statistics, Washington DC

Murray CJ et al (2012) Disability-adjusted life years (DALYs) for 291 diseases and injuries in 21 regions, 1990–2010: a systematic analysis for the Global Burden of Disease Study 2010. Lancet 380:2197–2223

National Center for Chronic Disease Prevention and Health (2016) At a glance 2016: heart disease and stroke preventing the nation's leading killer. Centers for Disease Control

Ndjaboue R, Brisson C, Vezina M, Blanchette C, Bourbonnais R (2014) Effort–reward imbalance and medically certified absence for mental health problems: a prospective study of white-collar workers. Occup Environ Med 71:40–47. https://doi.org/10.1136/oemed-2013-101375

Nielsen ML, Rugulies R, Smith-Hansen L, Christensen KB, Kristensen TS (2006) Psychosocial work environment and registered absence from work: estimating the etiologic fraction. Am J Ind Med 49:187–196. https://doi.org/10.1002/ajim.20252

Nielsen MB, Indregard AM, Overland S (2016) Workplace bullying and sickness absence: a systematic review and meta-analysis of the research literature. Scand J Work Environ Health 42:359–370. https://doi.org/10.5271/sjweh.3579

Rosch PJ (2001) The quandary of job stress compensation. Health Stress 3:1–4

Rosskam E (2007) Excess baggage: leveling the load and changing the workplace. Baywood, Amityville

Rugulies R, Christensen K, Borritz M, Villadsen E, Bultmann U, Kristensen T (2007) The contribution of the psychosocial work environment to sickness absence in human service workers: results of a 3-year follow-up study. Work Stress 21:293–311

Rugulies R, Aust B, Madsen IE (2017) Effort-reward imbalance at work and risk of depressive disorders. A systematic review and meta-analysis of prospective cohort studies. Scand J Work Environ Health 43:294–306. https://doi.org/10.5271/sjweh.3632

Schnall PL, Dobson M, Landsbergis P (2016) Globalization, work, and cardiovascular disease. Int J Health Serv 46:656–692

Shain S (2008) Stress at work, mental injury and the law in Canada: a discussion paper for the mental health commission of Canada. Available at: http://www.mentalhealthcommission.ca/SiteCollectionDocuments/Key_Documents/en/2009/Stress%20at%20Work%20MHCC%20V%203%20Feb%202009.pdf

Stewart W, Ricci J, Chee E, Hahn S, Moganstein D (2003) Cost of lost productive work time among US workers with depression. JAMA 289:3135–3144

Sundstrup E, Hansen Å, Mortensen E et al (2017) Cumulative occupational mechanical exposures during working life and risk of sickness absence and disability pension: prospective cohort study. Scand J Work Environ Health 43:415–425

Theorell T, Aronsson G (2015) A systematic review including meta-analysis of work environment and depressive symptoms. BMC Public Health 15:738

Theorell T, Jood K, Jarvholm LS, Vingard E, Perk J, Ostergren PO, Hall C (2016) A systematic review of studies in the contributions of the work environment to ischaemic heart disease development. Eur J Pub Health 26:470–477

Tokyo Declaration (2013) The Tokyo Declaration on Prevention and Management of Work-Related Cardiovascular Disorders. Adopted by the Plenary of the Sixth ICOH International Conference on Work Environment and Cardiovascular Diseases under the auspices of the ICOH Scientific Committee on Cardiology in Occupational Health in Tokyo, Japan on 30 March 2013. December 2013 V. 11 No. 2,3

UK Health and Safety Executive (2007) Managing the causes of work-related stress: a step-by-step approach using the management standards. UK Health and Safety Executive, London

Vézina M, Cloutier E, Stock S, Lippel K, Fortin E et al (2011) Summary report. Québec survey on working and employment conditions and occupational health and safety (EQCOTESST). Institut de recherche Robert-Sauvé en santé et sécurité du travail/Institut national de santé publique du Québec and Institut de la statistique du Québec, Québec

Weinberger AH, Gbedemah M, Martinez AM, Nash D, Galea S, Goodwin RD (2018) Trends in depression prevalence in the USA from 2005 to 2015: widening disparities in vulnerable groups. Psychol Med 48:1308–1315. https://doi.org/10.1017/s0033291717002781

Westerlund H, Ferrie J, Hagberg J, Jeding K, Oxenstierna G, Theorell T (2004) Workplace expansion, long-term sickness absence, and hospital admission. Lancet 363:1193–1197. https://doi.org/10.1016/S0140-6736(04)15949-7

Xu T et al (2018) Workplace bullying and workplace violence as risk factors for cardiovascular disease: a multi-cohort study. Eur Heart J. https://doi.org/10.1093/eurheartj/ehy683

Surveillance, Monitoring, and Evaluation 15

Regulatory and Voluntary Approaches on Health, Safety, and Well-Being

Stavroula Leka and Aditya Jain

Contents

Introduction	274
Health, Safety, and Well-Being Approaches at Macro and Meso Levels	275
Regulatory Approaches to Health, Safety, and Well-Being at Work	275
Voluntary Approaches to Health, Safety, and Well-Being at Work	280
Finding Balance Between Regulatory and Voluntary Approaches to Promote Health, Safety, and Well-Being	283
Conclusion	285
Cross-References	286
References	286

Abstract

The aim of this chapter is to present key policy approaches to surveillance, monitoring, and evaluation of health, safety, and well-being at work in terms of hard law (binding) and soft law (voluntary) approaches. Both hard and soft laws are important for employed people with a disability or those being at risk of disability. The chapter will first examine regulatory approaches, followed by voluntary approaches. It will present examples of both these types of approaches at the international, regional, and national levels while considering outcomes achieved. Finally the chapter will conclude by critically examining challenges in implementing these approaches for effective surveillance, monitoring, and evaluation.

S. Leka (✉)
Department of Marketing and Management, Cork University Business School, University College Cork, Cork, Ireland

School of Medicine, University of Nottingham, Nottingham, UK
e-mail: stavroula.leka@ucc.ie; stavroula.leka@nottingham.ac.uk

A. Jain
Management Division, Nottingham University Business School, University of Nottingham, Nottingham, UK
e-mail: aditya.jain@nottingham.ac.uk

© Springer Nature Switzerland AG 2020
U. Bültmann, J. Siegrist (eds.), *Handbook of Disability, Work and Health*, Handbook Series in Occupational Health Sciences, https://doi.org/10.1007/978-3-030-24334-0_14

Keywords

Policy · Regulatory · Voluntary · Standards · Surveillance · Monitoring · Evaluation

Introduction

Policy is defined in the Oxford English Dictionary as "a course or principle of action adopted or proposed by an organization or individual." Policies can be proposed or adopted at the macro level, meso level, or micro level. Macro level refers to the international, regional (such as European), or national level; meso level refers to the provincial or sectoral level; while micro level refers to the organizational level. This chapter focuses on approaches at the first two levels as important parts of surveillance and monitoring efforts.

Policy instruments have typically been differentiated as "hard law" or "soft law" (Kirton and Trebilcock 2004). Both of these types of instruments are important for employed people with a disability or those being at risk of disability. While hard law clearly delineates employer legal obligations, soft law offers additional guidance and tools to implement good practice.

Hard law is defined as a policy relying primarily on the authority and power of the State in the construction, operation, and implementation, including enforcement, of arrangements at international, national, or subnational level (Kirton and Trebilcock 2004). Hard law is also used to refer to legally binding obligations that are precise (or can be made precise through adjudication or the issuance of detailed regulations) and that delegate authority for interpreting and implementing the law (Abbott and Snidal 2000). Statutes or regulations in developed national legal systems are examples of hard law (Abbott et al. 2000). At the intergovernmental level, examples include legally binding treaties, conventions, and directives.

In soft law in contrast, the formal legal, regulatory authority of governments is not relied upon and may not be even contained in institutional design and operation (Ikenberry 2001). Furthermore, there is voluntary participation in soft law instrument construction, operation, and continuation and reliance on consensus-based decision-making for action. In such a regime, any participant is free to leave at any time and to adhere to the regime or not, without invoking the sanctioning power of State authority (Ikenberry 2001).

State and non-State actors can achieve many of their goals through soft law that is more easily attained or sometimes preferable. It can provide a basis for efficient international "contracts," and it helps create normative "covenants" and discourses (Abbott and Snidal 2000). Soft law instruments range from treaties, which include only soft obligations (legal soft law), to non-binding or voluntary resolutions, and codes of conduct formulated and accepted by international and regional organizations (nonlegal soft law) to statements prepared by individuals in a nongovernmental capacity, but which purport to lay down international principles. They also include voluntary standards designed and adopted by businesses and civil society to guide their shared understanding (Chinkin 1989; Kirton and Trebilcock 2004).

Health, Safety, and Well-Being Approaches at Macro and Meso Levels

In developing policy approaches, the ideal is for complementarity to exist across various initiatives whether they are focusing on public or occupational health issues, economic issues, social security, or sustainability. However, it has been widely acknowledged that such complementarity rarely exists due to different priorities and perspectives among policy makers (Iavicoli et al. 2014). This concerns also policies of relevance to health, safety, and well-being (HSW). In addition, the development and implementation of policy approaches are dependent on the context in which they take place. This means that approaches will vary across countries, both within the developed country cluster and between them and developing countries. The next section first examines some examples of regulatory approaches developed at macro level (international, regional, and national) in relation to HSW and considers their effectiveness.

Regulatory Approaches to Health, Safety, and Well-Being at Work

Regulation at international, regional, and national level is seen as a significant driver when it comes to HSW at work. A global example of international hard law comes from the International Labour Organization (ILO) through the issuing of occupational safety and health (OSH)-related conventions. These instruments seek to establish basic standards to ensure workers' health and safety. If ratified, a convention comes into force 1 year after the date of ratification and is legally binding. Ratifying countries commit to applying the convention in local legislation and practice and to regularly reporting on its application. While conventions No. 155, No. 161, and No.187 are recognized as the three key OSH conventions, there are several conventions of relevance to HSW. Table 1 presents ILO-OSH-related conventions (International Labour Organization [ILO] 2016; Wilson et al. 2007) that are relevant to HSW.

Table 1 highlights that many countries have chosen not to make use of specific conventions. However, there is evidence that, if adopted, conventions can influence health and safety standards. Wilson et al. (2007) showed a negative relationship between ratification status of OSH-related ILO conventions and reported fatalities, taking into consideration several confounds (including length of ILO membership and income level). However, it should be noted that while this suggests that such policies can translate into meaningful HSW outcomes, it may also be the case that countries only ratify relevant conventions once they have established sufficient initiatives at the policy level.

Several regional examples of hard law come from the European Union (EU). A target of the EU is the harmonization of standards across all its member states. To achieve this, legislation is developed in the form of directives. A European Directive is a legislative act of the EU which is binding in its entirety. The Council and the European Parliament under the "ordinary legislative procedure" adopts European Directives (European Agency for Safety and Health at Work

Table 1 ILO conventions of relevance to health, safety, and well-being

Convention	Name of convention	Year of adoption	Ratification[a] (no. of countries, 187 total)
13	White Lead (Painting)	1921	63
14	Weekly Rest (Industry)	1921	120
17	Workmen's Compensation (Accidents)	1925	74
18	Workmen's Compensation of Occupational Diseases	1925	68
29	Forced Labour	1930	178
45	Underground Work (Women)	1935	98
87	Freedom of Association and Protection of the Right to Organize	1948	154
98	Right to Organize and Collective Bargaining	1949	165
100	Equal Remuneration	1951	173
103	Maternity Protection, Revised	1952	41
105	Abolition of Forced Labour	1957	175
111	Discrimination (Employment and Occupation)	1958	175
115	Radiation Protection	1960	50
119	Guarding of Machinery	1963	52
120	Hygiene (Commerce and Offices)	1964	51
127	Maximum Weight	1967	29
135	Workers' Representatives	1971	85
136	Benzene	1971	38
138	Minimum Age	1973	170
139	Occupational Cancer	1974	41
148	Working Environment (Air Pollution, Noise and Vibration)	1977	46
155	Occupational Safety and Health	1981	66
161	Occupational Health Services	1985	33
162	Asbestos	1986	35
167	Safety and Health in Construction	1988	31
170	Chemicals	1990	21
174	Prevention of Major Industrial Accidents	1993	18
175	Part-Time Work Convention	1994	17
176	Safety and Health in Mines	1995	32
182	Worst Forms of Child Labour	1999	181
184	Safety and Health in Agriculture	2001	16
187	Promotional Framework for Occupational Safety and Health Convention	2006	42

[a]Correct as of December 2018

[EU-OSHA] 2016), first proposed as drafts by the European Commission. Following this, member states are given between 18 and 36 months to ensure that the intentions of the directive are reflected (or transposed) in their national legislation (Gold and Duncan 1993). This has three components: the establishment of rights and obligations as described in the directive; the amendment of any contradictory national legislation; and the creation of necessary structures to ensure that the terms of the directive are carried out. Following this, there is a requirement to ensure that the implemented legislation is complied with (Gold and Duncan 1993). If a member state fails to follow these steps, they can be tried in the European Court of Justice.

Directive 2000/78/EC establishes a general framework for equal treatment in employment and occupation. The purpose of the Directive is to lay down a general framework for combating discrimination on the grounds of religion or belief, disability, age, or sexual orientation as regards employment and occupation, with a view to putting into effect in the Member States the principle of equal treatment. Furthermore, the Framework Directive 89/391/EEC on safety and health of workers at work lays down employers' general obligations to ensure workers' health and safety regarding work, addressing all types of risk. To target more specific aspects of safety and health at work, a series of individual directives were also adopted, although the Framework Directive continues to apply to all areas of work. Where the provisions in individual directives are more specific and/or stringent, these provisions prevail. Individual directives tailor the principles of the Framework Directive to specific tasks, specific hazards at work, specific workplaces and sectors, specific groups of workers, and certain work-related aspects (European Commission 2004). The individual directives define how to assess these risks. Over 60 individual EU directives which set minimum health and safety requirements for the protection of workers have been adopted and implemented in the EU. Any standards established in individual directives are the minimum standards deemed necessary to protect workers; however, member states are allowed to maintain or establish higher levels of protection.

The European Commission published a report on the practical implementation of the provisions of the Health and Safety at Work Directives (European Commission [EC] 2004) indicating that EU legislation has had a positive influence on national standards for occupational health and safety. In Greece, Ireland, Portugal, Spain, Italy, and Luxembourg, the Framework Directive had considerable legal consequences due to the fact that these countries had outdated or inadequate legislation on the subject when the Directive was adopted. In Austria, France, Germany, the UK, the Netherlands, and Belgium, the Directive served to complete or refine existing national legislation, and, finally, in the case of Denmark, Finland, and Sweden, transposition did not require major adjustments, since these countries already had rules in place that were in line with the Directives concerned (EC 2004). Table 2 provides an overview of the Directive evaluation at that time. Since 2004, new countries have joined the EU. In these cases, the Framework Directive was part of the negotiation for joining the EU which meant the approximation of national laws to EU law before membership (Hämäläinen 2006).

National laws may conform to criteria established in international (e.g., if the country has ratified an ILO convention) and regional regulation (e.g., EU directives); however, there are large variations in the scope and coverage of national health and safety laws (ILO 2004). To implement national legislation, most countries have

Table 2 Evaluation of the impact of Framework Directive 89/391 in 15 EU member states

Area of impact	Effect of implementation
Legal impact in member states	In Greece, Ireland, Portugal, Spain, Italy, and Luxembourg, the Framework Directive had considerable legal consequences, since these countries had antiquated or inadequate national legislation on health and safety when the Directive was adopted In Austria, France, Germany, the UK, the Netherlands, and Belgium, the Directive served to complete or refine existing national legislation In Denmark, Finland, and Sweden, transposition of the Directive did not require major adjustments, since they already had national legislation in place that was in line with the Directive
Positive effects of implementation	Decrease in the number of accidents at work Increase in employers' awareness of health and safety concerns Emphasis on a prevention philosophy Broadness of scope, characterized by the shift from a technology-driven approach toward a policy of occupational safety and health that focused on the individuals' behavior and organizational structures Obligation for the employer to perform risk assessments and provide documentation Obligation for the employer to inform and train workers Increased emphasis on rights and obligations of workers Consolidation and simplification of exiting national regulations
Main difficulties of implementation	Increased administrative obligations and formalities, financial burden, and the time needed to prepare appropriate measures Lack of participation by workers in operational processes Absence of evaluation criteria for national labor inspectorates Lack of harmonized European statistical information system on occupational accidents and diseases; although this has been addressed to an extent Problems in implementing certain provisions in SMEs
Specific issues	Most existing risk assessment practices characterized as superficial, schematic procedures where the focus is put on obvious risks. Long-term effects (e.g., mental factors) as well as risks that are not easily observed were reported to be neglected Concerning the practical implementation of the provisions related to risk assessment, there is hardly any consideration of psychosocial risk factors and work organizational factors Significant deficits in ensuring a broad coverage of preventive services relating to psychological aspects were identified

Source: Adapted from Leka et al. 2010

designated occupational health and safety authorities and inspection systems to ensure compliance. In several countries, particularly developed countries, there are mechanisms for national surveillance (collection and analysis of data) on health and safety, tripartite (employers, trade unions, and government) consultation mechanisms or bodies, access to occupational health and safety services, occupational health and safety research institutions, and links with worker injury insurance schemes and institutions.

Table 3 Overview of "the six pack" regulations (UK)

Regulation	Brief description
Management of Health and Safety at Work Regulations 1992	Specify a range of management exercises (e.g., risk assessment) that should be carried out in all businesses
Workplace (Health, Safety and Welfare) Regulations 1998	Cover requirements regarding the internal environment, accident preventions, provision of facilities, and maintenance
Provision and Use of Work Equipment Regulations 1992	Cover the general duties and specific hazards
Personal Protective Equipment at Work Regulations 1992	Cover the provision, maintenance, storage, and proper use of equipment
Manual Handling Operations Regulations 1992	Set out a framework of basic responsibilities
Health and Safety (Display Screen Equipment) Regulations 1992	Set standards required of display equipment, furniture, and surrounding work areas

In Italy the employer European enterprise survey on new and emerging risks (ESENER) by the European Agency for Safety and Health at Work has been used as a surveillance tool after OSH legislation changed in the country to specifically refer to work-related stress. The term "work-related stress" was introduced for the first time into the regulatory framework in June 2008, when the European Framework Agreement on work-related stress was implemented into policy through the new updated normative framework concerning the health and safety at work, namely, Legislative Decree 81/2008 (Persechino et al. 2013). Using data collected through ESENER immediately after (2009) and 6 years after (2014) the implementation of this new legislation, Di Tecco et al. (2017) found a reported improvement in the management of work-related stress and its prevention.

Another example of national level legislation comes from the UK. On the 1st of January 1993, the EU Framework Directive and five subsidiary directives were implemented in the UK by six new regulations (the "six pack," see Table 3). Along with this new legislation, any laws pre-dating the 1974 Health & Safety at Work Act were also revised (e.g., provisions of the Factories Act 1961) (Barrett and Howells 1997). This allowed the simplification of approximately 40 pieces of legislation.

The Health and Safety Executive (HSE) in a review of their activities concluded that "legislation and associated guidance is a major form of leverage over employers in terms of bringing about change in their health and safety policies and practices. Most employers are motivated to change their practices to comply with the law" (Health and Safety Executive [HSE] 2001).

Another example of national level legislation of relevance to HSW comes from Australia where the Work Health and Safety Act, which is supported by relevant regulations, and several codes of practice (Safe Work Australia 2016) establish the general duties that are placed on various parties involved in the conduct of work. The relevant regulations focus on various aspects pertaining to health and safety at work including falls, driving, electrical safety, as well as plant and structures, construction work, hazardous chemicals, asbestos, major hazard fatalities, mines, and a review of decisions, exemptions, and prescribed serious illnesses. In 2011, a Model WHS Act was adopted, aiming at harmonization of existing legislation in Australia, in which health is conceptualized as being both physical and psychological in nature. Johnstone (2008) noted a positive impact of the Work Health and Safety Act although he noted that due to their control over aspects of work, various parties (including employers, persons in control of workplaces, employees, and designers, manufacturers, and suppliers) have a significant influence on HSW outcomes.

The next section will present examples of voluntary policy approaches that have been implemented to address HSW at macro level.

Voluntary Approaches to Health, Safety, and Well-Being at Work

Global initiatives also exist within the "soft law" approach. Examples include ILO recommendations or standards set by international standardization bodies. As with ILO conventions, recommendations are drawn up by representatives of governments, employers, and workers. Recommendations are designed to establish standards through the provision of guidance usually (although not necessarily) related to an existing convention. For example, recommendation 164 on Occupational Safety and Health (1981) is directly relevant to the convention of the same title.

Other examples of voluntary policies of relevance to HSW are international standards. The International Organization for Standardization (ISO) is the main international body for the creation and promotion of international standards. ISO 45001 is an OSH management standard published in 2018 that aims to promote a comprehensive approach in this area. This recent development follows years of consultation on the need for an international standard on health and safety which also spurred the development of national such initiatives. For example, the British Standards Institution (BSI) collaborated with OSH experts and stakeholders from around the world to create the OHSAS 18001:1999 (O'Connell 2004). A second partner document, the OHSAS 18002:2000, was established as a guideline for implementation of 18001. The aim of the series was to identify a structured approach to the implementation of a health and safety management system, the assessment of controls, and the management of improvement.

Sparey (2010) investigated 788 organizations and 81 auditors to consider whether users of BS OHSAS 18001 have evidence of performance improvement and whether BS OHSAS 18001 helps promote a positive approach to the management of health and safety and improve health and safety culture within organizations. The survey findings reported significant improvements in health and safety performance and that the standard helped to promote a positive approach to the management of health and safety and improve health and safety culture within organizations. However, it should be noted that other research has not found similar positive benefits (e.g., Robson et al. 2007). This discrepancy in findings might be explained by the goals/objectives organizations set to achieve. Some might set very ambitious goals, while others might only wish to follow minimum requirements. Since implementing a management standard means implementing a tool of management to realize an organization's objectives, studies on their effectiveness might not always show the desired benefits (Hasle and Zwetsloot 2011).

Apart from standards, other forms of examples of soft law include social partner agreements or guidance and tools available at regional, national, or sectoral level. For example, in Europe, participants in European social dialogue – ETUC (trade unions), BUSINESSEUROPE (private sector employers), UEAPME (small businesses), and CEEP (public employers) – have concluded a number of "voluntary" or autonomous agreements including framework agreements on telework (2002), work-related stress (2004), harassment and violence at work (2007), and inclusive labor markets (2010). An autonomous agreement signed by the European social partners creates a contractual obligation for the affiliated organizations of the signatory parties to implement the agreement at each appropriate level of the national system of industrial relations instead of being incorporated into a directive. Social partners then have to report implementation activities in each EU country to the European Commission.

The European Commission published its report on the implementation of the European social partners' framework agreement on work-related stress in 2011 (EC 2011). Table 4 presents key findings.

The main activities that followed the signing of the agreement were its translation in national languages and its use as an awareness raising tool. It is also interesting to note that additional activities took place mostly in countries where there was already high awareness in relation to the issue of work-related stress. The implementation of the agreement was reported to be a significant step forward and added real value in most member states, while some shortcomings in coverage, impact of measures, and the provision of a comprehensive action-oriented framework were identified (EC 2011). The implementation of the framework agreement on harassment and violence at work was monitored for 3 years from 2008 to 2010, and similar actions were reported in member states. Ertel et al. (2010) noted that both the framework agreements on work-related stress and on harassment and violence at work are broad and do not provide any guidance at the enterprise level on how to design, implement, and sustain programs for psychosocial risk management. Furthermore, differences in perception (in terms of perspectives, priorities, and interests) of psychosocial risks between social actors are a challenge for effective social dialogue on psychosocial risk management and for the effective implementation of the agreements (Ertel et al. 2010).

Other voluntary approaches include sectoral policies which are comprehensive, integrated, and coordinated initiatives targeted to address a sector's specific objectives. As in the case of macro level policies, the development of meso sectoral policies usually involves consultations with several stakeholders (both public and private) and user groups at the national and supranational (e.g., European) levels; however only sector-specific stakeholders are involved. The Work and Health Covenants in the Netherlands are an example of a sectoral policy approach at the national level.

Table 4 Results of the implementation of the European framework agreement on work-related stress

Social partners' involvement Instrument	Substantial joint efforts of social partners	Moderate or unilateral efforts of social partners	Limited social partners initiatives	No social partners initiative so far
National collective agreement or social partner action based on explicit legal framework	Netherlands, Finland, Sweden, Belgium, Denmark, UK,[a] France,[b] Iceland, Norway	Italy	Greece, Romania	
Non-binding instrument based on general legal provisions	Spain (agreement), Luxemburg, Austria (recommendations)	Ireland (recommendations), Czech Republic, Germany[c]		
Mainly legislation	Latvia[d]	Hungary[d], Slovakia[d] (social partner initiated), Portugal[d]		Lithuania[d], Bulgaria, Estonia
No action reported or declaration with limited follow-up			Cyprus[e], Poland, Slovenia	Malta

Source: Adapted from EC 2011
Notes: Situation in early 2010. This overview necessarily simplifies differences within categories
[a]Recognized as occupational health risk in common law
[b]National agreement, persistent problems at company level led to government intervention
[c]Joint action indirectly through statutory self-governed accident insurance bodies that have a preventive mission
[d]Regulation following European Framework Agreement
[e]Formal, joint recognition of pertinence of the general legal framework

From 1998 until 2007, the Dutch Ministry of Social Affairs and Employment actively encouraged and subsidized a sectoral approach to OSH risk management. The overall aim was to achieve a reduction of about 10% in exposure to sector-specific OSH risks over a period of approximately 3 years. These sectoral risk management projects were called Work and Health Covenants. A covenant can be described as an agreement between employer and employee representatives of a sector who – in the presence and with the advice of the Ministry – agree on the risks to tackle, the approach or measures to take, and the specific goals to be formulated at sectoral level. About 50 high-risk sectors (i.e., sectors in which either 40% of workers or at least 50,000 workers were exposed to primary work risks, including high job demands, high physical demands, and working with health damaging chemicals) participated in the initiative (Taris et al. 2010). Sectors did not start with the covenants at the same time. The covenants that were agreed in later years more often included goals related to absence reduction.

At the end of the "Work and Health Covenant period," two large evaluations took place, initiated by the Ministry of Social Affairs and Employment. One was mainly directed at absence (and cost) reduction, whereas the other was more directed at risk reduction at the national level, comparing risk change in sectors that did and did not participate in the covenants. The evaluation that considered absence (and cost) reduction resulted in a quite positive message since absence and related costs were reduced (Veerman et al. 2007). However, the study considering risk exposure was not so positive, as no differences were found (Blatter et al. 2007).

At national level, an example of soft law approach comes from Japan. The Mental Health Action Checklist is a list of 30 action items which could be useful in improving the psychosocial work environment (Yoshikawa et al. 2007). It is a tool developed for facilitating worker participation and it is a guide for improving work environments for worker mental health based on collecting, sorting and classifying more than 250 good practices obtained from successful cases among Japanese workplaces. It focuses on six technical areas: sharing work planning, work time and organization, ergonomic work methods, workplace environment, mutual support in the workplace, and preparedness and care (Yoshikawa et al. 2007). It has been extensively used in workplaces in Japan and has been shown to be effective in reducing depression and sick leave among workers. For example, an intervention study demonstrated that a worker participatory approach using the Checklist was effective in reducing job stressors and depression among while-collar workers (Kobayashi et al. 2008).

Finally, there are numerous examples of guidelines addressing HSW developed by actors at international, national, sectoral and organizational level. For example, the World Health Organization has produced guidance on key HSW issues through its Protecting Workers' Health series which have been translated in several languages. Topics covered include musculoskeletal disorders, harassment at work, manual handling etc. At national level, guidelines are often accompanied by tools that organizations can use to implement good practice. For example, the Management Standards for Work-related Stress, developed by the HSE in the UK (Mackay et al. 2004) and adapted by INAIL in Italy (Iavicoli et al. 2014) and Ireland (Work Positive) include guidance and tools that allow organizations to benchmark their practice against good practice standards (see Iavicoli et al. 2014 for a discussion of the evaluation of the Italian approach).

Finding Balance Between Regulatory and Voluntary Approaches to Promote Health, Safety, and Well-Being

As we have discussed in this chapter, both hard law (binding) and soft law (voluntary) policy approaches have been developed and implemented to address HSW in the workplace. Both of these approaches have several advantages and disadvantages.

Hard law offers the legitimacy, the strong surveillance and enforcement mechanisms and the guaranteed resources that soft law often lacks. Hard law has been reported to be one of the most important motivators for organizations to engage with HSW (EU-OSHA 2010). However, a hard law approach, promoted alone, may have some drawbacks. OSH regulation in the EU and other developed countries covers traditional health risks (e.g., physical risks) and emerging risks (e.g., psychosocial risks). However, in practice, actions mostly target traditional hazards (HSE 2005), as these are perceived to have the greatest potential to disable or kill (WHO 2010). As the focus has moved away from this, toward the prevention of ill health, the regulatory approach has been found to be less effective due to lack of specific coverage of risks and unclear terminology. This has brought about confusion among experts, policy makers and other key actors like employers, employees, and occupational health services (HSE 2005; Leka et al. 2011).

Additionally, a regulatory approach is most likely to be effective in developed countries, where a more advanced framework is available to effectively translate policy into practice. Indeed in developing countries, OSH legislation often does not meet international standards (e.g., Nyam 2006) and is often not enforced (Joubert 2002). Furthermore, most workers are not covered by these laws. However, even in developed nations, there have been ongoing challenges in relation to law enforcement since enforcement agencies (e.g., labor inspectorates) have found their resources cut in light of budget reviews (Leka et al. 2015).

A further issue is that nations might choose not to make use of legislative policy initiatives where available. As discussed earlier, many countries (both developed and developing) choose not to ratify ILO-OSH conventions. Furthermore, there is a desire to minimize the regulatory burden placed on organizations, especially SMEs (HSE 2005). Additionally, if dissatisfied with the state of legislation, business can lobby for changes in legislation (Bain 1997). Similarly, if deterrents are not established properly, this may fail to regulate organizational behavior, and organizations may view fines as "operational licenses" to be paid (McBarnet 2009). Businesses have also become extremely adept at dealing with legal burdens through the art of "creative compliance" where legislation is adhered to but only superficially and not in "spirit" (Gold and Duncan 1993). In these cases, enforcement is not an option because in the strictest of senses, these organizations have not violated any laws. A further issue is that regulation is designed to target minimum requirements (EU-OSHA 2010). Thus, even if one envisioned a scenario where organizations were compliant with these requirements, it is unlikely that goals established by organizations like the WHO and ILO could be achieved.

In contrast, soft law offers advantages such as timely actions when governments are stalemated; bottom-up initiatives that bring additional legitimacy, expertise, and other resources for making and enforcing new norms and standards and an effective means for direct civil society participation in global governance. These benefits are particularly important at a time when the demands of intensifying globalization may outstrip capacities of national governments (Kirton and Trebilcock 2004). Soft law has also been found to be more precise and user-friendly than hard law in relation to HSW (Leka et al. 2015).

Nonetheless, the soft law approach comes with its own challenges. It may lack the legitimacy and strong surveillance and enforcement mechanisms offered by hard law. With a broader array of stakeholders, soft law may promote compromise, or even compromised standards, less stringent than those delivered by governments acting with their full authority (Chinkin 1989). Soft law can also lead to uncertainty, as competing sets of voluntary standards struggle for dominance and as actors remain unclear about the costs of compliance or its absence and about when governments might intervene to impose a potentially different mandatory regime (Kirton and Trebilcock 2004).

There are also some overarching issues that concern both approaches. One of them relates to the fact that policies are made and implemented in multi-actor contexts, and the various stakeholders frequently view problems and solutions differently, and some will try to influence the aim and direction of a policy all the way through the policy process. Such situations call for more attention to be paid to different rationalities and lines of argument (Hanberger 2001). The economic argument includes, for example, availability and provision of resources, unemployment rates, labor productivity, as well as social factors such as freedom of association and union participation in public policy. The political argument relates to the system of governance (federal, central, unitary, intergovernmental), political stability, etc. The context has a direct impact on the policy framework for HSW, the actors who are included or excluded from the development of policies and their perception of HSW risks, the process of negotiation, development and implementation of these policies, and policy outcomes. These have an impact on the actions taken by governments, regions, and organizations to manage HSW and alleviate possible negative outcomes in terms of incidence of accidents, diseases, health conditions, and related business outcomes (e.g., absenteeism, presenteeism, and human error). In order for balance to be achieved between different approaches to be implemented, it is important to align perspectives across key stakeholders and across different types of policies, and social and economic agendas.

Conclusion

This chapter presented key policy approaches to surveillance, monitoring, and evaluation of health, safety, and well-being at work in terms of hard law (binding) and soft law (voluntary) approaches. Both hard and soft laws are important for employed people with a disability or those being at risk of disability. Examples of both these types of approaches at the international, regional and national levels were discussed, considering outcomes achieved. Furthermore, a number of critical issues surrounding the implementation of these approaches for effective surveillance, monitoring, and evaluation were highlighted. It should be underlined that effective support of people with, or at risk of, disability requires a comprehensive policy framework across areas such as health, safety and well-being, equal opportunities, and employment. For example, to address increasing mental health disability issues, there has been a move toward antidiscrimination policies to include and address mental ill health concerns. Furthermore, HSW and equal treatment and opportunities have been promoted through a human rights agenda. Examples include the Seoul

Declaration for safety and health at work, the Health in All Policies (HiAP) agenda, and the Sustainable Development Goals (SDGs) (Jain et al. 2018). A human rights approach to worker HSW requires not only adopting effective intervention strategies but also respect for basic human rights principles such as antidiscrimination, non-interference, participation, and the interdependency of rights (Hilgert 2013). The HiAP approach makes the case for the development and implementation of value-based policies (Rantanen et al. 2013). The SDGs are aligned with the human rights principles of universality, transparency, participation, equality and non-discrimination, and accountability (Frey and MacNaughton 2016). Their realization requires that not only governments but also non-state actors including the private sector support and complement the activities of one another in order to achieve desirable outcomes. This also applies to all surveillance, monitoring and evaluation efforts to address health, safety, and well-being. The policy context is rich in initiatives; however it is essential that alignment of perspectives and action coordination should be further pursued to achieve desired outcomes.

Cross-References

- A Human Rights Perspective on Work Participation
- Implementing Best Practice Models of Return to Work
- Policies of Reducing the Burden of Occupational Hazards and Disability Pensions

References

Abbott KW, Snidal D (2000) Hard and soft law in international governance. Int Organ 54:421–456
Abbott KW, Keohane RO, Moravcsik A, Slaughter AM, Snidal D (2000) The concept of legalization. Int Organ 54:401–419
Bain P (1997) Human resource malpractice: the deregulation of health and safety at work in the USA and Britain. Ind Relat J 28(3):176–191
Barrett B, Howells R (1997) Occupational health and safety law. Pitman Publishing, London
Blatter B, de Vroome E, van Hooff M, Smulders P (2007) Wat is de meerwaarde van de arboconvenanten? Een vergelijkende kwantitatieve analyse op basis van bestaand cijfermateriaal. TNO, Hoofddorp
Chinkin CM (1989) The challenge of soft law: development and change in international law. Int Comp Law Q 38:850–866
Di Tecco C, Jain A, Valenti A, Iavicoli S, Leka S (2017) An evaluation of the impact of a policy-level intervention to address psychosocial risks on organisational action in Italy. Saf Sci 100(1):103–109
Ertel M, Stilijanow U, Iavicoli S, Natali E, Jain A, Leka S (2010) European social dialogue on psychosocial risks at work: benefits and challenges. Eur J Ind Relat 16(2):169–183
European Agency for Safety and Health at Work (EU-OSHA) (2016) European directives. Retrieved from: http://osha.europa.eu/en/legislation/directives. Accessed 15 Dec 2017
European Agency for Safety and Health at Work (EU-OSHA) (2010) European survey of enterprises on new and emerging risks – Managing safety and health at work. Publications Office of the European Communities, Luxembourg

European Commission (EC) (2004) Communication from the Commission to the European Parliament, the Council, the European Economic and Social Committee and the Committee of Regions on the practical implementation of the provisions of the Health and Safety at Work Directives 89/391 (Framework), 89/654 (Workplaces), 89/655 (Work Equipment), 89/656 (Personal Protective Equipment), 90/269 (Manual Handling of Loads) and 90/270 (Display Screen Equipment) (COM(2004) 62 final). European Commission, Brussels

European Commission (EC) (2011) Report on the implementation of the European social partners – Framework Agreement on Work-related Stress. SEC(2011) 241 final, Commission staff working paper. European Commission, Brussels

Frey DF, MacNaughton G (2016) A human rights lens on full employment and decent work in the 2030 Sustainable Development Agenda. J Work Rights 6(2):1–13

Gold M, Duncan M (1993) EC health and safety policy – better safe than sorry. Eur Bus J 5(4):51–56

Hämäläinen R-M (2006) Workplace health promotion in Europe – The role of national health policies and strategies. Finnish Institute of Occupational Health, Helsinki

Hanberger A (2001) What is the policy problem? Evaluation 7(1):45–62

Hasle P, Zwetsloot GIJM (2011) Occupational health and safety management systems: issues and challenges. Saf Sci 49(7):961–963

Health and Safety Executive (HSE) (2001) Reducing risks, protecting people. HMSO, Norwich

Health and Safety Executive (HSE) (2005) Occupational health and safety support systems for small and medium sized enterprises. HSE Books, Sudbury

Hilgert J (2013) The future of workplace health and safety as a fundamental human right. Comp Labor Law J Policy J 34:715–736

Iavicoli S, Leka S, Jain A, Persechino B, Rondinone BM, Ronchetti M, Valenti A (2014) Hard and soft law approaches to addressing psychosocial risks in Europe: lessons learned in the development of the Italian approach. J Risk Res 17(7):855 869

Ikenberry J (2001) After victory: institutions, strategic restraint and the rebuilding order after major wars. Princeton University Press, Princeton

International Labour Organization (ILO) (2004) Promotional framework for occupational safety and health. International Labour Organization, Geneva

International Labour Organization (ILO) (2016) Conventions and Recommendations. Retrieved from: http://www.ilo.org/global/standards/introduction-to-international-labour-standards/conventions-and-recommendations/lang%2D%2Den/index.htm. Accessed 15 Dec 2017

Jain A, Leka S, Zwetsloot G (2018) Managing health safety and well-being: ethics, responsibility and sustainability. Springer, Dordrecht

Johnstone R (2008) Harmonising occupational health and safety regulation in Australia: the first report of the national OHS review. J Appl Law Policy 1:35–58

Joubert DM (2002) Occupational health challenges and success in developing countries: a South African perspective. Int J Occup Environ Health 8:119–124

Kirton JJ, Trebilcock MJ (eds) (2004) Hard choices, soft law: voluntary standards in global trade, environment and social governance. Ashgate, Aldershot

Kobayashi Y, Kaneyoshi A, Yokota A, Kawakami N (2008) Effects of a worker participatory program for improving work environments on job stressors and mental health among workers: a controlled trial. J Occup Health 50(6):455–470

Leka S, Jain A, Zwetsloot GIJM, Cox T (2010) Policy-level interventions and work-related psychosocial risk management in the European Union. Work Stress 24:298–307

Leka S, Jain A, Widerszal-Bazyl M, Żołnierczyk-Zreda D, Zwetsloot GIJM (2011) Developing a standard for psychosocial risk management: PAS1010. Saf Sci 49(7):1047–1057

Leka S, Jain A, Iavicoli S, Di Tecco C (2015) An evaluation of the policy context on psychosocial risks and mental health in the workplace in the European Union: achievements, challenges and the future. Biomed Res Int. https://doi.org/10.1155/2015/213089. Special issue on Psychosocial Factors and Workers' Health & Safety

Mackay CJ, Cousins R, Kelly PJ, Lee S, McCaig RH (2004) Management standards and work-related stress in the UK: policy background and science. Work Stress 18:91–112

McBarnet D (2009) Corporate Social Responsibility: beyond law through law for law. University of Edinburgh School of Law Working Paper No. 2009/03

Nyam A (2006) National occupational safety and health profile of Mongolia. Geneva: International Labour Organization

O'Connell R (2004) Making the case for OHSAS 18001. Occup Hazards 66(6):32–33

Persechino B, Valenti A, Ronchetti M, Rondinone BM, Di Tecco C, Vitali S, Iavicoli S (2013) Work-related stress risk assessment in Italy: a methodological proposal adapted to regulatory guidelines. Saf Health Work 4(2):95–99

Rantanen J, Benach J, Muntaner C, Kawakami T, Kim R (2013) Introduction to health in all policies and the analytical framework of the book. In: Leppo K, Ollila E, Peña S, Wismar M, Cook S (eds) Health in all policies: seizing opportunities, implementing policies. Ministry of Social Affairs and Health, Finland, Helsinki, pp 125–163

Robson L, Clarke J, Cullen K, Bielecky A, Severin C, Bigelow P et al (2007) The effectiveness of occupational health and safety management systems: a systematic review. Saf Sci 45:329–353

Safe Work Australia (2016) Guide to the model Work Health and Safety Act. Retrieved from: https://www.safeworkaustralia.gov.au/system/files/documents/1702/guide-to-the-whs-act-at-21-march-2016.pdf. Accessed 15 Dec 2017

Sparey T (2010) Does BS OHSAS 18001 work? The British Standards Institution. Retrieved from: https://www.bsigroup.com/LocalFiles/en-GB/bs-ohsas-18001/whitepapers/BSI-OHSAS-18001-Whitepaper-Does-BS-OHSAS-18001-work-UK-EN.pdf. Accessed 15 Dec 2017

Taris TW, van der Wal I, Kompier MAJ (2010) Large-scale job stress interventions: the Dutch experience. In: Houdmont J, Leka S (eds) Contemporary occupational health psychology: global perspectives in research and practice, vol 1. Wiley-Blackwell, Chichester, pp 77–97

Veerman TJ, de Jong PH, de Vroom B, Bannink DBD, Mur SG, Ossewaarde MRR, . . . Vellekoop N (2007) Arboconvenant. Convenanten in context. Aggregatie en analyse van de werking en opbrengsten van het beleidsprogramma Arboconvenanten Ministerie van SZW, Den Haag

Wilson DJ, Takahashi K, Sakuragi S, Yoshino M, Hoshuyama T, Imai T, Takala J (2007) The ratification status of ILO conventions related to occupational safety and health and its relationship with reported occupational fatality rates. J Occup Health 49:72–29

World Health Organization (WHO) (2010) Healthy workplaces: a WHO global model for action. World Health Organization, Geneva

Yoshikawa T, Kawakami N, Kogi K, Tsutsumi A, Shimazu M, Nagami M, Shimazu A (2007) Development of a mental health action checklist for improving workplace environment as means of job stress prevention. J Occup Health 49(4):127–142

Promoting Workplace Mental Wellbeing

16

A Rapid Review of Recent Intervention Research

Angela Martin, Clare Shann, and Anthony D. LaMontagne

Contents

Introduction	290
Review of Workplace Mental Wellbeing Interventions	291
Methodology	291
Results: Intervention Reviews Published 2013–2017	292
Results: Review of Selected Primary Level Intervention Studies Published 2013–2017	297
Factors Influencing the Success of Interventions	300
Caveats and Limitations	302
Intervention Review Summary and Discussion	303
Cross-References	304
References	305

Abstract

This chapter presents the results of a rapid review of intervention research on the promotion of workplace mental wellbeing in the past 5 years (2013–2017).

Based on published systematic reviews, there is evidence to support intervention in the following areas: bullying prevention, stress prevention, depression

---

A. Martin
Menzies Institute for Medical Research and Tasmanian School of Business and Economics, University of Tasmania, Hobart, TAS, Australia

C. Shann
University of Tasmania, Hobart, TAS, Australia

Shann Advisory, Preston, Geelong, VIC, Australia

Determinants of Health Domain, Institute for Health Transformation, Deakin University, Geelong, VIC, Australia

A. D. LaMontagne (✉)
Determinants of Health Domain, Institute for Health Transformation, Deakin University, Geelong, VIC, Australia
e-mail: tony.lamontagne@deakin.edu.au

© Springer Nature Switzerland AG 2020
U. Bültmann, J. Siegrist (eds.), *Handbook of Disability, Work and Health*, Handbook Series in Occupational Health Sciences, https://doi.org/10.1007/978-3-030-24334-0_15

prevention, suicide prevention and system-wide multicomponent organizational approaches to health, safety, and wellbeing. Mindfulness is an intervention that also shows evidence for promoting employee wellbeing. Stigma reduction interventions also appear effective in changing attitudes toward employees with mental illness. This review highlights the need for more studies that aim to improve the positive aspects of work itself, either solely or in combination with employee-directed strategies.

Evidence for intervention studies published in the last 5 years but not yet subjected to systematic review or meta-analysis that show some promise are working time control, job crafting, stress management, wellbeing focused manager training, recovery strategies, positive psychology-based approaches, and psychological capital.

A variety of intervention related, contextual, individual, and delivery-based characteristics were also shown to be associated with intervention effectiveness; thus wellbeing impacts observed in replication and/or implementation of these approaches may vary.

The development of strategies to promote the positive aspect of work as well as worker strengths and positive capacities remains an underserved area in workplace mental health and wellbeing, particularly with respect to programs that in some way are integrated with harm prevention and problem management/reactive strategies. Further work in this regard is warranted to demonstrate and realize the potential of fully integrated strategies to protect and promote workplace mental health and wellbeing.

Keywords

Workplace · Work · Wellbeing · Positive · Promote · Mental health · Intervention · Review

Introduction

Mental health problems commonly found in the working population represent a growing concern because of potential impacts on workers (e.g., discrimination), organizations (e.g., sickness absence, lost productivity), workplace health and compensation authorities (e.g., rising job stress-related claims), and social welfare systems (e.g., rising working age disability pensions for mental disorders). This concern has been paralleled by the rapid expansion of workplace mental health and wellbeing interventions over the last couple of decades.

Numerous reviews of this body of evidence have been conducted previously, but they have tended to focus on either preventing harm to mental health or responding to mental health problems and illness, with relatively less attention paid to promoting mental health via the positive aspects of work and worker strengths and positive capacities. More recently, interest has grown in taking "an integrated approach to workplace mental health" (Fig. 1), which includes promoting the positive aspects of work and worker strengths alongside preventing harm and responding to

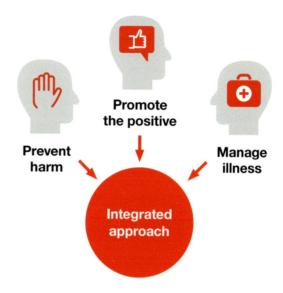

Fig. 1 An integrated approach to workplace mental health

mental health problems (LaMontagne et al. 2014). Accordingly, a review of the scientific literature related to studies of workplace mental wellbeing interventions, aligned with a more integrated approach, was conducted. The review is focused in particular on:

- The aims/objectives/approach of these interventions.
- The evaluation methods used, including the mental wellbeing outcomes assessed.
- The evidence of effectiveness of interventions, including any specific factors associated with success or failure to achieve their objectives.

Previous authors in this area have noted a relative paucity of randomized-controlled trials (RCTs) (Tan et al. 2014) in part due to feasibility and ethical challenges (Nielsen and Abildgaard 2013). Accordingly, we have chosen to be inclusive of various study designs while acknowledging the limitations with regard to strength of evidence.

Review of Workplace Mental Wellbeing Interventions

Methodology

Rapid Review

A "rapid review" methodology was employed. This method stems from the knowledge to action framework which seeks to facilitate collaboration between researchers and knowledge users by producing "evidence summaries" that inform decision-making by practitioners and policy makers. This is considered a suitable approach

(Ganann et al. 2010) to conducting a rigorous and critical appraisal in a short time frame (approximately 5 weeks compared with 6–24 months for a full systematic review). Emphasis is placed on locating and summarizing evidence from relevant systematic reviews and meta-analyses in order to limit unnecessary duplication, minimize resources needed to screen, summarize primary level evidence, and minimize the potential bias and/or error which could be incurred by reviewing primary evidence rapidly.

In relation to pertinent areas of literature in which recent systematic reviews were not available, our synthesis of the literature was supplemented with a review of recent primary intervention studies found in the search process.

Inclusion/Exclusion Criteria

To be included in this rapid review, a study must have met *each* of the following criteria:

1. Published in a peer-reviewed journal in the past 5 years (2013–2017).
2. Employed a systematic review or meta-analysis of intervention studies, delivered or facilitated via the workplace, that aimed to:
   (a) Prevent harm to mental wellbeing.
   (b) Promote positive mental wellbeing.
   (c) Promote mental wellbeing among those with a mental illness.

Reviews were excluded if they were clinical (treatment by a psychiatrist or psychologist in a health setting) or were solely PTSD focused.

Search Strategy, Results, and Study Selection

Figure 2 provides details of the databases searched and search terms used. Sixty-two review studies were identified and assessed resulting in 22 being selected for inclusion. An additional 24 primary intervention studies were selected for inclusion if they met all criteria above except being a systematic review/meta-analysis. All studies reviewed are described in an Appendix where they are listed alphabetically by author within groupings by each of the three pillars of the integrated approach (available on request from the lead author).

Results: Intervention Reviews Published 2013–2017

Twenty-two review studies published since 2013 were considered in scope for knowledge synthesis; of these 13 reviewed interventions that aimed to prevent harm to mental wellbeing, 6 reviewed interventions that aimed to promote positive mental wellbeing, and 3 reviewed interventions that aimed to promote the wellbeing of employees with a mental illness.

Databases	Search Terms		
	Mental wellbeing AND	Workplace AND	Intervention
Restricted search to 2013-2017 (June) and publications in English	OR Wellbeing Mental health Psychological health	OR Work Job Team Occupation*	OR (review studies) Systematic review Narrative review Evidence review Rapid review
Cochrane Library (reviews and trials)	Psychological distress Psychosocial	Organis/zation* Business* Compan*	OR (primary studies) Trial
Mega search (Pub Med, PsychINFO, Scopus, ProQuest, CINAHL, Dissertation abstracts)	Burnout Depression Anxiety Stress Resilience Coping	Employ* Leader* Supervisor* Industr* Personnel Human resources	RCT Experiment Evaluation Program* Training
Google Scholar	Positive affect Self-efficacy		Strategy Policy
Research Gate	Job satisfaction Work engagement		Meta-analy*
Communication via personal networks			

*searches word

Fig. 2 Search strategy

Preventing Harm to Mental Wellbeing: Bullying Prevention

Bullying and incivility are prominent psychosocial risks to workplace mental wellbeing. Two reviews examined interventions to prevent these behaviors. Gillen et al. (2017) reviewed five intervention studies and concluded that organizational and individual interventions may prevent bullying behaviors in the workplace, although the evidence was of very low quality. Hodgins et al. (2014) reviewed 12 intervention studies including 4 of high quality and 3 of moderate quality and concluded that multicomponent, organizational level interventions appear to have a positive effect in reducing levels of incivility.

Preventing Harm to Mental Wellbeing: Stress Prevention

Two meta-analytic reviews examined interventions designed to reduce stress in health professionals. Regehr et al. (2014) synthesized results from 12 studies, concluding that cognitive, behavioral, and mindfulness interventions were effective in reducing anxiety and burnout symptoms among physicians. Ruotsalainen et al. (2015) synthesized results from 58 studies to conclude that there is mixed evidence that cognitive behavioral therapy and relaxation interventions reduced stress. Changing work schedules was associated with reduced stress in two studies. A systematic review by Naghieh et al. (2015) examined four interventions to improve wellbeing and reduce work-related stress in teachers and found low quality evidence that organizational interventions lead to improvements in teacher wellbeing and retention rates.

Preventing Harm to Mental Wellbeing: Depression Prevention
Tan et al. (2014) reviewed nine intervention studies, finding good quality evidence that universally delivered workplace mental health interventions can reduce the level of depression symptoms among workers (particularly those that use Cognitive Behaviour Therapy techniques).

Preventing Harm to Mental Wellbeing: Suicide Prevention
Milner et al. (2015) reviewed 13 interventions from published and gray literature, of those that had been evaluated, results suggest beneficial effects. The same group of authors conducted a more recent systematic review and meta-analysis of suicide prevention program for emergency and protective services workers (Witt et al. 2017) finding some evidence of effectiveness in reducing suicide rates in those studies with adequate data to support meta-analysis (6/13 studies).

Preventing Harm to Mental Wellbeing: Physical Activity
Seventeen intervention studies of physical activity and yoga were reviewed by Chu et al. (2014). Of eight high-quality trials, two provided strong evidence for a reduction in anxiety, one reported moderate evidence for an improvement in depression symptoms, and one provided limited evidence on relieving stress. The remaining trials did not provide evidence on improved mental wellbeing.

Preventing Harm to Mental Wellbeing: Multi-Foci and Organizational Interventions
The National Institute for Occupational Safety and Health in the United States promotes "Total Worker Health" (TWH) interventions to integrate occupational health and safety with wellness and wellbeing interventions. Anger et al. (2015) reviewed 17 studies with this dual protection/promotion approach and all but 1 showed a positive impact on wellbeing outcomes. The authors suggest that TWH interventions can improve workforce health.

Daniels et al. (2017) reviewed 33 intervention studies and concluded that improvements in wellbeing and performance may be associated with system-wide approaches that simultaneously enhance job design and introduce a range of other employment practices that focus on worker welfare. They also noted that training may help when initiating job redesign by augmenting the effects of good job design on wellbeing.

Joyce et al. (2015) reviewed 140 studies stating they were workplace mental health interventions. Only 20 of these were considered to represent high quality evidence. Authors concluded that there is moderate evidence for enhancing employee control and promoting physical activity, strong evidence for CBT-based stress management and lesser evidence for counselling. They found strong evidence *against* the use of debriefing following trauma. Return to work interventions for employees showed a strong evidence base in relation to reducing mental illness symptomatology. The authors concluded that there are empirically supported interventions that workplaces can utilize to aid in the prevention of common mental illness as well as to facilitate recovery of employees diagnosed with depression and/or anxiety.

Montano et al. (2014) reviewed 39 organizational level interventions that aimed to promote employee health by altering working conditions (e.g., work time, work intensity, job demands/control, team organization, etc.). Nine studies looked at mental wellbeing indicators. The majority of interventions were of medium quality, and four studies had a high level of evidence. About half of the studies (19) reported significant positive effects. Success rates were higher and more likely to report an effect on burnout for more comprehensive interventions tackling material, organizational, and working time-related conditions simultaneously.

Haby et al. (2016) collated evidence from 14 systematic reviews regarding interventions that aim to facilitate "sustainable jobs" and positively impact the health (including mental health) of health sector employees. Interventions showing a positive impact on employee health included enforcing health and safety obligations, workers' compensation process improvements, provision of flexible work arrangements, changes to work schedules, and employee participation in decision-making. Interventions that showed negative impacts on health were downsizing and restructuring, temporary and insecure work arrangements, outsourcing and home-based work arrangements, and some forms of task restructuring. Authors recommend regulation of practices that showed negative impacts on health.

Promoting Positive Mental Wellbeing: Mindfulness
Bartlett et al. (2019) reviewed 27 RCTs examining the efficacy of mindfulness training for mental wellbeing and performance outcomes. While there are a wide variety of conceptualizations and methodologies used in this field for both delivery and evaluation, results point toward positive and protective outcomes for employees who participate in mindfulness training at work. However, claims of work-related benefits that go beyond personal mental health and wellbeing of employees are not yet supported by the evidence. Jamieson and Tuckey's (2017) review of 40 studies of mindfulness interventions in the workplace also reports consistent positive effects for stress, mental health, and wellbeing.

Promoting Positive Mental Wellbeing: Positive Psychology
Meyers et al. (2013) reviewed 15 studies that examined the effects of positive psychology interventions in organizational contexts (cultivating positive subjective experiences, building positive traits, or building positive institutions). The review found strong evidence of enhanced employee wellbeing, some evidence of alleviation of symptoms of mental health problems, and limited evidence of enhanced work performance (Meyers et al. 2013). Interventions were predominantly individual-directed (e.g., promoting resilience and psychological capital), with a minority focused on promoting positive organizations (e.g., strengths-based leadership coaching). None were explicitly work-directed (e.g., enhancing job quality,

designing jobs for positive mental wellbeing). The review found evidence of positive interventions countering mental ill health as well as promoting positive mental health and wellbeing. This review highlights the need for more studies that aim to improve the positive aspects of work, either solely or in combination with individual-directed strategies.

Promoting Positive Mental Wellbeing: Resilience
One meta-analysis and one systematic review looked at resilience training programs. Robertson et al. (2015) reviewed 14 studies and concluded that the evidence is tentative, although the impact on mental health and subjective wellbeing appeared to be one of the more prominent effects. They noted that no firm conclusions can be drawn about the most effective content or format for this type of training. Vanhove et al. (2015) synthesized results from 37 studies, demonstrating the overall effect of such programs is small and that the effects diminish over time (except where participants were initially at high risk of stress and lacking core protective factors). They found that programs using a coaching format were most effective, followed by classroom delivery. Online and train-the-trainer formats were least effective.

Promoting Positive Mental Wellbeing: Coaching
One meta-analysis (Theeboom et al. 2014) pooling results from 18 studies of coaching interventions that included mental wellbeing outcomes showed positive impacts on coping and wellbeing. These coaching interventions were based on cognitive behavioral solution-focused coaching and goal attainment within an organizational context. Evidence quality was generally low, and it was not possible to examine the sustainability of these effects.

Promoting the Mental Wellbeing of Employees with a Mental Illness: Workers on Sick Leave for Mental Health Problems
Ahola et al. (2017) reviewed 18 studies evaluating the effects of interventions to reduce burnout symptoms, 14 of which were individually focused and 4 were combined individual and organizational approaches. They found mixed results to support these interventions. A meta-analysis was able to be performed on four individually focused RCTs which did not demonstrate effects on exhaustion and cynicism.

Promoting the Mental Wellbeing of Employees with a Mental Illness: Stigma Reduction
Hanisch et al. (2016) reviewed 16 studies of workplace anti-stigma interventions, concluding that these interventions can lead to improved employee knowledge and supportive behavior toward employees with mental health problems. Effects on attitudes were more mixed but generally positive. Evidence quality was variable across these studies.

Results: Review of Selected Primary Level Intervention Studies Published 2013–2017

As outlined in methods, 24 primary intervention studies published since 2013 were also reviewed; of these 13 evaluated interventions that aimed to prevent harm to mental wellbeing and 11 evaluated interventions that aimed to promote positive mental wellbeing. Discussion of the key findings from these studies, grouped by intervention foci, is provided below.

Preventing Harm to Mental Wellbeing: Working Time Control Interventions

Two studies examined the impact of allowing employees increased control over working time. Moen et al. (2016) tested the STAR intervention, an organizational intervention designed to promote greater use of flexible work arrangements and increase supervisor support for workers' personal lives. They reported reduced burnout, perceived stress and psychological distress, and increased job satisfaction. These effects were mediated by declines in work-family conflict and burnout. The quality of this evidence is good given it was drawn from a cluster RCT.

Albertsen et al. (2014) assessed the effect of computer-based tools for planning rosters among shiftworkers. An overall positive effect of the implementation of self-rostering was found on the balance between work and private life with indicators of work-family conflict decreasing and work-family facilitation increasing. The quality of this evidence is reasonable, given the quasi-experimental design and use of comparison groups.

Preventing Harm to Mental Wellbeing: Participatory Interventions

Three studies used participatory approaches to improving working conditions. Schelvis et al. (2017) used a two-step process of needs analysis to identify actions for happy, healthy workers and implementation of changes by management teams. No positive intervention effects were found, and two negative effects were found (lower on absorption – a work engagement indicator and lower on organizational efficacy). The authors suggest that the intervention in its current form is not eligible for intervention and that it be modified to include an implementation strategy, more focus on stressors in the needs analysis phase, and used in combination with individual focused stress management interventions. Uchiyama et al. (2013) found that a participatory intervention to improve the psychosocial working environment was effective in improving co-worker support and goals and marginally effective in improving job control. No impact on mental health was observed. Sorensen and Holman (2014) assessed a participative organizational level intervention to improve working conditions and psychological wellbeing and showed significant improvements in relational job characteristics and burnout symptoms; however this study was uncontrolled.

The evidence for these specific participatory interventions is weak, and it has been noted that an unintended consequence of increasing discretion among knowledge workers is that it may also increase already problematic levels of task and role ambiguity.

Preventing Harm to Mental Wellbeing: Job Crafting

Three studies examined the effects of job crafting, a type of intervention involving employee-initiated design/redesign of work characteristics. Sakuraya et al. (2016) suggest that job crafting appears to be a way of increasing work engagement and decreasing psychological distress; however this was an uncontrolled study. Van Wingerden et al. (2017) found evidence that job crafting increased "need satisfaction" (defined as a sense of self-determination, e.g., competence, belongingness, and control) and indicators of work engagement in the intervention group but not in the control group. Heuvel et al. (2015) did not find a significant effect of the intervention in comparison with a control group; however sub-analyses revealed higher self-efficacy, less negative affect, more development opportunities, and closer ties to their leader in the intervention group pre- to post-assessment. These results are mixed, and the quality of evidence needs to be considered. Although quasi-experiments were used in two of the three studies, RCT evidence is not available to date.

Preventing Harm to Mental Wellbeing: Stress Management

Two studies investigated stress management programs. Lloyd et al. (2017) assessed the impact of a stress management training program showing reductions in psychological strain, emotional exhaustion, and depersonalization. These effects were stronger for employees who were low in self-efficacy and high in work motivation prior to the training. Müller et al. (2015) evaluated an intervention based on the selection, optimization, and compensation (SOC) model, a lifespan psychology approach, focused on coping with a job demand and activating a job resource. While the intervention showed a positive impact on mental wellbeing, particularly when job control was low at baseline, it did not impact work ability. The quality of this evidence is good given both studies applied cluster RCT methods.

Preventing Harm to Mental Wellbeing: Management Skills Training

Stansfeld et al. (2015) evaluated an intervention on Guided e-Learning for Managers (GEM) focused on work-related stress. Overall results showed that the manager intervention was only partially implemented among those who could be recruited, and the impacts on employee wellbeing were not significant overall. However, when the effectiveness analysis was restricted to only those employees whose managers adhered to the intervention (completed the manager training program), there was a small, statistically significant improvement in wellbeing. Data from employees of these managers demonstrated a positive impact of the intervention on mental wellbeing even though only approximately half of the participating mangers adhered to the training. The quality of this evidence is good given it was drawn from a cluster RCT.

Preventing Harm to Mental Wellbeing: Mental Health Screening and Online Intervention

Bolier et al. (2014) studied the impact of a worker health surveillance module that offers screening, tailored feedback and online interventions targeting both positive mental health and mental health complaints. The intervention significantly enhanced positive mental health but not mental health symptoms or work engagement. Uptake and compliance was very low at around 16% logging in and 5% starting an intervention module. The authors concluded that the intervention needed modification in relation to the screening tool, the technology format and provision of guidance to support engagement and compliance. The quality of the evidence is good given the cluster RCT approach.

Preventing Harm to Mental Wellbeing: Recovery Strategies

De Bloom et al. (2017) conducted two intervention trials using lunch breaks for recovery activities, one used park walks and the other relaxation activities, run in both spring and autumn. Impacts were assessed at different time points throughout the day. Both intervention groups reported less tension after lunch breaks after the intervention than before. The most consistent positive effects on recovery experiences (detachment, relaxation, enjoyment) and recovery outcomes (restoration, fatigue and job satisfaction) were reported by the park walking group, but it was noted that the effects were weak, short lived, and dependent on the season. Ebert et al. (2015) evaluated the efficacy of an internet-based recovery training intervention focused on teaching healthy restorative behavior for dealing with work strain. Intervention participants reported significant reductions in insomnia severity, work-related rumination and worrying, and depression symptoms, all maintained at 6-month follow-up. Both studies provided good quality evidence using RCTs.

Promoting Positive Mental Wellbeing: Psychological Capital

Psychological capital (PsyCap) is a positive individual capacity representing hope, efficacy, resilience, and optimism. Following initial support for a procedure for improving individuals' PsyCap (Luthans et al. 2006), recent replications by della Russo and Stoykova (2015) and Zhang et al. (2014) support the efficacy of PsyCap with effects demonstrating stability for up to 1 and 3 months, respectively. Another study by Harty et al. (2015) showed it is possible to increase PsyCap, positive emotions, self-efficacy, and job satisfaction of members of a working team by using a learned optimism group intervention. The level of evidence is good, with two of these three studies using RCT designs.

Promoting Positive Mental Wellbeing: Gratitude and Social Connectedness

Two studies compared the impact of a gratitude intervention with a social connectedness intervention. Kaplan et al. (2014) found the gratitude intervention resulted in significant increases in affective wellbeing and gratitude but did not impact negative affective wellbeing or social connectedness. The social connectedness exercise did not impact any of the outcome measures. The authors concluded that gratitude interventions may be a potentially useful component of workplace wellness initiatives although it should be noted that this study was uncontrolled. In a more rigorous test using an RCT, Winslow et al. (2017) found neither intervention showed a main effect on affective wellbeing indicators. Subgroup analyses showed that participant agreeableness, conscientiousness, and job tenure were moderators of intervention effectiveness.

Promoting Positive Mental Wellbeing: Wellbeing Education
Three studies on wellbeing education interventions were reviewed. Page and Vella-Brodrick (2013) used positive psychology principles to design an employee wellbeing program and demonstrated a positive impact on subjective wellbeing and psychological wellbeing, but effects were reduced at 6 months post-intervention. Shaghaghi et al. (2016) tested Seligman's wellbeing education program showing increased job satisfaction. No effects on psychological wellbeing or happiness were detected. No follow-up was reported. West et al. (2014) examined the impact of facilitated small group discussions incorporating elements of mindfulness, reflection, and shared experience. Empowerment, meaning, and engagement increased, and depersonalization decreased in the intervention group (sustained at 12 months), but no effects on stress, depression symptoms, quality of life, or job satisfaction were observed. The level of evidence for these three studies is good as they all utilized an RCT.

Promoting Positive Mental Wellbeing: Psychological Flexibility
Psychological flexibility, the ability to persist or change behavior even in the presence of challenging psychological events, is considered an important determinant of mental wellbeing and performance at work. Deval et al. (2017) tested an intervention based on Acceptance and Commitment Therapy which demonstrated a moderate improvement in psychological flexibility although no improvement in wellbeing was observed (possibly because the sample reflected a high functioning group at baseline). The quality of this evidence is good as an RCT was utilized.

Promoting Positive Mental Wellbeing: Strengths Intervention
Meyers and van Woerkom (2017) assessed the impact of an intervention which used activities that target the identification, development, and use of individual strengths. The study showed the intervention creates short-term increases in positive emotions and longer-term (1 month) increases in psychological capital. No impact on satisfaction with life, work engagement, or burnout was detected. This quality of this evidence is good given the RCT design.

Factors Influencing the Success of Interventions

Calls for greater attention to the question of "what works for whom in which circumstances" (Nielsen and Miraglia 2016) have drawn attention to the need for intervention evaluation studies to try to better understand the factors that influence their observed outcomes.

Of the studies reviewed above, findings regarding moderators of intervention effect, sub-group analyses, or process evaluation are briefly summarized below.

Intervention Characteristics
More comprehensive or multicomponent interventions reviewed tended to produce greater impact. Montano et al. (2014) observed that interventions were more likely to report an effect on burnout if they were more comprehensive, e.g., tackling material, organizational, and working time-related conditions simultaneously. The Total Worker Health interventions review by Anger et al. (2015) also supports this notion.

The extent to which interventions are greater in "dose" or length of time participants are engaged in an intervention may also be associated with effects. Theeboom et al. (2014) reported that although the difference in the number of sessions did not seem to impact the mean effect size, variability estimates suggest the robustness of the effects of coaching seems to increase with the number of sessions.

Contextual Characteristics
Literature on occupational health interventions consistently identifies the importance of "business champions" as crucial. As noted by Robinson et al. (2013), champions can proactively coordinate project strands, embed the project, encourage participation, raise awareness, encourage changes to work procedures, and strengthen networks and partnerships needed to facilitate changes in organizational culture. They can also achieve leverage with senior management and understand what is needed to handover ownership of interventions to fellow employees for sustainability. Champions' potential to make a difference depends on their existing roles, skills work setting, and motivation.

Daniels et al. (2017) found that successful implementation of job design and employment practice interventions was associated with worker involvement and engagement with interventions, managerial commitment to interventions, and integration of interventions with other organizational systems. Harty et al. (2015) stated that intervention results were more pronounced when reinforcement of the resources and positive aspects of the workplace environment were provided. Sorensen and Holman (2014) noted that the scale of intervention implementation "depended upon employee commitment, timely support from senior management, provision of information, change process expertise and appreciation of the social meanings and relational implications of job change initiatives" (p. 67). Page and Vella-Brodrick (2013) noted a lack of on-the-job support for changes is a barrier to intervention success. West et al. (2014) also observed that regular protected paid work time to participate in interventions is helpful.

Individual Characteristics
Participants commitment to and engagement with interventions is a critical factor. Müller et al. (2015) observed that training was more effective when participant's commitment to the intervention was strong. Stansfeld et al. (2015) noted uptake from

65% of managers and of those less than 50% adhered to intervention protocol. They note that future studies should include strategies for active encouragement of manager motivation, reflection, and behavior change. Bolier et al. (2014) also noted very low uptake, compliance, and attrition from follow-up surveys can impact results. Winslow et al. (2017) showed that participant agreeableness, conscientiousness, and job tenure were moderators of intervention effectiveness.

Participant characteristics also interact with intervention methods showing different profiles and impacts. These can be personal or job characteristics. The intervention studied by Müller et al. (2015) showed greater impact on participants whose baseline job control was low. Harty et al. (2015) noted that their intervention had a greater influence on those persons who at the start of the study reported a low level of self-enhancement. Lloyd et al. (2017) found reductions in emotional exhaustion and depersonalization at certain time points were experienced only by those who had low baseline levels of work-related self-efficacy and high baseline levels of intrinsic work motivation. Winslow et al. (2017) found personality characteristics of agreeableness, conscientiousness, and job tenure were significant moderators of intervention effectiveness. Vanhove et al. (2015) showed that among participants who were at high risk of stress at baseline, resilience training effects were more sustained.

Training Delivery Characteristics

While no clear trends in intervention delivery formats can be observed across such a diverse range of approaches, several studies did highlight delivery format as a factor. Vanhove et al. (2015) found that resilience training using coaching or face-to-face formats was superior to online or train the trainer formats. Bartlett et al. (2019) showed the effect estimate for the impact of mindfulness training on stress was marginally stronger if training was delivered flexibly, required under 8-h class time, and included stress physiology, micro-practices, and 20-min daily meditation.

Caveats and Limitations

It should be acknowledged that interventions to promote mental wellbeing in the workplace are not always evaluated, and even among those that are, the conclusions from evaluations using weak study design are often speculative. For those that are evaluated, randomized control trials (RCTs) are the gold standard, providing the strongest evidence that observed differences between intervention and comparison groups are attributable to the intervention and not something else. Some RCTs are not published or made publically available. In some cases, RCTs are not feasible to conduct or unable to be resourced. It should be noted that systematic reviews and meta-analyses rely on published evaluations. Potentially efficacious interventions may not have been captured by the identified systematic reviews.

In addition, interventions that do not demonstrate evidence of efficacy can, in some cases, be attributed to implementation failure. That is, it may not be that an intervention "doesn't work" but rather it may have not been implemented or only partially implemented as planned, or contextual factors may have limited its success. Implementation science is a growing field in which it is recommended that both the process and outcomes of interventions be examined.

Intervention Review Summary and Discussion

Interventions that appear to be clearly recommended by recent systematic evidence reviews examined in this report include bullying prevention, stress prevention, depression prevention, suicide prevention, and system-wide multicomponent organizational approaches to health, safety, and wellbeing. Mindfulness is an intervention that also shows evidence for promoting employee wellbeing. Stigma reduction interventions also appear effective in improving knowledge and supportive behavior toward employees with mental illness.

Evidence for newer intervention studies not yet subjected to review or meta-analysis that show some promise include working time control, job crafting, stress management, wellbeing focused manager training, recovery strategies, positive psychology-based approaches, and psychological capital. With the exception of psychological capital, the evidence on positive approaches and mindfulness interventions evidence is not as strong for improved work performance outcomes as it is for mental wellbeing. The evidence around this is currently being developed, but at this point it is important not to overstate the economic/business case but rather to justify on best practice or corporate social responsibility grounds.

A variety of intervention related, contextual, individual, and delivery-based characteristics were also shown to be associated with intervention effectiveness, and thus benefits gained in replication and/or implementation of these approaches may vary. It is critical to pay attention to these factors in designing and implementing interventions. Process evaluation in this area of research is arguably as important as efficacy evaluation. RCTs provide the best quality evidence of whether an intervention is effective or not, but implementation science tells us that contextual factors, adherence to protocols, and participant engagement are equally important in achieving outcomes.

There is some indication that face-to-face coaching and resilience training interventions may be more effective than online ones. Hence, it is recommended that consideration be given to the potential motivating role of interpersonal factors as supporting the implementation of workplace wellbeing interventions. More research is needed in this area, particularly in light of the rapid growth of online interventions.

In a recent review of the field of occupational health psychology research, Tetrick and Winslow (2015) noted that we may have focused too much on "red cape interventions," which are interventions designed to redress negative experiences, and not enough on "green cape interventions", which are interventions designed to grow positive experiences. Le Blanc and Oerlemans (2016) recently introduced the term amplition, after the Latin word amplio, meaning to enlarge, increase, or magnify. Interventions focused on amplition aim to enhance positive work-related wellbeing. The authors argue that the essential ingredients for these interventions are at hand through existing empirical knowledge on positive psychology and related interventions, though further work is required to adapt them to the workplace context.

While there is a rapidly growing body of research on positive approaches to promote wellbeing, it is disproportionately individual-directed (e.g., mindfulness). This highlights the need to expand the development and evaluation of work-directed approaches (e.g., job design, job crafting, positive work cultures, positive leadership) to complement and extend individual-level strategies. That being said, it should also be noted that positive mental health and wellbeing can buffer (protect) individuals from the harmful impacts of job stressors (Page et al. 2014). Thus a focus on positive wellbeing in this sense has a double value, protecting from the negative while simultaneously promoting the positive.

Looking toward the future in this area, two workplace health and wellbeing models seem particularly germane to provide frameworks encompassing the literature reviewed. Bakker and Demerouti's job demands-resources (JDR) model is one (Bakker and Demerouti 2007). The JDR model includes positive motivational and negative resource depletion mechanisms (Tetrick and Winslow 2015). It recognizes multiple domains (work, family, and other non-work domains) and different kinds of resources (job resources, personal resources, family resources, etc.) in understanding employee wellbeing. It also enables the integration of recovery interventions as well as health promotion programs, without treating negative experiences at work and positive experiences at work as simple opposite ends of the same continuum. The second model is an "integrated approach" to workplace mental health, distilled at its essence to argue that workplace mental wellbeing interventions need to integratively prevent harm, promote the positive, and react to mental health and wellbeing problems as they manifest through work (LaMontagne et al. 2014). While research is progressing rapidly in each of these three domains of workplace intervention, much of the research still sits within disciplinary silos. Greater focus on industry partnered, interdisciplinary research is needed to enable the design of feasible, synergistic interventions like the rigorously evaluated multicomponent interventions in this review.

As this review shows, the development of policies and strategies to promote the positive aspect of work and worker strengths and positives capacities remains an underserved area in the workplace mental health and wellbeing field, particularly with respect to programs that in some way are integrated with harm prevention and problem management/reactive strategies. Further work in this regard is warranted to demonstrate and realize the potential of fully integrated strategies to protect and promote workplace mental health and wellbeing.

Cross-References

- ▶ Occupational Determinants of Affective Disorders
- ▶ Surveillance, Monitoring, and Evaluation
- ▶ The Changing Nature of Work and Employment in Developed Countries

▶ Work-Related Burden of Absenteeism, Presenteeism, and Disability: An Epidemiologic and Economic Perspective

References

Ahola K, Toppinen-Tanner S, Seppänen J (2017) Interventions to alleviate burnout symptoms and to support return to work among employees with burnout: systematic review and meta-analysis. Burn Res 4:1–11

Albertsen K, Garde AH, Nabe-Nielsen K et al (2014) Work-life balance among shift workers: results from an intervention study about self-rostering. Int Arch Occup Environ Health 87:265

Anger WK, Elliot DL, Bodner T, Olson R, Rohlman DS, Truxillo DM, Kuehl KS, Hammer LB, Montgomery D (2015) Effectiveness of Total worker health interventions. J Occup Health Psychol 202:226–247

Bakker AB, Demerouti E (2007) The job demands-resources model: state of the art. J Manag Psychol 223:309–328

Bartlett L, Martin AJ, Neil A, Memish K, Otahal P, Kilpatrick M, Sanderson K (2019) A systematic review and meta-analysis of workplace mindfulness training randomised controlled trials. J Occup Health Psychol 24:108–126

Bolier L, Ketelaar S, Nieuwenhuijsen K, Smeets O, Fartner FR, Sluiter JK (2014) Workplace mental health promotion online to enhance wellbeing of nurses and allied health professionals: a cluster-randomized controlled trial. Internet Interv 14:196–204

Chu AHY, Koh D, Moy F, Müller-Riemenschneider F (2014) Do workplace physical activity interventions improve mental health outcomes? Occup Med 64(4):235–245

Daniels K, Gedikli C, Watson D, Semkina A, Vaughn O (2017) Job design, employment practices and wellbeing: a systematic review of intervention studies. Ergonomics 60(9):1–20

de Bloom J, Sianoja M, Korpela K, Tuomisto M, Lilja A et al (2017) Effects of park walks and relaxation exercises during lunch breaks on recovery from job stress: two randomized controlled trials. J Environ Psychol 51:14–30

della Russo S, Stoykova P (2015) Psychological capital intervention (PCI): a replication and extension. Hum Resour Dev Q 26(3):329–347

Deval C, Bernard-Curie S, Monestes JL (2017) Effects of an acceptance and commitment therapy intervention on leaders' and managers' psychological flexibility. Journal de Therapie Comportementale et Cognitive 27:34–42

Ebert DD, Thiart H, Laferton JAC, Berking M, Riper H, Cuijpers P, Sieland B, Lehr D (2015) Restoring depleted resources: efficacy and mechanisms of change of an internet-based unguided recovery training for better sleep and psychological detachment from work. Health Psychol 34:1240–1251

Ganann R, Ciliska D, Thomas H (2010) Expediting systematic reviews: methods and implications of rapid reviews. Implement Sci 5:56

Gillen PA, Sinclair M, Kernohan WG, Begley CM, Luyben AG (2017) Interventions for prevention of bullying in the workplace. Cochrane Database Syst Rev 1:CD009778

Haby MM, Chapman E, Clark R, Galvao LAC (2016) Interventions that facilitate sustainable jobs and have a positive impact on workers' health: an overview of systematic reviews. Pan Am J Public Health 40(5):332–340

Hanisch SE, Twomey CD, Szeto ACH, Birner UW, Nowak D, Sabariego C (2016) The effectiveness of interventions targeting the stigma of mental illness at the workplace: a systematic review. BMC Psychiatry 16(1):1

Harty B, Gustafsson JA, Björkdahl A, Möller A (2015) Group intervention: a way to improve working teams' positive psychological capital. Work 5(32):387–398

Heuvel M, Demerouti E, Peeters C (2015) The job crafting intervention: effects on job resources, self-efficacy, and affective wellbeing. J Occup Organ Psychol 88(3):511–532

Hodgins M, MacCurtain S, Mannix-McNamara P (2014) Workplace bullying and incivility: a systematic review of interventions. Int J Workplace Health Manag 7(1):54–72

Jamieson SD, Tuckey MR (2017) Mindfulness interventions in the workplace: a critique of the current state of the literature. J Occup Health Psychol 222:180–193

Joyce S, Modini M, Christensen H, Mykletun A (2015) Workplace interventions for common mental disorders: a systematic meta-review. Psychol Med 46(4):683–697

Kaplan S, Bradley-Geist JC, Ahmad A et al (2014) A test of two positive psychology interventions to increase employee wellbeing. J Bus Psychol 29:367–380

LaMontagne AD, Martin A, Page KM, Reavley N, Noblet AJ, Milner AJ, Keegal T, Smith PM (2014) Workplace mental health: developing an integrated intervention approach. BMC Psychiatry 14:131

Le Blanc PM, Oerlemans WGM (2016) Amplition in the workplace: building a sustainable workforce through individual positive psychological interventions. Psychol Papers 373:185–191

Lloyd J, Bond W, Flaxman P (2017) Work-related self-efficacy as a moderator of the impact of a worksite stress management training intervention: intrinsic work motivation as a higher order condition of effect. J Occup Health Psychol 22:115–127

Luthans F, Avey JB, Avolio BJ, Norman SM, Combs GM (2006) Psychological capital development: towards a micro-intervention. J Organ Behav 27:387–393

Meyers MC, van Woerkom MJ (2017) Effects of a strengths intervention on general and work-related wellbeing: the mediating role of positive affect. J Happiness Stud 18:671–689

Meyers MC, van Woerkom M, Bakker AB (2013) The added value of the positive: a literature review of positive psychology interventions in organisations. Eu J Work Organ Psychol 22(5):618–632

Milner A, Page K, Spencer-Thomas S, LaMontagne A (2015) Workplace suicide prevention: a systematic review of published and unpublished activities. Health Promot Int 30(1):29–37

Moen P, Kelly E, Fan W, Lee SR, Almeida D, Kossek EE, Buxton OM (2016) Does a flexibility/support organisational initiative improve high-tech employees' wellbeing? Evidence from the work, family, and health network. Am Sociol Rev 81(1):134–164

Montano D, Hoven H, Siegrist J (2014) Effects of organisational-level interventions at work on employees' health: a systematic review. BMC Public Health 14(1):135

Müller A, Heiden B, Herbig B, Poppe F, Angerer P (2015) Improving well-being at work: a randomized controlled intervention based on selection, optimization, and compensation. J Occup Health Psychol 21:169–181

Naghieh A, Montgomery P, Bonell CP, Thompson M, Aber JL (2015) Organisational interventions for improving wellbeing and reducing work-related stress in teachers. Cochrane Database Syst Rev 4:CD002892

Nielsen K, Abildgaard JS (2013) Organisational interventions: a research-based framework for the evaluation of both process and effects. Work Stress 27:278–297

Nielsen K, Miraglia M (2016) What works for whom in which circumstances? On the need to move beyond the 'what works?' question in organisational intervention research. Human Relations, 70(1), 40–62. https://doi.org/10.1177/0018726716670226

Page KM, Vella-Brodrick DA (2013) The working for wellness program: RCT of an employee well-being intervention. J Happiness Stud 143:1007–1031

Page KM, Milner AJ, Martin A, Turrell G, Giles-Corti B, LaMontagne AD (2014) Workplace stress: what is the role of positive mental health? J Occup Environ Med 568:814–819

Regehr C, Glancy D, Pitts A, LeBlanc VR (2014) Interventions to reduce the consequences of stress in physicians: a review and meta-analysis. J Nerv Ment Dis 202(5):353–359

Robertson IT, Cooper CL, Sarkar M, Curran T (2015) Resilience training in the workplace from 2003 to 2014: a systematic review. J Occup Organ Psychol 88:533–562

Robinson M, Tilford S, Branney P, Kinesella K (2013) Championing mental health at work: emerging practice from innovative projects in the UK. Health Promot Int 293:583–595

Ruotsalainen JH, Verbeek JH, Mariné A, Serra C (2015) Preventing occupational stress in healthcare workers. Cochrane Database Syst Rev 4:CD002892

Sakuraya A, Shimazu A, Imamura K, Namba K, Kawakami N (2016) Effects of a job crafting intervention program on work engagement among Japanese employees: a pretest-posttest study. BMC Psychol 4:49

Schelvis RMC, Wiezer NM, van der Beek AJ, Twisk JWR, Bohlemijer ET, Oude Hengel KM (2017) The effect of an organisational level participatory intervention in secondary vocational education on work-related health outcomes: results of a controlled trial. BMC Public Health 17:141

Shaghaghi F, Abedian Z, Forouhar M, Asgharipour N, Esmaily H (2016) Effectiveness of wellbeing interventions on job satisfaction of midwives: a randomized clinical trial. Iran J Obstet Gynecol Infertilit 19(32):1–11

Sorensen OH, Holman D (2014) A participative intervention to improve employee wellbeing in knowledge work jobs: a mixed-methods evaluation study. Work Stress 28:67–86

Stansfeld SA, Kerry S, Chandola T et al (2015) Pilot study of a cluster randomised trial of a guided e-learning health promotion intervention for managers based on management standards for the improvement of employee wellbeing and reduction of sickness absence: GEM study. BMJ Open 5:e007981

Tan L, Wang MJ, Modini M, Joyce S, Mykletun A, Christensen H, Harvey SB (2014) Preventing the development of depression at work: a systematic review and meta-analysis of universal interventions in the workplace. BMC Med 12:74

Tetrick L, Winslow C (2015) Workplace stress management interventions and health promotion. Ann Rev Organ Psychol Organ Behav 2:583–603

Theeboom T, Beersma B, van Vianen AEM (2014) Does coaching work? A meta-analysis on the effects of coaching on individual level outcomes in an organisational context. J Posit Psychol 9(1):1–18

Uchiyama A, Odagiri Y, Ohya Y, Takamiya T, Inoue S, Shimomitsu T (2013) Effect on mental health of a participatory intervention to improve psychosocial work environment: a cluster randomized controlled trial among nurses. J Occup Health 553:173–183

van Wingerden J, Bakker AB, Derks D (2017) Fostering employee wellbeing via a job crafting intervention. J Vocat Behav 100:164–174

Vanhove AJ, Herian MN, Perez AL, Harms PD, Lester PB (2015) Can reliance be developed at work? A meta-analytic review of resilience building programme effectiveness. J Occup Organ Psychol 89:278–307

West CP, Dyrbye LN, Rabatin JT, Call TG, Davidson JH et al (2014) Intervention to promote physician wellbeing, job satisfaction, and professionalism: a randomized clinical trial. JAMA Intern Med 1744:527–533

Winslow CJ, Kaplan S, Bradley-Geist JC, Lindsey AP, Ahmad AS, Hargrove AK, Kaplan SA (2017) An examination of two positive organisational interventions: for whom do these interventions work? J Occup Health Psychol 222:129–137

Witt K, Milner A, Allisey A, Purnell L, LaMontagne AD (2017) Effectiveness of suicide prevention programs for emergency and protective services employees: a systematic review and meta-analysis. Am J Ind Med 60:394–407

Zhang X, Li YL, Ma SH, Huang J, Jiang L (2014) A structured reading materials-based intervention program to develop the psychological capital of Chinese employees. Soc Behav Pers 42(3):503–515

Reducing Inequalities in Employment of People with Disabilities

The Impact of National Labour and Social Protection Policies

17

Ben Barr, Philip McHale, and Margaret Whitehead

Contents

Introduction	310
The Scale of the Problem	311
What Role for Active Labour Market Policies?	313
A Typology of Active Labour Market Policies for People with Disabilities	313
Examples and Effectiveness of Different Types of ALMPs	315
What About Activation Strategies to Counteract Disincentives to Work?	322
Ongoing Challenges and Forward View	324
Cross-References	325
References	325

Abstract

Across the OECD, the situation for working age people not in employment, or on long-term sick leave, through disability or chronic illness is a serious issue for public health policy. The employment gap between people with disabilities and those without is a common feature of many OECD countries. It is a gap that is widening in many cases and is particularly marked between disabled people in low skilled, manual occupations and their more privileged counterparts in professional occupations. This chapter presents a typology of active labour market policies (ALMPs) that have been introduced in high-income countries to help sick and disabled people into work, thereby reducing their risk of poverty and social exclusion. There are two distinct orientations for these policies: a focus on the employment environment to make it more "disability friendly" and a focus on increasing the employability of the individual. These approaches are illustrated by examples from the UK, Sweden, Denmark, and Canada. The chapter outlines the evidence base for the effectiveness of the different types of ALMPs and what some of the key implications and future challenges are.

B. Barr · P. McHale · M. Whitehead (✉)
Department of Public Health and Policy, University of Liverpool, Liverpool, UK
e-mail: benbarr@liverpool.ac.uk; p.mchale@liverpool.ac.uk; mmw@liverpool.ac.uk

© Springer Nature Switzerland AG 2020
U. Bültmann, J. Siegrist (eds.), *Handbook of Disability, Work and Health*, Handbook Series in Occupational Health Sciences, https://doi.org/10.1007/978-3-030-24334-0_16

We conceptualize ALMPs as one key component of broader "activation strategies." These strategies also encompass attempts to promote the employment of people with disabilities through changes to the disability-related social protection system and wider labour market policies. We therefore go on to outline evidence on the impact and consequences of another key component of recent activation strategies – changes to disability benefits that aim to reduce potential disincentives to work for disabled or chronically ill people. The chapter ends with an overview of future challenges that are relevant to this issue and aspects which should be considered when designing policy to improve employment opportunities for disabled people.

Keywords

Disability employment · Work environment · Labour market policies · Activation strategies · Social inequalities

Introduction

Across the OECD, the employment of people with disabilities or chronic illness is a serious issue for public health and social welfare policy. In most countries people with disabilities are less likely to be employed than people who are not disabled (OECD 2003, 2010), and this puts them at greater risk of poverty. To address this issue, most OECD countries have developed social protection systems that provide earnings replacement benefits to people who cannot work due to disability. In many OECD countries, there are large numbers of people in receipt of these disability benefits, with these numbers having increased rapidly over recent decades.

These developments have stimulated countries to introduce so-called activation strategies with the general aim of getting working-age people off benefits and into work, including those with disability or limiting longstanding illness (Martin 2014; European Commission 2016). A major component of these activation strategies has been the introduction of a range of active labour market policies (ALMPs), aimed at enhancing incentives to seek employment, improving job readiness, help in finding suitable employment, and expanding employment opportunities (OECD 2013). A second major component of activation strategies in recent decades has been the introduction of measures in the welfare benefit system designed to counteract potential disincentives to work for disabled or chronically ill people (Martin 2014). This chapter deals with both components.

The welfare systems we have today were originally set up to provide an essential income for people who were too sick to work and otherwise faced destitution. The systems have come a long way since then and have many more objectives, but this central goal of the social protection system remains the same. Two key challenges therefore exist for policy makers when designing national labour market and social protection policies. First, policies need to help as many people with disabilities as possible into appropriate work and to help retain them in the workforce once they have jobs. Second, policies should ensure that the social protection system really does protect the incomes of people with disabilities and chronic illness, so that they have an adequate standard of living for their health and well-being even when they cannot work, and that the lack of employment does not lead to poverty. Associated with this, extra effort is needed to improve living conditions and life chances for the most disadvantaged in society and help reduce the marked inequalities. In all this, labour market and social protection policies are intertwined and need to be considered together.

For public health, the issue is intricately linked to health inequalities. Being in poor health is an important risk factor for non-employment, poverty, and social exclusion. The exclusion that comes from being outside the labour market relates not only to the work environment but to exclusion from close social relationships and the opportunity to participate in society in many arenas. Crucially, the adverse consequences of health problems are not evenly spread across the population, but rather become more severe with decreasing social position. This tendency has the potential to generate further inequalities in health. Helping chronically ill and disabled people return to work can, therefore, be viewed as an important part of a strategy to tackle health inequalities.

The aims of this chapter are fivefold. Firstly, we outline the scale of the problem across selected countries – the UK, Denmark, Sweden, and Canada – all of which have universal health care and advanced welfare systems. Secondly, we give an overview of the main types of ALMPs that have been employed by national governments in these countries to help people return to work or maintain their jobs when they have ill-health. Thirdly, we outline some of the evidence on how effective, if at all, the various types of ALMPs have been in boosting employment chances of people with disabilities or chronic ill-health. Fourth, we go on to cover activation strategies aimed at intervening in the welfare benefit system to counteract potential disincentives to work for disabled or chronically ill people. In this context, we present some empirical evidence from our own research on the impact of punitive reforms aimed at tightening eligibility and adequacy of disability-related benefits. The final section flags up further ongoing challenges and policy implications for the future.

The Scale of the Problem

In most OECD countries, people with disabilities experience lower employment than people without disabilities. This gap is a feature of labour markets throughout the OECD; however, there is significant variation in the size of the gap (Geiger et al. 2017). People with disabilities from more disadvantaged socioeconomic groups – for example, those with lower levels of education – experience even lower employment chances. Figure 1 shows the employment rate of men and women with and without a limiting illness in Canada, Sweden, Denmark, and the UK and how this differs by educational level. While employment chances decrease with lower levels of education, this social gradient is even more marked among people with a disability. This

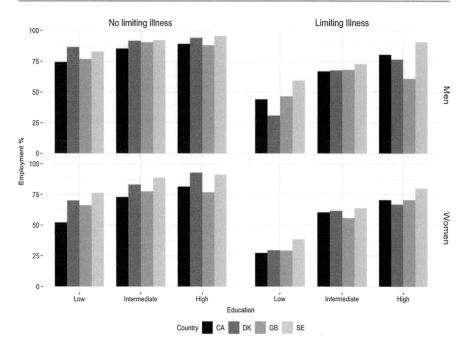

Fig. 1 The employment rate for people with and without a limiting illness by educational group for 35–64 year olds in Canada, Sweden, the UK, and Denmark. Datasets: Canadian Community Health Survey, 2014 (CA), European Social Survey 2012–2016 (SE, DK, GB). (Source: Barr, McHale and Whitehead: authors' own analyses)

means, for example, that women with limiting long-standing illness in Canada, Denmark, and the UK have employment rates on average of around 25% if they have low education, but around 70% if they are at a higher educational level. Some countries such as Sweden tend to maintain higher employment rates for people with and without disabilities.

Social protection systems have come under increasing strain in recent decades. In the UK, there was a significant and rapid expansion of claimant numbers for disability benefits between 1970 and 1995, claimants accounted for 7% of the workforce and 1.6% of GDP in 1995. Subsequent reforms, beginning in 1996, to these benefits led to a halting of the increasing trend, but only a small reduction in claimant numbers by 2010 and beyond. These reforms included introducing stricter eligibility criteria and reduced adequacy of disability benefits (e.g., employment and support allowance) and the introduction of welfare-to-work programmes. (Barr and McHale 2018).

Sweden also faced a rapid expansion of claimants during this period, experiencing a peak of claiming in 2005 of 9.6% (McVicar et al. 2019). Reforms to the Swedish system included tightening of medical eligibility criteria for long-term disability benefits (Cohen Birman and Andersson 2014; Hagelund and Bryngelson 2014) and increased focus on rehabilitation for sickness benefit claimants.

In Denmark, receipt of disability benefits increased more gradually, reaching a peak of around 8% of the working-age population in 1999, with the rate falling slightly since that time (Bingley et al. 2011). The Danish disability pension programme was reformed in 2013 to reduce availability for people under 40 and to increase focus on rehabilitation. The rehabilitation programme was extended to sickness benefits claimants in 2014 (OECD 2015) and the provision of wage subsidies for disabled people was expanded through the Flexjobs programme. These reforms were followed by a halving of new claimants and a steady reduction in total claimant numbers.

A recognized policy dilemma moving forward is that the aging population will exacerbate the health inequalities issue still further. Recently, many countries are in the process of extending retirement ages, requiring individuals to work longer before receiving a state pension. One consequence of extending working lives in this way is that there will be a higher prevalence of disability and comorbidity in the older workforce to contend with, as the prevalence of health conditions increase with increasing age. In addition, as rates of limiting longstanding illness are higher in socioeconomically disadvantaged groups and sickness sets in at younger ages, the adverse effects of this extension of working life is likely to be greater for low educated, less skilled workers.

What Role for Active Labour Market Policies?

Many countries have introduced active labour market policies (ALMPs) in response to the low employment rates of chronically ill people and people with disabilities and the rise in the receipt of disability benefits. What are the different types of ALMPs in the context of disability? What is known about the effectiveness of the ALMPs that have been tried so far?

A Typology of Active Labour Market Policies for People with Disabilities

The purpose of a typology of ALMPs is to facilitate cross-country comparison of the impact of seemingly diverse policies that have been initiated in different countries, but which, nonetheless, share underlying characteristics. In Table 1, we present a typology of these different ALMPs, based on their underpinning "theory of change," sometimes termed "programme logic" (Whitehead et al. 2009). The programme logic is the explicit or implicit reasoning about how the intervention will operate to bring about the desired change in the perceived problem (Whitehead 2007).

Conceptually, ALMPS for people with disabilities fall into two principal policy orientations. One has a focus on the employment environment, attempting to make it more "disability-friendly." The second is a focus on the disabled people themselves – attempting to develop their skills, education, or health condition, in order to increase their employability.

Table 1 Typology of interventions to help chronically ill and disabled people into work

Focus	Intervention type and programme logic	Examples of interventions
Work environment	**i. Tackling discrimination** Legislate to outlaw discrimination by employers against disabled/chronically ill in recruitment and retention of staff	*Human Rights Act/Employment Equity Act 1996* (Can), *Act on Prohibition of Discrimination in the labour market 2004* (Den), *Working Environment Act 1977/2005* (Nor), *Prohibition of Discrimination in Working Life of People with Disability Act 1999* (Swe), *Disability Discrimination Act 1995* (UK)
	ii. Improving workplace and employment accessibility Legal or financial measures to remove or reduce barriers to accessibility of work and employment for the disabled/chronically ill	Duties in various legislative acts (Can, Den), *Provisions in Working Environment Act 1977* (Nor), *Working Life Fund/duties in Work Environment Act 1977* (Swe), *Access to Work* (UK)
	iii. Offering financial incentives to employers Job creation or financial incentives to employers to employ disabled and chronically ill to increase employment opportunities	*Opportunities Fund* (Can), *Icebreaker, Flexjob* (Den), *Job Introduction Scheme, Work Trial* (UK)
	iv. Enhancing return to work planning Improve provision for planned return to work and for agencies to cooperate and integrate services offered	*Active Sick Leave* (Nor). *Finsam, Socsam, Frisam* (Swe)
Individual employability	**v. Individualized case management and job search assistance** Individualized vocational advice/job search assistance on a case management basis	*Canada Pension Plan Disability Vocational Rehabilitation Program* (Can), *New Deal for Disabled People, Pathways to Work, Work Programme* (UK)
	vi. Education, training, and work trial Improve claimants' skills, education, and training to increase "employability"	*Labour Market Agreement for Persons with Disabilities* (Can), *Employers' duty to provide* (Den), *Residential Training, Work Trial* (UK)
	vii. Health condition/impairment management Medical rehabilitation and/or advice on health condition management to improve fitness to work	Medical/vocational rehabilitation (Can, Den, Nor, Sweden), *Dagmar* (Swe), *Rehabilitation Chain* (Swe); *Condition Management Programme* (UK)
	viii. Offering financial incentives for welfare claimants Financial incentives to gain employment and to ease the transition from benefits to work	Tax credits (Can, UK) *Job Grant, Return to Work Credit, Job Preparation Premium; Permitted Work Rules* (UK); *Resting Disability Pension* (Swe); *Continuous Deduction Programme* (Swe)

Source: Adapted from Whitehead et al. 2009, Table 5.1

ALMPs attempting to make the employment environment "disability-friendly," depicted in Table 1 (types i–iv), are aimed at stimulating job opportunities and removing barriers in the labour market and the work environment, for example, through job creation, regulating and offering incentives to employers, regulating physical accessibility while in, and traveling to, the work environment, providing more flexible work patterns to better suit individual needs, and so on. The underlying programme logic here is that the removal of barriers to employment that exist in the labour market and working environment will result in increased employment opportunities for people with disabilities.

ALMPs with an individual orientation focus on improving the "employability" of chronically ill and disabled people themselves. This may be through education, training, vocational rehabilitation, or medical interventions which aim to increase individuals' capabilities and motivation to return to work. These ALMPs are underpinned by the notion of the problem being located within the individual, rather than the environment. They are therefore focused on strengthening the individual's knowledge, skills, or capabilities to help them move into work.

Examples and Effectiveness of Different Types of ALMPs

This typology in Table 1 has been employed in a series of systematic reviews to synthesize the evidence on how effective, if at all, the various types of ALMPs are in boosting employment chances of people with disabilities or chronic ill-health (Whitehead et al. 2009; Barr et al. 2010; Clayton et al. 2011, 2012). Each approach has its advantages but also disadvantages and, in some cases, unintended adverse effects, which have been confirmed in recent empirical research. The evidence base highlights above all that the impacts of the various ALMPs are highly context specific, depending, for example, on how large a financial incentive is, the level of awareness of voluntary schemes in the population, and what other strategies are being employed at the same time which may be pulling in the opposite direction and cancelling out any positive effects.

There is also the backdrop of the economic situation in a country at any one time, influencing the availability and degree of competition for jobs. Even the most promising interventions at the pilot stage can fail to improve employment chances for people with disabilities if they are implemented when there are no jobs to go to. Context needs to be taken into account when interpreting findings. Pointers from evaluations so far include the following:

Type I – Legislating Against Disability Discrimination
One factor said to contribute to the poorer employment chances of disabled people is that employers discriminate against them when recruiting staff, when deciding on redundancies and when identifying what is a reasonable adjustment to the working environment. Anti-discrimination legislation is one strategy that aims to tackle this barrier to employment. Countries including Canada, Sweden, and the UK have all enacted national anti-discrimination legislation, specifically outlawing

discrimination against disabled people in relation to employment. The UK introduced the *Disability Discrimination Act in 1995*, which has since been superseded by the *Equality Act 2010* (UK Government 2010). In Canada, protection against discrimination for disabled people is provided under the *Canadian Charter of Rights and Freedoms*.

Until recently, Denmark represented a complete contrast, in that not only was there an absence of specific legislation governing rights for disabled people in Denmark but there was debate about whether such legislation was desirable or would run counter to other welfare state equity principles. Denmark first introduced anti-discrimination legislation in 2004; however this was criticized for being too narrow in both the definition of disability and what qualifies as a reasonable adjustment. This was extended in 2013 as a response to statements from the EU Court of Justice (Lane and Videbaek Munkholm 2015).

In terms of effectiveness, it is difficult to detect an effect of legislation to combat discrimination by employers. The emphasis of rights-based legislation has been on prohibiting discrimination, i.e., only taking action when discrimination has been legally demonstrated. This is a slow and laborious approach, in which only a small minority of disabled people are helped by the courts. There is no evidence from the UK studies, for example, that the *Disability Discrimination Act* had any wider effects on employment rates among disabled people of a magnitude that could be picked up at the population survey level. Evidence suggested that there was a negative impact of the *Disability Discrimination Act* in the UK on employment outcomes (Bambra and Pope 2007). Notably, there is evidence that awareness of legislation, and the requirements it places on employers, is lacking (Clayton et al. 2012). Legislation of this nature may be a necessary, but not sufficient, strategy. The absence of a population-level effect is no reason, however, to abandon such legislation; arguably, the passing of such legislation signals the unacceptability of some of the discriminatory practices that were taken for granted previously and helps to bring about a slow shift in public and employers' behavior in the desired direction.

Type II – Improving Physical Accessibility of Workplaces

Accessibility measures are designed to facilitate the take up of employment and improve job retention by reducing workplace and employment barriers which disabled and chronically ill people may face. These can include legislation or regulations to adapt the work environment, through adaptations to buildings or workplace reorganization, and financial incentives or other support to enable employers to carry out these adjustments. Accessibility measures have been employed in many countries, although there are clear differences in the extent to which accessibility is viewed as a physical or specialized equipment issue and where it is viewed as a matter of adapting the wider organization of the work environment.

In the UK, the programme which relates to this policy area is *Access to Work*. Introduced in 1994, this is a government programme that provides financial support for employers to make workplace adjustments. There are five main areas of support that can be provided: communication support, aids and equipment, support worker, travel to work, and travel in work. Since 2011, support has been extended to mental health conditions (Department for Work and Pensions 2017). Denmark provides funding support for accessibility on a municipal level. In Canada, the proposed *Accessible Canada Act* will allow the Canadian government to take a proactive approach to removing accessibility barriers (Government of Canada 2018).

In terms of effectiveness, workplace adjustments have been shown to have a positive impact on employment but low uptake. Evidence suggests that where adjustments are made by employers, particularly where employers can be flexible with work schedules, and give employees greater control over work demands, they may produce some promising results in terms of improved employment chances for disabled people (Nevala et al. 2015). To have an impact on overall levels of employment of people with disabilities, however, workplace adjustments need to take place on a much larger scale and be accessible to less skilled groups in the population. Although there is evidence that the UK's *Access to Work* scheme, for example, was highly valued by the recipients, only a small minority of people with disabilities received support, and those tended to be in non-manual and professional jobs (Sayce 2011). It is the people in low-skilled jobs, however, that are most likely to suffer from a disability and be out of work because of it.

Type III – Offering Incentives to Employers to Employ Disabled Workers

There is some evidence that employers have the perception that it is more costly to employ a disabled worker or that their disability will render them less productive (Simm et al. 2007). One ALMP that aims to overcome these perceptions has been to offer employers financial incentives to employ disabled workers, usually on a trial basis, for example, by offering wage subsidies to cover the initial costs of employment. This allows time for employers to assess the suitability of the applicant at no cost to their firm and is designed to break down barriers of uncertainty about workplace abilities.

The most widespread use of wage subsidies has been in Denmark through the *Flexjobs* scheme introduced in 1986, which offers subsidized jobs to people who are not able to carry out a normal full time job due to impairments. Employers who hire eligible workers are entitled to a wage subsidy of between one third and two thirds of their wages graduated according to the degree of reduction of working capacity. The 2013 disability pension reforms in Denmark expanded the *Flexjob* scheme to include more part-time jobs of fewer than 12 h, which was the former threshold (Datta Gupta et al. 2015). There are now around 70,000 people in Denmark on a *Flexjobs* scheme. Similar schemes have been introduced on a smaller scale in Sweden through the *New-start* job programme in 2007, while in the UK, two schemes with relatively small wages subsidies have been implemented: the *Work Trial* and *Job Introduction Scheme*.

There is some evidence that financial incentives for employers, such as wage subsidies, can work if they are sufficiently generous but can have unintended side effects (Clayton et al. 2012). To a certain extent, the level of wage subsidies presents a dilemma. If they are too low, they do not act as a strong enough incentive. If they are too high, they can create a segregated form of employment for people with disabilities, which is outside the competitive labour market. Some of the evidence from evaluations of the *Flexjobs* programme in Denmark indicates that this may be disempowering and result in further social exclusion (Clayton et al. 2012); however when the subsidies provided by the scheme were reduced, there was an associated reduction in hiring of disabled people (Datta Gupta et al. 2015). Evaluations of UK-based interventions found that subsidies were generally associated with low-paid jobs and low work satisfaction, and while the influence was positive on short-term employment outcomes, there was no influence on long-term outcomes, e.g., job retention (Bambra et al. 2005). In general, much of the qualitative evidence highlights how providing support, whether in terms of subsidies or changes to working conditions, for people with disabilities, can have both positive and negative effects. In introducing new policies, attention needs to be paid to the effects of support on the self-esteem and status of the recipients of this support, as well as on employment outcomes.

Type IV – Enhancing Employers' and Employees' Responsibilities in Return-to-Work Planning

This type of ALMP focuses on early intervention to actively manage return to work plans for sick-listed individuals. It requires employees and employers to actively engage in helping sick-listed people back into work. The purpose of this is to reduce the numbers of people who move from short-term into long-term sickness and subsequent detachment from the labour market. In both Sweden and Denmark, the requirement for employers to engage in return to work planning has been enhanced in recent reforms. Since 2009 in Denmark, employers are required to conduct sickness absence interviews with employees within 4 weeks of sickness absence, the employer and employee have a duty to attend this interview, and the employees are entitled to ask for a return-to-work plan at any point in the process if they expect to be off sick for more than 8 weeks.

Similar to the Danish model, Sweden attempts to take a prevention and early intervention approach to return-to-work planning, with strong employer responsibility, multidisciplinary coordination, and inclusive rehabilitation services. The 2008 sickness and disability benefit reforms introduced various requirements for people to engage in rehabilitation, referred to as the *Rehabilitation Chain*. In particular, in the first 90 days of sickness absence, the employer and employee engage in an assessment to identify what workplace adjustments or alternative adjustments would be needed to keep the employee in work. A return to work and rehabilitation plan is established providing an overview of the measures and interventions necessary to enable them to regain their work capacity. The plan is used to coordinate rehabilitation support between employer, healthcare, and social insurance. Those participating in rehabilitation as part of this plan can receive a rehabilitation allowance to cover travel costs, study resources, and course fees.

In Canada there is a well-developed process for coordinating return to work with employers through the workers compensation system; however this only applies to people with disabilities or injuries caused by their work. Provincial workers compensation boards such as the Ontario Workplace Safety and Insurance

Board have introduced various schemes to improve coordination and communication throughout the process (Institute for Work and Health 2018). In the UK there are very limited requirements for employers to engage in return to work planning, and hence limited coordination of the process, meaning that intervention for workers who do not have occupational health services provided by their employers only comes after they have lost their jobs. The need for greater coordinated system, similar to the Danish and Swedish models, has been noted in several reviews of UK policy; however limited progress has been made (Belin et al. 2016).

The evidence suggests that involving employers in return to work planning can reduce subsequent sick leave and be appreciated by employees, but this type of policy has not been taken up with the level of intensity that is likely to make a difference. There is conflicting evidence on the effect of employer led return to work interventions on employment outcomes. A meta-analysis found these interventions to have a small, positive effect on employment outcomes for individuals using sickness benefits, with increased likelihood of return to work (Schandelmaier et al. 2012), while a Cochrane systematic review found no evidence of benefit (Vogel et al. 2017). When combined with workplace accommodations, there was evidence that return to work interventions reduced duration of sickness absence (Vargas-Prada et al. 2016). All reviews noted there was a lack of high-quality evidence. Another potential reason for the lack of supporting evidence for return to work interventions is incomplete access to these services. A systematic review of Swedish vocational rehabilitation programmes found that there was inconsistent access to such programmes, especially for workers from lower socioeconomic backgrounds. This is notable because these access issues exist in the presence of legislation requiring the equitable access to such programmes (Burstrom et al. 2011). Clearly, more attention needs to be paid to awareness-raising and encouraging take-up of promising approaches.

Type V – Individual Support and Advice in Locating and Obtaining Work

Most high-income welfare states have adopted ALMPs aimed at helping people move into employment by providing general support in finding work. These include efforts to enhance job search skills, match individuals to jobs, arrange access to training and education schemes, offer information about in-work benefits, and provide other forms of vocational advice and support, such as return to work planning. This is often provided on an individualized, case management basis. The increased use of case management approaches has often entailed the reorganization of those agencies responsible for providing these services, e.g., the merger of those parts of the social welfare and employment services responsible into a single agency. Another aspect of this reorganization of services in some countries is the subcontracting of service provision to the private or voluntary sectors. The countries differ, however, in the degree to which they target disabled people or provide a universal system that does not distinguish by disability status. Examples of this approach include the *New Deal for Disabled People*, introduced in the UK in 1998 (Stafford 2005), *Pathways to Work*, and the *Work Programme* (a subcontracted service in the UK, introduced in 2011). In Canada, the national government fund territories and provinces to provide such services through *Labour Market Agreements*, with a specific agreement for disabled people (Government of Canada 2017).

Personalized support in seeking employment can be effective under certain conditions. There is evidence from several studies that the use of personal advisors and individual case management in schemes to support disabled people in their job search and interview skills did help some participants back to work. Qualitative studies, however, reveal that time pressures and job outcome targets influence some advisors to select "easier-to-place" claimants into programmes and also inhibit the development of mutual trust, which is needed for individual case management to work effectively (Clayton et al. 2011).

Type VI – Education, Training, and Work Placements for Disabled People

This type of ALMP recognizes that disabled people will be at a disadvantage in the labour market if they do not have the required educational level or vocational skills or if they need re-training for a job that is more suitable for their changed situation. Education, training, and work placement schemes have been introduced with the aim of increasing employment opportunities by boosting skills and training. This approach tends to be packaged with the previous intervention type, for example, both UK programmes (*New Deal for Disabled People* and the *Work Programme*) incorporate this intervention type. The 2013 and 2014 Danish reforms introduced mandatory vocational rehabilitation, which includes coordinated employment and educational measures and usually lasts between 1 and 5 years.

There is a dearth of robust evidence investigating the effect of education and training on its own – most studies involve multicomponent interventions that may include some training (Clayton et al. 2011). The findings of the evaluations that have been carried out on this type of ALMPs are equivocal, finding both positive and negative employment outcomes (Whitehead et al. 2009). The interventions that have been studied tend to suffer from major defects concerned with selection bias, which make interpretation of results difficult. Some studies, for example, have found evidence of selection into the programmes of people who are more work-ready and easier to place in jobs (known as "cream-skimming"), resulting in better labour market outcomes. Conversely, studies have found that some forms of educational rehabilitation worsened reemployment chances compared with no rehabilitation. On further inspection, researchers have attributed these negative results in part to recruitment into the programmes of participants who had the worst prospects and were more difficult to place (e.g., with high previous sick leave). Some seemingly negative effects of rehabilitation programmes have also been shown by subgroup analyses to be artefacts of the system: the registered sickness spell was prolonged while the participant completed the rehabilitation, thus erroneously making it seem that the rehabilitation programme itself was to blame for the observed longer periods of being off work in the intervention group (Whitehead et al. 2009).

Type VII – Health Condition/Impairment Management

A further strategy for getting chronically ill and disabled people back into work is to attend to their particular health problem: to improve the health condition or prevent a decline. Medical rehabilitation to improve physical fitness and mobility, for example, may widen the range of jobs and work environments that disabled people can participate in. Preventive initiatives to halt further declines in health could be hypothesized to improve chances of keeping a job or of earlier return to work. The Nordic countries and Germany have taken the lead in experimenting with such strategies, and the UK is also beginning to take more interest in this approach. In the UK, the *Condition Management Programme* was part of the wider *Pathways to Work* programme.

There is some evidence that the management of health conditions/medical rehabilitation can be effective in assisting participants to manage their particular health condition better and thereby reducing its work-limiting effect. There is evidence that return to work outcomes are improved for individuals with musculoskeletal conditions by extensive rehabilitation or behavioral approaches combined with physiotherapy (Whitehead et al. 2009). Qualitative evidence for the UK *Condition Management programme* found there were positive views about the intervention and that it was useful in helping claimants make steps toward the labour market; however there was a common theme that lack of expertise among advisors limited the effectiveness (Clayton et al. 2011). A systematic review for musculoskeletal and mental health conditions found that these interventions were effective when combined with workplace modifications and coordination interventions (Cullen et al. 2018).

Type VIII – Financial Incentives to Help the Transition from Benefits to Work

Policy makers have experimented with several types of incentive – for example, by providing additional income for those making the transition from welfare benefits to a job – to make up for potential, or perceived fears of, loss of income. This has often been through allowing people to undertake some work while still receiving benefits. In Sweden, for example, since 2000, disability benefit recipients have had the opportunity to work for a limited time without losing their benefit status, within a system called *resting benefits*. As there was lower than expected take up of this opportunity in 2009, the *Continuous Deduction Programme* was introduced. Under this new scheme there is a gradual reduction or "taper" in benefits as a person's income from employment increases ensuring they are financially better off when doing more work (Andersson 2018). Similar schemes have been implemented in the UK through the provision of in-work benefits – such as *Working Tax Credit* – and plans to combine multiple welfare benefits into a single scheme (called *Universal Credit*) will involve a tapered reduction in benefit as employment income increases (Clayton et al. 2011).

A systematic review of the evidence concluded that financial incentives for disabled people, such as tax credits, can help with lasting transitions into work.

Qualitative evidence from UK schemes suggest the schemes have a positive effect on employment outcomes but the take up of such schemes was low (Clayton et al. 2011). Evidence from Norway also suggests incentives are positively associated with employment outcomes (Kostol and Mogstad 2014). The incentives, however, are often set too low or are too short-term to have an effect. Many evaluative studies suffer from selection bias into these programmes, recruiting more work-ready claimants. In addition, even though financial incentives are based on national programmes, they often have very low awareness and take-up rates, making it unlikely that a population-level impact would be achieved even if effective for individual participants.

What About Activation Strategies to Counteract Disincentives to Work?

Alongside efforts to implement ALMPS, the second major component of activation strategies in recent decades has been the introduction of measures in the welfare benefit system aimed at counteracting potential disincentives to work, including those aimed at disabled or chronically ill people. Since the early 1990s, for example, irrespective of the adequacy of their welfare benefit schemes, many countries have increasingly restricted the level of, and eligibility to, their earnings replacement welfare benefits for disabled people. Justifications for these financial penalties or "sticks" include (a) to limit escalating costs of welfare provision and (b) to act as a disincentive to "welfare dependency." Indeed, one of the justifications for having low, flat-rate benefit levels with tight eligibility criteria in countries such as Canada and the UK in the first place is the notion that if the standard of living achievable through benefits is too close to that achievable through paid work, then people who can work will not want to.

In recent decades, such activation strategies have gained more prominence. One recent assessment for the OECD concluded that while there was some evidence from individual OECD countries that such measures can be effective in increasing return to work for unemployment benefit recipients in general, that was not the case for recipients of disability-related benefits, for whom the measures were much less successful in all countries (Martin 2014). Our studies on these measures have also demonstrated adverse consequences for health and living standards of disabled people, at the same time as having little or no effect on employment chances (Barr et al. 2010, 2015a, b).

In the UK, reforms to the disability income replacement benefits have included increasing restrictiveness of eligibility through new standardized assessments, reducing adequacy of replacement rates, and making benefits contingent on participating in work-related activity for some claimants (Barr and McHale 2018). These changes have been introduced through multiple reforms to the main disability benefits. In 1995 the Invalidity Benefit was replaced by the Incapacity Benefit, which was then further superseded by the Employment and Support Allowance (ESA) in 2008. The increased restrictiveness of eligibility criteria was initiated through the introduction of the "All Work Test" in 1996, and the test was made stricter still with the introduction of the "Work Capability Assessment" which came with the ESA in 2008. ESA grouped claimants into those assessed as unable to work and those who had capacity to prepare for work (work-related activity group). Benefits for the work-related activity group were only available if claimants participate in programmes to support employment finding, such as a "work-focused interview."

Similarly, Sweden has introduced reforms to the disability and sickness benefits to reduce adequacy and restrict eligibility. Between 2003 and 2008, reforms were introduced which reduced the adequacy of sickness benefits and restricted the length of time they are available to less than one year, and restrictions were placed on the eligibility criteria for disability benefits (Cohen Birman and Andersson 2014; Hagelund and Bryngelson 2014). The reforms to sickness benefit also introduced the *Rehabilitation Chain* which involved an assessment of claimant work capacity at specific time points, extended beyond their current work situation to wider work at later points.

Much like the Swedish example, Denmark has introduced significant reforms to both the disability pension (for individuals who permanently lose work capability) and sickness benefits. In 2013, age restrictions were placed on the disability pension; claimants under 40 years old were excluded from the benefit unless severe functional limitations were present which precluded any future opportunity for work. For claimants who were deemed as having a chance of return to work, obligatory vocational rehabilitation was introduced. In 2014, assessments were introduced for sickness benefit claimants at 5 months which included the vocational rehabilitation if further sickness absence is likely (OECD 2015).

The effectiveness of the punitive approach on claimant numbers and employment is equivocal. There is little evidence to support the effectiveness of restricting access to these benefits through stricter eligibility criteria, or reducing the adequacy of the replacement rates, in improving employment outcomes for disabled people. A systematic review of studies from five OECD countries with advanced health and welfare systems found that there was some evidence that increasing the adequacy of disability benefits had a small negative effect on the employment of people with disabilities, while tightening disability benefit eligibility criteria tended to move people onto other welfare benefits (e.g., unemployment) rather than into employment (Barr et al. 2010). A further study from the UK has evaluated the employment effects of reassessing the eligibility of 1.5 million existing claimants of the main out of work disability benefit with the stricter "*Work Capability Assessment*." This was shown to be ineffective in increasing the transitions of people with disabilities into employment, but, instead, it moved people with mental health problems from disability benefits into unemployment benefits (Barr et al. 2015a). Not only did this process fail to have an impact on the employment of people with disabilities, it also appears to have had severe adverse consequences for mental health. Barr et al. (2015b), for example, estimated that the application of this stricter assessment process led to an increase in mental health problems, antidepressant prescribing, and suicides. The policy was estimated to have led to an additional 600 suicides.

A further potential unintended consequence of restricting access to disability benefits is that it could increase risk of poverty among people with disabilities who are not able to work. In the UK the risk of poverty has been increasing among people with disabilities following recent reforms, particularly among those who are out of work (Barr and McHale 2018).

Ongoing Challenges and Forward View

This chapter demonstrates that there are many disparate approaches to improving employment among people with disabilities and chronic health conditions and improving return to work outcomes for individuals who are long-term absent from work with sickness.

There are several important aspects of the current policy picture that warrant further attention. Firstly, it is notable that, despite reforms throughout the OECD, the employment gap for disabled people is particularly difficult to reduce. This has important implications for the inequalities picture: deprivation and disability are closely linked with each making the other more likely, and employment is an intrinsic aspect of socioeconomic status. Given we are seeing a reduction in the adequacy of disability benefits without an associated improvement in employment outcomes, and that disabled people are more likely to be in poverty already, there is legitimate concern that inequalities will increase for this vulnerable group. It is vital that the potential negative consequences of activation strategies that reduce eligibility and adequacy of benefits are considered, particularly when implementing punitive welfare reforms. Considering the evidence for adverse outcomes associated with such reforms, approaches are needed to prevent these if the punitive changes are implemented.

The second issue concerns inequalities within the cohort of disabled people. Some of the interventions discussed are more accessible to, and more successful for, disabled people from a more affluent socioeconomic position and those closer to the labour market. Evidence from the UK *Access to Work* programme, for example, indicated that the pattern of take-up favored people who had sensory or mobility impairments, younger people, and those in professional or public sector occupations. People with mental health conditions and those in less skilled jobs were least likely to receive support from the scheme (Sayce 2011). Another important factor for inequalities is that some interventions led to low paid, unskilled employment. This means that policy interventions may not be effective in reducing the socioeconomic inequalities that disabled people face, and a subset of this cohort who are particularly vulnerable may not have sufficient access to interventions from which they could benefit. This indicates a need to be vigilant about interventions, to ensure that particular subgroups are not left behind by the way that policies are implemented.

The third issue surrounds the future of labour markets in countries such as those discussed. Demographic change means future population projections are of a rapidly increasing older (over 65) cohort and a relatively smaller working-age population. There is thus an economic imperative to extend working lives.

The current policy response is to increase retirement ages for state pensions. Given the disability employment gap, however, and the higher prevalence of health problems in older ages, this is unlikely to be a sufficient response. The potential policy interventions discussed here are likely to be important to this issue. Given evidence that some interventions have higher take-up among younger people, there is a need to ensure that interventions are successful in supporting older people into employment.

It is clear from the continuing issues of lower employment for people with disabilities, as demonstrated by the persisting disability employment gap, and the increased risk of poverty in this group, that continuing efforts to improve equity for disabled people are required. This chapter highlights both a typology of approaches and the evidence that more work is needed to identify the most effective approaches. Policy makers should consider a comprehensive mix of environmental and individual ALMPs to improve employment opportunities. Careful consideration should be given to potential adverse consequences of activation strategies, and ensuring policies are accessible to all appropriate disabled people. Finally, it is important to evaluate these interventions for differential impact by socioeconomic status, to help identify which measures or combination of measures work best for disabled people in the most disadvantaged socioeconomic circumstances.

Cross-References

▶ Investing in Integrative Active Labour Market Policies
▶ Policies of Reducing the Burden of Occupational Hazards and Disability Pensions
▶ Reducing Inequalities in Employment of People with Disabilities
▶ Regulatory Contexts Affecting Work Reintegration of People with Chronic Disease and Disabilities

References

Andersson J (2018) Financial incentives to work for disability insurance recipients – Sweden's special rules for continuous deduction. Institute for Evaluation of Labour Market and Education Policy, Uppsala

Bambra C, Pope D (2007) What are the effects of anti-discriminatory legislation on socioeconomic inequalities in the employment consequences of ill health and disability? J Epidemiol Community Health 61:421–426. https://doi.org/10.1136/jech.2006.052662

Bambra C, Whitehead M, Hamilton V (2005) Does "welfare-to-work" work? A systematic review of the effectiveness of the UK's welfare-to-work programmes for people with a disability or chronic illness. Soc Sci Med 60:1905–1918. https://doi.org/10.1016/j.socscimed.2004.09.002

Barr B, McHale P (2018) The rise and fall of income replacement disability benefit receipt in the United Kingdom. In: MacEachen E (ed) The science and politics of work disability prevention. Routledge, New York

Barr B, Clayton S, Whitehead M et al (2010) To what extent have relaxed eligibility requirements and increased generosity of disability benefits acted as disincentives for employment?

A systematic review of evidence from countries with well-developed welfare systems. J Epidemiol Community Health 64:1106–1114. https://doi.org/10.1136/jech.2010.111401

Barr B, Taylor-Robinson D, Stuckler D et al (2015a) Fit-for-work or fit-for-unemployment? Does the reassessment of disability benefit claimants using a tougher work capability assessment help people into work? J Epidemiol Community Health 70:452–458. https://doi.org/10.1136/jech-2015-206333

Barr B, Taylor-Robinson D, Stuckler D et al (2015b) 'First, do no harm': are disability assessments associated with adverse trends in mental health? A longitudinal ecological study. J Epidemiol Community Health 70:339–345. https://doi.org/10.1136/jech-2015-206209

Belin A, Dupont C, Oulès L et al (2016) Rehabilitation and return to work: analysis report on EU and member states policies, strategies and programmes. European Agency for Safety and Health at Work, Bilbao

Bingley P, Datta Gupta N, Pedersen P (2011) Disability programme, health and retirement in Denmark since 1960: working paper 1713. National Bureau of Economic Research, Cambridge, MA

Burstrom B, Nylen L, Clayton S, Whitehead M (2011) How equitable is vocational rehabilitation in Sweden? A review of evidence on the implementation of a national policy framework. Disabil Rehabil 33:453–466. https://doi.org/10.3109/09638288.2010.493596

Clayton S, Bambra C, Gosling R et al (2011) Assembling the evidence jigsaw: insights from a systematic review of UK studies of individual-focused return to work initiatives for disabled and long-term ill people. BMC Public Health 11:170. https://doi.org/10.1186/1471-2458-11-170

Clayton S, Barr B, Nylen L et al (2012) Effectiveness of return-to-work interventions for disabled people: a systematic review of government initiatives focused on changing the behaviour of employers. Eur J Pub Health 22:434–439. https://doi.org/10.1093/eurpub/ckr101

Cohen Birman M, Andersson C (2014) Stricter sickness and disability insurance systems and early retirement. Swedish Social Insurance Inspectorate, Stockholm

Cullen KL, Irvin E, Collie A et al (2018) Effectiveness of workplace interventions in return-to-work for musculoskeletal, pain-related and mental health conditions: an update of the evidence and messages for practitioners. J Occup Rehabil 28(1):1–15. https://doi.org/10.1007/s10926-016-9690-x

Datta Gupta N, Larsen M, Thomsen LS (2015) Do wage subsidies for disabled workers reduce their non-employment? – evidence from the Danish Flexjob scheme. IZA J Labor Policy 4:10. https://doi.org/10.1186/s40173-015-0036-7

Department for Work and Pensions (2017) Access to work: factsheet for customers. https://www.gov.uk/government/publications/access-to-work-factsheet/access-to-work-factsheet-for-customers. Accessed 5 Sep 2017

European Commission (2016) European semester thematic factsheet: active labour market policies. European Commission, Brussels

Government of Canada (2017) Labour market agreements for persons with disabilities. https://www.canada.ca/en/employment-social-development/programs/labour-market-agreement-disability.html. Accessed 20 Dec 2018

Government of Canada (2018) Making an accessible Canada for people with disabilities. https://www.canada.ca/en/employment-social-development/programs/accessible-people-disabilities.html. Accessed 20 Dec 2018

Hagelund A, Bryngelson A (2014) Change and resilience in welfare state policy. The politics of sickness insurance in Norway and Sweden. Soc Policy Adm 48:300–318. https://doi.org/10.1111/spol.12009

Institute for Work & Health (2018) Integrating return-to-work principles in an occupational medicine service. https://www.iwh.on.ca/impact-case-studies/integrating-return-to-work-principles-in-occupational-medicine-service. Accessed 20 Dec 2018

Kostol AR, Mogstad M (2014) How financial incentives induce disability insurance recipients to return to work. Am Econ Rev 104:624–655. https://doi.org/10.1257/aer.104.2.624

Lane J, Videbaek Munkholm N (2015) Danish and British protection from disability discrimination at work – past, present and future. Int J Comp Labour Law Ind Relat 31:91–112

Martin J (2014) Activation and active labour market policies in OECD countries: stylized facts and evidence on their effectiveness: IZA Policy Paper No. 84. Geary institute University College Dublin, Dublin

McVicar D, Wilkins R, Ziebarth NR (2019) Four decades of disability benefit policies and the rise and fall of disability recipiency rates in five OECD countries. In: Besharov D, Call D (eds) Labor activation in a time of high unemployment: encouraging work while preserving the social safety net. Oxford University Press, Oxford

Nevala N, Pehkonen I, Koskela I et al (2015) Workplace accommodation among persons with disabilities: a systematic review of its effectiveness and barriers or facilitators. J Occup Rehabil 25:432–448. https://doi.org/10.1007/s10926-014-9548-z

OECD (2003) Transforming disability into ability policies to promote work and income security for disabled people. OECD Publishing, Paris

OECD (2010) Sickness, disability and work: breaking the barriers. Canada: opportunities for collaboration. OECD Publishing, Paris

OECD (2013) G20 task force on employment: activation strategies for stronger and more inclusive labour markets in G20 countries: key policy challenges and good practices. OECD Publishing, Paris

OECD (2015) Ageing and employment policies: Denmark 2015. OECD Publishing, Paris

Sayce L (2011) Getting in, staying in and getting on: disability employment support fit for the future. Department for Work and Pensions, London

Schandelmaier S, Ebrahim S, Burkhardt SCA et al (2012) Return to work coordination programmes for work disability: a meta-analysis of randomised controlled trials. PLoS One 7:e49760. https://doi.org/10.1371/journal.pone.0049760

Simm C, Aston J, Williams C et al (2007) Organisations' responses to the disability discrimination act: research report no. 410. Department for Work and Pensions, Leeds

Stafford B (2005) New deal for disabled people: what's new about new deal? University of Nottingham, Nottingham

UK Government (2010) Definition of disability under the Equality Act 2010. https://www.gov.uk/definition-of-disability-under-equality-act-2010. Accessed 18 Apr 2017

Vargas-Prada S, Demou E, Lalloo D et al (2016) Effectiveness of very early workplace interventions to reduce sickness absence: a systematic review of the literature and meta-analysis. Scand J Work Environ Health 42(4):261–272. https://doi.org/10.5271/sjweh.3576

Vogel N, Schandelmaier S, Zumbrunn T et al (2017) Return-to-work coordination programmes for improving return to work in workers on sick leave. Cochrane Database Syst Rev 3:CD011618. https://doi.org/10.1002/14651858.CD011618.pub2

Whitehead M (2007) A typology of actions to tackle social inequalities in health. J Epidemiol Community Health 61:473. https://doi.org/10.1136/jech.2005.037242

Whitehead M, Dahl E, Burstrom B, Diderichsen F, Ng E et al (2009) Helping chronically ill or disabled people into work: what can we learn from international comparative analyses? Final report to the Public Health Policy Research Programme of Department of Health. Public Health Research Consortium, London

Part II

Access/return to Work of Persons with Disabilities or Chronic Diseases

A Human Rights Perspective on Work Participation

18

Jerome Bickenbach

Contents

Introduction: Work, Disability, and Human Rights	332
Negative and Positive Human Rights	334
Positive Rights and the CRPD	334
CRPD Article 27 – Work and Employment	336
Positive Rights to Work and Political Equality	339
Article 27 and Work Capacity Determination	340
Conclusion	343
Cross References	343
References	343

Abstract

Participation in work has, at least since the 1948 *Universal Declaration of Human Rights*, been recognized to be a core human right; it has recently been entrenched as such for persons with disabilities in the UN Convention on the Rights of Persons with Disabilities. In this chapter, I explore the source, scope, rationale, and, in effect, the logic of this human right, as it applies to people with long-term health problems or permanent impairments. In particular, the debate whether the right to work is merely a negative right of non-discrimination or both that and a positive right i.e., the right to resources and services to enable, protect and promote work participation, a right that demands action on the part of state agencies. I argue that, to be meaningful, the right to work must incorporate these position elements – to ensure equality – and explore the potential impact of this approach to national policies and practices of work capacity determination.

J. Bickenbach (✉)
University of Lucerne and Swiss Paraplegic Research, Nottwil, Switzerland
e-mail: jerome.bickenbach@paraplegie.ch

> **Keywords**
>
> Accessibility · Accommodation · Human rights · Work/employment · Participation

Introduction: Work, Disability, and Human Rights

Whether one looks at standard quality of life indicators, the results of sociopsychological studies, or autobiographical accounts, all agree that work is a key life activity that defines us as social beings. Work is central to social inclusion and full participation and is the source of both our material and psychological well-being (see, e.g., Neff 1985; Moos 1986; Rothman 1998; Blustein 2008). Worldwide, unemployment and underemployment have been directly or indirectly linked to a wide variety of adverse mental and physical health problems (Benach and Muntaner 2013; Marmot and Bell 2010) as well as low levels of life satisfaction and happiness (Stiglitz et al. 2009; Siegrist and Marmot 2006; EUROSTAT 2018). Economic and social insecurity are obvious risks of unemployment but often more serious, although considerably more difficult to measure, are the loss of self-respect and the breakdown of social interactions, connectedness, and the sense of social belonging (Szymanski and Parker 2010). Although these facets of social connection associated with employment are important to everyone, they are especially crucial to those groups who are, for other reasons, already socially marginalized and stigmatized. Prominent among these groups are individuals with physical or mental disabilities (Fabian 2013).

We know that people with disabilities experience some of the highest levels of unemployment of any social group, around the world. Even taking account of the fact that nearly half of those experiencing disability are over age 65, those of working age are also unemployed. In the United States in 2016, for example, the employment rate for ages 18–64 was only 31% for people with disabilities, compared to 76% for those without. Given that the part-time employment rate is twice as high for people with disabilities, even those who do find work are underemployed (US 2017). In 2010, the OECD reported that, despite recent improvement in OECD high-income countries, the employment rate for people with a disability remains half that of people without a disability (OECD 2010); and in the case of disability associated with mental ill-health, the employment gap is even greater (OECD 2015). Labor statistics for low- and medium-resource countries, although not always well-developed, certainly confirm these results.

Whenever a fundamental human life activity is shown to have complex associations with basic psychological, sociological, and material human needs, and especially when the activity is not equally enjoyed across the population, society and its organizations are put on notice that it is fundamentally failing its population. To emphasize the importance of responding to this failure, it is common to translate the underlying values into the language of human rights.

Indeed, the so-called right to work figured prominently in the mid-nineteenth-century transformation of human rights from philosophical aspirations to legal guarantees. This trend culminated in Article 23.1 of the 1948 *Universal Declaration of Human Rights*, the originating document of the United Nations. The article states that "Everyone has the right to work, to free choice of employment, to just and favourable conditions of work and to protection against unemployment" (UN 1948). Like nearly every statement of the right to work since then, the Declaration grounds the right in the "inherent dignity of all members of the human family," which underscores the belief that some domains of human life – such as employment – are central to what it means to be human. More recently scientifically established linkages to health and well-being bring this somewhat vague normative language very much down to earth: people just don't flourish if they are systematically denied participation in areas of life that is characteristically human.

Since the first international recognition of the human right to work in 1948, there have been several reaffirmations and restatements. Article 6 of the United Nations' *International Covenant on Economic, Social and Cultural Rights* not only recognizes a right to work but also the obligation of states to provide "technical and vocational guidance and training programmes, policies and techniques" required to achieve the full realization of that right (UN 1976). The *European Social Charter* that entered into force in 1965 begins in Article 1 by expressing the obligation of each state to ensure that "there is work for all who are available for and seeking work" (EU 1965); and Article 15 of the *Charter of Fundamental Rights of the European Union* states that "everyone has the right to engage in work and to pursue a freely chosen or accepted occupation . . . and has the freedom to seek employment, to work, to exercise the right of establishment and to provide services in any Member State" (EU 2000).

It was more or less inevitable therefore that, when the United Nations' *Convention on the Rights of Persons with Disabilities* (CRPD) was debated and drafted in the early years of this century, the right to work and employment was one of the first to be included. Significantly, though the drafters of the CRPD, many of whom were long-time disability advocates themselves, felt nearly as strongly about the need to render into the human rights discourse other entitlements that were more closely tied – both historically and conceptually – to the nature of disability itself. There was in particular a keen desire to protect against discriminatory practices that arose, not only from fear and animus but also and more commonly from perverse and stigmatizing attitudes of inferiority, incapability, and the need for paternalistic protection. While, abstractly, it might be argued that people with disabilities do not need their own declaration of human rights – people with disabilities are, after all, humans like everyone else – the practical political need for the CRPD was urged on the argument that the manifestation of the denial of human rights for people with disabilities was sufficiently distinct that disability-specific social dynamics needed to be addressed. The CRPD, in short, is essentially a reaffirmation of basic human rights for people with disabilities.

Negative and Positive Human Rights

Human rights discourse, especially when operationalized in legal language, is grounded in the fundamental distinction between negative and positive human rights. Negative rights prohibit the intentional or indirect and systematic creation of obstacles to the enjoyment of the content of human rights (either very general rights to human dignity, life, liberty, and security or else specific rights to free speech and association, education, and work). The prohibition against discrimination in work is perhaps the most well-known of these negative rights. Positive rights by contrast require societies and their agencies to provide whatever essential resources and opportunities are needed so that individuals are enabled to enjoy these rights in practice. Positive rights, it might be said, create actual and achievable opportunities, not merely formal or theoretical opportunities. Like everyone else, people with disabilities are entitled to negative rights and to be free from the obstacles to be fully human. Historically, it is the realm of positive rights that has characterized the significance and impact of human rights for people with disabilities (see, e.g., Scotch 1989).

Positive rights are of such importance to people with disabilities because of the history of the societal response to disability and the very nature of disability itself. To be sure there have been historical examples in which people with disabilities have experienced direct and violent violations of their negative human rights. People with disabilities have experienced, and continue to experience, denials of inherent dignity and respect, denials of the necessities of life, and denials of life itself. That said, for the most part, the history of disability has been characterized by benign neglect grounded in misperceptions of inherent inferiority and uselessness that have given rise to pity and charity (Driedger 1989; Bickenbach 1993). Even when the need for provision of supports, services, and other resources to enhance opportunities has been acknowledged, these resources have been characterized as "special needs" outside of the mainstream. Special needs by definition pose an additional special burden on society, one that can arguably wait until the needs of "normal people" have been addressed. It was only recently, the last 40 years or so, that there has been a call for a "human rights approach" to disability in which the provision of empowering supports and resources has been understood as human rights – in particular – positive human rights (Kavka 2000).

Positive Rights and the CRPD

The language of the CRPD addresses positive rights in two distinct ways. Firstly, the CRPD explicitly includes disability-relevant positive rights of practical empowerment. The most obvious example of this is Article 9 on accessibility. In the disability context, accessibility is a general term that refers to those resources, opportunities, and accommodations that make it possible for people with disabilities to, in the words of the article, "live independently and participate fully in all aspects of life." Given the realities of the physical and mental impairments that underlie the experience of disability – limitations of mobility, of seeing and hearing, of cognition – ordinary features of the physical and social world may not take these differences into account, making it difficult to fully participate in activities of daily life. The physical and social world, in short, may need to be altered to respond to needs created by impairment-related differences: public buildings may need to be modified so that people in wheelchairs can use them; information may need to be provided in alternative formats so that people who are blind can access them; and, in general, assistive technology may need to be provided so that people with physical or mental limitations can perform the simple or complex actions that they need to do.

In short, because of the nature or severity of the impairments people experience, the equal enjoyment of the basic activities of daily life may require society to provide resources and modifications that make their world accessible to them. Accessibility – in all of its myriad forms – is therefore a positive human right closely associated with disability. The CRPD has been carefully drafted in order to fully integrate accessibility in all of its substantive provisions. In order for every state-provided service that is generally available to everyone (health care, rehabilitation, income security, informational and educational services, and so on) to be available to people with disabilities, the CRPD mandates that these supports and services need to be made accessible so that these are useable to the person.

The second, and more subtle way in which the CRPD addresses positive rights, involves the notion of accommodation. This notion has its origins in anti-discrimination law and policy as they developed, first in Anglo-American jurisprudence and then across the world. Although it had its origins in the law on religious freedom, the notion of accommodation soon became central to disability law and policy (see Stein et al. 2014). In essence, an accommodation is any modification or adjustment to an institution, service, or area of life that enables a person with a disability to fully participate in the benefits of the institution, service, or area of life. In legal jargon, especially as it is applied in the context of employment, the notion is usually termed "reasonable accommodation," reflecting the essential balancing act that is often required in practice to weigh, on the one hand the benefits of full participation, with on the other, the social cost of providing accommodation (Waddington and Hendricks 2002).

Conceptually, the right to accommodation is clearly a positive right – since it requires that positive actions be taken to make modifications or adjustments to the world. In the disability human rights literature, however, there has been a tradition of characterizing reasonable accommodation not as a separate and positive human right but as an aspect of the negative right of nondiscrimination. The reasons for this are historical and directly tied to unique features of the constitutional and administrative structure of the federal government of the United States and in particular to the judicial interpretation of the *Americans with Disabilities Act of 1990* the world's first – and still paradigmatic – disability anti-discrimination law (for a complete description of this context constitutional situation see Bagenstos 2009; Bickenbach 2012). Essentially, it would be constitutionally problematic in the United States for federal legislation to include actionable rights that were usually cast as forms of social welfare – specially the provision of resources and supports to individuals. The

Americans with Disabilities Act was constitutionally acceptable when viewed as a remedial statute – correcting a harm in the form of discrimination – but not as a statement of positive obligations on the part of the state to create entitlements. Lawyers and disability advocates overcame this legal hurdle by legally characterizing the intentional refusal or culpable failure to provide reasonable accommodation as itself a form of discrimination. This analysis – although unnecessary and even distorting outside of the United States – has been carried over into the interpretation of the CRPD (see, e.g., Stein et al. 2014; Bantekas et al. 2018).

Legal and historical technicalities aside, the important feature of the human right to accommodation is that, very much unlike the right to accessibility that points to relatively discrete and practical solutions to limitations related to impairments, accommodation is far more nuanced a remedy. This feature of accommodation is best seen in the area of the right to work for persons with disabilities, where historically, the legal notion of reasonable accommodation has made the greatest impact. And for this we need to turn to more specifically to the language of Article 27 of the CRPD.

CRPD Article 27 – Work and Employment

The full text of Article 27 of the CRPD is as follows:

1. *States Parties recognize the right of persons with disabilities to work, on an equal basis with others; this includes the right to the opportunity to gain a living by work freely chosen or accepted in a labour market and work environment that is open, inclusive and accessible to persons with disabilities. States Parties shall safeguard and promote the realization of the right to work, including for those who acquire a disability during the course of employment, by taking appropriate steps, including through legislation, to,* inter alia*:*

    (a) *Prohibit discrimination on the basis of disability with regard to all matters concerning all forms of employment, including conditions of recruitment, hiring and employment, continuance of employment, career advancement and safe and healthy working conditions;*
    (b) *Protect the rights of persons with disabilities, on an equal basis with others, to just and favourable conditions of work, including equal opportunities and equal remuneration for work of equal value, safe and healthy working conditions, including protection from harassment, and the redress of grievances;*
    (c) *Ensure that persons with disabilities are able to exercise their labour and trade union rights on an equal basis with others;*
    (d) *Enable persons with disabilities to have effective access to general technical and vocational guidance programmes, placement services and vocational and continuing training;*

(e) *Promote employment opportunities and career advancement for persons with disabilities in the labour market, as well as assistance in finding, obtaining, maintaining and returning to employment;*
(f) *Promote opportunities for self-employment, entrepreneurship, the development of cooperatives and starting one's own business;*
(g) *Employ persons with disabilities in the public sector;*
(h) *Promote the employment of persons with disabilities in the private sector through appropriate policies and measures, which may include affirmative action programmes, incentives and other measures;*
(i) *Ensure that reasonable accommodation is provided to persons with disabilities in the workplace;*
(j) *Promote the acquisition by persons with disabilities of work experience in the open labour market;*
(k) *Promote vocational and professional rehabilitation, job retention and return-to-work programmes for persons with disabilities.*

2. *States Parties shall ensure that persons with disabilities are not held in slavery or in servitude, and are protected, on an equal basis with others, from forced or compulsory labour.* (UN 2007).

It is important to cite the Article in full because its very length and level of detail is noteworthy. Far from an abstract or platitudinous expression of a "right to work," Article 27 sets out explicit preconditions for the right. A disability activist or advocate might put the point this way: The lesson of history is that it is quite useless to affirm that people with disabilities have a right to work; the full force and effect of recognizing this human right depends entirely on specific obligations both of accessibility and accommodation that together operationalize a society's commitment to political equality, supported by positive human rights.

The opening subsection of Section 1 highlights the classic negative right of nondiscrimination (and is explicit about its scope, "including conditions of recruitment, hiring and employment, continuance of employment, career advancement, and safe and healthy working conditions"). This negative right is of great significance given that discrimination (in its modern legal interpretation) addresses far more than the relatively rare case of overt and intentional discrimination and includes more subtle forms of hidden discriminatory barriers. Examples of these barriers include legislative requirements that people with disabilities need certifications of "fitness to work" from a doctor before being employed, or regulations that limit in the number of hours they can work, or require people to take out life insurance, or prevent them from benefiting from minimum wage legislation, or put limits on publically provided health insurance or income support if they work (see Bantekas et al. 2018). In all these, and many other instances, the state, often unintentionally, creates disincentives to work that apply only to people with disabilities. These disincentives are discriminatory and are prohibited by this subsection.

That said, the rest of Section 1 of Article 27 is entirely couched in the discourse of positive rights. To see this may require some decoding of legal language: when lawyers speak of "protecting" rights or "ensuring," "enabling," or "promoting" the detailed preconditions for the enjoyment of the right to work, they are using language that is understood to signal the need not only to removing obstacles (and of course, preventing the creation of new obstacles) but also the obligation to positively act in order to create the preconditions essential to the actual and concrete enjoyment of the right to work (or the material conditions conductive to sustaining the enjoyment of that right).

As an example, consider subsection 1(c). In order to successfully "ensure that persons with disabilities are able to exercise their labour and trade union rights," the state must enable and facilitate the exercise of these rights. If there were laws prohibiting the exercise of labor rights, that would be discriminatory and in contravention of Article 27. But explicit prohibitions like this are rare. What is more common is the failure to empower people to exercise their labor right. In other words, "ensuring" the exercise of rights may require the state to actively inform people with disabilities of these rights, or educate them in the processes of enforcing their rights, or even providing financial and legal resources to force state agencies to ensure that these rights are acknowledged. Similarly, enabling people to access technical and vocational guidance programs may require the creation and sustained funding of these programs, advertising their availability, providing individual financial support to defray their costs, or any number of other positive actions the point and objective of which is to enable people to enjoy these work-related benefits. Human rights require equal vigilance to secure both negative and positive rights; but it is more often that the positive rights are neglected.

As a general matter, a focus on positive rights demands a great deal from the state and its agencies and actors. Often it is a relatively simple matter to fulfil negative obligations: remove the offending obstacle. But it may not be clear what the state needs to do to live up to its positive obligations: Should it create a new program targeting the specific needs of people with disabilities for life skills, vocational rehabilitation services, or employment counselling (see, ILO 2013)? Should it invest in research to find the best way to encourage people with cognitive impairments or mental health problems to work when they may never have worked before? Should it pass laws requiring the private sector to institute flexible work measures (such as teleworking or flexible time schedules) to ensure job retention for persons with disabilities? Should it develop a comprehensive national strategy promoting the employment of persons with disabilities (see, EU Commission 2010)? Should it finance the development, piloting, and implementation of new format of self-employment, such as social enterprises (see, ILO 2012)? Should it institute a policy of targets or quotas for public sector hiring, with reporting obligations (see, NDA n.d.)? Again, the outcomes may be clear (enabling, ensuring, protecting), but the means may not be clear at all.

In short, once the human right obligation is expressed in terms of enabling, protecting, or promoting something, the state is engaged in the practical task of identifying and putting into place both workplace accessibility solutions but also realistic and feasible accommodations for people with disabilities to participate in work. The state must use its resources, authorities, and powers to reconfigure its institutions to practically achieve specific outcomes beneficial to the actual enjoyment of the right to work by people with disabilities.

Positive Rights to Work and Political Equality

But what, at the end of the day, is the significance of the fact that the CRPD's right to work is framed in terms of positive rights and accommodation? In particular, what is the added value of positive rights, over and above the protections provided by the negative right of nondiscrimination? A hint of the answer can be found in the slogan associated with the Madrid Declaration of the European Congress on People with Disabilities held in 2002: "Non-discrimination plus positive action results in social inclusion" (ECD 2002). The added value of positive rights is that they are essential for securing political equality for persons with disabilities.

As a political and legal value, equality and the social preconditions for securing equality are highly contestable. Does a social commitment to equality merely require that everyone is formally allowed to pursue their life goals unhindered by prohibitions or other legal obstacles, or does it require that people enjoy realistic capabilities to pursue these goals? Is it enough to remove barriers or is the state obliged to put into place facilitators and the resources that people need to take advantage of opportunities? Putting this enormous political-theoretical debate to one side, the CRPD, as a modern human rights document, provides a relatively clear conceptualization of what equality entails in practice, from the perspective of disability. Lawyers call it "substantive equality" – the maintenance of a social, political, and economic arrangement that actually empowers everyone to achieve their individual life goals. Perhaps ironically, the clearest evidence that the CRPD is committed to this powerful sense of political equality is a legal phrase that, on the face of it, appears to limit the practical impact of the CRPD as a legal mandate.

Throughout the CRPD and specifically in the openly sentence of Article 27, the human rights of persons with disabilities are said to be recognized "on an equal basis with others." What this seemingly innocuous phrase means, first of all, is that people with disabilities are not possessed of more, or additional or more impactful, rights to work than people without disabilities. Equal means equal. But it also entails – and has been consistently interpreted to mean – that if a particular country has only a minimal recognition of employment-related rights for the general population, then that level of recognition is the legal threshold of rights for people with disabilities as well. In other words, the human rights mandate of the CRPD applies nationally – not transnationally or universally – and seeks to ensure that people with disabilities are treated on an equal basis with others in that setting, whatever the actual contours of that setting happens to be. In contrast, other United Nations declarations – in particular the Sustainable Development Goals (UN n.d.) – seek to raise the level of the material and social well-being for all peoples of the world (including the recognition of human rights); but not so the CRPD. It does not mandate more or more effective rights than the general population enjoys; it is in effect a reaffirmation in the case of people with disabilities of the equality of the enjoyment of rights.

It is important to emphasize that this "on an equal basis with others" sense of political equality is not at all useless or inconsequential. A good example of its real-world impact in the context of employment is how the CRPD responds to what is usually called "sheltered employment." This is an alternative system of employment that is available only to people with disabilities – typically people with moderate or severe cognitive impairments or mental health problems – and tends to be exempt from general labor laws, including minimum wage provisions and health and safety legislation.

Although it remains controversial whether the CRPD explicitly prohibits alternative employment regimes (May-Simera 2018), the phrase "open labor market" is used twice in Article 27 to describe the scope of the right to work, making a clear contrast to any "closed" system of alternative employment restricted to people with disabilities. A 2012 thematic study of the right to work by the United Nations Office of the High Commissioner for Human Rights (OHCHR 2012), the agency in charge of interpreting and implementing the CRPD, goes further and states that sheltered employment exists only because "persons with disabilities are often seen as unfit for working life, incapable of carrying out tasks, as required in the open labour market" and recommends that "it is imperative that States parties move away from employment schemes and promote equal access for persons with disabilities in the open labour market". In other words, sheltered employment is implicitly a violation of the sense of equality embodied in the CRPD since it is not employment "on an equal basis with others."

Evidence of the impact of the "on an equal basis with others" sense of equality can be found in the explicit requirement of "equal work for equal value," safe and health working conditions, exercise of labor and trade union rights and other incidences of the right to work found in subsection 1 of Article 27. Of equal significance is the implicit commitment to what is often called 'affirmative action' in the employment sector. It is widely agreed among CRPD commentators that the thrust of Article 27 is that countries should use positive measures such as quotas or financial incentives to the private sector in order to 'positively' achieve the level of equality of employment outcome, measured by standard national level employment indicators, for persons with disabilities (Waddington 2016). Each of these provisions point to a commitment to a sense of political equality in which the goal is not merely to remove barriers and limitations but, with positive action, to achieve that level of equality that is enjoyed by everyone else.

Article 27 and Work Capacity Determination

There is another aspect of the right to work for persons with disabilities which Article 27 impacts that is often neglected but – in practice – has enormous consequences. For a substantial number of people with severe impairments who find themselves outside of the labor market, there is an essential administrative portal that directs them not only to the open labor market, but crucially to the supports and services that make it possible for the person to find work and maintain employment. This portal is usually termed "work capacity determination."

Work capacity determination is an instance of the more broader process found primarily in social welfare policy called disability determination, the object of which is to determine the eligibility of an individual (the "claimant") to some benefit, support, service, or protection. The kinds of benefits available vary from country to country, but in a high-resource country would comprise health and rehabilitation services (including access to assistive technology); social security cash benefits; disability pensions; health and social insurance (including short- and long-term sick leaves); specific benefits such access to transportation, housing, or educational services; social care services, at home or in an institution; personal assistant services; and subsidized utilities and assistance for independent living. When the object of the disability determination is to determine access to employment-related benefits, including access to vocational rehabilitation, the focus is on *work capacity*, the degree to which a person can work, given their impairments and underlying health conditions.

Work capacity determination is used for roughly two groups of individuals with impairments – those who have never worked in their lives and those who have a work history but because of illness or injury have had to leave the work force. The first group may have congenital or early onset health conditions or acquired an impairment before they got a chance to work. Typically, these are individuals with moderate or profound cognitive impairments who historically were deemed "unemployable" and often institutionalized. Increasingly, both because of human rights legislation and the enormous financial burden of keeping a substantial minority of potential workers out of the workplace, attempts have been made to increase work participation. For those who have a work history and acquired short- or long-term impairments through accidents at work or have acquired a disabling health problem, work capacity determinations are used to determine their capacity to return to work, either at their previous job or another.

In most medium- and high-resource countries, access to employment for persons with disabilities is strongly determined by the structure of the administrative process of determining work capacity (Bickenbach 2015; Bickenbach et al. 2015). Not only does an assessment of work capacity determine who will be eligible for a "return to work" or entry-level work preparation program, it will also determine whether a person is removed from the open market and given some form of permanent pension or social welfare payment. Evidence suggests that once removed from the job market, it is very difficult to return to it. A considerate amount of research has been done in this area to suggest that in many cases, work capacity determinations are unfair and arbitrary because the decision-maker is unaccountable, the process lacks transparency, or the decisions are neither evidence-based nor reliable (e.g., Dal Pozzo et al. 2002; Stobo et al. 2007; de Boer et al. 2007; Rudbeck and Fonager 2011).

Less frequently is it noticed that the criteria by which work capacity is determined are themselves barriers to the enjoyment of the right to work. In a recent WHO and World Bank study on worldwide approaches to disability assessment and work capacity determination for working age populations, it was noted that there are only three basic criteria that inform these administrative procedures (Bickenbach et al. 2015). Work capacity can focus either on (i) the individual's underlying health condition and the impairments associated with them; (ii) his or her functional limitations in basic or simple activities, understood independently of the context in which the person lives; or (iii) the overall disability experience conceptualized as the outcome of interactions between features intrinsic to the person (health conditions, impairments, and functional limitations) and the full range of environmental factors that, possibly uniquely, characterize the overall lived context of the individual. It is argued in that study that only the last approach – which is also the least commonly in place around the globe – can plausibly be claimed to satisfy the basic requirements of a human rights approach to work.

The argument is roughly this: Article 27 insists that people with disabilities enjoy the right to work "on an equal basis with others" and, at a minimum, that means that they are not presumed to be passive recipients of benefits rather than potentially active participants in all aspects of society, including the labor force. Yet both the purely medical or impairment approach and the functional limitation approaches focus on deficits and incapacities of the applicant and ignore, or downplay, his or her strengths and potential capacities. These approaches in effect see only half of the picture because they ignore two possibilities: that the impairments or functional deficits can be partially or fully accommodated by the provision of assistant technology and, more importantly, that the work place environment can be modified to accommodate functional deficits. Workplace modifications include making physical changes to the workplace to make them more accessible, altering the social or attitudinal environment by addressing stigmatizing views of co-workers or employers or providing better information about the needs and strengths of workers with disabilities. The requirements and demands of the job itself can be modified by way of accommodation. Making these environmental modifications and providing relevant assistive technology and other relevant supports, not only accommodate disability-related deficits, they also acknowledge and build on the potential assets of the disabled worker.

In a few of its analyses of the progress made by countries in implementing the provisions of the CRPD, the CRPD Committee has identified disability assessment procedures and work capacity criteria as being problematic by violating the spirit of Article 27. The Committee points to the fact that not only would better disability determination help to increase the level of work participation, new procedures may help to put to rest common prejudicial presumptions about what the impact of severe impairments has on a person's capacity to be employed. For almost as long as disability assessment has existed, some impairments have automatically been assessed as resulting in "total" or 100% work disability – blindness, for example. But if a broader and more asset-focused approach is taken seriously, this automatic response will need to be rethought. An individual may be blind, but if she or he has access to a full range of job-relevant assistive technology and other accommodations which make it possible to work at the level of any non-blind peer, then she or he may not have a work-related disability at all. Such a fundamental shift in how work capacity is assessed involves a shift in our perception of what disability is and what people with disabilities are capable of – a shift that is very much aligned with the human rights approach to employment.

Conclusion

The human rights approach to employment for persons with disabilities includes far more than the mere assertion of a "right to work." As this discussion has tried to make it clear, the detail and conceptual nuance found in the language of the CRPD – and in particular its explicit reliance on positive rights to empower people to successfully enter and remain in employment – ushers in a new era of disability employment policy. Tackling misconceptions about the ability of people with even the most severe impairments to hold down a job, fighting the assumption of inferiority and incapacity and, most operationally, assessing people's capacity in terms of their assets and strengths, all help to make the human rights approach possible. Given the importance of work to people's health, happiness, and their sense of self-worth and social belonging, a full and robust recognition of the human right to work for persons with disabilities is an essential precondition to the recognition of their dignity as equal human beings.

Cross-References

- Concepts and Social Variations of Disability in Working-Age Populations
- Reducing Inequalities in Employment of People with Disabilities
- Regulatory Contexts Affecting Work Reintegration of People with Chronic Disease and Disabilities

References

Bagenstos SR (2009) Law and the contradictions of the disability rights movement. Yale University Press, New Haven

Bantekas I, Pennilas F, Trömel S (2018) Work and employment. In: Bantekas I, Stein M, Anastasiou D (eds) The UN Convention on the Rights of Persons with Disabilities: A Commentary. Oxford University Press, New York, pp 764–801

Benach J, Muntaner C (2013) Employment, work and health inequalities: a global perspective. Employment Conditions Network; Commission on the Social Determinants of Health, World Health Organization. https://www.who.int/social_determinants/resources/articles/emconet_who_report.pdf?ua=1

Bickenbach J (1993) Physical disability and social policy. University of Toronto Press, Toronto

Bickenbach J (2012) Ethics, law, and policy. Volume 4 of The SAGE reference series on disability: key issues and future directions. Sage, Thousand Oaks

Bickenbach J (2015) Legal dimensions of disability evaluation: work disability and human rights. In: Escorpizo R et al (eds) Handbook of vocational rehabilitation and disability evaluation. Springer, New York, pp 141–160

Bickenbach J, Posarac A, Cieza A, Kostanjsek N (2015) Assessing disability in working age population a paradigm shift: from impairment and functional limitation to the disability approach. Report no: ACS14124. The World Bank, Washington, DC

Blustein DL (2008) The psychology of working: a new perspective for career development, counseling, and public policy. Erlbaum, Mahwah

Dal Pozzo C, Haines H, Laroche Y et al (2002) Assessing disability in Europe – similarities and differences. Council of Europe, Strasbourg

de Boer WEL, Besseling JJM, Willems JHBM (2007) Organization of disability evaluation in 15 countries. Pratiques et organisation des soins. 38:205–217

Driedger D (1989) The last civil rights movement. Hurst, London

ECD, European Congress on Disability (2002) The Madrid Declaration. http://www.angsalombardia.it/objects/madrid_declaration_eng.pdf

EU (1965) European Social Charter, 529 UNTS 89. https://rm.coe.int/168007cf93

EU (2000) Charter of Fundamental Rights of the European Union. http://eur-lex.europa.eu/en/treaties/dat/32007X1214/htm/C2007303EN.01000101.htm

EU Commission (2010) European disability strategy 2010–2020: a renewed commitment to a barrier-free Europe. http://eurlex.europa.eu/LexUriServ/LexUriServ.do?uri = COM:2010:0636:FIN:en:PDF

EUROSTAT (2018) Quality of life indicators – productive or main activity. Statistical office of the European Union (EUROSTAT): Luxembourg. http://ec.europa.eu/eurostat/statistics-explained/index.php/Quality_of_life_indicators

Fabian E (2013) Work and disability. In: Blustein DL (ed) Oxford library of psychology. The Oxford handbook of the psychology of working. Oxford University Press, New York, pp 185–200

ILO (2012) Issue brief: a cooperative future for people with disabilities. https://www.ilo.org/skills/pubs/WCMS_194822/lang%2D%2Den/index.htm

ILO, International Labour Office (2013) Inclusion of people with disabilities in vocational training: a practical guide. https://www.ilo.org/wcmsp5/groups/public/%2D%2D-dgreports/%2D%2D-gender/documents/publication/wcms_230732.pdf

Kavka G (2000) Disability and the right to work. In: Frances LP, Silvers A (eds) Americans with disabilities: exploring the implications for individuals and institutions. Routledge, New York, pp 174–192

Marmot M, Bell R (2010) Challenging health inequalities – implications for the workplace. Occup Med 60(3):162–164

May-Simera C (2018) Reconsidering sheltered workshops in light of the United Nations Convention on the Rights of Persons with Disabilities (2006). Laws 7(1):6–23

Moos RH (1986) Work as a human context. In: Pallak MS, Perloff R (eds) Psychology and work. American Psychological Association, Washington, DC, pp 9–52

National Disability Authority (n.d.) Employment of people with disabilities. http://nda.ie/Publications/Employment/Employment-of-people-with-disabilities-in-the-public-service

Neff WS (1985) Work and human behavior. Aldine, New York

OECD (2010) Sickness, disability and work: breaking the barriers. OECD Publishing, Paris. http://www.oecd.org/publications/sickness-disability-and-work-breaking-the-barriers-9789264088856-en.htm

OECD (2015) Fit mind, fit job: from evidence to practice in mental health and work. OECD Publishing, Paris. http://www.oecd.org/els/fit-mind-fit-job-9789264228283-en.htm

OHCHR (2012) Annual report: thematic study on the work and employment of persons with disabilities. UN Doc A/HRC/22/25 (17 December 2012). https://www.ohchr.org/EN/Issues/Disability/Pages/StudyonWorkandEmploymentofPersonswithDisabilities.aspx

Rothman RA (1998) Working: sociological perspectives, 2nd edn. Prentice Hall, Upper Saddle River, NJ

Rudbeck M, Fonager K (2011) Agreement between medical expert assessments in social medicine. Scand J Public Health 39(7):766–772

Scotch RK (1989) Politics and policy in the history of the disability rights movement. Milbank Q 67, Suppl 2 (Part 2):380–400
Siegrist J, Marmot M (2006) Social inequalities in health: new evidence and policy implications. Oxford University Press, Oxford
Stein MA et al (2014) Accommodating every body. Chic Law Rev 81:689–756
Stiglitz JE, Sen A, Fitoussi J-P (2009) Report by the Commission on the Measurement of Economic Performance and Social Progress. http://www.stiglitz-sen-fitoussi.fr/documents/rapport_anglais.pdf
Stobo JD, McGeary M, Barnes DK (eds) (2007) Improving the social security disability decision process. National Academic of Sciences, Washington, DC
Szymanski EM, Parker RM (2010) Work and disability: basic concepts. In: Szymanski EM, Parker RM (eds) Work and disability – contexts, issues, and strategies for enhancing employment outcomes for people with disabilities, 3rd edn. PRO-ED, Austin, pp 1–15
United Nations (1948) Universal Declaration of Human Rights. http://www.un.org/en/universal-declaration-human-rights/
United Nations (1976) International Covenant on Economic, Social and Cultural Rights. http://www.ohchr.org/EN/ProfessionalInterest/Pages/CESCR.aspx
United Nations (2007) Convention on the Rights of Persons with Disabilities, G.A. Res. 61/106. http://www.un.org/esa/socdev/enable/rights/convtexte.htm
United Nations (n.d.) Sustainable Development Goals. https://www.un.org/sustainabledevelopment/sustainable-development-goals/
United States (2017) Bureau of Labor statistics. News Release June 21, 2017: Persons with a Disability: Labor Force Characteristics – 2016. https://www.bls.gov/news.release/archives/disabl_06212017.pdf
Waddington L (2016) Positive Action Measures and the UN Convention on the Rights of Persons with Disabilities. Int Labour Rights Case Law 2:396–401
Waddington L, Hendricks A (2002) The expanding concept of employment discrimination in Europe: from direct and indirect discrimination to reasonable accommodation discrimination. Int J Comp Labour Law Ind Relat 18:403–427

Regulatory Contexts Affecting Work Reintegration of People with Chronic Disease and Disabilities

19

An International Perspective

Katherine Lippel

Contents

Introduction	348
Relevance of Legal Rules for the Science of Work Disability Prevention	349
Concepts and Beliefs That Are Commonly Used in the Science of Work Disability Prevention	350
Rules Affect Expectations, Behaviors, and Practices of Participants in the Return to Work Process	351
Rules of Relevance for Work Disability Prevention	353
Rules Governing Social Security, Compensation, and Sickness Insurance Systems	354
Rules Governing Employer-Employee Relations	356
Rules Governing Human Rights and Protections Against Discrimination	357
Conclusion	359
Cross-References	360
References	360

Abstract

This international overview of regulatory issues that determine the context in which work reintegration takes place provides tools for researchers and practitioners. We first address the relevance of legal rules for the science of work disability prevention, underlining the importance of local regulatory protections and processes when developing measures that aim to predict return to work and examining the ways in which these rules affect behaviors of participants in work reintegration processes. We then look at categories of legal rules that have an impact on employers, healthcare providers, insurers, and workers with chronic disease and disabilities who try to return to their pre-injury employment or to reenter the labor market. These include rules on workers' compensation and

---

K. Lippel (✉)
Faculty of Law (Civil Law Section), Canada Research Chair in Occupational Health and Safety Law, University of Ottawa, Ottawa, ON, Canada
e-mail: klippel@uottawa.ca

© Springer Nature Switzerland AG 2020
U. Bültmann, J. Siegrist (eds.), *Handbook of Disability, Work and Health*, Handbook Series in Occupational Health Sciences, https://doi.org/10.1007/978-3-030-24334-0_18

sickness insurance, employer-employee-union relations, and human rights protections against discrimination on the basis of disability. We conclude that in most systems, the economic value of the disabled worker is key to the return to work incentives placed on employers, yet systems that provide rehabilitation supports based on eventual costs to employers will not be successful in promoting re-employment of low-waged workers. This leads us to question the ethics of current regulatory models that may systemically exclude those in greatest need of support.

Keywords

Sickness insurance · Workers' compensation · Regulation · Employers · Healthcare providers · Work reintegration · Chronic illness · Disability prevention · Job security

Introduction

Disease and disability are universal, but the experience of individuals in engaging with the labor market when they are affected by chronic disease or disability will vary depending on the context and in particular the regulatory context applicable in the society in which they live. Every country, and in some countries every province, every state, and sometimes even every municipality, may have different regulations governing social insurance, employment relations, job security, discrimination, return to work policies, and access to healthcare. Specialists in work disability prevention are rarely lawyers, and most, as is the case with healthcare providers, employers and workers who are involved in the return to work process are at best vaguely aware of the legal rules affecting the relations between all the participants in that process. Yet the legal rules of the jurisdiction in which a study takes place will determine the behavior of the different participants, even though they are often unaware of the parameters at play.

A recent scoping review noted there is an increase of peer-reviewed studies "that address government laws, policies and programs designed to foster labour market integration of people who, due to illness or disability, face challenges entering or staying in the workforce" (MacEachen et al. 2017), and they noted a particular emphasis, in recent years, on work disability programs and policies related to mental health problems. While such studies are interesting for the purpose of tracking the evolution of regulatory discourse on work disability policies and the prevalence of methods used, they say nothing about the actual categories of legal rules that need to be understood: studies of rules that are not explicitly about disability will not emerge using scoping review methodology. For example, job security, supported by legal rules providing job protection, is a key driver of behavior of workers and employers; an employer who has free reign to terminate a worker with a disability will behave differently than an employer who can be fined or sued for terminating an employee. A worker who has job security may be more inclined to disclose needs associated with her or his disability, particularly if the nature of the disability is stigmatized, as is the case with many chronic diseases such as fibromyalgia (Oldfield et al. 2016), mental health problems (Moll et al. 2013), and other invisible disabilities (Prince 2017). Literature addressing rules governing termination of employees will not be identified in a scoping review focusing on disability policy, yet those rules play an important role in every facet of the relationship between an employer and an employee with a chronic health problem.

Needs of an aging workforce and of those suffering from chronic disease or disability include the ability to improve working conditions so that they are adjusted to the residual abilities of the worker. One study found that such adjustments are more likely to be made by the self-employed and are less accessible to employees (Fleischmann et al. 2018), which suggests that those workers with greater control over their own working conditions, and their working time, are more likely to successfully continue in the workforce after a diagnosis of chronic disease. Another study underlined the importance of adapting to the needs of those suffering from specific chronic illnesses, pointing out that incentives designed to promote return to work of those suffering from physical problems required different strategies than for those suffering from mental health problems (Vossen et al. 2017).

This chapter relies on an analysis using classic legal methodology, applied to regulatory frameworks in a variety of jurisdictions, the results of which are then linked to the literature on work disability prevention. It seeks to identify the areas of law/policy that can have an impact on work disability prevention in a given jurisdiction. It aims, firstly, to identify some of the reasons why scientists and practitioners should be conscious of the legal rules applicable in the jurisdiction of relevance to their study or their practice, in light of certain premises often assumed in the field of work disability prevention. It then turns to the categories of legal rules that can be of relevance for scientists and practitioners, as often as possible drawing on examples related to the situation of workers with chronic disease, to tease out the importance of differentiating the policy implications depending on the type of health problem affecting the worker involved in a return to work process. Regulatory provisions related to the initial integration of people with chronic illness into the labor market are beyond the scope of this chapter, which has as its focus workers who have been active in the labor market, whether or not that activity occurred prior to onset of the chronic health problem.

Relevance of Legal Rules for the Science of Work Disability Prevention

Rehabilitation science relies on scales and measures designed to identify workers at risk for work disability. It also focuses on the roles of key participants in the return to work process. Here we explain why an understanding of regulatory issues is useful in the design of measures and in the interpretation of results in studies applying those measures. We then turn to the examination of ways in which legal rules affect the behavior of different participants in the return to work process.

Concepts and Beliefs That Are Commonly Used in the Science of Work Disability Prevention

A broad range of scales and measures have been developed for the purpose of predicting return to work outcomes and identifying variables that increase duration of absence from work. Legal scholars interested in work disability prevention are drawn to discussions on several threads of research in the field because there are often conclusions drawn in studies and practices that would be more accurate if the authors had a better understanding of the relevant legal environment. These rules may be determinants of the results in a given study, yet authors may either ignore or oversimplify the importance of the context in which the study takes place. Such threads include studies examining compensation status as a variable in length of disability and research linking results drawn from the application of scales measuring variables understood to be associated with length of disability, such as perceived injustice, pain catastrophizing, and fear avoidance.

Fiona Clay and colleagues have documented the lack of attention paid to rules governing compensation systems in the disability prevention literature (Clay et al. 2014). Yet a body of epidemiological literature suggests that disability duration is prolonged when compensation is at stake or when access to compensation is contentious and a lawyer is involved (Harris et al. 2008). This literature has been criticized as being oversimplistic, not examining the actual nature of the compensation process or the factors associated with disability duration that could be affected by the reasons for disputes (Grant and Studdert 2009; Carroll et al. 2011; Lippel 2008; Swartzman et al. 1996).

In a systematic review of this literature, Spearing and colleagues concluded that although some studies have found associations between the compensation process and ill health, the direction of those associations had not been examined by the studies analyzed, and they concluded that "there is no clear evidence to support the idea that compensation and its related processes lead to worse health" (Spearing et al. 2012). A more recent "best evidence synthesis" found that while there was "limited evidence to suggest that receiving worker's compensation/disability benefit in itself is an obstacle to work participation...there is robust evidence to suggest that specific, unhelpful characteristics of compensatory systems are obstacles to work participation" (Bartys et al. 2017, p. 905).

Nonetheless there are many earlier studies and articles that oversimplify the issue and promote the discourse that compensation or involvement with a lawyer is a variable determining disability duration, sometimes equating disability duration by date of closure of the compensation claim, as was the case in a number of studies, including a classic study by Cassidy and colleagues, (Cassidy et al. 2000), that concluded that the elimination of the right to damages for pain and suffering would improve recovery times for patients suffering from whiplash. Although this study had a variety of measures, it is of note that if the legal environment eliminates the right to compensation associated with ongoing pain, thus shortening the period in which claims will be paid, it is problematic to measure the end of disability by the date of claim closure. Another study that failed to enquire as to the specificities of the compensation process, and that did not enquire as to possible disputes or conflicts associated with that process, concluded that "as with perceived disability, it is possible that patients with long-term compensation involvement have had their pain symptoms so strongly reinforced by the benefits of that compensation involvement that they are reluctant to report improvement regardless of the treatment used" (Rainville et al. 1997). Many of these studies that include the "lawyer" variable or the "compensation" variable fail to enquire as to the reasons why a lawyer's involvement was necessary, even though it is likely that claimants requiring a lawyer were those who had difficulty in the processing of their claim. Furthermore, it is highly likely that those with lawyer involvement were more likely to have their benefits reinstated retroactively if an appeal was successful, which would statistically prolong disability duration in studies measuring disability by duration of benefits.

Because these studies often address readers of the medical literature, they may affect the way in which physicians and other health professionals see injured workers. This in turn can contribute to prolonging disability if the doctor-patient relationship is permeated by distrust or if access to timely healthcare is compromised because doctors refuse to treat injured workers or victims of motor vehicle crashes involved in compensation claims (Brijnath et al. 2016; Lippel et al. 2016; MacEachen et al. 2010; Kilgour et al. 2015).

Scientists have developed scales, such as the "perceived injustice scale," to measure the extent to which a patient's perception of injustice is associated with disability outcomes (Sullivan et al. 2012). Perceived (in)justice of the compensation process is a determinant of successful return to work (Franche et al. 2009; Franche et al. 2005b; Giummarra et al. 2017), and some suggest that addressing the patient's beliefs regarding the injustice may reduce disability (Sullivan et al. 2012). Other scales use patients' belief that he or she will return to work as a measure to prioritize interventions, and while some include issues related to the work environment and the compensation system (Wilford et al. 2008; Beales et al. 2016), this is not the case in all studies. These scales and approaches may be useful in prioritizing interventions for work disability prevention, but they do not appear to consider the realism of the subject's perceptions. Legal scholars would suggest that realistic threats of dismissal in a workplace situated in a jurisdiction with no regulatory protections of job security will contribute to the worker's response to a question inquiring as to the likelihood of return to work.

Rules Affect Expectations, Behaviors, and Practices of Participants in the Return to Work Process

Patrick Loisel and colleagues developed the Sherbrooke model of work disability prevention and showed that the roles of insurers (including compensation and social insurance authorities), healthcare providers, employers, and workers were all key in determining successful return to work outcomes (Loisel et al. 2005). The experiences and behaviors of all these participants in the return to work process are determined in large part by the regulatory context guiding their relationships with each other, yet they are often unaware of the way regulation shapes their experiences (Hoefsmit et al. 2013).

For example, the opinions of the worker's treating physician on diagnosis, treatment plans, date of maximum medical recovery, functional limitations, and permanent impairment are all binding on the compensation authority in the Canadian province of Québec, although a formal dispute mechanism allows for the employer and the compensation authority to question those opinions; this is not the case in the neighboring province of Ontario. In a recent comparative study of doctors involved in workers' compensation cases in these two Canadian provinces, neither physicians nor compensation authorities were aware of this disparity between systems, yet the experience of doctors in Ontario, who complained of feeling ignored by the authorities, was very different from those of Québec doctors, who felt they were continuously being disputed by employers and the compensation authority (Lippel et al. 2016).

A study looking at system effects on the practice of physiotherapists in these same two provinces showed that Ontario WCB policy provides bonus remuneration for a physiotherapist whose patient returns to work before a set deadline, a practice said to provide an economic incentive to pressure patients into returning to work, perhaps prematurely. However, other study participants suggested that the absence of a set deadline for end of treatment by a physiotherapist in Québec prolonged treatment unnecessarily (Hudon et al. 2018). Thus, in both these examples, policy environments can be seen to affect behavior of healthcare providers.

Similarly, experience rating rules, rules providing economic incentives for employers to reduce the costs of compensation benefits, are supposedly meant to encourage employers to prevent work disability by accommodating workers with disabilities before they have attained maximum medical recovery. These workers may be less productive than they were prior to their injury, but the economic incentive in the compensation system may offset the reduction in productivity. However, these rules may also lead employers to dispute compensation claims in order to reduce the impact of cost incentives (Duncan 2019; Boden and Galizzi 2017), and disputing a claim, which also entails multiple medical assessments, may in itself increase workers' anxiety and decrease the chances of their reintegration into pre-injury employment (Grant et al. 2014; Lippel 2007), particularly if they distrust the employer because of the claims management/dispute process (Franche et al. 2005a). In New Zealand, where the compensation system covers all injury attributable to accidents, but experience rates only injuries attributable to work, employers have been shown to behave differently in their support of return to work, depending on whether or not the injury was found to be caused by work (Duncan 2019). Duncan (p. 97) suggests that in some cases, employers are "more motivated to reintegrate workers injured in their own workplaces," but he points out they may also encourage workers to declare that injuries were incurred outside of the workplace. Workers receive the same level of benefits in any case, and the employer has less incentive to bring the worker back to work early, an outcome that might also be perceived favorably by the worker. Experience rating rules (Harcourt et al. 2007) and extensive employer responsibility for sickness absence (de Rijk 2019; Mittag et al. 2018) have also been found to provide economic incentives to employers to screen out disabled workers looking for new employment.

System characteristics will necessarily color workers' experiences and their willingness to return to work before maximum medical recovery. Among the "unhelpful" characteristics of compensation systems identified by Bartys and colleagues was the rigidity of some systems. Citing evidence from a cross-country study comparing six countries (Anema et al. 2009), they found that "eligibility criteria should be less strict for long-term and/or partial disability benefits" (Bartys et al. 2017, p. 905). Workers need to be able to attempt return to work without adverse consequences, and this is particularly true for workers with chronic or episodic illnesses (Gewurtz et al. 2015).

Trust is a key factor in successful work reintegration (Ståhl 2010), yet studies have found that workers and employers distrust each other when the insurance system requires them to cooperate in return to work processes (Hoefsmit et al. 2013), a finding that is particularly problematic in small workplaces (Eakin and MacEachen 2003). Thus compensation systems may inadvertently undermine the trust between workers and employers by providing clumsy incentive tools based on punishment for non-compliance of the employer, the worker, or both, when support systems that are more sensitive to specific needs of the worker and the workplace could be more successful.

In the United States, where economists have a strong influence on the design of workers' compensation systems, each state's rules differ. Some state legislation limits the number of weeks a worker can receive benefits and actually prohibits employers from providing additional benefits to workers (Spieler 2017, p. 943). While some subscribe to the philosophy that low benefits provide an economic incentive for workers to return to work, others question the desirability of return to work when workers are "starved back to work" because of the low level of benefits available to them. As Boden and Galizzi note, "even to economists, higher benefits can be a good thing when they prevent people from being starved back to work. This is doubly true in workers' compensation: if workers face pressure to return to work before full recovery, they may jeopardize their immediate recovery, but also their longer-term productivity and performance" (Boden and Galizzi 2017). Statistics may confirm that a person with little or no economic support returns to work more quickly, but this is not necessarily a therapeutic outcome for the individual, nor is it an outcome that insures long-term productivity and sustainable return to work.

Rules of Relevance for Work Disability Prevention

Here we examine three categories of regulatory measures that can contribute to positive or negative experiences of workers with chronic illness in the return to work process. We first examine specificities of social security systems, including compensation and sickness insurance systems that can help or hinder effective recovery and return to work. We then turn to rules governing job security, trade unions, and the employment relationship, including protections from bullying and harassment. Finally, we examine issues related to human rights legislation.

Rules Governing Social Security, Compensation, and Sickness Insurance Systems

Elsewhere (Lippel and Lötters 2013) we have explored the important distinctions between public insurance systems that are cause-based, such as workers' compensation and motor vehicle insurance systems, and those based on disability regardless of the cause, such as the disability insurance system in the Netherlands (de Rijk 2019) and sickness insurance systems available in many European countries (Ståhl and Seing 2019; Martimo 2019). Within the cause-based systems, employers are involved when work is the cause of the disability, but they are not required to be involved in return to work processes when the disability is not caused by work, even if a compensation authority is responsible for providing economic support and rehabilitation for the worker who is injured (Lippel 2019). In those cases, only job security rules and human rights legislation will determine whether employers have incentives to reintegrate those suffering from chronic illness or disease.

Within the category of workers' compensation systems, studies have also identified key parameters for protection of claimants' dignity, which in turn protects claimants' mental health by diminishing stigma associated with claiming workers' compensation (Lippel 2012). Others have examined the rehabilitation effects of New Zealand's accident insurance system that does not distinguish between work-related and non-work-related injury when it comes to rehabilitation support provided by the compensation authority (Armstrong and Laurs 2007; Duncan 2019). In the United States, studies by legal scholars and economists have documented the deterioration of protections in workers' compensation since the initial "grand bargain" where workers relinquished the right to sue their employer for damages in exchange for workers' compensation "no-fault" coverage (Spieler 2017). The economic incentives placed on different participants in the system within the design of that legal framework have been found to be ineffective in promoting prevention of injury and reduction of long-term disability. This is particularly true in relation to the protections of workers against retaliation by employers who sanction them for claiming compensation, as the remedies available to workers are ineffective and costly (Morantz et al. 2017; Spieler 2017).

An Australian study examining suicide following work-related musculoskeletal disorders identified "three critical events: unsuccessful return to work; the development of chronic pain or disability and suicidal ideation in the context of chronic pain." Systemic factors related to the compensation and healthcare systems had a moderating influence (Davis et al. 2013). As we have seen, healthcare practitioners may treat patients differently, or even refuse to treat them, if they are claiming compensation of some kind for their injuries (Brijnath et al. 2016; Lippel et al. 2016; MacEachen et al. 2010; Kilgour et al. 2015).

In summary, a first series of issues related to compensation systems speaks to the process itself: Do system characteristics ensure that claimants are treated with dignity? Do they have access to the support of healthcare providers who want to be treating them and supporting them in their efforts to return to work? Are employers under economic pressure to reduce claims numbers by disputing claims or to return an injured worker to the workplace even though neither the employer nor the worker feel the arrangement to be appropriate to the worker's condition?

Beyond these issues, there are also technical characteristics of a disability insurance system that can increase the chances of workers returning to employment; one is accessibility of partial sick leave; the other relates to the determination of salary insurance benefits. Some European countries such as Finland have successfully experimented with a part-time sick leave whereby "employee's work hours can be reduced to 40% to 60% of the average number of hours on a daily or weekly basis" and the worker receives a part-time sickness allowance based on 50% of the full-time benefit for not more than 120 days. The authors concluded that "partial sick leave reduces the risk of a worker going on a full disability pension. Even if the risk for partial disability pension is increased the result is increased work participation" (Martimo 2019, p. 143). Partial earning incapacity benefits in one form or another are available in Belgium (Mairiaux 2019), the Netherlands (de Rijk 2019), Germany (Welti 2019), and Sweden (Ståhl and Seing 2019). However, a Swedish study also shows that employers were reticent to take workers back on a part-time basis, as the economic viability of their business was their primary priority and the legal obligations placed on them were apparently successfully resisted (Seing et al. 2015). Part-time sick leave is particularly important for workers suffering from chronic, episodic conditions, as the system allows them to work as much as they are able, rather than taking an all-or-nothing approach, as is common in many systems.

North American workers' compensation systems frequently determine the degree to which the insurer will invest in rehabilitation and return to work support by measuring the cost of doing nothing and paying out benefits to the worker for a long (er) period of time, comparing that cost to the cost of providing retraining or other vocational rehabilitation support. Low-wage earners and the precariously employed are particularly disadvantaged by this system, as in most jurisdictions the cost of their benefits will be based on their earnings at the time of their injury, even though their earning ability might well be far superior to their current earnings. An example drawn from a comparison of two Canadian provinces illustrates how legal rules can make an important difference in the determination of a rehabilitation program. In Québec, there is a minimum floor to compensation benefits that must be based on at least 40 hours a week at minimum hourly wage; in Ontario no such floor exists. The rehabilitation program for a precariously employed worker will be designed to permit the worker to earn full-time minimum wage in Québec; in Ontario the target will be pre-injury earnings even if they are based on employment for a few hours a week at minimum hourly wage (Lippel 2019).

When workers are no longer eligible for benefits under a dedicated compensation scheme, they may be eligible for social security supports. A major difference between the European systems and those available in North America, Australia, and New Zealand is that in the latter countries, the social security benefits available for those who are unable to work because of illness or disability are often means tested in a way that takes into consideration family income. Benefits are said to be "of last resort" and are both very low and require evidence of, in some cases, extreme poverty. While benefits for sickness absence may be slightly lower in European countries with parallel systems for work-related injury and sickness absence insurance, in North America, the contrast between coverage under a "no-fault" system and coverage under the universally accessible social security system is stark.

In the United States, even access to healthcare may not be taken for granted if a workers' compensation claim is denied or access to benefits is delayed (Spieler 2017). In Canada, while healthcare coverage is far more accessible than in the United States, universal coverage does not include timely access to physiotherapists, occupational therapists, psychologists, or even to medication prescribed by a doctor outside of a hospital setting. Furthermore, with only 15 weeks of low-level sickness benefits provided to those who have contributed to the Employment Insurance scheme, workers whose claims are denied are obliged to enter the means tested "welfare" schemes (Lippel 2019). Those whose spouses or children are working or those who own their houses or have retirement savings may well be ineligible. It is relatively common, for example, in the province of Québec, to find workers' compensation claimants who have dilapidated their savings or even separated from their families during the lengthy appeals process if their claim is denied (Lippel 2007, 2012). When their appeal is ultimately successful, the worker receives retroactive benefits some of which will be used to reimburse the social security system. They may have lost their house or their car in the process. They then must commence supported rehabilitation and return to work processes, often years after the initial incident that led to their disability, sometimes targeting re-employment by the employer who contested their claim. Retroactive payment will raise the overall cost of their claim, so that those scientists measuring disability by claims costs will indeed find that compensation is associated with longer disability periods or that lawyers are associated with more costly claims, but the reasons for these increased costs may well be the psychosocial consequences of having to contest claim denials or to answer arguments of employers who have disputed claims. Those psychosocial consequences can include family disintegration, development of mental health problems in workers whose initial injury was physical in nature, and mental health problems that can be linked to the consequences of loss of benefits, including the experience of having to resort to a very minimalist and often stigmatizing social security system.

Rules Governing Employer-Employee Relations

Disclosure is a key element in ensuring that reasonable accommodations are made in the workplace, so that the workplace and work organization, including scheduling, can be adapted to the needs of the individual with a disability (Oldfield et al. 2016).

Incentives to disclose or to not disclose a disability will depend on the individual's perception of his or her job security, which will be determined in large part by the regulatory and organizational context. Does the law guarantee job protection for disabled workers in her jurisdiction, as is the case in many European countries, including the Netherlands, where the employer cannot fire an employee because of illness without obtaining permission from administrative bodies or the courts (Lippel and Lötters 2013)? Are protections available under labor standards legislation, as in Québec, Canada, or may the employer fire the employee at will, as is the case in many American states (Morantz et al. 2017)? Does the answer depend on whether the worker is unionized with protections in a collective agreement or are all workers protected from dismissal? Are the workers in precarious employment working through a temporary employment agency or a sub-contractor or are they hired under indeterminate contracts? All these factors will affect the practices of employers and workers and in some cases healthcare providers.

Denmark adopted the flexicurity model (Madsen 2013) which provides low job protection but greater protection from the social insurance system in the event of unemployment or disability, and research has suggested that this model actually improves employment participation of workers with chronic disease (Pedersen et al. 2012). Despite the ability of Danish employers to terminate disabled workers, one study comparing experiences in Denmark and the Netherlands found that several Danish employers did not terminate their disabled employees even if they could, and the authors suggest that mandatory rules for maintaining the employment relationship may lead to early return to work for the Dutch employees but also increase distrust that may impair the employment relationship and the sustainability of return to work (Vossen et al. 2017). Beyond the legislative protections against unjust dismissal, presence of a trade union whose role is to protect workers' job security may affect the behavior of all participants in a return to work process. A collective agreement that promotes reintegration of workers with disabilities will strengthen the worker's ability to negotiate adequate conditions and will protect them from dismissal in the case of episodic disability (Aversa and Carlan 2014); it is also possible that the rigidity of provisions in the collective agreement could limit options of managers in offering alternative employment within the organization (Kristman et al. 2014).

Several countries have protection against bullying and harassment in the workplace, while others do not. Studies in the United Kingdom have found that workers with disabilities are disproportionately targeted by bullies (Fevre et al. 2013) and strategic bullying, used to encourage less productive workers to leave the workplace, may be left unchecked if no regulation specifically addresses workplace bullying.

Rules Governing Human Rights and Protections Against Discrimination

In most countries of the Organisation for Economic Co-operation and Development (OECD), discrimination on the basis of disability is illegal, and employers are usually required to demonstrate that the continued employment of a disabled worker would impose undue hardship on the organization. While these protections look sound on paper, most countries rely on a complaints-based system that requires the worker to proactively take action against the employer, which aside from being both costly and time-consuming undermines the relationship with the employer (Allen 2010). Recent regulatory approaches in the Canadian province of Ontario have encouraged design of work organization in a way that reduces the need for individuals with disabilities to file complaints or to request accommodation of their individual needs by requiring design of work spaces and working conditions that are easily adaptable to the needs of all workers, including those with disabilities (Ontario 2011). For example, s. 30 includes specifications required of employers engaged in performance management. It reads as follows:

> **30.** (1) An employer that uses performance management in respect of its employees shall take into account the accessibility needs of employees with disabilities, as well as individual accommodation plans, when using its performance management process in respect of employees with disabilities. O. Reg. 191/11, s. 30 (1).
>
> (2) In this section,
> "performance management" means activities related to assessing and improving employee performance, productivity and effectiveness, with the goal of facilitating employee success. O. Reg. 191/11, s. 30 (2).

This type of legislation encourages organizations to develop policies that are designed to accommodate workers with a broad range of needs related to acute or chronic disability. A study on organizations in that province found that workers suffering from chronic illness whose accommodation needs were exceeded by existing workplace accommodation practices reported better job outcomes than those whose accommodation needs had been unmet or merely met without being exceeded. The authors conclude that work context rather than health conditions was the source of unmet accommodation needs and that better accommodation policies and practices were key to maintaining older workers and those with chronic conditions in the workforce (Gignac et al. 2018).

Some countries, such as Sweden (Swedish Work Environment Authority 2015), not only provide for protection against discrimination and victimization but also require that employers regularly conduct occupational health and safety risk assessments that include evaluation of psychosocial hazards in all but the very smallest workplaces in order to promote a healthy work environment that is accessible to all workers, not just the least vulnerable. Such approaches could go far in improving working conditions for all workers, which would facilitate return to work for those with chronic illnesses.

In this section we have seen different regulatory categories that may determine whether and to whom employers will offer support in the work reintegration process. These regimes may include positive and negative incentives to encourage employers to actively manage return to work in a timely manner. However, when an injury is compensable in one of the cause-based systems, issues may arise to undermine the relationship between the employer and the worker, including costly surcharges imposed on employers through experience rating and associated disputes of claims;

constraints placed on both employers and workers to force workers back to work very rapidly despite their shared desire to allow the worker more time to heal, and to become more useful to the workplace; and system proceedings that promote distrust. These systems may also affect the behavior of other participants in the return to work process, including that of healthcare practitioners and claims adjudicators working for the insurers. We then turn to other types of regulation that are not related to the compensation process, including labor legislation affecting job security and the role of unions, as well as legislation promoting healthy workplaces that are free from bullying and harassment. Finally, we consider human rights legislation designed to protect workers with disabilities, as well as more modern provisions that promote workplaces that are accommodating for all workers, eliminating the need for disclosure of disabilities by providing accommodations to all workers.

Other regulatory frameworks that are important to our understanding of work disability prevention include those governing occupational health and safety and access to healthcare and health services within and outside the workplace. While these categories of legislation are important, comparative analysis of approaches around the world goes beyond the scope of this chapter. This said, a fundamental question to be asked in relation to these frameworks is that relating to the types of health problems that fall within the scope of these provisions. More specifically, it is important to be aware of the scope of occupational health and safety legislation: Does it aim to protect workers' mental health in the jurisdiction studied or only their physical health? Similarly, do healthcare services provided to a population include coverage of mental health problems? If they do not, the dynamics of return to work interactions will be adversely affected.

Conclusion

For scientists and knowledge users, we have described in the first part of this chapter the ways in which the regulatory context in which research or interventions take place determines a broad range of factors that must be considered in the design and interpretation of studies. Geography matters, because rules differ depending on the geographical location of a study. Time also matters; legal rules or compensation system characteristics applicable during a study conducted in 2000 may no longer exist in 2019, so that it is key, for appropriate design and understanding, to continually track the temporal and geographic context and the regulatory environment associated with a study on return to work.

In the second part of this chapter, we have examined three categories of regulatory environments that are key to understanding the behavior of participants in the return to work process: rules associated with social security, compensation, and sickness insurance systems, various measures to protect job security, and the protection of workers from discrimination on the basis of disability.

In examining the sickness insurance system, it is clear that many countries have integrated economic incentives placed on employers to encourage retention of workers who are sick-listed or injured at work. Yet the mechanisms at play in those systems are predicated on the cost of doing nothing, and one may conclude that workers who cost little, such as those in precarious employment, will not be as effectively returned to the workplace or the labor market as those who will prove to be costly to the system or the employer if sustainable return to work is not achieved. In many regulatory/policy systems, the economic value of the disabled worker is key to the successful implementation of return to work incentives for employers. Systems that provide rehabilitation supports based on eventual costs to employers, such as experience rating systems, will not be successful in promoting re-employment of low-waged workers. This is ironic given that employers are less likely to require an incentive to reinstate a valued employee (Seing et al. 2015). The challenge for the future lies in insuring that low-waged and precarious workers with disabilities have equal access to support in their quest to return to sustainable work despite chronic illness or disability. If they are not better protected, current regulatory models may systemically exclude those in greatest need of support.

Cross-References

▶ Policies of Reducing the Burden of Occupational Hazards and Disability Pensions

References

Allen D (2010) Strategic enforcement of antidiscrimination law: a new role for Australia's equality commissions. Monash Univ Law Rev 36(3):103–137

Anema J, Schellart A, Cassidy J, Loisel P, Veerman T, Van der Beek A (2009) Can cross country differences in return-to-work after chronic occupational back pain be explained? An exploratory analysis on disability policies in a six country cohort study. J Occup Rehabil 19(4):419–426

Armstrong H, Laurs R (2007) Vocational Independence: outcomes for ACC claimants: a follow up study of 160 claimants who have been deemed vocationally independent by ACC and case law analysis of the vocational independence process. Department of Labour, Wellington, New Zealand

Aversa T, Carlan N (2014) Navigating chronic injuries in the workplace: five workers' experiences with systems and relationships. In: Stone SD, Owen MK, Crooks VA (eds) Working bodies: chronic illness in the Canadian workplace. McGill-Queens University Press, Montreal, pp 71–88

Bartys S, Fredericksen P, Bendix T, Burton K (2017) System influences on work disability due to low back pain: an international evidence synthesis. Health Policy (Amsterdam Neth) 121:903–912. https://doi.org/10.1016/j.healthpol.2017.05.011

Beales D, Fried K, Nicholas M, Blyth F, Finniss D, Moseley GL (2016) Management of musculoskeletal pain in a compensable environment: implementation of helpful and unhelpful models of care in supporting recovery and return to work. Best Pract Res Clin Rheumatol 30(3):445–467

Boden LI, Galizzi M (2017) Blinded by moral hazard. Rutgers Univ Law Rev 69:1213–1231

Brijnath B, Mazza D, Kosny A, Bunzli S, Singh N, Ruseckaite R, Collie A (2016) Is clinician refusal to treat an emerging problem in injury compensation systems? BMJ Open 6(1):1–7. https://doi.org/10.1136/bmjopen-2015-009423

Carroll LJ, Connelly LB, Spearing NM, Côté P, Buitenhuis J, Kenardy J (2011) Complexities in understanding the role of compensation-related factors on recovery from whiplash-associated disorders. Spine 36(25S):S316–S321. https://doi.org/10.1097/BRS.0b013e3182388739

Cassidy JD, Carroll LJ, Cote P, Lemstra M, Berglund A, Nygren A (2000) Effect of eliminating compensation for pain and suffering on the outcome of insurance claims for whiplash injury. N Engl J Med 342(16):1179–1186. https://doi.org/10.1056/nejm200004203421606

Clay FJ, Berecki-Gisolf J, Collie A (2014) How well do we report on compensation systems in studies of return to work: a systematic review. J Occup Rehabil 24(1):111–124. https://doi.org/10.1007/s10926-013-9435-z

Davis M-C, Ibrahim JE, Ranson D, Ozanne-Smith J, Routley V (2013) Suicide following work-related injury in Victoria, Australia. J Law Med 21(1):13

de Rijk A (2019) Work disability in the Netherlands: a key role for employers. In: MacEachen E (ed) The science and politics of work disability prevention. Routledge/Taylor & Francis, New York/London, pp 223–241

Duncan G (2019) The New Zealand universal accident scheme. In: MacEachen E (ed) The science and politics of work disability prevention. Routledge/Taylor & Francis, New York/London, pp 88–101

Eakin JM, MacEachen E (2003) Playing it smart' with return to work: small workplace experience under Ontario's policy of self-reliance and early return. Policy Pract Health Saf 1(2):19–42

Fevre R, Robinson A, Lewis D, Jones T (2013) The ill-treatment of employees with disabilities in British workplaces. Work Employ Soc 27(2):288–307. https://doi.org/10.1177/0950017012460311

Fleischmann M, Carr E, Xue B, Zaninotto P, Stansfeld SA, Stafford M, Head J (2018) Changes in autonomy, job demands and working hours after diagnosis of chronic disease: a comparison of employed and self-employed older persons using the English longitudinal study of ageing (ELSA). J Epidemiol Community Health 72(10):951–957. https://doi.org/10.1136/jech-2017-210328

Franche R-L, Baril R, Shaw W, Nicholas M, Loisel P (2005a) Workplace-based return-to-work interventions: optimizing the role of stakeholders in implementation and research. J Occup Rehabil 15(4):525–542. https://doi.org/10.1007/s10926-005-8032-1

Franche R-L, Cullen K, Clarke J, Irvin E, Sinclair S, Frank J, The Institute for Work & Health (IWH) Workspace-Based RTW Intervention Literature Review Research Team (2005b) Workplace-based return-to-work interventions: a systematic review of the quantitative literature. J Occup Rehabil 15(4):607–631. https://doi.org/10.1007/s10926-005-8038-8

Franche R-L, Severin CN, Lee H, Hogg-Johnson S, Hepburn CG, Vidmar M, MacEachen E (2009) Perceived justice of compensation process for return-to-work: development and validation of a scale. Psychol Inj Law. https://doi.org/10.1007/s12207-009-9053-4

Gewurtz RE, Cott C, Rush B, Kirsh B (2015) How is unemployment among people with mental illness conceptualized within social policy? A case study of the Ontario disability support program. Work 51(1):121–133. https://doi.org/10.3233/WOR-141843

Gignac MAM, Kristman V, Smith PM, Beaton DE, Badley EM, Ibrahim S, Mustard CA (2018) Are there differences in workplace accommodation needs, use and unmet needs among older workers with arthritis, diabetes and no chronic conditions? Examining the role of health and work context. Work Aging Retire 4(4):381–398. https://doi.org/10.1093/workar/way004

Giummarra MJ, Cameron PA, Ponsford J, Ioannou L, Gibson SJ, Jennings PA, Georgiou-Karistianis N (2017) Return to work after traumatic injury: increased work-related disability in injured persons receiving financial compensation is mediated by perceived injustice. J Occup Rehabil 27:173–185

Grant G, Studdert D (2009) Poisoned chalice? A critical analysis of the evidence linking personal injury compensation processes with adverse health outcomes. Melb Univ Law Rev 33(3):1–25

Grant G, O'Donnell ML, Spittal MJ, Creamer M, Studdert D (2014) Relationship between stressfulness of claiming for injury compensation and long-term recovery: a prospective cohort study. JAMA Psychiat. https://doi.org/10.1001/jamapsychiatry.2013.4023

Harcourt M, Lam H, Harcourt S (2007) The impact of workers' compensation experience-rating on discriminatory hiring practices. J Econ Issues 41(3):681–699

Harris I, Young J, Jalaludin B, Solomon M (2008) The effect of compensation on general health in patients sustaining fractures in motor vehicle trauma. Publ Med 22(4):216–220

Hoefsmit N, De Rijk A, Houkes I (2013) Work resumption at the price of distrust: a qualitative study on return to work legislation in the Netherlands. BMC Public Health 13(1):1–14

Hudon A, Hunt M, Ehrmann Feldman D (2018) Physiotherapy for injured workers in Canada: are insurers' and clinics' policies threatening good quality and equity of care? Results of a qualitative study. BMC Health Serv Res 18(1):682. https://doi.org/10.1186/s12913-018-3491-1

Kilgour E, Kosny A, McKenzie D, Collie A (2015) Healing or harming? Healthcare provider interactions with injured workers and insurers in workers' compensation systems. J Occup Rehabil 25(1):220–239. https://doi.org/10.1007/s10926-014-9521-x

Kristman VL, Shaw W, Williams-Whitt K (2014) Supervisors' perspectives on work accommodation for chronically ill employees. In: Working bodies: chronic illness in the Canadian workplace. McGill-Queen's University Press, Montreal, pp 114–137

Lippel K (2007) Workers describe the effect of the workers' compensation process on their health: a Québec study. Int J Law Psychiatry 30(4–5):427–443

Lippel K (2008) La place des juristes dans la recherche sociale et la place de la recherche sociale en droit: réflexions sur la «pratique de la recherche» en matière de droit à la santé au travail. In: Noreau P, Rolland L (eds) Mélanges Andrée Lajoie. Éditions Thémis, Montréal, pp 251–284

Lippel K (2012) Preserving workers' dignity in workers' compensation systems: an international perspective. Am J Ind Med 55(6):519–536. https://doi.org/10.1002/ajim.22022

Lippel K (2019) Strengths and weaknesses of regulatory systems designed to prevent work disability after injury or illness: an overview of mechanisms in a selection of Canadian compensation systems. In: MacEachen E (ed) The science and politics of work disability prevention. Routledge/Taylor & Francis, New York/London, pp 50–71

Lippel K, Lötters F (2013) Public insurance systems: a comparison of cause-based and disability-based income support systems. In: Loisel P, Anema JR (eds) Handbook of work disability prevention and management. Springer, New York, pp 183–202

Lippel K, Eakin JM, Holness DL, Howse D (2016) The structure and process of workers' compensation systems and the role of doctors: a comparison of Ontario and Québec. Am J Ind Med 59(12):1070–1086. https://doi.org/10.1002/ajim.22651

Loisel P, Buchbinder R, Hazard R, Keller R, Scheel I, Tulder M, Webster B (2005) Prevention of work disability due to musculoskeletal disorders: the challenge of implementing evidence. J Occup Rehabil 15(4):507–524. https://doi.org/10.1007/s10926-005-8031-2

MacEachen E, Kosny A, Ferrier S, Chambers L (2010) The "toxic dose" of system problems: why some injured workers don't return to work as expected. J Occup Rehabil 20(3):349–366. https://doi.org/10.1007/s10926-010-9229-5

MacEachen E, Du B, Bartel E, Ekberg K, Tompa E, Kosny A, Petricone I, Stapleton J (2017) Scoping review of work disability policies and programs. Int J Disabil Manag 12(1):1–11. https://doi.org/10.1017/idm.2017.1

Madsen K (2013) Shelter from the storm?- Danish flexicurity and the crisis. J Eur Labor Stud 2(6):1–19

Mairiaux P (2019) Disability prevention policies in Belgium: navigating between scientific and socioeconomic influences. In: MacEachen E (ed) The science and politics of work disability prevention. Routledge/Taylor & Francis, New York/London, pp 205–222

Martimo K-P (2019) Work disability prevention in Finland: promoting work ability through occupational health collaboration. In: MacEachen E (ed) The science and politics of work disability prevention. Routledge/Taylor & Francis, New York/London, pp 141–158

Mittag O, Kotkas T, Reese C, Kampling H, Groskreutz H, de Boer W, Welti F (2018) Intervention policies and social security in case of reduced working capacity in the Netherlands, Finland and Germany: a comparative analysis. Int J Public Health. https://doi.org/10.1007/s00038-018-1133-3

Moll S, Eakin JM, Franche R-L, Strike C (2013) When health care workers experience mental ill health: institutional practices of silence. Qual Health Res 23(2):167–179

Morantz A, Levine SM, Palsson MV (2017) Economic incentives in workers' compensation: a holistic international perspective. Rutgers Univ Law Rev 69:1015–1080

Oldfield M, MacEachen E, Kirsh B, MacNeill M (2016) Impromptu everyday disclosure dances: how women with fibromyalgia respond to disclosure risks at work. Disabil Rehabil 38(15):1442–1453

Ontario (2011) Integrated Accessibility Standards, O Reg. 191/11, regulations adopted under Accessibility for Ontarians with Disabilities Act, 2005, S.O. 2005, c. 11

Pedersen J, Bjorner JB, Burr H, Christensen KB (2012) Transitions between sickness absence, work, unemployment, and disability in Denmark 2004–2008. Scand J Work Environ Health 38(6):516–526. https://doi.org/10.2307/23558287

Prince MJ (2017) Persons with invisible disabilities and workplace accommodation: findings from a scoping literature review. J Vocat Rehabil 46(1):75–86. https://doi.org/10.3233/JVR-160844

Rainville J, Sobel J, Hartigan C, Wright A (1997) The effect of compensation involvement on the reporting of pain and disability by patients referred for rehabilitation of chronic low back pain. Spine 22(17):2016–2024

Seing I, MacEachen E, Ekberg K, Ståhl C (2015) Return to work or job transition? Employer dilemmas in taking social responsibility for return to work in local workplace practice. Disabil Rehabil 37(19):1760–1769. https://doi.org/10.3109/09638288.2014.978509

Spearing NM, Connelly LB, Gargett S, Sterling M (2012) Does injury compensation lead to worse health after whiplash? A systematic review. Pain 153:1274–1282. https://doi.org/10.1016/j.pain.2012.03.007

Spieler EA (2017) (Re) assessing the grand bargain: compensation for work injuries in the United States, 1900–2017. Rutgers Univ Law Rev 69:891–1014

Ståhl C (2010) In cooperation we trust: Interorganizational cooperation in return-to-work and labour market reintegration. National Centre for work and rehabilitation. Linköping University, Linköping, Sweden

Ståhl C, Seing I (2019) Reforming activation in Swedish work disability policy. In: MacEachen E (ed) The science and politics of work disability prevention. Routledge/Taylor & Francis, New York/London, pp 125–140

Sullivan MJL, Scott W, Trost Z (2012) Perceived injustice: a risk factor for problematic pain outcomes. Clin J Pain 28(6):484–488

Swartzman LC, Teasell RW, Shapiro AP, McDermid AJ (1996) The effect of litigation status on adjustment to whiplash injury. Spine 21(1):53–58

Swedish Work Environment Authority (2015) Regulations and general recommendations on organisational and social work environment, AFS 2015-4 adopted under The Swedish Work Environment Act (1977, 1160) WEA. www.av.se

Vossen E, Van Gestel N, Van der Heijden BIJM, Rouwette EAJA (2017) "Dis-able bodied" or "dis-able minded": stakeholders' return-to-work experiences compared between physical and mental health conditions. Disabil Rehabil 39(10):969–977. https://doi.org/10.3109/09638288.2016.1172675

Welti F (2019) Work disability policy in Germany. In: MacEachen E (ed) The science and politics of work disability prevention. Routledge/Taylor & Francis, New York and London, pp 171–188

Wilford J, McMahon AD, Peters J, Pickvance S, Jackson A, Blank L, Craig D, O'Rourke A, Macdonald EB (2008) Predicting job loss in those off sick. Occup Med 58(2):99–106

Employment as a Key Rehabilitation Outcome

20

Kerstin Ekberg and Christian Ståhl

Contents

Introduction	366
The Value of Work	367
Rehabilitation Outcomes in the Literature	369
Getting and Keeping a Job: The Matter of Employability	371
Employment for Whom?	374
Changing Labor-Market Conditions	376
Policies and Regulations	378
Conclusions	380
Cross-References	381
References	381

Abstract

Preventing sick leave and helping people to return to work (RTW) is a major challenge in many societies. Different definitions and perspectives of RTW have led to a lack of agreement about what constitutes a successful RTW outcome. Commonly used outcome measures of RTW interventions capture only parts of the process to sustainable participation in the labor market. In this chapter we discuss theoretical and empirical research on inclusion and exclusion from the labor market for long-term sick-listed or people with disabilities. Work disability policy based on activation principles that restrict benefits for the sick-listed and

---

K. Ekberg (✉)
Community Medicine, Department of Health, Medicine and Caring Sciences, Linköping University, Linköping, Sweden
e-mail: kerstin.ekberg@liu.se

C. Ståhl
Unit of Education and Sociology, Department of Behavioural Sciences and Learning, Linköping University, Linköping, Sweden
e-mail: christian.stahl@liu.se

© Springer Nature Switzerland AG 2020
U. Bültmann, J. Siegrist (eds.), *Handbook of Disability, Work and Health*, Handbook Series in Occupational Health Sciences, https://doi.org/10.1007/978-3-030-24334-0_20

unemployed in favor of active work reintegration may serve to increase the inequality gap in the labor market, since they tend to focus on individual responsibilities and agency rather than resource-generation. Increased demands on flexibility seem to promote opportunities and employability for people who have good resources. For those with less resources, the labor market is restricted to temporary or precarious jobs, increasing the inequality gap. This dynamic development creates new challenges for work disability prevention research. The notion of equality needs to be reinterpreted from looking at outcomes to taking a broader perspective on equality of opportunity. Employment in any job is questioned as the best outcome unless the quality of the job is taken into account, providing resources for sustainable participation in the labor market.

Keywords

Value of work · Employability · Sustainability · Activation · Work conditions

Introduction

What is a good or relevant rehabilitation outcome? This question has no simple answer; rather, the answer will differ depending on whom you ask. A physician, a psychologist, a politician, a representative of an insurance company, or an employer will all be likely to give different answers depending on their different perspectives and roles in the return-to-work (RTW) or labor-market integration process. According to traditional definitions, rehabilitation is a matter of restoring physical and/or mental capacities to enable the individual to participate in social life, including the labor market. In essence, the goal is to restore capacities and to adjust contextual factors to provide opportunities for a disabled person to participate in normal daily and working life. For the sick-listed and the unemployed, this means providing opportunities to return to work, either to the job they previously occupied or to a new job.

For most people, employment and work constitute a desirable goal, but not irrespective of working conditions. A decent job, acceptable employment conditions, opportunities for individual development, and the consideration of disabilities are all reasonable requirements. This opens up questions about *how* to consider employment as a relevant rehabilitation outcome – what type of employment, for whom, and under what conditions? We also need to ask questions about the relationship between individuals and the labor market, where issues of employability and labor-market policies come into play.

Interventions designed to promote return to work (RTW) for sick-listed workers have moved from unidimensional methods to alleviate symptoms of ill-health to multidimensional interventions encompassing both the individual and the workplace. The outcome measures in intervention studies vary, but the implicit goal is usually employment, although the measures do not always achieve this goal. The outcome measures in empirical studies are therefore important for understanding what we can reasonably expect to learn from the effects of interventions, and whether they are associated with actual labor-market participation.

In this chapter, we discuss theoretical and empirical research on inclusion in or exclusion from the labor market for the long-term sick-listed or people with disabilities. We will also discuss the ways in which employment and inclusion in the labor market can be considered rehabilitation goals and the extent to which the existing outcomes of intervention studies relate to the conditions for employment, work, and health in real life.

The Value of Work

The concept of work and what it means to humans and human societies has been under scrutiny for thousands of years. For instance, Rawls (1971) provides a reading of Aristotle which implies that human beings enjoy the exercise of their realized capacities and that this enjoyment increases the more the capacity is realized, or the greater the complexity. In a similar conceptualization, Marx describes work as something that defines us as humans – it is unique among animals that we produce our own means of subsistence, and as a free, creative activity, it is a natural part of being human (Karlsson and Månson 2017). Marx's later analyses of capitalism and work as alienated labor show specifically how social structures restrict work from being such a free and creative activity, and his vision of a postcapitalist society serves the purpose of liberating work from compulsion. A different conception of work can be found in Weber's interpretation of the protestant work ethic. Here, work is considered a duty, based on spiritual or ascetic virtues, and serves to shield people from sinful living and to work for the glory of God (Karlsson and Månson 2017). This perspective on work is radically different, since it is based on a strong moral imperative, illustrated by the aphorism "he who does not work shall not eat" (originally from the Bible, but also repeated as a maxim by Lenin in the Soviet Union; in the latter use, it was primarily directed against the bourgeoisie, while the work-incapacitated should be provided for through social security). In later social science, the value of work is to a large degree considered a *social* rather than an intrinsic value. The value of work was stressed by Jahoda in her study of Marienthal in the 1930s, focusing on the consequences for people and their living after becoming unemployed (Jahoda et al. 1971). Prolonged unemployment led to a state of apathy in which the victims did not utilize even the few opportunities left to them. They did not miss the work per se, but rather the social structure and sense of participation it gave.

These different conceptualizations of work also have implications for how we consider the *value* of work. If we conceptualize it as a virtue and a creative endeavor, we may consider it as having value as an activity in itself, independent of what it may bring in terms of monetary returns or social standing. If we consider work as a moral imperative, or as an alienated activity forced upon us by a coercive social structure, the value of work will be radically different; here, it is a means of subsistence, or a way of avoiding moral condemnation. The perspective of work as a social value focuses on the work context primarily as a means to an end – given the social structure of our societies, work is the most common arena for social relations and by which we can gain status and recognition.

What is considered work is not consistent over time. In Aristotle's society, the exercise of capacities was not considered "work," and only slaves performed manual labor. Likewise, activities we today consider to be work were a few decades ago seen as domestic chores not worthy of being paid a salary, such as caring for children or the elderly, which have now become professions in their own right. Even activities recently considered to be leisure, for example, making online videos or posting pictures on social media platforms, may today be considered work if the people doing it are able to make a living through sponsorships or commercial revenue. The line between work and other activities is hence under constant negotiation, where the dividing line is whether somebody is willing to pay for it being done or not. While artistic activities or community engagement may have a high social value, they are not considered legitimate outcomes for labor-market policies since these activities are not tied to financial remuneration and hence are not valued in economic terms.

Whichever conceptualization of work we subscribe to, we will need to consider the conditions under which work is performed, since this will determine whether it leads to positive or negative health outcomes (Harvey et al. 2017). These conditions are affected by organizational structures as well as conditions in the labor market. We have seen a steady increase in stress-related disorders in most Western countries over the last few decades, concurrent with the development of increasing demands for a flexible and contingent workforce and high productivity. As a consequence, preventing sick leave and helping people return to work have been recognized as challenges in many societies, which is one reason for the rapid increase in work disability prevention research over the last few decades.

Long-term sickness absence is a major predictor for all types of exit from the labor market, including unemployment, disability pension (OECD 2010), and early retirement (Aranki and Macchiarelli 2013). The social exclusion process resulting from long-term or chronic illness is strongly mediated by access to paid work. Evaluated on an epidemiological basis, the evidence suggests a strong, positive association between unemployment and many adverse health outcomes. Whether unemployment causes these adverse outcomes is less straightforward, since there are likely to be many mediating and confounding factors which may be social, economic, or clinical (Jin et al. 1995). The causal relationship between increased work and improved health probably runs in both directions. Employment improves health status, and healthy people are more likely to seek and maintain employment. However, longitudinal studies provide reasonably good evidence that unemployment itself is detrimental to health (Paul and Moser 2009) and has an impact on health outcomes – it increases premature mortality rates and causes physical and mental ill-health and greater use of health services (Mathers and Schofield 1998). The negative effects of not having a job are not necessarily tied to work being healthy but are also a consequence of the conditions for the unemployed and the social consequences of being placed outside the strong working norm: the welfare system is heavily oriented toward promoting employment, and stigmatizing measures are taken against those who do not comply. Given this social structure, and since the unemployed often lack other arenas for social coherence, almost any job becomes positive compared to the alternative of being unemployed.

These different perspectives on the nature and value of work and its position in society are relevant to account for when considering if and why work may be considered a relevant rehabilitation outcome, why work is important to people given the societal structure they live in, and which conditions to consider when assessing what types of work may be positive or negative to a person's health and well-being. Hence, it is relevant to look in more detail into how different types of studies conceptualize and measure work and employment, which we will consider in the next section.

Rehabilitation Outcomes in the Literature

The debate regarding how to view and measure work-related rehabilitation outcomes reflects different perspectives both in practice and in research. The concept of RTW is generally poorly defined, and there is a lack of agreement about what constitutes a successful RTW outcome (Pransky et al. 2005). In many studies, notably within epidemiology, the perspective on work disability is primarily descriptive, with the aim of identifying certain factors and determining the causal relationships between them. In intervention studies, the purpose is to develop and test specific interventions in which work is one of the outcomes. Quality criteria in such outcomes focus on the validity and reliability of the measurements used. In an article appropriately entitled "Measuring Return to Work," it is stated that one of the factors limiting the understanding of RTW following work disability is that measurement tools do not capture a "complete picture of workers' RTW experiences" (Wasiak et al. 2007, p. 766). From a system-oriented perspective, however, work disability is not primarily related to the work-disabled person; it is rather constantly reconstructed through social relations between different actors, who in this process attribute different meanings to it. A "complete picture of workers' RTW experiences" is, from this perspective, extremely hard to arrive at through the use of a quantitative measure.

Still, several studies have tried to determine which measures and outcomes are most relevant for determining the success of rehabilitation processes. For instance, Elfering (2006) discussed traditional measures, for example, work status and sickness absence, in addition to other work-related outcome assessment instruments. Work status may mean, for example, that a person is employed in their usual job, a light-duty job, with reduced working hours, in a supported job, a new job, or is unemployed, a student, retired, or on a disability pension. These outcomes may, however, merely reflect demographic or cultural factors, and it is not always clear that such outcomes actually measure how successful the RTW intervention was.

Sickness absence is another concept that comprises a number of different aspects, and may be measured in different units. Usually, RTW in this literature is measured as the point when sick leave benefits end. It is, however, rarely reported whether the end of sick leave is due to the regulations, i.e., an upper limit on the number of permitted sick leave days, the end of a job contract due to sickness absence, return to the current or another job, unemployment, studies, a pension, or other reasons. Therefore, measuring the end of sick leave days does not tell us whether RTW was successful or whether it was sustainable. The number of days of sickness absence may also be associated with different measures of health but also with such factors as job satisfaction, psychosocial and physical working conditions, job insecurity, work-home interference, and contextual factors.

Relapse into sick leave is rarely measured, although it is important for determining the sustainability of RTW. The contextual factors at work, or how the individual values their work, may be more important than health measures if we want to assess sustainability in work capacity and labor-market participation.

The complexity associated with the two traditional outcomes of work status and sick leave has led to discussions about how to standardize outcome measures to make studies comparable. Hensing et al. (1998) suggested five measures of sick leave (frequency, length, incidence rate, cumulative incidence, duration) that have become widely used in epidemiological studies. They emphasize the need to choose outcome measures depending on the purpose of the study. In studies of RTW, the purpose is usually to assess whether interventions lead to participation in the labor market, i.e., employment, either continued employment in the job from which they were sick-listed, or another job. Likewise, employment is the key outcome in studies of reintegration into the labor market of unemployed or disabled people.

Recent etiological models are multifactorial and emphasize environmental conditions at work, the social climate, and support at the workplace and in the life situation as important determinants for the individual's motivation, expectations, and decision to return to work or not. A review of RTW outcomes emphasized that "RTW is not merely a state: rather it is a multi-phase process, encompassing both a series of events, transitions, and phases as well as interactions with other individuals and the environment" (Wasiak et al. 2007, p. 767). This conceptualization hence represents a more comprehensive view of RTW, encompassing the sickness absence and the phases of work reentry, maintenance, and advancement, i.e., also characteristics of the employment conditions. The authors reviewed existing instruments for their use as measures of the different phases in RTW and found measures of RTW-related tasks and actions (such as vocational participation, work preparation, job seeking, job securing, work participation, evaluation, work maintenance/durability, and career advancement), and instruments measuring context-dependent outcomes in the personal and environmental domains of ICF and RTW process outcomes.

The huge number of instruments measuring very specific parts of the RTW domains and processes clarifies the complexity and the need for a better theoretical basis for instruments and a model for what interventions actually aim to achieve. The importance of choosing the right outcome measure was empirically supported in a mixed method study (Hees et al. 2012). Key stakeholders (employees, supervisors, occupational physicians) responded to what constitutes successful RTW after sickness absence due to common mental disorders. All three stakeholder groups considered sustainability of work capacity to be important, but supervisors and physicians regarded at-work functioning to be more important, while the workers considered job satisfaction, work-home balance, and mental functioning to be most important, i.e., aspects that constitute important domains of a worker's valuation of work. This means that, from a worker's perspective, other measures of outcome than the traditional sick leave days and work status are important in assessing RTW and employability.

The rehabilitation outcomes reported in the literature are generally quantitative, most often measuring individual competencies or attitudes, and usually made at a single point in time. The perspectives and outcome measures of successful interventions commonly used in RTW studies may be questioned, as they fail to capture aspects that are important for the actual process. RTW is a complex process involving the individual, the workplace, and different stakeholders. At the center of this process is the sick-listed worker with his or her resources, skills, and goals. Recent research highlights the importance of incorporating the contextual conditions as determinants when evaluating interventions to promote RTW (Cullen et al. 2018). According to Pransky et al. (2005), the greatest barriers and opportunities to achieving improved RTW outcomes are in the workplace. Returning to a job that the worker knows is harmful to her/his health has limited prospects of being successful. To return to a job where accommodations are made that are suited to the worker's condition may, on the other hand, have a positive impact on the individual worker's value of work. How stakeholders interact with the worker, which rehabilitation opportunities they offer, and how the workplace acts are critical factors for a successful process toward work and for sustained work capacity and job satisfaction. Very little is known about gender differences in how men and women value work, and how the value of work may differ between different branches, over time, or in different cultures (Conen and de Beer 2017).

In sum, the quantitative literature on RTW has struggled to find measures that can represent a realistic conceptualization of work or employment as an outcome. Thus, we can conclude that many of the traditional measures are too simplistic, measuring RTW as a dichotomized variable – working or not working, on sick leave or not. Attempts to include more aspects into the measures, on the other hand, can result in overcomplex and highly context-specific variables. Hence, in the ambition to capture all the nuances of work and employment as an outcome in research, there is a risk that the measures arrived at become difficult to use in a relevant manner. Another approach is to combine cruder measures with qualitative outcomes that may imbue the figures with more content and retain RTW as a complex social process involving many actors in different phases.

Getting and Keeping a Job: The Matter of Employability

The concept of employability is widely used in local, regional, national, and international contexts to describe the objectives of labor-market and social welfare policies. A basic requirement for being employed is that the individual her/himself, a workplace, and in some cases the social welfare authorities think that the individual is employable. Employability is often defined as a characteristic of the individual, or as a characteristic of both the individual and labor-market conditions (McQuaid and Lindsay 2005). Traditionally, the assessment of whether a worker is able to work, and hence is available for continued or new employment, is based on measures of the individual's physical, and sometimes mental, capacity. Researchers and policy makers have used a narrow concept of employability focusing upon "employability skills and attributes," often resulting in purely supply-side employability policies, such as activating and "up-skilling" the individual (McQuaid and Lindsay 2005).

The concept of interactive employability was proposed by Gazier (1998), who reflected that employability is about overcoming a number of different barriers to work and that employability policies should therefore also focus on the labor market. In line with the concept of interactive employability, McQuaid and Lindsay (2005) proposed a broad or holistic model encompassing three main interrelated components that influence a person's employability: (a) individual factors such as skills, qualifications, work experience, labor-market attachment, demographics, health and well-being, active job seeking, adaptability, and mobility; (b) personal circumstances, e.g., caring responsibilities, work culture in the family, access to resources such as transportation, financial support, and access to social capital; and (c) external factors, e.g., labor-market demand factors and enabling support factors, which may be related to labor-market policies. How the interactions between each of the components evolve is of fundamental importance, emphasizing the importance of both demand- and supply-side factors, where a question is whether the demand side includes good-quality jobs with flexible working arrangements, and which social norms are influencing employers' willingness to employ people.

The changing labor market and the increased educational level of populations have entailed increasing numbers of self-employed people who work on temporary projects, exercising the often-called-for flexibility in today's labor-market policies. The traditional value of occupying life-long employment is questioned by many, in particular younger and well-educated people. The value of work among these people is less tied to having a specific job and more oriented toward individual agency and self-fulfillment and having control over their lives. Accordingly, van der Klink et al. (2016) argue that present-day workers require a wider range of valued outcomes from their work than income alone. They propose a model for how resources, context, sustainable employability, and values are related, based on the concept of capability developed by Sen (1993). An individual's sustainable employability, according to this model, is determined by how her or his resources are converted into capabilities, and subsequently into work, functioning in such a way that values such as security, recognition, and meaning are met. The major thesis is that people are more likely to remain sustainably employed if their work is not only a means of generating income but is also intrinsically valuable; i.e., they consider sustainability in the labor market to be an individual choice. Health in this model is not per se an outcome only but also a determinant for participation, a condition that is necessary to enable people to accomplish valuable goals in their lives. Work is conceptualized as a creative endeavor for people with agency, having merits as an activity, with less emphasis on what it may bring in terms of monetary returns or social standing.

The context contributes to the opportunities and conditions affecting employees' capacity to participate in the labor market.

The model reflects changing labor-market conditions, with increasing numbers of people working as entrepreneurs or intrapreneurs on time-limited projects, with an emphasis on initiative and agency by the individual. Thus, a successful career no longer equates to achieving objective (extrinsic) career success such as promotions, status, and higher salaries, but is rather a matter of attaining subjective (intrinsic) career success – which concerns job (life) satisfaction, increasing employability, and the feasibility of combining family life with work (Shockley et al. 2016). This self-government of people's employability is, however, not a feasible opportunity for everyone, but only primarily for those with sufficient financial or educational resources to make such choices. For poorly educated workers on long-term sick leave or unemployed in socioeconomically strained situations, access to secure employment may be of greater importance than self-fulfillment. Hence, the model proposed by van der Klink et al. (2016) has problems in describing how to reach sustainable employability for the long-term sick-listed or unemployed.

The development toward flexibility is reflected in the development of policies, e.g., in the flexicurity systems that tend to focus more on employment security than job security, i.e., making it easy to hire and fire, while maintaining a reasonable social security through active labor-market policies to bridge the gaps between jobs (Bekker et al. 2008). In such systems, employability is a central concept, since it describes what is guaranteed by the policy – employment, rather than financial compensation. It is not clear, however, how the employability promoted by such policies will be made sustainable for those who have harsh working conditions or who are involuntarily working in temporary jobs. Following the lines of the interactive model of employability, societal responsibilities may need to incorporate requirements for decent jobs with both intrinsic and extrinsic value in order to achieve sustainability in labor-market participation for vulnerable groups.

To ensure sustainable RTW, Nielsen et al. (2018) argue that the integration of resources needs to be accomplished at five levels: the individual, the group, the leader, the organizational, and the overarching contextual level. Their proposed IGLOO model aims to promote an understanding of how resources in the work and nonwork contexts are integrated. The model has its theoretical foundations in the conservation of resources (COR) theory proposed by Hobfoll (1989). This theory describes the motivation that drives humans to both maintain their current resources and pursue new resources. People will invest resources in order to protect against resource loss, to recover from losses, and to gain resources. Personal resources help people to gain additional resources, suggesting that employees with high perceived employability hold a powerful negotiating position and thus can accumulate further resources from their employer, for instance, more training. The IGLOO model also incorporates the nonwork domain and the overarching social context, such as compensation systems, national legislation, and social welfare policy as possible resource-generating determinants of RTW. The concept of sustainability is not explicitly defined; rather, it is assumed that sustainable participation in the labor market is a consequence of strategies and actions at all levels and that a positive interaction between the domains generating resources for the individual will ensure a sustainable ability to work and the motivation to do so. A consequence of this model is that outcome measures should focus on the degree to which interventions at different levels are generating resources for the individual, thus motivating them to invest in employability.

These policy- and research-based conceptualizations of employability suggest that the concept needs to be explored in more depth in terms of the conditions that support the sustainability of work capacity and employability. The results reflect the need to develop multi-domain models for employability and sustainable employment in the labor market and to measure adequate outcomes. The various definitions of employability emphasize the importance of looking at both the supply side and the demand side, i.e., the individual's skills and resources, their personal life situation, and the contextual factors at the workplace and among stakeholders. The proposed models have the merit of approaching today's flexible working conditions, but they are generally less capable of analyzing the complexities for groups with varied backgrounds and social positions to accomplish intrinsically rewarding or resource-generating employment. The models need to acknowledge the structural conditions that offer very different starting points for people in their struggle to gain and maintain resources, where their position in the social order determines what type of jobs are available for different groups. We know from epidemiological research that there is a social gradient in which differences in health and social status are connected to education and the types of jobs people occupy (Marmot and Bell 2012). Furthermore, people with disabilities may be seen as a group experiencing specific barriers to employment.

Employment for Whom?

People with disabilities have lower labor-market participation than people without disabilities, and the unemployment rate among people with mental health problems is twice as high as for those without. The recurrence rate among people with common mental disorders is high, and sickness absence is longer for this group than for other disorders (Nielsen et al. 2018). People with intellectual disabilities and mental health illnesses compose the most discriminated against groups in the population (Hogan et al. 2012) due to factors such as lower skill levels and misconceptions about their capabilities. The employment rate varies considerably for people with different disabilities, with individuals with mental health difficulties or intellectual impairments experiencing the lowest employment rates (Thornicroft 2006). Research in the USA has shown that 44% of workers with disabilities are in some contingent or part-time employment arrangement, compared with 22% of those without disabilities (Schur 2003). Across 14 EU countries, more than 50% of those with basic activity difficulties (such as sight, hearing, walking, communicating) were inactive in 2011. For people limited in work because of a long-standing health problem and/or a basic activity difficulty, the employment rate recorded at EU-28 level was 38.1%, nearly 30 percentage points lower than people who did not declare a limitation in work. Analyzing the personal or environmental factors limiting access to work, the lack of suitable job opportunities was the biggest factor in the EU, quoted by 31% of the working age population (Eurofound 2017), indicating that the problem is primarily an environmental one with limited opportunities for people with disabilities, rather than explicitly dependent on the disability itself.

There are common myths that people with disabilities are unable to work and that accommodating a person with a disability in the workplace is expensive. Contrary to these notions, many companies have found that people with disabilities are contributing to the workplace climate and are reliable in the same capacity as any other worker. Disability does not in itself mean ill-health or that a person is doomed to unemployment. Yelin and Trupin (2003) report that, in a California survey, 54% of people with disabilities who reported that they were in "excellent, very good, or good" health were employed compared to only 26% of those who reported that they were in "fair or poor" health. Another survey found that employed individuals with any disability experience mental distress less frequently than those with a disability who are not employed (18% vs. 40%). This relationship held up even when controlling for demographics and individual characteristics, including age, sex, race/ethnicity, education, marital status, health-risk behaviors, body mass index, healthcare coverage, and self-rated general health (Okoro et al. 2007). A systematic review of observational studies showed that entering paid employment reduces the risk of depression and improves general mental health (van der Noordt et al. 2014). Luciano et al. (2014) similarly found that entering paid employment was associated with decreased psychiatric treatment and increased self-esteem. In the Black report (2008), it was stated that "Work, *matched to one's knowledge and skills and undertaken in a safe, healthy environment*, can reverse the harmful effects of prolonged sickness or long-term unemployment, and promote health, well-being and prosperity" (italics added). Employment is hence associated with better health and well-being, independent of whether the individual has disabilities or not; it is, however, important to focus on the conditions of employment, and how these interact with the specific type of disability.

Extensive literature has identified social barriers faced by persons with disabilities, such as negative attitudes, lack of accessibility, lack of coordination of services, and an unfair distribution of resources to support employment (Shaw et al. 2014). Barriers at the workplace include employers who are reluctant to hire people with disabilities as employers lack knowledge and understanding about how to assess performance and skills, and how to accommodate these workers in the workplace. It is also common to find a lack of integration of services and policies to promote the hiring and retention of persons with disabilities. Employers may want to prevent possible unplanned expenses in terms of accommodation, mentorship, support, etc. Employers may also see a risk in employing someone who is different from the rest of the workforce or who does not fit into the existing work culture. Several studies have also shown that employers' lack of knowledge or experience of disabilities is associated with prejudices and myths. Furthermore, lack of support from the authorities for both the prospective employer and the disabled individual may be a problem. Similar findings were reported by Strindlund et al. (2019), who found that employers perceived disabled people as hard to match with job demands and that they were considered as having reduced work ability and motivation, implying that hiring them would be time-, energy-, and resource-demanding for the employer without adequate support from the authorities. Strindlund et al. (2019) also found that some employers could have other perspectives, from which disability was not seen as directly affecting work ability or was even seen as a resource. The need for labor increased the incentive to focus on abilities rather than disabilities, and employees with disabilities were considered as adding value to the workplace. In such cases, authority support could facilitate employment, but was not seen as necessary or important.

As discussed above, not having a job in modern Western societies is often linked to socioeconomic inequalities, social stigma, and ill-health. In almost all countries, the employment situation is worse for disabled people compared to people without disabilities. It is also apparent that people with mental disorders, women, the poorly educated, and minorities have fewer opportunities than others to get into the labor market, in particular if they are disabled. The fact that people may simultaneously belong to more than one disadvantaged group calls for intersectional approaches to analyze how different grounds for discrimination may interact to create additional burdens for specific groups, e.g., disabled women, disabled with few socioeconomic resources, or belonging to minority groups.

Changing Labor-Market Conditions

Leveling up from the individual or the employer level to a structural or societal level provides a broader perspective on employment conditions for long-term sick-listed and disabled people. On the labor market, the traditional criteria for employment are changing. One of the key features of labor-market developments over the last 25 years has been an increase in the share of temporary and contingent employment in most industrially advanced countries, and also in emerging countries (Cazes and de Laiglesia 2015). Many occupations are being automated, and specific competences are becoming obsolete (Méda 2016), while other skills, such as the ability to communicate, to find new solutions, and to be social and innovative, are increasingly in demand. The evolving labor market provides opportunities for workers with competitive work skills (e.g., high education, IT competence, social skills) and the ability to be flexible, but it also creates challenges, especially for vulnerable groups, such as the lower-educated, immigrants, the chronically ill, and individuals with disabilities (Ekberg et al. 2016). Requirements placed on workers change as the labor market changes; continuous learning of new skills, adaptation to technical developments, social abilities, and teamwork are common requirements. On the demand side, measurements and evaluations of performance using quantitative measures are common to keep productivity at high levels, according to the principles of the New Public Management policies. The evolving labor market creates new barriers for some people with disabilities to get a job or to RTW after long-standing sick leave, unless working conditions are accommodated and inclusive. The qualification demands in the labor market are challenging for those who have fewer personal resources, due to factors such as ill-health, a limited education, another native language, or a strained financial situation. These groups may often end up in precarious work situations with looser employment relations linked to greater levels of job insecurity.

The consequences for workers include growing job insecurity and work intensification (EU-OSHA 2013). According to Virtanen et al. (2005), these developments are assumed to follow a core-periphery structure. The core employees with relatively secure labor-market status are surrounded by sectors of a "buffer workforce" with various types of unstable and insecure work arrangements. In the growing gig economy, temporary positions are common, and organizations contract with independent workers for short-term engagements. The results of a gig economy are cheaper services for those willing to use them, but insecure positions in the labor market for the workers. Several studies highlight the need for better regulations for temporary workers. In several countries, there are regulations that do not permit employers to dismiss employees during sick leave. For temporary workers, these regulations seem to be frequently disregarded, if at all applicable (Flach et al. 2013). Therefore, temporary workers often go to work while ill as they otherwise risk unemployment. Negative expectations of job stability, combined with limited resources to compete in the labor market, seem to lead to longer sick leave, possibly due to a gradual depletion of personal resources due to problematic interactions with rehabilitation stakeholders or limited support from the workplace (MacEachen et al. 2010). Research is needed to disentangle the employer's responsibilities for temporary employment in order to secure reasonable employment and welfare conditions.

Individuals who do not proactively take charge of their careers, or who lack the resources to do so, may end up in unwanted positions or become marginalized over time. As a consequence of these changes, those with fewer resources will be forced to stay in undesired work situations. This corresponds to the circumstances described by Siegrist (2005), in which individuals have to stay in non-desirable situations because of few alternatives on the labor market and therefore are at risk of being laid off or facing downward mobility. The changing labor market thus creates new challenges for RTW or work integration attempts, especially in the context of job security no longer being a matter of course in many welfare systems (as discussed in relation to the flexicurity model above). For this group, interventions to promote sustainable work ability may benefit from incorporating support for the prospect of changing profession or job to promote work ability over the long term. It has been suggested that intervention programs to reduce long-term sick leave should include measures to facilitate job mobility for some sick-listed people (Ekberg et al. 2011). To improve employability and sustainable employment, it is necessary to move from standardized interventions toward differentiating RTW interventions based on knowledge about the sick-listed person's resources in relation to the labor market and the workplace, and their expectations of future employment. Such employability-oriented measures would, however, need to be geared toward strengthening the positive aspects of activation, such as the development of skills, rather than providing negative incentives through increasingly restrictive benefit structures.

Policies and Regulations

A general trend in many Western countries over the last few decades has been to implement activation policies, under which the rhetoric focuses on the individual's capacity to work rather than the disability. Through such policies, the focus is also shifted from demand-side policies to supply-side interventions and actions centered on the individual. More often than not, the policies are designed toward what we may call "negative" activation, that is, making unemployment or sick leave less attractive by restricting the generosity or increasing the conditionality connected to benefits. Under such policies, the responsibilities of individuals are underlined, rather than their rights. Given the complexities outlined above relating to the social dimensions of disability, the social gradient in resources and the potential intersectional discrimination against specific groups, we need to carefully consider the question of equity in relation to such policies. Those with few resources, or those who lose their resources by losing their job or becoming ill, will, according to Hobfoll (1989), experience stress and more resource loss in the future. If policies and structures at the societal level are not resource-generating, the prospects of employability and sustainable employment for people starting with limited resources will be bleak, and the negative activation policies may actually work to increase inequity rather than compensating for it. Hence, social policy is at risk of becoming subordinated to the needs of labor-market flexibility, whereby the activation measures serve to redefine the relationship between rights and responsibilities in ways that may be detrimental to certain groups.

In most countries, there are regulations preventing discrimination against disabled people and supporting their right to gain employment. Still, as disabled people have a much lower employment rate than those without disabilities, it may be questioned how well anti-discrimination laws work in practice. Article 27 of The UN Convention on the Rights of People with Disabilities (UNCRPD) recognizes:

> the right of persons with disabilities to work, on an equal basis with others; this includes the right to the opportunity to gain a living by work freely chosen or accepted in a labour market and work environment that is open, inclusive and accessible to persons with disabilities. (United Nations 2008)

Similarly, the Americans with Disabilities Act (ADA) prohibits discrimination on the basis of disability in employment, state and local government, public accommodation, commercial facilities, transportation, and telecommunications (ADA 1990). Other jurisdictions have similar protections against discrimination for the disabled, as well as for other groups (e.g., based on religion, sexual orientation, gender, or age). These regulations are mostly concerned with discrimination in relation to employers' hiring procedures and state that a person with disability cannot be denied a job on the basis of that disability. Discrimination is also relevant, however, when discussing the design of labor-market policies. As discussed above, policies that are blind to people's different resources risk exacerbating rather than ameliorating the personal struggles involved when someone loses their job or becomes ill or disabled. Policies that are based on overly standardized measures will therefore discriminate against those who are already worse off.

One argument for the introduction of activation policies is the assumption that work has an enabling effect, leading to good health and well-being. This development reflects a shift in focus from passive compensation paid to those unable to work toward active work reintegration. Sick-listed or unemployed people are expected to be active, and, instead of disability or impairment, the focus is on the individual's ability to work (Seing et al. 2015). A basic idea underlying such policies is that all citizens (including most disabled people) should contribute to society's development. Activation policies are a combination of policy tools that provide support and incentives for people to engage in searching for and finding jobs that lead to independence from public support benefits, where a large responsibility is placed on the individual to become employable. The OECD considers activation policy to contribute to greater social integration for people with work disabilities (OECD 2010).

The complexity of most national systems of welfare policy, social insurance, rehabilitation, and workplace health makes it difficult to gain a thorough overview of how they work in practice. The results of activation policies, as they are currently designed, are not, however, very encouraging. Generally, they have not been successful in relation to long-term sickness/disability benefit recipients, especially not for those with mental health problems, with whom employers are reluctant to engage. Raffass concludes, after looking through empirical studies, that:

> implementation of welfare-to-work policies has not resulted in bringing down the rates of unemployment (independently of the business cycle), combating long-term unemployment, reducing (in-work) poverty or empowering job-seekers as consumers of public services, which were all goals of the reformed "activating state." (Raffass 2017, p. 349)

A problem with activation policies seems to be that unemployed individuals are driven into low-skilled, low-paid jobs, or temporary jobs, in which they continue to remain partly dependent on the state (through in-work benefits). Such jobs are also unstable, making repeated returns to unemployment highly probable (Arni and Schiprowski 2015). While agency may be a responsibility of the individual, it is also a responsibility of society to provide the support needed for labor-market inclusion. Activation through policies promoting early RTW after sick-leave may instead lead to presenteeism, i.e., showing up for work when one is ill (Johns 2010), unless the workplace is accommodated to the individual's needs and resources. Presenteeism may be either positive or negative – for some chronic health conditions, integration into the labor market can be beneficial, while in other cases, it is important to fully recover first, and presenteeism may seriously affect sustainable work capacity.

An embedded assumption in activation-oriented work disability policy is that there is a receptive labor market for people seeking jobs and that work, irrespective of the type of job, is good for people's health. However, policies that drive workers toward any job, regardless of quality, can be considered irresponsible, given what we know about the potential negative health effects of poor working conditions (Harvey et al. 2017); rather, policies should advance decently paid and sustainable work under fair conditions (MacEachen and Ekberg 2018).

Conclusions

Is employment a key rehabilitation outcome? The answer to this question, we would propose, is dependent to a large extent on the type of job, the person's resources, the available options, and the conditions under which a person lives and works. We have seen how the commonly used outcome measures of RTW interventions only capture parts of the process, and sometimes aspects that are of less relevance than the final goal of rehabilitation, which we would argue is sustainable participation in the labor market. The goal of many policies, and unfortunately also of some RTW interventions, seems to be work at any cost. Activation policies based on negative financial incentives indicate this, as do interventions that only evaluate their results based on whether or not a person is still on sickness benefits. We know from the literature that work remains a meaningful goal for work-disabled people (Saunders and Nedelec 2014; Ståhl and Stiwne 2014), and, given that society values work as the primary arena for social networks, identity, social position, and economic subsistence, employment is a relevant rehabilitation outcome. What the discussion in this chapter clearly indicates, however, is the need to consider the *quality* of work as a central aspect of the rehabilitation process and to place explicit emphasis on the conditions for different groups. Today's flexible labor market may imply for resourceful groups that work offers intrinsic values, such as opportunities for agency, career success, and life satisfaction, which in turn may lead to the gaining of more resources in an upward spiral. For those without the necessary resources, however, having to return to a job with poor working conditions may be the very opposite of a rehabilitation goal – it may be a factor that leads to relapses and recurrent periods of work disability. People in such a situation are also at risk of being forced into temporary or precarious jobs combined with job insecurity, which in turn may accentuate ill-health and deplete their resources, i.e., a negative spiral that may lead to long-term disability and social exclusion.

Work disability policy based on activation principles that restrict benefits for the sick-listed and unemployed in favor of active work reintegration may serve to increase the inequality gap in the labor market, since they tend to focus on individual responsibilities and agency rather than resource-generation. It therefore seems questionable whether RTW to just any job is a good outcome of societal efforts. Rather, policies should advance decently paid and sustainable employment. Relevant policies on employment, health, social security, and equality need to be integrated and coherent in order to prevent social exclusion. To do so, the notion of equality needs to be reinterpreted from simply looking at outcomes to taking a broader perspective on equality of opportunity. This requires a change in the social contract whereby society needs to be more proactive, using long-term social investment policies to reduce inequalities.

It seems clear that outcome measures in intervention studies aiming to promote sustainable RTW or sustainable participation in the labor market need to capture other aspects than the traditional measures do. Employment as an outcome needs to take the quality of the job into account, and, in order to include sustainability, other measures are needed that capture the individual worker's valuation of work and how the workplace and stakeholders work to generate and promote the individual's resources.

In the end, we will need to revisit the foundations of how we consider work as a human activity. The idea of work having a value in itself needs to be put into the context of the structural conditions for performing it. We need to see the difference between the well-off person in an attractive job and the person sick-listed from a poor working environment who is pushed to return by repressive activation policies and that the latter does not constitute the idea of work as a resource-providing activity. Work in itself cannot be considered as either positive or negative; the structural conditions and the characteristics of the person will determine whether it is or not. If we think that work is merely a moral duty and that enduring harsh conditions is part of the virtue of work, we may be comfortable with RTW policies that promote work at any cost. If, on the other hand, we think that work should be a healthy, creative, and self-developing activity, we need to be attentive to what the work means for the person and make sure that it does not lead to illness rather than health. Hence, employment as such is not relevant as an outcome of rehabilitation; rather, we need to consider what that actually implies for the specific person, in the specific context. The ultimate goal may then be sustainable participation in the labor market.

Cross-References

▶ IGLOO: A Framework for Return to Work Among Workers with Mental Health Problems
▶ Investing in Integrative Active Labour Market Policies
▶ The Changing Nature of Work and Employment in Developed Countries

References

ADA (1990) Americans with Disabilities Act. https://www.eeoc.gov/eeoc/history/35th/thelaw/ada.html. Accessed 11 Oct 2018
Aranki T, Macchiarelli C (2013) Employment duration and shifts into retirement in the EU. LEQS paper, vol 58/2013. London School of Economics and Political Science, London
Arni P, Schiprowski A (2015) The effects of binding and non-binding job search requirements. IZA discussion papers, vol 8951. IZA Institute of Labor Economics, Bonn

Bekker S, Wilthagen T, Kongshøj Madsen P, Zhou J, Rogowski R, Keune M, Tangian A (2008) Flexicurity – a European approach to labour market policy. Intereconomics 43(2):68–111. https://doi.org/10.1007/s10272-008-0244-0

Black C (2008) Working for a healthier tomorrow. TSO (The Stationary Office), London

Cazes S, de Laiglesia J (2015) Temporary contracts, labour market segmentation and wage inequality. In: Berg J (ed) Labour markets, institutions and inequality: building just societies in the 21st century. ILO, Geneva

Conen W, de Beer P (2017) The value of work in a changing labour market: a review and research agenda. Goldschmeding Foundation, Amsterdam

Cullen KL, Irvin E, Collie A, Clay F, Gensby U, Jennings PA, Hogg-Johnson S, Kristman V, Laberge M, McKenzie D, Newnam S, Palagyi A, Ruseckaite R, Sheppard DM, Shourie S, Steenstra I, Van Eerd D, Amick BC 3rd (2018) Effectiveness of workplace interventions in return-to-work for musculoskeletal, pain-related and mental health conditions: an update of the evidence and messages for practitioners. J Occup Rehabil 28(1):1–15. https://doi.org/10.1007/s10926-016-9690-x

Ekberg K, Wåhlin C, Persson J, Bernfort L, Öberg B (2011) Is mobility in the labor market a solution to sustainable return to work for some sick listed persons? J Occup Rehabil 21(3):355–365. https://doi.org/10.1007/s10926-011-9322-4

Ekberg K, Pransky GS, Besen E, Fassier J-B, Feuerstein M, Munir F, Blanck P, Hopkinton Conference Working Group on Workplace Disability Prevention (2016) New business structures creating organizational opportunities and challenges for work disability prevention. J Occup Rehabil 26(4):480–489. https://doi.org/10.1007/s10926-016-9671-0

Elfering A (2006) Work-related outcome assessment instruments. Eur Spine J 15(1):S32–S43. https://doi.org/10.1007/s00586-005-1047-7

EU-OSHA (2013) Priorities for occupational safety and health research in Europe: 2013–2020. Publications Office of the European Union, Luxembourg

Eurofound (2017) Reactivate: employment opportunities for economically inactive people. Publications Office of the European Union, Luxembourg

Flach PA, Groothoff JW, Bültmann U (2013) Identifying employees at risk for job loss during sick leave. Disabil Rehabil 35(21):1835–1841. https://doi.org/10.3109/09638288.2012.760657

Gazier B (1998) Employability – definitions and trends. In: Gazier B (ed) Employability: concepts and policies. European Employment Observatory, Berlin, pp 37–71

Harvey SB, Modini M, Joyce S, Milligan-Saville JS, Tan L, Mykletun A, Bryant RA, Christensen H, Mitchell PB (2017) Can work make you mentally ill? A systematic meta-review of work-related risk factors for common mental health problems. Occup Environ Med 74(4):301–310. https://doi.org/10.1136/oemed-2016-104015

Hees HL, Nieuwenhuijsen K, Koeter MWJ, Bültmann U, Schene AH (2012) Towards a new definition of return-to-work outcomes in common mental disorders from a multi-stakeholder perspective. PLoS One 7(6). https://doi.org/10.1371/journal.pone.0039947

Hensing G, Alexanderson K, Allebeck P, Bjurulf P (1998) How to measure sickness absence? Literature review and suggestion of five basic measures. Scand J Soc Med 26(2):133–144. https://doi.org/10.1177/14034948980260020201

Hobfoll SE (1989) Conservation of resources: a new attempt at conceptualizing stress. Am Psychol 44(3):513–524. https://doi.org/10.1037/0003-066X.44.3.513

Hogan A, Kyaw-Myint SM, Harris D, Denronden H (2012) Workforce participation barriers for people with disability. Int J Disabil Manag 7:1–9. https://doi.org/10.1017/idm.2012.1

Jahoda M, Lazarsfeld PF, Zeisel H (1971) Marienthal; the sociography of an unemployed community. Aldine, Atherton/Chicago

Jin RL, Shah CP, Svoboda TJ (1995) The impact of unemployment on health: a review of the evidence. CMAJ 153(5):529–540

Johns G (2010) Presenteeism in the workplace: a review and research agenda. J Organ Behav 31(4):519–542. https://doi.org/10.1002/job.630

Karlsson JC, Månson P (2017) Concepts of work in Marx, Durkheim, and Weber. Nord J Work Life Stud 7(2):107–119. https://doi.org/10.18291/njwls.v7i2.81597

Luciano A, Bond GR, Drake RE (2014) Does employment alter the course and outcome of schizophrenia and other severe mental illnesses? A systematic review of longitudinal research. Schizophr Res 159(2):312–321. https://doi.org/10.1016/j.schres.2014.09.010

MacEachen E, Ekberg K (2018) Science, politics, and values in work disability policy: a reflection on trends and the way forward. In: MacEachen E (ed) The science and politics of work disability prevention. Routledge, New York, pp 261–283

MacEachen E, Kosny A, Ferrier S, Chamber L (2010) The "toxic dose" of system problems: why some injured workers don't return to work as expected. J Occup Rehabil 20(3):349–366. https://doi.org/10.1007/s10926-010-9229-5

Marmot M, Bell R (2012) Fair society, healthy lives. Public Health 126:S4–S10. https://doi.org/10.1016/j.puhe.2012.05.014

Mathers CD, Schofield DJ (1998) The health consequences of unemployment: the evidence. Med J Aust 168(4):178–182. https://doi.org/10.5694/j.1326-5377.1998.tb126776.x

McQuaid RW, Lindsay C (2005) The concept of employability. Urban Stud 42(2):197–219. https://doi.org/10.1080/0042098042000316100

Méda D (2016) The future of work: the meaning and value of work in Europe. Research paper no 18. ILO, Geneva

Nielsen K, Yarker J, Munir F, Bültmann U (2018) IGLOO: an integrated framework for sustainable return to work in workers with common mental disorders. Work Stress 32(4):400–417. https://doi.org/10.1080/02678373.2018.1438536

OECD (2010) Sickness, disability and work: breaking the barriers. A synthesis of findings across OECD countries. Organisation for Economic Co-operation and Development (OECD), Paris

Okoro C, Strine T, McGuire L, Balluz L, Mokdad A (2007) Employment status and frequent mental distress among adults with disabilities. Occup Med 57(3):217–220. https://doi.org/10.1093/occmed/kql177

Paul KI, Moser K (2009) Unemployment impairs mental health: meta-analyses. J Vocat Behav 74(3):264–282. https://doi.org/10.1016/j.jvb.2009.01.001

Pransky G, Gatchel R, Linton SJ, Loisel P (2005) Improving return to work research. J Occup Rehabil 15(4):453–457. https://doi.org/10.1007/s10926-005-8027-y

Raffass T (2017) Demanding activation. J Soc Policy 46(2):349–365. https://doi.org/10.1017/S004727941600057X

Rawls J (1971) A theory of justice. Harvard University Press, Cambridge

Saunders SL, Nedelec B (2014) What work means to people with work disability: a scoping review. J Occup Rehabil 24(1):100–110. https://doi.org/10.1007/s10926-013-9436-y

Schur LA (2003) Barriers or opportunities? The causes of contingent and part-time work among people with disabilities. Ind Relat 42(4):589–622. https://doi.org/10.1111/1468-232X.00308

Seing I, MacEachen E, Ståhl C, Ekberg K (2015) Early-return-to-work in the context of an intensification of working life and changing employment relationships. J Occup Rehabil 25(1):74–85. https://doi.org/10.1007/s10926-014-9526-5

Sen AK (1993) Capability and well-being. In: Nussbaum M, Sen AK (eds) The quality of life. Oxford University Press, Oxford

Shaw L, Daraz L, Bezzina MB, Patel A, Gorfine G (2014) Examining macro and meso level barriers to hiring persons with disabilities: a scoping review. Environmental contexts and disability. Res Soc Sci Disabil 8:185–210. https://doi.org/10.1108/S1479-354720140000008011

Shockley KM, Ureksoy H, Rodopman OB, Poteat LF, Dullaghan TR (2016) Development of a new scale to measure subjective career success: a mixed-methods study. J Organ Behav 37(1):128–153. https://doi.org/10.1002/job.2046

Siegrist J (2005) Social reciprocity and health: new scientific evidence and policy implications. Psychoneuroendocrinology 30(10):1033–1038. https://doi.org/10.1016/j.psyneuen.2005.03.017

Ståhl C, Stiwne EE (2014) Narratives of sick leave, return to work and job mobility for people with common mental disorders in Sweden. J Occup Rehabil 24(3):543–554. https://doi.org/10.1007/s10926-013-9480-7

Strindlund L, Abrandt-Dahlgren M, Ståhl C (2019) Employers' views on disability, employability, and labor market inclusion: a phenomenographic study. Disabil Rehabil 41(24):2910–2917. https://doi.org/10.1080/09638288.2018.1481150

Thornicroft G (2006) Shunned: discrimination against people with mental illness. Oxford University Press, New York

United Nations (2008) Convention on the Rights of Persons with Disabilities. www.un.org/disabilities/default.asp?id=150. Accessed 1 Oct 2018

van der Klink JJL, Bültmann U, Burdorf A, Schaufeli WB, Zijlstra FRH, Abma FI, Brouwer S, van der Wilt GJ (2016) Sustainable employability – definition, conceptualization, and implications: a perspective based on the capability approach. Scand J Work Environ Health 1:71–79. https://doi.org/10.5271/sjweh.3531

van der Noordt M, Ijzelenberg H, Droomers M, Proper KI (2014) Health effects of employment: a systematic review of prospective studies. Occup Environ Med 71(10):730. https://doi.org/10.1136/oemed-2013-101891

Virtanen M, Kivimäki M, Joensuu M, Virtanen P, Elovainio M, Vahtera J (2005) Temporary employment and health: a review. Int J Epidemiol 34(3):610–622. https://doi.org/10.1093/ije/dyi024

Wasiak R, Young AE, Roessler RT, McPherson KM, Van Poppel MNM, Anema JR (2007) Measuring return to work. J Occup Rehabil 17(4):766–781. https://doi.org/10.1007/s10926-007-9101-4

Yelin EH, Trupin L (2003) Disability and the characteristics of employment. Mon Labor Rev 126:20–31

21 Personal and Environmental Factors Influencing Work Participation Among Individuals with Chronic Diseases

Ranu Sewdas, Astrid de Wind, Femke I. Abma, Cécile R. L. Boot, and Sandra Brouwer

Contents

Introduction	386
Theoretical Model and Approach	387
Overview of the Literature	388
Personal Factors	388
Environmental Factors	390
Considerations and Knowledge Gaps	391
Knowledge Gaps	392
Conclusions and Future Directions	394
Recommendations	394
Cross-References	395
References	395

Abstract

Recent policy reforms aim at encouraging workers, including those with chronic diseases, to prolong their working life. However, the employment rates of individuals with chronic diseases are still lower than those of healthy individuals. Therefore, it is important to gain insight into factors that hinder or facilitate individuals with chronic diseases to participate in work while maintaining work productivity. In this chapter, we searched for relevant literature reviews to provide an overview of the current knowledge on the personal and environmental determinants of work participation among individuals with chronic diseases. We found personal and environmental

---

R. Sewdas · A. de Wind · C. R. L. Boot
Department of Public and Occupational Health, Amsterdam Public Health Research Institute, Amsterdam UMC, VU University, Amsterdam, The Netherlands
e-mail: r.sewdas@amsterdamumc.nl; a.dewind@amsterdamumc.nl; crl.boot@vumc.nl

F. I. Abma · S. Brouwer (✉)
Department of Health Sciences, Community and Occupational Medicine, University of Groningen, University Medical Center Groningen, Groningen, The Netherlands
e-mail: f.i.abma@umcg.nl; sandra.brouwer@umcg.nl

© Springer Nature Switzerland AG 2020
U. Bültmann, J. Siegrist (eds.), *Handbook of Disability, Work and Health*, Handbook Series in Occupational Health Sciences, https://doi.org/10.1007/978-3-030-24334-0_21

factors that enable individuals with chronic diseases to work sustainably. Examples of these factors are good health as well as healthy behavior, having adequate psychological resources, a supportive social environment, low job demands, adequate job resources, presence of organizational policies at work aiming at an open communication, and a positive and supporting work environment. In particular older women with chronic diseases in a low socioeconomic position seem to be at risk for decreased work participation. Employers and governments are encouraged to pay more attention to these personal and environmental factors in order to facilitate employees with chronic diseases to continue working sustainably. Researchers are encouraged to investigate these factors related to early retirement and presenteeism. Employers, governments, and researchers are also encouraged to take into account labor market developments, as the labor market becomes more flexible and more insecure, in combination with an increasing demand to work longer and to provide informal care.

Keywords

Personal factors · Environmental factors · Work participation · Chronic disease · Aging · Prolonged working

Introduction

Due to an *aging* population in most European countries, the number of individuals suffering from *chronic diseases* is increasing (Eurostat 2015). Other factors contributing to a rising number of individuals with chronic diseases relate to better prevention and improved medical care, i.e., (i) health promotion initiatives have enhanced lifestyles (e.g., healthy diet or physical activity), (ii) enhanced screening methods have resulted in earlier detection of diseases, and (iii) better treatments have led to delayed death from severe diseases (Remington and Brownson 2011). Individuals aged 55 years and older face an additional challenge since the co-occurrence of more than one disease, i.e., *multi-morbidity*, is becoming more common as well (Börsch-Supan et al. 2013).

Many countries have raised the statutory retirement age and have taken measures to discourage *early exit from the workforce* via disability pension or early retirement schemes (Sigg and De-Luigi 2007). These policy reforms aim at encouraging workers, including those with chronic diseases, to prolong their working life. However, the employment rates of individuals with chronic diseases are still lower than those of healthy individuals. It has been shown that they experience more difficulties in finding a job and have a higher risk of job loss because of work disability (Schuring et al. 2007; van Rijn et al. 2014). This implies that workers with chronic diseases may need specific support to prolong their working life.

Work is a major determinant of health and well-being (Milner et al. 2014; Schuring et al. 2011). Involvement in work may help people building confidence and self-esteem, and it is financially rewarding. Being healthy, in turn, helps people to be productive at work and to enjoy retirement. This might be different for individuals with chronic diseases when they do not find a job that matches their needs and wishes. Not being involved in paid work coincides with economic consequences both at micro-level (i.e., lower income for an individual), meso-level (i.e., productivity losses for employers), and macro-level (i.e., costs as a result of work disability and unemployment) (Koopmanschap et al. 2013). To tackle these health and economic consequences, it is important to gain insight into factors that hinder or facilitate individuals with chronic diseases to participate in work, i.e., remain and/or reenter work while maintaining work productivity.

Several models underline the importance of personal and environmental factors in supporting work participation among individuals with chronic diseases. According to *the model of illness flexibility*, employment outcomes are dependent on someone's capacity, skills, knowledge, and adjustment latitude, i.e., the opportunity to adjust work tasks to the health situation (Johansson and Lundberg 2004). *The capability approach* describes the ability of an individual to convert her/his personal resources (e.g., health situation, skills required to work) and environmental resources (e.g., access to transportation to get to work, work accommodations) into the capability to work (Sen 1993; van der Klink et al. 2016). Both personal and environmental factors play a role in work participation and, therefore, offer opportunities to enable individuals with chronic diseases to continue employment.

The aim of this chapter is to synthesize the existing evidence in the scientific literature on the influence of personal and environmental factors on work participation among individuals with chronic diseases. We focus our chapter on literature describing the most prevalent and disabling chronic diseases, i.e., cancer and cardiovascular diseases, including diabetes, mental diseases, musculoskeletal diseases, rheumatoid arthritis, and respiratory diseases (Murray et al. 2012).

Theoretical Model and Approach

In this chapter, we use *the International Classification of Functioning, Disability and Health (ICF)* as a theoretical framework to classify personal and environmental factors influencing work participation of individuals with chronic diseases (WHO 2001). The ICF is a framework that describes the functioning and disability of individuals whose body functions and body structures may be impaired, activities may be limited, and participation may be restricted. Examples of personal factors are demographic factors, psychological factors, health-related personal factors, and work-related personal factors (Geyh et al. 2011). Environmental factors include social and occupational factors (Heerkens et al. 2004).

To provide an overview of the current knowledge on individual and environmental determinants of work participation in individuals with chronic diseases, we searched for relevant literature reviews on observational studies while excluding literature reviews on intervention studies.

Work participation was operationalized as loss of productivity (i.e., presenteeism), sickness absence (i.e., sick leave or absenteeism), return to work, and early exit from work (i.e., via disability pension, unemployment, or early retirement). Reviews that did not specify work participation, but included multiple definitions, were grouped under "sustained work participation," which refers to "staying at work" in this chapter.

Overview of the Literature

This section summarizes information from 24 literature reviews on personal and environmental factors and work participation among individuals with chronic diseases. (The results table that provides an overview of the factors and the corresponding literature review(s) can be obtained by the corresponding author by request.)

Personal Factors

The categories classified under *personal factors* are sociodemographic factors, socioeconomic status, health and health behavior, and psychological resources (see Fig. 1).

Sociodemographic Factors

Age and gender are the most commonly studied *sociodemographic factors*. Younger age is associated with sustained work participation, less sickness absence, earlier return to work, and lower risk of work disability among individuals with cancer, cardiovascular diseases, mental diseases, musculoskeletal diseases, rheumatoid

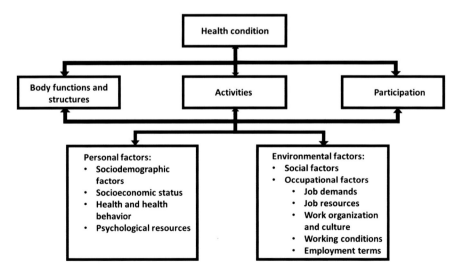

Fig. 1 Overview of personal and environmental factors in the ICF model

arthritis, and respiratory diseases (Cornelius et al. 2011; De Croon et al. 2004; Detaille et al. 2009; de Vries et al. 2017; Hansson and Jensen 2004; Lagerveld et al. 2010; Van Muijen et al. 2013; Steenstra et al. 2017; Vooijs et al. 2015; Dekkers-Sanchez et al. 2008). Thus, younger age is a favorable factor when it comes to work participation among individuals with chronic diseases.

For sex, some reviews showed that men with chronic diseases have a higher probability of sustained work participation, shorter sick leave episodes, and a lower risk of work disability, compared to women with chronic diseases (Achterberg et al. 2009; Detaille et al. 2009; Hansson and Jensen 2004; Hensing and Wahlström 2004; Van Muijen et al. 2013; Vooijs et al. 2015). This accounts for individuals with cancer, cardiovascular diseases, mental diseases, musculoskeletal diseases, rheumatoid arthritis, and respiratory diseases. However, other reviews that studied the same type of chronic diseases did not find differences between men and women regarding sustained work participation and sick leave (Blank et al. 2008; Lagerveld et al. 2010; Van Muijen et al. 2013; de Vries et al. 2012, 2017; Laisné et al. 2012; Peters et al. 2007; Spelten et al. 2002; Hansson and Jensen 2004; Kuijer et al. 2006; De Croon et al. 2004).

Socioeconomic Status

Socioeconomic status is often operationalized as educational level, income position, or job type (blue vs. white collar). A higher socioeconomic position is beneficial for sustained work participation among individuals with chronic diseases; individuals with chronic diseases having a higher educational level, a higher income, and working in white collar jobs have a higher probability of sustained work participation, including shorter sick leave episodes and a lower risk of work disability (Achterberg et al. 2009; Detaille et al. 2009; De Croon et al. 2004; de Vries et al. 2017; Lagerveld et al. 2010; Van Muijen et al. 2013; Peters et al. 2007). This accounts for individuals with cancer, cardiovascular diseases, mental diseases, rheumatoid arthritis, and respiratory diseases.

Health and Health Behavior

This subcategory of personal factors describes the influence of general *health* factors, for example, self-perceived health status, multi-morbidity, and health behavior. A better health (i.e., better general health, no multi-morbidity, less depressive symptoms, and no sleeping problems) reduces sick leave, results in earlier return to work following sick leave, and reduces the risk of work disability for individuals with chronic diseases, including individuals with mental diseases and musculoskeletal diseases (Detaille et al. 2009; de Vries et al. 2017; Rashid et al. 2017; Spelten et al. 2002; de Wit et al. 2018). The effects of better health on work participation are strong as, for example, in a study by Van der Giezen and colleagues, individuals with musculoskeletal diseases reporting a good self-perceived health status were 1.5 times more likely to return to work compared to individuals with musculoskeletal diseases reporting a poor self-perceived health status (van der Giezen et al. 2000). Regarding *health behavior*, not smoking reduces sick leave and results in earlier return to work following sick leave among individuals with musculoskeletal diseases (de Vries et al. 2017).

Psychological Resources
Several *psychological resources*, such as positive recovery beliefs, being ready for change and willing to utilize health strategies, are associated with sustained work participation, including shorter sick leave episodes and a lower risk of work disability (Kuijer et al. 2006; Laisné et al. 2012; Rashid et al. 2017; Thisted et al. 2017; de Wit et al. 2018). This applies for individuals with chronic diseases, including individuals with mental diseases and individuals with musculoskeletal diseases. Among individuals with musculoskeletal diseases, coping, self-efficacy, self-esteem, and somatization were not associated with work participation (de Vries et al. 2012; Laisné et al. 2012). However, there is an indication that a higher self-efficacy is associated with sustained work participation among individuals with chronic diseases in general (de Wit et al. 2018). Furthermore, locus of control was not associated with work participation among individuals with chronic diseases in general (de Wit et al. 2018) nor among individuals with mental diseases and individuals with musculoskeletal diseases (Laisné et al. 2012; Hensing and Wahlström 2004).

Environmental Factors

With regard to *environmental factors*, we distinguish social and occupational factors (see Fig. 1).

Social Factors
Social factors describe the influence of the living situation, perceived support from and attitude of significant others, and perceived support at work regarding working with a health problem. Several social factors were studied in the literature, such as social support and opinion of relatives, life events, social network, and family-related problems. A positive attitude, encouragement, motivation, and communication of significant others relate with sustained work participation, including shorter sick leave episodes of individuals with chronic diseases (Snippen et al. 2019). Among individuals with musculoskeletal diseases, more positive expectations of a significant other about illness and condition reduce sick leave and result in earlier return to work following sick leave (Kuijer et al. 2006).

Occupational Factors
Occupational factors are classified as follows: job demands, job resources, work organization and culture, working conditions, and employment terms.

Job demands – Lower job demands, such as lower job strain, no physically heavy work, and no difficulties in handling work tasks, were found to reduce sick leave, reduce the risk of work disability, and result in earlier return to work following sick leave (De Croon et al. 2004; de Vries et al. 2017; Hansson and Jensen 2004;

Van Muijen et al. 2013; Spelten et al. 2002; Steenstra et al. 2017; Thisted et al. 2017). This was studied in individuals with cancer, mental diseases, musculoskeletal diseases, and rheumatoid arthritis. For instance, in a study by Young et al. (2002), individuals with rheumatoid arthritis who did manual work had a five times higher risk of work disability compared to individuals with rheumatoid arthritis who did sedentary work.

Job resources – Examples of job resources facilitating work participation are job control, co-worker and supervisor support, and a positive attitude of co-workers regarding working with a health problem. We found that having more resources at work is associated with a higher probability of sustained work participation and shorter sick leave episodes among individuals with cancer, mental diseases, and musculoskeletal disease (de Vries et al. 2017; Greidanus et al. 2018; Spelten et al. 2002; Thisted et al. 2017; Campbell et al. 2013).

Work organization and culture – For individuals with cancer and individuals with mental diseases, the presence of organizational policies aiming at an open communication, and a positive and supporting work environment, relates to sustained work participation, including shorter sick leave episodes and a lower risk of work disability (de Vries et al. 2017; Greidanus et al. 2018; Thisted et al. 2017).

Working conditions – More variations in work reduce sick leave and result in earlier return to work following sick leave among individuals with musculoskeletal disease (Kuijer et al. 2006). However, no associations were found for other working conditions, such as company type (i.e., private or self-employed), organization size, and vibrations at work, with work participation among individuals with mental diseases and musculoskeletal diseases (de Vries et al. 2017; Hansson and Jensen 2004; Lagerveld et al. 2010; Kuijer et al. 2006).

Employment terms – Among individuals with cancer, musculoskeletal diseases, and rheumatoid arthritis, no associations were found between employment terms such as less working hours, job tenure, or flexible working hours with work participation (De Croon et al. 2004; de Vries et al. 2012; Van Muijen et al. 2013).

Considerations and Knowledge Gaps

We showed that *sustainable work participation* among individuals with chronic diseases is influenced by a wide range of personal and environmental factors. In Box 1, we present a case description illustrating how personal and socio-environmental factors can make a positive difference regarding work participation.

> **Box 1 Case description**
> Edward is 30 years old, has chronic low back pain, and works as a construction worker. Edward does not smoke, he is physically active during leisure time, and his partner has positive expectations regarding functioning with his low back pain. Edward is a manager of a team with 18 highly motivated

(continued)

Box 1 (continued)
professionals, and he experiences freedom to manage his team as he sees best. He likes his job, and his colleagues are very supportive regarding his back pain; they relieve him when it is necessary, and he can work from home. Although Edward has been experiencing chronic low back pain for 2 years, he does not take up more sick leave days compared to his colleagues without back pain.

Similar to the general population, individuals with chronic diseases with a higher *level of education* experience fewer work participation problems compared to individuals with a lower level of education. Furthermore, young male individuals with chronic diseases are more likely to prolong work participation. Therefore, among individuals with chronic diseases, specific groups are extra vulnerable with regard to work participation, i.e., women, older individuals, lower educated individuals, and those with poor working conditions. These groups need specific attention from professionals and policy makers.

Psychological factors playing an important role in work participation are readiness for change and positive recovery beliefs. Information about these factors provide promising input for the development of interventions for work participation with chronic diseases, such as behavioral interventions focusing on return to work. Occupational factors important for work participation with chronic diseases are job demands and influence at work. A healthy lifestyle and positive attitude toward work from significant others are important as well. Following this, examples of possible interventions are investing in the development of skills and knowledge where possible and improving support regarding access to work for those with a lower socioeconomic position. Work adjustments and strengthening social support at work and at home should be encouraged to enable empowerment through *self-management* of individuals with chronic diseases (Huber et al. 2011).

Knowledge Gaps

In this section, we will address some knowledge gaps in the scientific literature on the personal and environmental factors that may hinder or facilitate sustained work participation of individuals with chronic diseases. The first gap is that not all employment outcomes were studied in the available reviews. To illustrate, reviews focusing on *work disability* are scarce, and we did not find any reviews focusing on presenteeism (i.e., productivity loss due to health problems) and early retirement specifically of individuals with chronic diseases. Although single studies on presenteeism and *early retirement* among individuals with chronic diseases are available in the literature (Haglund et al. 2015; Karoly et al. 2013; Boot et al. 2018; Leijten et al. 2015), more literature reviews focusing on these employment outcomes are required. In the context of an increasing retirement age, it is important to determine why individuals with chronic diseases retire early and how they could be supported to remain in the labor market for a longer period of time. Furthermore, it is important to gain more insight into factors influencing presenteeism for individuals with chronic diseases. That is, presenteeism is a consequence of health problems but may also lead to further deterioration of self-rated health, and it may be a precursor of sickness absence as well (Skagen and Collins 2016). Additionally, it is important to gain insight into the process beyond participation in work, for example, how individuals with chronic diseases function at work (Abma et al. 2018), what kind of struggles they experience during work performance, and to what extent their chronic condition impacts their ability to meet the demands of their work. This may show possibilities and directions for interventions to facilitate sustainable work participation and improve productivity at work of these vulnerable workers with poor health.

The second gap was that the majority of the identified systematic reviews focused on musculoskeletal disorders, followed by mental diseases. We argue that the personal and environmental factors related to work participation are independent of diagnosis or chronic disease; therefore, we should not distinguish between different types of chronic diseases. It is possible that *disease-specific factors* have a greater impact on work participation among individuals in the acute phase of a disease, whereas personal and environmental factors may have a greater impact on work participation among individuals in the chronic phase of a disease (Baanders et al. 2002; Loisel 2014). In addition, the prevalence of multi-morbidity increases. From an intervention point of view, one approach targeting disease-generic factors might thus be more relevant than separate approaches targeting disease-specific factors. Furthermore, implementing interventions targeting individuals with chronic diseases in general is more practical compared to targeting every specific disease with specific interventions.

Third, several trends are observed in the labor market that are not yet taken into account in the reviews. First, our workforce is aging. Since the risk of chronic disease and multi-morbidity increases with age, it is also important to focus on the vulnerable group of older workers with health problems. Moreover, an aging population increases the need for *informal caregiving*. Following this, individuals in general as well as individuals with chronic diseases may more often have to combine paid work with providing care to a family member which could affect someone's work-life balance (Carmichael et al. 2008). Furthermore, individuals with chronic diseases have to cope with several other developments in the labor market. For example, the labor market is becoming more flexible. Traditionally, organizations had a large proportion of workers with a permanent contract and a small proportion of workers with *temporary contracts*. Currently, a transition has taken place in the labor market from permanent contracts to temporary contracts. This particularly affects young professionals entering the labor market. Those with chronic diseases may become extra vulnerable since they already experience difficulties in finding a job (Schuring et al. 2007). In addition, there has been an increase in self-employment in the labor market. Self-employed workers differ from employees regarding job characteristics and social security and may require a different approach in return to work or work disability prevention strategies (Bjuggren et al. 2012; Hatfield 2015; Schonfeld and Mazzola 2015).

Conclusions and Future Directions

In this chapter, we described the influence of personal and environmental factors on work participation of individuals with chronic diseases, and these factors were disease generic instead of disease specific. Those who are women, older, and having a low *socioeconomic status* (including lower educational level) besides having a chronic disease seem to be extra vulnerable when it comes to work participation. Good health as well as healthy behavior, having adequate psychological resources, a supportive social environment, low job demands, adequate job resources, the presence of organizational policies at work aiming at an open communication, and a positive and supporting work environment enable individuals with chronic diseases to work sustainably.

Recommendations

- Healthcare professionals are encouraged to pay more attention to work participation as a *patient-reported outcome* of treatment. They should focus on empowerment (i.e., discussing work adjustments with employer) of their patients with chronic diseases to improve work participation.
- Employers are encouraged to pay more attention to balance job demands and job resources, to improve social support at work, and to implement organizational policies aiming at an open communication and a positive and supporting work environment in order to facilitate employees with chronic diseases to work sustainably.
- Governments are encouraged to pay more attention to specific *vulnerable groups* among individuals with chronic diseases in the labor market. Vulnerable groups are older workers, women, workers with low socioeconomic status, and those with poor working conditions.
- Researchers should investigate personal and environmental factors that play a role in work participation among individuals with chronic diseases related to early retirement and presenteeism and take into account the flexible labor market as a contextual factor that might increase vulnerability.
- All stakeholders, i.e., (occupational) healthcare professionals, employers, governments, and researchers, should take into consideration how developments in the labor market influence health and employment outcomes. Specific challenging developments involve the increasing demand to work longer, increasing demand to provide informal care, and a labor market that is becoming more and more flexible.

Cross-References

▶ Concepts of Work Ability in Rehabilitation
▶ Employment as a Key Rehabilitation Outcome
▶ Reducing Inequalities in Employment of People with Disabilities
▶ Shifting the Focus from Work Reintegration to Sustainability of Employment

References

Abma FI, Bültmann U, Amick I BC, Arends I, Dorland HF, Flach PA, van der Klink JJL, van de Ven HA, Bjørner JB (2018) The work role functioning questionnaire v2.0 showed consistent factor structure across six working samples. J Occup Rehabil 28(3):465–474. https://doi.org/10.1007/s10926-017-9722-1

Achterberg T, Wind H, De Boer A, Frings-Dresen M (2009) Factors that promote or hinder young disabled people in work participation: a systematic review. J Occup Rehabil 19(2):129–141

Baanders AN, Rijken PM, Peters L (2002) Labour participation of the chronically ill: a profile sketch. Eur J Public Health 12(2):124–130

Bjuggren CM, Johansson D, Stenkula M (2012) Using self-employment as proxy for entrepreneurship: some empirical caveats. Int J Entrep Small Bus 17(3):290–303

Blank L, Peters J, Pickvance S, Wilford J, MacDonald E (2008) A systematic review of the factors which predict return to work for people suffering episodes of poor mental health. J Occup Rehabil 18(1):27–34

Boot CRL, de Wind A, van Vilsteren M, van der Beek AJ, van Schaardenburg D, Anema JR (2018) One-year predictors of presenteeism in workers with rheumatoid arthritis: disease-related factors and characteristics of general health and work. J Rheumatol 45(6):766–770. https://doi.org/10.3899/jrheum.170586

Börsch-Supan A, Brandt M, Hunkler C, Kneip T, Korbmacher J, Malter F, Schaan B, Stuck S, Zuber S (2013) Data resource profile: the Survey of Health, Ageing and Retirement in Europe (SHARE). Int J Epidemiol 42(4):992–1001

Campbell P, Wynne-Jones G, Muller S, Dunn KM (2013) The influence of employment social support for risk and prognosis in nonspecific back pain: a systematic review and critical synthesis. Int Arch Occup Environ Health 86(2):119–137. https://doi.org/10.1007/s00420-012-0804-2

Carmichael F, Hulme C, Sheppard S, Connell G (2008) Work – life imbalance: Informal care and paid employment in the UK. Fem Econ 14(2):3–35. https://doi.org/10.1080/13545700701881005

Cornelius L, Van der Klink J, Groothoff J, Brouwer S (2011) Prognostic factors of long term disability due to mental disorders: a systematic review. J Occup Rehabil 21(2):259–274

De Croon E, Sluiter J, Nijssen T, Dijkmans B, Lankhorst G, Frings-Dresen M (2004) Predictive factors of work disability in rheumatoid arthritis: a systematic literature review. Ann Rheum Dis 63(11):1362–1367

de Vries HJ, Reneman MF, Groothoff JW, Geertzen JH, Brouwer S (2012) Factors promoting staying at work in people with chronic nonspecific musculoskeletal pain: a systematic review. Disabil Rehabil 34(6):443–458

de Vries H, Fishta A, Weikert B, Sanchez AR, Wegewitz U (2017) Determinants of sickness absence and return to work among employees with common mental disorders: a scoping review. J Occup Rehabil 28(3):393–417 de Wit M, Wind H, Hulshof CTJ, Frings-Dresen MHW (2018) Person-related factors associated with work participation in employees with health problems: a systematic review. Int Arch Occup Environ Health 91(5):497–512. https://doi.org/10.1007/s00420-018-1308-5

Dekkers-Sanchez PM, Hoving JL, Sluiter JK, Frings-Dresen MH (2008) Factors associated with long-term sick leave in sick-listed employees: a systematic review. Occup Environ Med 65 (3):153–157. https://doi.org/10.1136/oem.2007.034983

Detaille SI, Heerkens YF, Engels JA, Van Der Gulden JW, Van Dijk FJ (2009) Common prognostic factors of work disability among employees with a chronic somatic disease: a systematic review of cohort studies. Scand J Work Environ Health 35:261–281

Eurostat (2015) Population by type of longstanding health problem, sex and age. Eurostat. http://appsso.eurostat.ec.europa.eu/nui/show.do?dataset=hlth_dp020&lang=en. Accessed 06 Aug 2018

Geyh S, Peter C, Muller R, Bickenbach JE, Kostanjsek N, Ustun BT, Stucki G, Cieza A (2011) The Personal Factors of the International Classification of Functioning, Disability and Health in the literature – a systematic review and content analysis. Disabil Rehabil 33(13–14):1089–1102. https://doi.org/10.3109/09638288.2010.523104

Greidanus M, de Boer A, de Rijk A, Tiedtke C, Dierckx de Casterlé B, Frings-Dresen M, Tamminga S (2018) Perceived employer-related barriers and facilitators for work participation of cancer survivors: a systematic review of employers' and survivors' perspectives. Psychooncology 27 (3):725–733

Haglund E, Petersson IF, Bremander A, Bergman S (2015) Predictors of presenteeism and activity impairment outside work in patients with spondyloarthritis. J Occup Rehabil 25(2):288–295. https://doi.org/10.1007/s10926-014-9537-2

Hansson T, Jensen I (2004) Chapter 6. Sickness absence due to back and neck disorders. Scand J Public Health 32(63_suppl):109–151

Hatfield I (2015) Self-employment in Europe. Institute for Public Policy Research, London

Heerkens Y, Engels J, Kuiper C, Van der Gulden J, Oostendorp R (2004) The use of the ICF to describe work related factors influencing the health of employees. Disabil Rehabil 26 (17):1060–1066. https://doi.org/10.1080/09638280410001703530

Hensing G, Wahlström R (2004) Chapter 7. Sickness absence and psychiatric disorders. Scand J Public Health 32(63_suppl):152–180

Huber M, Knottnerus JA, Green L, van der Horst H, Jadad AR, Kromhout D, Leonard B, Lorig K, Loureiro MI, van der Meer JW (2011) How should we define health? BMJ 343:d4163

Johansson G, Lundberg I (2004) Adjustment latitude and attendance requirements as determinants of sickness absence or attendance. Empirical tests of the illness flexibility model. Soc Sci Med 58(10):1857–1868

Karoly P, Ruehlman LS, Okun MA (2013) Psychosocial and demographic correlates of employment vs disability status in a national community sample of adults with chronic pain: toward a psychology of pain presenteeism. Pain Med (Malden) 14(11):1698–1707. https://doi.org/10.1111/pme.12234

Koopmanschap MA, Burdorf A, Lötters FJB (2013) Work absenteeism and productivity loss at work. In: Handbook of work disability. Springer, New York. 31–41

Kuijer W, Groothoff JW, Brouwer S, Geertzen JH, Dijkstra PU (2006) Prediction of sickness absence in patients with chronic low back pain: a systematic review. J Occup Rehabil 16 (3):430–458

Lagerveld S, Bültmann U, Franche R, Van Dijk F, Vlasveld M, Van der Feltz-Cornelis C, Bruinvels D, Huijs J, Blonk R, Van Der Klink J (2010) Factors associated with work participation and work functioning in depressed workers: a systematic review. J Occup Rehabil 20(3):275–292

Laisné F, Lecomte C, Corbière M (2012) Biopsychosocial predictors of prognosis in musculoskeletal disorders: a systematic review of the literature (corrected and republished). Disabil Rehabil 34(22):1912–1941

Leijten FR, de Wind A, van den Heuvel SG, Ybema JF, van der Beek AJ, Robroek SJ, Burdorf A (2015) The influence of chronic health problems and work-related factors on loss of paid employment among older workers. J Epidemiol Community Health 69(11):1058–1065. https://doi.org/10.1136/jech-2015-205719

Loisel PAJ (2014) Handbook of work disability: prevention and management. Springer, New York

Milner A, LaMontagne AD, Aitken Z, Bentley R, Kavanagh AM (2014) Employment status and mental health among persons with and without a disability: evidence from an Australian cohort study. J Epidemiol Community Health 68(11):1064–1071. https://doi.org/10.1136/jech-2014-204147

Murray CJ, Vos T, Lozano R, Naghavi M, Flaxman AD, Michaud C, Ezzati M, Shibuya K, Salomon JA, Abdalla S, Aboyans V, Abraham J, Ackerman I, Aggarwal R, Ahn SY, Ali MK, Alvarado M, Anderson HR, Anderson LM, Andrews KG, Atkinson C, Baddour LM, Bahalim AN, Barker-Collo S, Barrero LH, Bartels DH, Basanez MG, Baxter A, Bell ML, Benjamin EJ, Bennett D, Bernabe E, Bhalla K, Bhandari B, Bikbov B, Bin Abdulhak A, Birbeck G, Black JA, Blencowe H, Blore JD, Blyth F, Bolliger I, Bonaventure A, Boufous S, Bourne R, Boussinesq M, Braithwaite T, Brayne C, Bridgett L, Brooker S, Brooks P, Brugha TS, Bryan-Hancock C, Bucello C, Buchbinder R, Buckle G, Budke CM, Burch M, Burney P, Burstein R, Calabria B, Campbell B, Canter CE, Carabin H, Carapetis J, Carmona L, Cella C, Charlson F, Chen H, Cheng AT, Chou D, Chugh SS, Coffeng LE, Colan SD, Colquhoun S, Colson KE, Condon J, Connor MD, Cooper LT, Corriere M, Cortinovis M, de Vaccaro KC, Couser W, Cowie BC, Criqui MH, Cross M, Dabhadkar KC, Dahiya M, Dahodwala N, Damsere-Derry J, Danaei G, Davis A, De Leo D, Degenhardt L, Dellavalle R, Delossantos A, Denenberg J, Derrett S, Des Jarlais DC, Dharmaratne SD, Dherani M, Diaz-Torne C, Dolk H, Dorsey ER, Driscoll T, Duber H, Ebel B, Edmond K, Elbaz A, Ali SE, Erskine H, Erwin PJ, Espindola P, Ewoigbokhan SE, Farzadfar F, Feigin V, Felson DT, Ferrari A, Ferri CP, Fevre EM, Finucane MM, Flaxman S, Flood L, Foreman K, Forouzanfar MH, Fowkes FG, Fransen M, Freeman MK, Gabbe BJ, Gabriel SE, Gakidou E, Ganatra HA, Garcia B, Gaspari F, Gillum RF, Gmel G, Gonzalez-Medina D, Gosselin R, Grainger R, Grant B, Groeger J, Guillemin F, Gunnell D, Gupta R, Haagsma J, Hagan H, Halasa YA, Hall W, Haring D, Haro JM, Harrison JE, Havmoeller R, Hay RJ, Higashi H, Hill C, Hoen B, Hoffman H, Hotez PJ, Hoy D, Huang JJ, Ibeanusi SE, Jacobsen KH, James SL, Jarvis D, Jasrasaria R, Jayaraman S, Johns N, Jonas JB, Karthikeyan G, Kassebaum N, Kawakami N, Keren A, Khoo JP, King CH, Knowlton LM, Kobusingye O, Koranteng A, Krishnamurthi R, Laden F, Lalloo R, Laslett LL, Lathlean T, Leasher JL, Lee YY, Leigh J, Levinson D, Lim SS, Limb E, Lin JK, Lipnick M, Lipshultz SE, Liu W, Loane M, Ohno SL, Lyons R, Mabweijano J, MF MI, Malekzadeh R, Mallinger L, Manivannan S, Marcenes W, March L, Margolis DJ, Marks GB, Marks R, Matsumori A, Matzopoulos R, Mayosi BM, McAnulty JH, McDermott MM, McGill N, McGrath J, Medina-Mora ME, Meltzer M, Mensah GA, Merriman TR, Meyer AC, Miglioli V, Miller M, Miller TR, Mitchell PB, Mock C, Mocumbi AO, Moffitt TE, Mokdad AA, Monasta L, Montico M, Moradi-Lakeh M, Moran A, Morawska L, Mori R, Murdoch ME, Mwaniki MK, Naidoo K, Nair MN, Naldi L, Narayan KM, Nelson PK, Nelson RG, Nevitt MC, Newton CR, Nolte S, Norman P, Norman R, O'Donnell M, O'Hanlon S, Olives C, Omer SB, Ortblad K, Osborne R, Ozgediz D, Page A, Pahari B, Pandian JD, Rivero AP, Patten SB, Pearce N, Padilla RP, Perez-Ruiz F, Perico N, Pesudovs K, Phillips D, Phillips MR, Pierce K, Pion S, Polanczyk GV, Polinder S, Pope CA 3rd, Popova S, Porrini E, Pourmalek F, Prince M, Pullan RL, Ramaiah KD, Ranganathan D, Razavi H, Regan M, Rehm JT, Rein DB, Remuzzi G, Richardson K, Rivara FP, Roberts T, Robinson C, De Leon FR, Ronfani L, Room R, Rosenfeld LC, Rushton L, Sacco RL, Saha S, Sampson U, Sanchez-Riera L, Sanman E, Schwebel DC, Scott JG, Segui-Gomez M, Shahraz S, Shepard DS, Shin H, Shivakoti R, Singh D, Singh GM, Singh JA, Singleton J, Sleet DA, Sliwa K, Smith E, Smith JL, Stapelberg NJ, Steer A, Steiner T, Stolk WA, Stovner LJ, Sudfeld C, Syed S, Tamburlini G, Tavakkoli M, Taylor HR, Taylor JA, Taylor WJ, Thomas B, Thomson WM, Thurston GD, Tleyjeh IM, Tonelli M, Towbin JA, Truelsen T, Tsilimbaris MK, Ubeda C, Undurraga EA, van der Werf MJ, van Os J, Vavilala MS, Venketasubramanian N, Wang M, Wang W, Watt K, Weatherall DJ, Weinstock MA, Weintraub R, Weisskopf MG, Weissman MM, White RA, Whiteford H, Wiebe N, Wiersma ST, Wilkinson JD, Williams HC, Williams SR, Witt

E, Wolfe F, Woolf AD, Wulf S, Yeh PH, Zaidi AK, Zheng ZJ, Zonies D, Lopez AD, AlMazroa MA, Memish ZA (2012) Disability-adjusted life years (DALYs) for 291 diseases and injuries in 21 regions, 1990-2010: a systematic analysis for the Global Burden of Disease Study 2010. Lancet (Lond) 380(9859):2197–2223. https://doi.org/10.1016/s0140-6736(12)61689-4

Peters J, Pickvance S, Wilford J, MacDonald E, Blank L (2007) Predictors of delayed return to work or job loss with respiratory ill-health: a systematic review. J Occup Rehabil 17(2):317–326

Rashid M, Kristofferzon M-L, Nilsson A, Heiden M (2017) Factors associated with return to work among people on work absence due to long-term neck or back pain: a narrative systematic review. BMJ Open 7(6):e014939

Remington PL, Brownson RC (2011) Fifty years of progress in chronic disease epidemiology and control. MMWR Surveill Summ 60(Suppl 4):70–77

Schonfeld IS, Mazzola JJ (2015) A qualitative study of stress in individuals self-employed in solo businesses. J Occup Health Psychol 20(4):501

Schuring M, Burdorf L, Kunst A, Mackenbach J (2007) The effects of ill health on entering and maintaining paid employment: evidence in European countries. J Epidemiol Community Health 61(7):597–604

Schuring M, Mackenbach J, Voorham T, Burdorf A (2011) The effect of re-employment on perceived health. J Epidemiol Community Health 65(7):639–644. https://doi.org/10.1136/jech.2009.103838

Sen A (1993) Capability and well-being. The quality of life. Oxford University Press, Oxford

Sigg R, De-Luigi V (2007) The success of policies aimed at extending working life. In Developments and trends supporting dynamic social security. International Social Security Association, Switzerland. 51

Skagen K, Collins AM (2016) The consequences of sickness presenteeism on health and wellbeing over time: a systematic review. Soc Sci Med 161:169–177. https://doi.org/10.1016/j.socscimed.2016.06.005

Snippen NC, de Vries HJ, van der Burg-Vermeulen SJ, Hagedoorn M, Brouwer S (2019) Influence of significant others on work participation of individuals with chronic diseases: a systematic review. BMJ Open 9(1):e021742. https://doi.org/10.1136/bmjopen-2018-021742

Spelten ER, Sprangers MA, Verbeek JH (2002) Factors reported to influence the return to work of cancer survivors: a literature review. Psychooncology 11(2):124–131

Steenstra IA, Munhall C, Irvin E, Oranye N, Passmore S, Van Eerd D, Mahood Q, Hogg-Johnson S (2017) Systematic review of prognostic factors for return to work in workers with sub acute and chronic low back pain. J Occup Rehabil 27(3):369–381

Thisted CN, Nielsen CV, Bjerrum M (2017) Work participation among employees with common mental disorders: a meta-synthesis. J Occup Rehabil 28(3):452–464

van der Giezen AM, Bouter LM, Nijhuis FJ (2000) Prediction of return-to-work of low back pain patients sicklisted for 3–4 months. Pain 87(3):285–294

van der Klink JJ, Bültmann U, Burdorf A, Schaufeli WB, Zijlstra FR, Abma FI, Brouwer S, van der Wilt GJ (2016) Sustainable employability-definition, conceptualization, and implications: a perspective based on the capability approach. Scand J Work Environ Health 42(1):71–79

Van Muijen P, Weevers N, Snels IA, Duijts S, Bruinvels DJ, Schellart AJ, Van Der Beek AJ (2013) Predictors of return to work and employment in cancer survivors: a systematic review. Eur J Cancer Care 22(2):144–160

van Rijn RM, Robroek SJ, Brouwer S, Burdorf A (2014) Influence of poor health on exit from paid employment: a systematic review. Occup Environ Med 71(4):295–301. https://doi.org/10.1136/oemed-2013-101591

Vooijs M, Leensen MC, Hoving JL, Daams JG, Wind H, Frings-Dresen MH (2015) Disease-generic factors of work participation of workers with a chronic disease: a systematic review. Int Arch Occup Environ Health 88(8):1015–1029

WHO (2001) International classification of functioning, disability and health: ICF. WHO, Geneva

Young A, Dixey J, Kulinskaya E, Cox N, Davies P, Devlin J, Emery P, Gough A, James D, Prouse P (2002) Which patients stop working because of rheumatoid arthritis? Results of five years' follow up in 732 patients from the Early RA Study (ERAS). Ann Rheum Dis 61(4):335–340

Cancer Survivors at the Workplace

22

Anja Mehnert-Theuerkauf

Contents

Cancer as a Chronic Disease	400
Cancer Survivorship and the Burden of Health Problems	400
Employment and Return to Work	403
Prevalence of Employment and Return to Work	403
Factors Related to Employment and Return to Work	403
Barriers Related to Not Returning to Work and to Job Loss	405
Sick Leave and Length of Absence from Work	406
Reduction in Work Hours, Wages, and Work Changes	407
Work Ability	408
Career Changes	409
Quality of Life Issues	409
Interventions to Promote Return to Work	411
Cross-References	411
References	412

Abstract

Retaining or returning to working life is playing an increasingly important role for cancer patients through improved survival rates. Whether patients succeed in working with and after cancer depends on a variety of societal, economic, and individual medical and psychosocial factors. Many cancer patients have a high motivation to return to work when their physical and mental ability is given. However, research also shows the high prevalence of long term and late effects of multimodal cancer therapies during cancer survivorship. Prevalent health problems in cancer survivors that adversely impact work include psychological distress, pain, fatigue, depression, as well as a poor health condition and limited quality of life. In addition to physical and psychosocial health problems, a variety

A. Mehnert-Theuerkauf (✉)
Department of Medical Psychology and Medical Sociology, University Medical Center Leipzig, Leipzig, Germany
e-mail: anja.mehnert@medizin.uni-leipzig.de

© Springer Nature Switzerland AG 2020
U. Bültmann, J. Siegrist (eds.), *Handbook of Disability, Work and Health*, Handbook Series in Occupational Health Sciences, https://doi.org/10.1007/978-3-030-24334-0_22

of barriers and facilitators have been identified as factors that affect return to work such as a low socioeconomic status as well as insufficient education and training, heavy physical work, and adverse working conditions with regard to the possibility of flexible working arrangements and support. Cancer survivorship programs and self-management interventions need to address these late and long-term health problems in order to better facilitate retaining or returning to work. Interdisciplinary occupational intervention programs involving physical, psychosocial, and occupational components are effective in terms of return to work.

Keywords

Cancer survivorship · Return to work · Employment/unemployment · Rehabilitation · Quality of life · Work ability

Cancer as a Chronic Disease

Cancer Survivorship and the Burden of Health Problems

Cancer is among the most common causes of mortality and morbidity worldwide. Overall, there were 14 million new cancer cases worldwide in 2012 and 20 million new cancer cases are predicted by 2025 (Ferlay et al. 2015). The most commonly diagnosed cancers are lung, breast, prostate, and colorectal cancer. The improved clinical diagnostics and multimodal medical treatments of cancer have led to a longer survival time for many patients, as epidemiological studies show (Ferlay et al. 2015). And although the cancer incidence is increasing with higher age, a significant number of patients are diagnosed during working age (Oortwijn et al. 2011).

With life expectancy steadily rising in countries with a higher Human Development Index (United Nations 2018), older people will increasingly continue to work longer. Thus, the short-, medium-, and long-term follow-up problems and long-term consequences of cancer and its treatments are of high importance for the employment prognosis of individual patients as well as for the society as a whole. A population-based analysis of the cost of all cancers in Europe shows that 60% of the economic burden stems from non-healthcare costs, namely informal costs including unpaid care and costs associated with lost productivity, sick leave, and lost working days (Luengo-Fernandez et al. 2013).

The variety of physical and psychosocial consequences of cancer can have a negative impact on returning to work and remaining in work despite improved medical treatment options (de Boer et al. 2009; Mehnert 2011; Dorland et al. 2018a, 2018b). Cancer survivors face a variety of biological and psychosocial stressors during the disease trajectory. The high physical burden and neurobiological changes adversely affect patients' quality of life and emotional well-being. Patients experience a variety of affective states, including anxiety and depression that closely interact with biologic stressors such as pain and fatigue. Psychological problems are also associated with changes in social roles, increasing dependency, the need to adjust to impaired functional status, and existential concerns such as the search for meaning in life.

Epidemiological studies on mental comorbidity in cancer patients show that the 4-week prevalence for any mental disorder is 32% (Mehnert et al. 2014), with a high variance between the different tumor entities, ranging from 20% to 42%. The most common mental disorders in cancer patients include adjustment disorders, anxiety disorders, and affective disorders such as depression (Mitchell et al. 2011; Mehnert et al. 2014, 2018; Hartung et al. 2017). Almost every second cancer patient (52%) feels emotionally distressed and reports an average of eight problems, most frequently fatigue, pain, and problems getting around. Patients also have to deal with difficult treatment decisions as well as a changed life situation and life goals. Individual characteristics such as age or education, personality patterns, coping strategies, family functioning, and social support can affect both the perception of stressors and the onset of psychosocial distress and mental disorders.

Cancer survivorship research seeks to identify, examine, prevent, and control adverse cancer diagnosis and treatment-related outcomes such as long-term and late effects of treatment, second cancers, and quality of life, and provide broad knowledge regarding optimal follow-up care and surveillance of cancer survivors. Major aspects of medium- and long-term survival include chronic pain, cancer-specific fatigue, psychosocial stress, infertility, quality of life, health literacy, and lifestyle change, as well as employment and work-related issues (Aaronson et al. 2014). With an increasing prevalence of cancer in the working-age population worldwide, more evidence is needed to better understand factors both promoting and limiting employment and work-related aspects in cancer patients. Key research areas with regard to employment comprise the investigation of risk and prognostic factors for adverse work-related events including unemployment and unintended early retirement in cancer in different cancer populations and the development and evaluation of effective employer or employee specific interventions and occupational rehabilitation programs to support patients stay employed or return to work.

Previous research has indicated the significance of work in cancer survivorship. The motivation to continue work during treatment or to return to work after treatment completion seems strong in many cancer patients when their physical ability is given (Mahar et al. 2008; Mehnert and Koch 2013; Stergiou-Kita et al. 2014). Many patients associate employment with the return to normalcy. In addition to financial incentives, work in cancer survivors has been mainly linked to meaning, the maintenance of personal identity, social relationships and social roles, daily structure, self-esteem, and life satisfaction (Peteet 2000; Hoffman 2005; Isaksson et al. 2016).

Work, and in particular meaningful work, can be described as an activity through which an individual uses his talents, learns and grows, creates new relations, develops his/her identity and a sense of belonging, worth, and dignity (Morin 2004). To work can provide the opportunity for individuals to accomplish things in life, to surpass oneself, and to achieve a sense of self-fulfillment and legacy. However, work can also become problematic and lead to adverse personal consequences when an individual cannot relate to it and does experience labor exploitation, excessive mental and/or physical demands, job discrimination, an increasing exposure to demands for flexibility and mobility at work, or a sense of alienation.

According to Morin (2004), there are three approaches to the study of meaning of work:

- Significance of work can be defined as the importance and individual attributes to work, its representations of work, and the individually attributed principles and values of work.
- Orientation of work can be defined as an individual's orientation toward work, what he/she is seeking in his/her work, and the intents that guide his/her action such as autonomy, social advancement, self-achievement, social interactions, and risk-taking.
- Coherence of work can be defined as the coherence between the individual and the work he/she does; the level of harmony and balance he/she achieves in the relationship to work including expectations, values, and daily actions at work.

Peteet (2000) has specifically focused on the meaning of work in cancer survivors. He emphasized the importance of work for the maintenance of a sense of personal identity. For many cancer survivors, work is not only important to express and to realize core values, such as creating new knowledge and contributing to a community or the society, but to maintain or regain a social role which is often linked to work or specifically to a certain profession. The financial remuneration can help patients to define or redefine his/her role at home and within the family. Work furthermore has been found to play a key role in facilitating and maintaining social relationships which provide the individual with psychosocial support (Hoffman 2005; Chan et al. 2008). The experience of a cancer diagnosis can lead to a loss of sense of normalcy, intactness, or control (Peteet 2000). Return to work after or during treatment offers patients a sense of normalcy, the sense of being valued and of being a part of the community and the society.

The following quotation of a full-time retail owner does enlighten the importance of work for the personal identity as well as for the social life of an individual and the family: "I sold my retail business (23 years) because I would not have been able to perform my duties because of the demands of the treatment schedule. Personally, I was devastated by the loss of my business and the loss of any daily contacts, conferences etc. I was severely depressed by this – not by my cancer...Subsequently the loss of earnings impacted severely on us" (Bennett et al. 2009, p. 1060).

In addition to the individual meaning of work, employment for many cancer survivors provides several practical benefits including financial remuneration, health insurance, and health benefits, as well as daily structure to a patient's routine and formal social support at the workplace (Feuerstein et al. 2007; Earle et al. 2010).

Employment and Return to Work

Prevalence of Employment and Return to Work

Occupational aspects in cancer survivorship can be considered from different perspectives: (1) the cancer survivor (e.g., health, quality of life, work ability, employment or return to work, dealing with the cancer in the workplace, job satisfaction, discrimination, career prospects, or (early) retirement); (2) the caregiver and the family (e.g., the burden of care, partnership issues, financial problems, risk for poverty); (3) the employer and coworkers (e.g., working conditions, work load, working arrangements); (4) the healthcare provider (e.g., supportive care and rehabilitation needs, effective support programs and interventions); and (5) the community or society (e.g., economic and policy changes) (Mehnert et al. 2013).

Early return to work is a desirable goal for many patients (Kennedy et al. 2007; Lilliehorn et al. 2013). International reviews show that 1 year after diagnosis, an average of 62% of those affected by cancer return to work (or keep working during cancer treatments) with a huge range between 39% and 93% (Spelten et al. 2002; Mehnert 2011; Islam et al. 2014; Paltrinieri et al. 2018). Approximately 1 year after cancer rehabilitation, return rates are slightly higher with 76–79% (Böttcher et al. 2013; Mehnert and Koch 2013). The median interval between diagnosis and documented return to work was 2 years (Paltrinieri et al. 2018).

Despite a high level of motivation and willingness among cancer patients to return to work, a meta-analysis shows that cancer patients are at an increased risk of unemployment compared to healthy individuals (33.8% vs. 15.2%) (de Boer et al. 2009). Empirical studies also indicate numerous work-related changes in cancer patients. These include reduced monthly working hours, reduced likelihood of full-time work, reduction in income, reduced physical and mental work ability, changes in professional roles, less chance of promotion, and changes in relationships with colleagues and supervisors (Spelten et al. 2002; Mehnert 2011; Sun et al. 2017; Torp et al. 2017; Paltrinieri et al. 2018). A Danish registry study shows that cancer patients have an increased risk of early retirement (Carlsen et al. 2008a). The observed risk factors for early retirement included increased age, metastasis, manual labor, sick leave, physical and mental comorbidity, low education, and low income.

Factors Related to Employment and Return to Work

Figure 1 presents a model of factors influencing the occupational activity of cancer patients (Mehnert et al. 2013). This model first includes the legal framework as well as economic factors that determine the working conditions in a specific country. However, the work environment is also influenced by individual and interpersonal factors on the one hand and the consequences of cancer and treatment on the other hand. Vocational intervention and specific rehabilitation programs can influence these factors and improve the return to work or career of cancer patients.

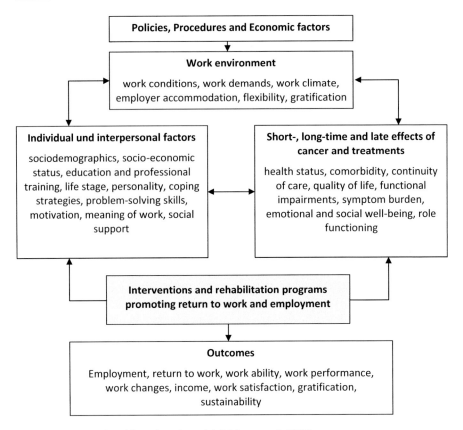

Fig. 1 Cancer survivorship and work model (Mehnert et al. 2013)

An early review by Spelten et al. (2002) found perceived employer accommodation for cancer and treatment as a strong and significant predictor for return to work. Recent studies and literature reviews seem to strengthen these findings (Mehnert 2011; Roelen et al. 2011a; Islam et al. 2014; Sun et al. 2017; Torp et al. 2017; Paltrinieri et al. 2018). Pryce et al. (2007) found a return to work meeting with employer as well as advice from doctor about work as factors significantly positive associated with return to work in cancer survivors. Moreover, counseling, miscellaneous training services, job replacement services, job search assistance, and maintenance services (Chan et al. 2008), as well as perceived employer accommodation (Bouknight et al. 2006) were significantly associated with a greater likelihood of being employed.

Further factors related to return to work are younger age and cancer sites of younger persons; higher levels of education, overall physician's performance, and continuity of care; absence of surgery, less physical symptoms, and the length of sick-leave as well as male gender (Mehnert 2011; Paltrinieri et al. 2018). Cancer types with a greater proportion of survivors working are genitourinary, melanoma, and Hodgkin's disease (Mehnert 2011). One important factor associated with working during treatment is the possibility of flexible working arrangements (Pryce et al. 2007; Mehnert 2011). Moreover, lower fatigue and higher value of work, work ability, and job self-efficacy of cancer survivors are associated with earlier return to work, particularly in breast cancer patients. Work ability and job self-efficacy seem to be key predictors (Wolvers et al. 2018).

Overall, reviews show the following fostering factors for return to work and employment of cancer patients (Mehnert 2011; van Muijen et al. 2013; Islam et al. 2014; Stergiou-Kita et al. 2014; Sun et al. 2017).

- **Work-related factors**: Perceived support from the employer, flexible working conditions, supportive working environment, type of work/nonmanual work, and higher income
- **Individual and medical factors**: Younger age, male gender, higher education and socioeconomic status, early cancer stage, less invasive therapies, better physical functioning, less symptoms, coping, shorter sick leave absence, higher work motivation, and work abilities
- **Factors related to environmental supports**: Partner and family, workplace, and professionals
- **Interventions**: Job-related counseling, rehabilitation, training and continuing education, and job-search assistance

Barriers Related to Not Returning to Work and to Job Loss

The majority of research reveals that a non-supportive work environment, perceived employer discrimination because of cancer and treatment, heavy manual work, low socioeconomic status, certain cancer types such as head and neck cancer, as well as the presence of functional impairments and symptom burden including fatigue and pain have been reported as barriers for returning to work (Spelten et al. 2002; Mehnert 2011; Rottenberg et al. 2016; Paltrinieri et al. 2018). Cancer survivors were found to have a significantly increased risk for unemployment both short term and longer term and were less likely to be reemployed (Park et al. 2008a; Syse et al. 2008; de Boer et al. 2009; Mehnert 2011; Paalman et al. 2016; Rottenberg et al. 2016; den Bakker et al. 2018; Grinshpun and Rottenberg 2018).

Several findings show that between 47% and 53% of cancer survivors lost their job or quitted working over a 12 months respectively 72 months period; and 26–50% of survivors lost their job or quitted working within the first year post diagnosis (Short et al. 2005; Choi et al. 2007; Park et al. 2008a, b; Mehnert 2011). However, between 23% and 75% of patients who lost their job were reemployed. Park et al. (2008a) showed that the mean time to job loss was 41 months, significantly lower in cancer patients than in non-cancer controls (50 months). The mean time to reemployment was 46 months (Park et al. 2008b). Likewise, the mean time to reemployment was significantly longer in cancer patients than in the non-cancer comparison group (47 months vs. 32 months) (Park et al. 2008b).

Risk for unemployment and for work disability was associated with extensive surgery, advanced tumor stage, higher age, female gender, lower levels of education, and lower socioeconomic status (Short et al. 2005; Bouknight et al. 2006; Choi et al. 2007; Chan et al. 2008; Park et al. 2008a; Mehnert 2011; Rottenberg et al. 2016; Paalman et al. 2016; Bennett et al. 2018; den Bakker et al. 2018).

A range of cancer sites has been associated with a higher risk for unemployment and job loss. These cancer sites include liver cancer, lung cancer, advanced blood cancer and lymph malignancies, brain and central nervous system cancers, gastrointestinal cancers including pancreatic cancer, and head and neck cancers (Short et al. 2005; Choi et al. 2007; Park et al. 2008a, b; Mehnert 2011; Paltrinieri et al. 2018). Results furthermore revealed the significant impact of socioeconomic and work-related factors on unemployment such as low income (Mehnert 2011; Paltrinieri et al. 2018).

A large body of research shows that the working environment, the nature of work as well as physically exhaustion and fatigue, poor health, and disablement as most frequent reasons for not returning to work or stop working. Particularly the presence of comorbid diseases and depression have been found as risk factors for unemployment (Spelten et al. 2002; Carlsen et al. 2008b; Mehnert 2011; Roelen et al. 2011a; Islam et al. 2014; Sun et al. 2017; Torp et al. 2017; den Bakker et al. 2018; Paltrinieri et al. 2018). A Danish study by Carlsen et al. (2008a) showed that cancer survivors had a significantly increased risk of early retirement pension compared to cancer-free controls. Risk factors for early retirement included older age; dissimilated disease, manual job, and sickness leave the year before taking early retirement pension, physical and psychological comorbidity, low education, and low income, as well as cancer sites containing leukemia, prostate cancer, and ovary cancer.

Sick Leave and Length of Absence from Work

Sick leave is an employee benefit in the form of paid leave which can be provided by the employer during periods of sickness to attend doctor visits or to care for family members. Overall, findings suggest call for increased awareness and evaluation of reasons for long-term work disability and sick leave absence in cancer survivors (Glimelius et al. 2015). Studies indicate a wide range of the length of sickness absence in cancer survivors from averagely 27 days in prostate cancer patients to averagely 11 months in early-stage breast cancer survivors. On the basis of the reported sick leave periods, the mean duration of absence from work is 151 days (Mehnert 2011). Short et al. (2005) reported that 41% of male and 39% female patients with mixed cancer sites who were working at the time of diagnosis stopped during cancer treatment. Older age, elementary school education, comorbidities, and presence of sequelae, as well as disease stage IV and having lung cancer were significantly associated with sick leave (Mehnert 2011). No significant differences in current sick leave between cancer survivors and (gender and age matched) non-cancer controls were found by Gudbergsson et al. (2007). Here, disease-free women had no longer length of sickness absence than women in the comparison group 3 years post diagnosis. Duration of absence from work was significantly longer in patients who underwent chemotherapy or multimodal treatment, who belonged to the most economically deprived group, who reported higher levels of fatigue, physical complaints, and higher workload, who were older, and who reported work changes due to cancer (Mehnert 2011).

Reduction in Work Hours, Wages, and Work Changes

The majority of studies that concentrated on working time report a reduction in work hours – at least partially or time limited – in cancer survivors (Mehnert 2011). Slightly more than 50% of survivors reduced their work schedule at least one time, although 86% of survivors returned to former work schedules (Bradley and Bednarek 2002). Compared with the general population, cancer survivors reported reduced working hours and had significantly more difficulties with reduced working hours (Mehnert 2011). Roelen et al. (2011a) showed that the proportion of full return to work decreased in the Netherlands in breast cancer survivors. Possible explanations include changes in disability policy, economic decline, and resulting decreases in work latitude and workplace accommodations (Roelen et al. 2011b).

For both genders, significant effects of survivorship on the probability of full-time employment and hours were found. However, it is noteworthy that again for both genders, these effects were primarily attributable to new cancers. There were no significant effects on the employment of cancer-free survivors (Mehnert 2011). Likewise, Peuckmann et al. (2008) found a similar extent of employment (paid by the hour, temporary work, and average weekly hours) between patients and the general women population. However, cancer survivors of both genders worked an average of 3–5 h less per week than non-cancer controls (Short et al. 2008). The majority of the cancer survivors who remained employed after treatment reduced work by more than 4 h per week with a mean reduction of 16 h per week (Steiner et al. 2008). In a further study, the mean hours per week were 49 h for full-time workers and 20 h for part-time workers (Bradley and Bednarek 2002). A reduction in work hours is significantly associated with advanced stages, more physical symptoms (specifically lack of energy), and with more psychological symptoms such as anxiety and depression (Mehnert 2011).

A significant proportion of patients had changed work due to cancer such as job change. Patients who reported work changes due to cancer were significantly more frequently female and worked part time. Furthermore, patients who had changed work had significantly poorer current work ability, reduced physical and mental work ability, as well as significantly higher anxiety and depression (Mehnert 2011).

Research shows that the impact of cancer on the employment status of cancer survivors is significantly negative for both genders. The employment pathways indicate that 88% of female cancer survivors employed upon diagnosis continue to work during the full 12 months after diagnosis. Further analyses on earnings demonstrate the possibility of cancer survivors retaining their job but at lower pay (Lo 2019). Pearce et al. (2018) also confirm that unemployment due to cancer is significantly associated with financial toxicity and that those with limited financial resources are most at risk.

Syse et al. (2008) found cancer to be associated with a 12% decline in overall earnings. On average, working women lost 27% of their projected usual annual wages (median = 19%) after compensations received had been taken into account (Lauzier et al. 2008). A higher percentage of lost wages was significantly associated with a lower level of education (Lauzier et al. 2008; Syse et al. 2008), lower social support, chemotherapy, self-employment, shorter tenure in the job, and part-time work. Furthermore, Syse et al. (2008) found that leukemia; lymphomas; lung, brain, bone, colorectal, and head-and neck cancer resulted in the largest reductions in employment and earnings.

Work Ability

The concept of work ability emphasizes that individual work ability is a process of human resources in relation to work (Ilmarinen 2001). Thus, work ability can be defined as an individual's physical, psychological, and social resources for participation in any kind of paid work or self-employment. Work ability is dependent on mental and somatic health status as well as on social skills, level of education, motivation, work demands, the work environment, and the organization of the work (Ilmarinen 2001).

Several studies have investigated work ability following the diagnosis and treatment of cancer and found a significant reduction in physical or mental work ability (Mehnert 2011). Even 4 years post diagnosis, studies showed that breast cancer survivors reported higher levels of age-adjusted work limitations compared to a non-cancer group of employed workers. In contrast, work ability improved significantly over time in a study by de Boer et al. (2008). In this study, the work ability of women improved more over time in comparison to male employees. Work ability at 6 months after sick leave strongly predicted return to work at 18 months (de Boer et al. 2008).

Risk for reduced work ability is associated with hematological neoplasias, chemotherapy, older age among women, diseases or injuries, as well as with work changes due to cancer. In contrast, better work ability was found to be related to genitourological and gastrointestinal cancers, to a higher level of education, and to better social climate at work and greater commitment to the work organization among both genders (de Boer et al. 2008; Mehnert 2011; van Muijen et al. 2017). Sociodemographic, health- and work-related factors were associated with fatigue and work ability in cancer survivors on long-term sick leave. As fatigue and poor work ability are important risk factors for work disability, addressing the identified predictive factors may assist in mitigation of work disability in cancer survivors (van Muijen et al. 2017).

Career Changes

The majority of cancer survivors who returned to work report one or more changes in occupational roles (Steiner et al. 2008; Mehnert 2011). In a cross-sectional study among breast cancer survivors, who were assessed 9 years post diagnosis, about a quarter of patients reported a career change, 12.5% retired early as a result of cancer, 41% felt the cancer had altered their priorities and ambitions at work, and 12% reported that they were unable to fulfill their work or career potential. However, another 26% of the women felt that cancer had made them more goal focused and 6.5% reported a positive career change (Stewart et al. 2001). Coping style, support systems, and changing perspectives about work and life in general were influential on career decisions among young adult cancer survivors (Stone et al. 2017).

The majority of patients disclosed the cancer diagnosis to their employer as well as to co-workers (Villaverde et al. 2008), whereas Stewart et al. (2001) reported that 41% of the sample had told their cancer diagnosis to their boss or supervisor at work. Bouknight et al. (2006) showed that 87% of breast cancer patients reported that their employer was accommodating to their cancer illness and treatment. Similar results were found by Steiner et al. (2008), who showed that cancer survivors reported only few workplace barriers on returning to work. In the study by Villaverde et al. (2008), 29% of cancer survivors noticed changes in their relationship with co-workers and managers, however, usually in a supportive way. Job discrimination was not reported.

Few studies, however, indicate difficulties in returning to work. Workplace discrimination may include hiring discrimination, harassment, job reassignment, job loss, denied promotion, and limited career advancement. Strategies to mitigate stigma and workplace discrimination include education, advocacy, and anti-discrimination policies (Mehnert 2011; Stergiou-Kita et al. 2017).

Quality of Life Issues

The impact of cancer and cancer treatments may be particularly evident at the workplace. Cancer survivors are significantly more likely as non-cancer controls to report fair or poor health, psychosocial distress, limitations of activities of daily living, functional limitations, and, among those under the age of 65, being unable to work because of a health condition (Mehnert 2011; Islam et al. 2014).

Many studies show cancer-related disabilities in a significant proportion of survivors and many of the patients with disabilities are working. For both genders, the rate of work disability is significantly higher in the cancer sample compared to non-cancer controls (Aaronson et al. 2014; Mehnert 2011). The increase in disability for survivors with any new cancers is significantly stronger than the increase in disability for cancer-free survivors. Cancer survivors were found to be more likely to have comorbid diseases than controls. This was particularly evident among male patients, who had a significantly worse subjective health status and higher somatic symptom levels than non-cancer controls. Gudbergsson et al. (2008) found statistically lower rates of vigor domains among cancer patients, and a significantly poorer health status, greater numbers of disease symptoms, more anxiety, and reduced physical quality of life. Limitations were most frequently reported by long-term breast cancer survivors in the following activities: managing "heavier work at home, taking a short walk" with a "rather healthy speed, climbing stairs, doing the grocery, and taking the bus" (Peuckmann et al. 2008). In addition, going outside the house, walking around at home, getting out of bed, taking a bath, getting dressed, and managing light work at home were reported by 65% of patients as troublesome (Peuckmann et al. 2008).

Cancer-related fatigue is a profound fatigue related to cancer or its treatment and has been recognized as a common and debilitating complaint among cancer survivors (Aaronson et al. 2014). The most prevalent problems in cancer survivors are fatigue (56%), sleep problems (51%), and problems getting around (47%) (Mehnert et al. 2018). Fatigue has a strong impact on both housework and gainful work and is strongly associated with work limitations in cancer survivors. A study by Gonzalez et al. (2018) reveals that the worse outcomes observed among employees receiving treatment for breast and prostate cancer were partially explained by the impacts of cancer and treatment for cancer on sleep disturbance. These findings suggest that preventing or addressing sleep disturbance may result in economic benefits in addition to improvements in health and quality of life.

Psychosocial issues such as emotional distress, anxiety, and depression play a significant role in employment and return to work in cancer survivors. Inhestern et al. (2017) showed that approximately 40% of the cancer survivors of working-age reported moderate to high anxiety scores and approximately 20% reported moderate to high depression scores. The authors found higher anxiety levels in cancer survivors of working-age than in the general population.

The lowest level of psychosocial distress and the highest levels of physical and mental functioning, and Quality of Life (QoL) were found in women who continued to work through treatment, followed by women who discontinued to work through treatment but returned to work (Mahar et al. 2008). Likewise, the highest level of psychosocial distress and the lowest levels of physical and mental functioning, and quality of life were found in women who stopped working at all after the diagnosis of cancer (Mahar et al. 2008). Among fully employed patients with hematological malignancies, 73% reported good QoL compared to 22% of those on disability insurance and 28% of those on part-time work.

A systematic review about the physical and psychosocial problems in cancer survivors beyond return to work indicated that cognitive limitations, coping issues, fatigue, depression, and anxiety were reported to influence cancer survivor's work ability. Physical problems were frequently described to affect functioning at work. Thus, ongoing physical and/or psychosocial problems are present in occupationally active cancer survivors, which may cause serious difficulties at work (Duijts et al. 2014).

Interventions to Promote Return to Work

Many studies indicate the need for psychosocial screening and psycho-oncological support, e.g., in survivorship programs for working-age cancer survivors. Given the importance of occupational activity for cancer patients, it is necessary to provide interventions to patients that improve their ability to work and support their return to work. Over the past two decades, a number of work-related intervention programs have been developed internationally that focus on the mental and physical consequences of cancer mainly affecting work-related issues such as work ability (Mehnert et al. 2013).

Overall, the state of research on evidence-based interventions on a variety of work-related traits is limited. A systematic review included 15 randomized controlled-trials (RCTs) mostly conducted in high-income countries and most studies were aimed at breast cancer or prostate cancer patients. The interventions including psycho-educational interventions and multidisciplinary interventions in which vocational counseling was combined with patient education, patient counseling, and biofeedback-assisted behavioral training or physical exercises are very broad with mixed outcome criteria. De Boer et al. (2015) found moderate quality evidence that multidisciplinary interventions enhance the return to work rate in cancer patients.

Internationally, cancer rehabilitation programs play a central role to the restoration of physical and mental health. The improved survival rates of cancer patients are also increasingly leading to vocational reintegration programs. These programs include, for example, special workplace training and group trainings for improving job-related behavior and experiences. Typical occupational counseling issues include work-related motivation, job-related problems and health complaints, dealing with stress and problems returning to work, job satisfaction and conflicts at the workplace, unemployment and skills training, as well as comprehensive career and social counseling.

Intervention research has so far focused primarily on patients. Future interventions should also include the perspective of employers and co-workers on the structuring of work organization. This perspective implies the appropriate use of human resources and particularly of those with disabilities, work and skills training, education, and the development of an adaptive approach to new needs and unfamiliar work situations with chronically ill workers.

Cross-References

▶ A Human Rights Perspective on Work Participation
▶ Employment as a Key Rehabilitation Outcome
▶ Investing in Integrative Active Labour Market Policies
▶ Shifting the Focus from Work Reintegration to Sustainability of Employment

References

Aaronson NK, Mattioli V, Minton O, Weis J, Johansen C, Dalton SO, Verdonck-de Leeuw IM, Stein KD, Alfano CM, Mehnert A, de Boer A, van de Poll-Franse LV (2014) Beyond treatment – psychosocial and behavioral issues in cancer survivorship research and practice. EJC Suppl 12:54–64. https://doi.org/10.1016/j.ejcsup.2014.03.005

Bennett JA, Brown P, Cameron L, Whitehead LC, Porter D, McPherson KM (2009) Changes in employment and household income during the 24 months following a cancer diagnosis. Support Care Cancer 17:1057–1064. https://doi.org/10.1007/s00520-008-0540-z

Bennett D, Kearney T, Donnelly DW, Downing A, Wright P, Wilding S, Wagland R, Watson E, Glaser A, Gavin A (2018) Factors influencing job loss and early retirement in working men with prostate cancer-findings from the population-based Life After Prostate Cancer Diagnosis (LAPCD) study. J Cancer Surviv 12:669–678. https://doi.org/10.1007/s11764-018-0704-x

Böttcher HM, Steimann M, Ullrich A, Rotsch M, Zurborn KH, Koch U, Bergelt C (2013) Evaluation of a vocationally oriented concept within inpatient oncological rehabilitation. Rehabilitation 52:329–336. https://doi.org/10.1055/s-0032-1329961

Bouknight RR, Bradley CJ, Luo Z (2006) Correlates of return to work for breast cancer survivors. J Clin Oncol 24:345–353

Bradley CJ, Bednarek HL (2002) Employment patterns of long-term cancer survivors. Psychooncology 11:188–198

Carlsen K, Oksbjerg Dalton S, Frederiksen K, Diderichsen F, Johansen C (2008a) Cancer and the risk for taking early retirement pension: A Danish cohort study. Scand J Public Health 36:117–125. https://doi.org/10.1177/1403494807085192

Carlsen K, Oksbjerg Dalton S, Diderichsen F, Johansen C (2008b) Risk for unemployment of cancer survivors: A Danish cohort study. Eur J Cancer 44:1866–1874. https://doi.org/10.1016/j.ejca.2008.05.020

Chan F, Strauser D, da Silva Cardoso E, Xi Zheng L, Chan JY, Feuerstein M (2008) State vocational services and employment in cancer survivors. J Cancer Surviv 2:169–178. https://doi.org/10.1007/s11764-008-0057-y

Choi KS, Kim EJ, Lim JH, Kim SG, Lim MK, Park JG, Park EC (2007) Job loss and reemployment after a cancer diagnosis in Koreans – prospective cohort study. Psychooncology 16(3):205–213

de Boer AG, Verbeek JH, Spelten ER, Uitterhoeve AL, Ansink AC, de Reijke TM, Kammeijer M, Sprangers MA, van Dijk FJ (2008) Work ability and return-to-work in cancer patients. Br J Cancer 98:1342–1347. https://doi.org/10.1038/sj.bjc.6604302

de Boer AG, Taskila T, Ojajärvi A, van Dijk FJ, Verbeek JH (2009) Cancer survivors and unemployment: a meta-analysis and meta-regression. JAMA 301:753–762. https://doi.org/10.1001/jama.2009.187

de Boer AG, Taskila TK, Tamminga SJ, Feuerstein M, Frings-Dresen MH, Verbeek JH (2015) Interventions to enhance return-to-work for cancer patients. Cochrane Database Syst Rev 9:CD007569. https://doi.org/10.1002/14651858.CD007569.pub3

den Bakker CM, Anema JR, Zaman AGNM, de Vet HCW, Sharp L, Angenete E, Allaix ME, Otten RHJ, Huirne JAF, Bonjer HJ, de Boer AGEM, Schaafsma FG (2018) Prognostic factors for return to work and work disability among colorectal cancer survivors; a systematic review. PLoS One 13:e0200720. https://doi.org/10.1371/journal.pone.0200720

Dorland HF, Abma FI, Van Zon SKR, Stewart RE, Amick BC, Ranchor AV, Roelen CAM, Bültmann U (2018a) Fatigue and depressive symptoms improve but remain negatively related to work functioning over 18 months after return to work in cancer patients. J Cancer Surviv 12:371–378. https://doi.org/10.1007/s11764-018-0676-x

Dorland HF, Abma FI, Roelen CAM, Stewart RE, Amick BC, Bültmann U, Ranchor AV (2018b) Work-specific cognitive symptoms and the role of work characteristics, fatigue, and depressive symptoms in cancer patients during 18 months post return to work. Psychooncology 27:2229–2236. https://doi.org/10.1002/pon.4800. Epub 2018 Jul 12

Duijts SF, van Egmond MP, Spelten E, van Muijen P, Anema JR, van der Beek AJ (2014) Physical and psychosocial problems in cancer survivors beyond return to work: a systematic review. Psychooncology 23:481–492. https://doi.org/10.1002/pon.3467

Earle CC, Chretien Y, Morris C, Ayanian JZ, Keating NL, Polgreen LA, Wallace R, Ganz PA, Weeks JC (2010) Employment among survivors of lung cancer and colorectal cancer. J Clin Oncol 28:1700–1705. https://doi.org/10.1200/JCO.2009.24.7411

Ferlay J, Soerjomataram I, Dikshit R, Eser S, Mathers C, Rebelo M, Parkin DM, Forman D, Bray F (2015) Cancer incidence and mortality worldwide: sources, methods and major patterns in GLOBOCAN 2012. Int J Cancer 136:E359–E386. https://doi.org/10.1002/ijc.29210

Feuerstein M, Luff GM, Harrington CB, Olsen CH (2007) Pattern of workplace disputes in cancer survivors: a population study of ADA claims. J Cancer Surviv 1:185–192. https://doi.org/10.1007/s11764-007-0027-9

Glimelius I, Ekberg S, Linderoth J, Jerkeman M, Chang ET, Neovius M, Smedby KE (2015) Sick leave and disability pension in Hodgkin lymphoma survivors by stage, treatment, and follow-up time–a population-based comparative study. J Cancer Surviv 9:599–609. https://doi.org/10.1007/s11764-015-0436-0

Gonzalez BD, Grandner MA, Caminiti CB, Hui SA (2018) Cancer survivors in the workplace: sleep disturbance mediates the impact of cancer on healthcare expenditures and work absenteeism. Support Care Cancer 26:4049–4055. https://doi.org/10.1007/s00520-018-4272-4

Grinshpun A, Rottenberg Y (2018) Unemployment following breast cancer diagnosis: A population-based study. Breast 44:24–28. https://doi.org/10.1016/j.breast.2018.12.013

Gudbergsson SB, Fosså SD, Sanne B, Dahl AA (2007) A controlled study of job strain in primary-treated cancer patients without metastases. Acta Oncol 46:534–544

Gudbergsson SB, Fosså SD, Dahl AA (2008) Is cancer survivorship associated with reduced work engagement? A NOCWO Study. J Cancer Surviv 2:159–168

Hartung TJ, Brähler E, Faller H, Härter M, Hinz A, Johansen C, Keller M, Koch U, Schulz H, Weis J, Mehnert A (2017) The risk of being depressed is significantly higher in cancer patients than in the general population: Prevalence and severity of depressive symptoms across major cancer types. Eur J Cancer 72:46–53. https://doi.org/10.1016/j.ejca.2016.11.017

Hoffman B (2005) Cancer survivors at work: a generation of progress. CA Cancer J Clin 55:271–280. Review

Ilmarinen J (2001) Aging workers. Occup Environ Med 58:546–552

Inhestern L, Beierlein V, Bultmann JC, Möller B, Romer G, Koch U, Bergelt C (2017) Anxiety and depression in working-age cancer survivors: a register-based study. BMC Cancer 17:347. https://doi.org/10.1186/s12885-017-3347-9

Isaksson J, Wilms T, Laurell G, Fransson P, Ehrsson YT (2016) Meaning of work and the process of returning after head and neck cancer. Support Care Cancer 24:205–213. https://doi.org/10.1007/s00520-015-2769-7

Islam T, Dahlui M, Majid HA, Nahar AM, Mohd Taib NA, Su TT, MyBCC study group (2014) Factors associated with return to work of breast cancer survivors: a systematic review. BMC Public Health 14(Suppl 3):S8. https://doi.org/10.1186/1471-2458-14-S3-S8

Kennedy F, Haslam C, Munir F, Pryce J (2007) Returning to work following cancer: A qualitative exploratory study into the experience of returning to work following cancer. Eur J Cancer Care 16(1):17–25

Lauzier S, Maunsell E, Drolet M, Coyle D, Hébert-Croteau N, Brisson J, Mâsse B, Abdous B, Robidoux A, Robert J (2008) Wage losses in the year after breast cancer: extent and determinants among Canadian women. J Natl Cancer Inst 100:321–332. https://doi.org/10.1093/jnci/djn028. Epub 2008 Feb 26

Lilliehorn S, Hamberg K, Kero A, Salander P (2013) Meaning of work and the returning process after breast cancer: a longitudinal study of 56 women. Scand J Caring Sci 27:267–274. https://doi.org/10.1111/j.1471-6712.2012.01026.x

Lo JC (2019) Employment pathways of cancer survivors-analysis from administrative data. Eur J Health Econ 20(5):637–645. https://doi.org/10.1007/s10198-018-1025-8

Luengo-Fernandez R, Leal J, Gray A, Sullivan R (2013) Economic burden of cancer across the European Union: a population-based cost analysis. Lancet Oncol 14:1165–1174. https://doi.org/10.1016/S1470-2045(13)70442-X

Mahar KK, BrintzenhofeSzoc K, Shields JJ (2008) The impact of changes in employment status on psychosocial well-being: a study of breast cancer survivors. J Psychosoc Oncol 26:1–17

Mehnert A (2011) Employment and work-related issues in cancer survivors. Crit Rev Oncol Hematol 77:109–130. https://doi.org/10.1016/j.critrevonc.2010.01.004

Mehnert A, Koch U (2013) Predictors of employment among cancer survivors after medical rehabilitation–a prospective study. Scand J Work Environ Health 39:76–87. https://doi.org/10.5271/sjweh.3291

Mehnert A, de Boer A, Feuerstein M (2013) Employment challenges for cancer survivors. Cancer 119(Suppl 11):2151–2159. https://doi.org/10.1002/cncr.28067

Mehnert A, Brähler E, Faller H, Härter M, Keller M, Schulz H, Wegscheider K, Weis J, Boehncke A, Hund B, Reuter K, Richard M, Sehner S, Sommerfeldt S, Szalai C, Wittchen HU, Koch U (2014) Four-week prevalence of mental disorders in patients with cancer across major tumor entities. J Clin Oncol 32:3540–3546. https://doi.org/10.1200/JCO.2014.56.0086

Mehnert A, Hartung TJ, Friedrich M, Vehling S, Brähler E, Härter M, Keller M, Schulz H, Wegscheider K, Weis J, Koch U, Faller H (2018) One in two cancer patients is significantly distressed: prevalence and indicators of distress. Psychooncology 27:75–82. https://doi.org/10.1002/pon.4464

Mitchell AJ, Chan M, Bhatti H, Halton M, Grassi L, Johansen C, Meader N (2011) Prevalence of depression, anxiety, and adjustment disorder in oncological, haematological, and palliative-care settings: a meta-analysis of 94 interview-based studies. Lancet Oncol 12:160–174. https://doi.org/10.1016/S1470-2045(11)70002-X

Morin E (2004) The meaning of work in modern times. https://uiamaket.files.wordpress.com/2015/03/estelle-2004-the-meaning-of-work-in-modern-times-pdf.pdf. Accessed 11 Jan 2019

Oortwijn W, Nelissen E, Adamini S, van den Heuvel S, Geuskens G, Burdof L (2011) Social determinants state of the art reviews – health of people of working age – summary report. European Commission Directorate General for Health and Consumers, Luxembourg. ISBN 978-92-79-18527-4

Paalman CH, van Leeuwen FE, Aaronson NK, de Boer AG, van de Poll-Franse L, Oldenburg HS, Schaapveld M (2016) Employment and social benefits up to 10 years after breast cancer diagnosis: a population-based study. Br J Cancer 114:81–87. https://doi.org/10.1038/bjc.2015.431

Paltrinieri S, Fugazzaro S, Bertozzi L, Bassi MC, Pellegrini M, Vicentini M, Mazzini E, Costi S (2018) Return to work in European Cancer survivors: a systematic review. Support Care Cancer 26:2983–2994. https://doi.org/10.1007/s00520-018-4270-6

Park JH, Park EC, Park JH, Kim SG, Lee SY (2008a) Job loss and re-employment of cancer patients in Korean employees: a nationwide retrospective cohort study. J Clin Oncol 26:1302–1309. https://doi.org/10.1200/JCO.2007.14.2984

Park JH, Park JH, Kim SG (2008b) Effect of cancer diagnosis on patient employment status: a nationwide longitudinal study in Korea. Psychooncology 18:691–699. https://doi.org/10.1002/pon.1452

Pearce A, Tomalin B, Kaambwa B, Horevoorts N, Duijts S, Mols F, van de Poll-Franse L, Koczwara B (2018) Financial toxicity is more than costs of care: the relationship between employment and financialtoxicity in long-term cancer survivors. J Cancer Surviv 13(1):10–20. https://doi.org/10.1007/s11764-018-0723-7

Peteet JR (2000) Cancer and the meaning of work. Gen Hosp Psychiatry 22:200–205

Peuckmann V, Ekholm O, Sjøgren P, Rasmussen NK, Christiansen P, Møller S, Groenvold M (2008) Health care utilisation and characteristics of long-term breast cancer survivors: Nationwide survey in Denmark. Eur J Cancer 45:625–633. https://doi.org/10.1016/j.ejca.2008.09.027

Pryce J, Munir F, Haslam C (2007) Cancer survivorship and work: symptoms, supervisor response, co-worker disclosure and work adjustment. J Occup Rehabil 17:83–92

Roelen CA, Koopmans PC, van Rhenen W, Groothoff JW, van der Klink JJ, Bültmann U (2011a) Trends in return to work of breast cancer survivors. Breast Cancer Res Treat 128:237–242. https://doi.org/10.1007/s10549-010-1330-0

Roelen CA, Koopmans PC, Groothoff JW, van der Klink JJ, Bültmann U (2011b) Return to work after cancer diagnosed in 2002, 2005 and 2008. J Occup Rehabil 21:335–341. https://doi.org/10.1007/s10926-011-9319-z

Rottenberg Y, Ratzon NZ, Cohen M, Hubert A, Uziely B, de Boer AG (2016) Unemployment risk at 2 and 4 years following colorectal cancer diagnosis: a population based study. Eur J Cancer 69:70–76. https://doi.org/10.1016/j.ejca.2016.09.025

Short PF, Vasey JJ, Tunceli K (2005) Employment pathways in a large cohort of adult cancer survivors. Cancer 103:1292–1301

Short PF, Vasey JJ, Moran JR (2008) Long-term effects of cancer survivorship on the employment of older workers. Health Serv Res 43:193–210. https://doi.org/10.1111/j.1475-6773.2007.00752.x

Spelten ER, Sprangers MA, Verbeek JH (2002) Factors reported to influence the return to work of cancer survivors: a literature review. Psychooncology 11:124–131

Steiner JF, Cavender TA, Nowels CT, Beaty BL, Bradley CJ, Fairclough DL, Main DS (2008) The impact of physical and psychosocial factors on work characteristics after cancer. Psychooncology 17:138–147

Stergiou-Kita M, Grigorovich A, Tseung V, Milosevic E, Hebert D, Phan S, Jones J (2014) Qualitative meta-synthesis of survivors' work experiences and the development of strategies to facilitate return to work. J Cancer Surviv 8:657–670. https://doi.org/10.1007/s11764-014-0377-z

Stergiou-Kita M, Qie X, Yau HK, Lindsay S (2017) Stigma and work discrimination among cancer survivors: a scoping review and recommendations. Can J Occup Ther 84:178–188. https://doi.org/10.1177/0008417417701229

Stewart DE, Cheung AM, Duff S, Wong F, McQuestion M, Cheng T, Purdy L, Bunston T (2001) Long-term breast cancer survivors: confidentiality, disclosure, effects on work and insurance. Psychooncology 10:259–263

Stone DS, Ganz PA, Pavlish C, Robbins WA (2017) Young adult cancer survivors and work: a systematic review. J Cancer Surviv 11:765–781. https://doi.org/10.1007/s11764-017-0614-3

Sun Y, Shigaki CL, Armer JM (2017) Return to work among breast cancer survivors: a literature review. Support Care Cancer 25:709–718. https://doi.org/10.1007/s00520-016-3446-1

Syse A, Tretli S, Kravdal Ø (2008) Cancer's impact on employment and earnings – a population-based study from Norway. J Cancer Surviv 2:149–158. https://doi.org/10.1007/s11764-008-0053-2

Torp S, Syse J, Paraponaris A, Gudbergsson S (2017) Return to work among self-employed cancer survivors. J Cancer Surviv 11:189–200. https://doi.org/10.1007/s11764-016-0578-8

United Nations Human Development Indices and Indicators 2018 Statistical Update (2018) http://hdr.undp.org/sites/default/files/2018_human_development_statistical_update.pdf. Accessed 9 Jan 2019

van Muijen P, Weevers NL, Snels IA, Duijts SF, Bruinvels DJ, Schellart AJ, van der Beek AJ (2013) Predictors of return to work and employment in cancer survivors: a systematic review. Eur J Cancer Care 22:144–160. https://doi.org/10.1111/ecc.12033.

van Muijen P, Duijts SFA, Bonefaas-Groenewoud K, van der Beek AJ, Anema JR (2017) Predictors of fatigue and work ability in cancer survivors. Occup Med 67:703–711. https://doi.org/10.1093/occmed/kqx165

Villaverde MR, Batlle FJ, Yllan VA, Gordo JAM, Sánchez RA, Valiente SJB, Baron GM (2008) Employment in a cohort of breast cancer patients. Occup Med 58:509–511. https://doi.org/10.1093/occmed/kqn092

Wolvers MDJ, Leensen MCJ, Groeneveld IF, Frings-Dresen MHW, De Boer AGEM (2018) Predictors for earlier return to work of cancer patients. J Cancer Surviv 12:169–177. https://doi.org/10.1007/s11764-017-0655-7

Return to Work After Spinal Cord Injury

23

Marcel W. M. Post, Jan D. Reinhardt, and Reuben Escorpizo

Contents

Introduction	418
Spinal Cord Injury	419
Epidemiology	420
Impairments and Activity Limitations	420
Secondary Health Problems	421
Employment	422
Employment Rates	423
Return to Work Rates	423
Determinants of Labor Market Participation and Return to Work	424
Vocational Rehabilitation in SCI	424
Vocational Rehabilitation as Part of SCI Rehabilitation	425
Evidence-Based VR Interventions	426

M. W. M. Post
Center of Excellence for Rehabilitation Medicine, UMC Utrecht Brain Center, University Medical Center Utrecht and De Hoogstraat Rehabilitation, Utrecht, The Netherlands

Department of Rehabilitation Medicine, University of Groningen, University Medical Center Groningen, Groningen, The Netherlands
e-mail: m.post@dehoogstraat.nl

J. D. Reinhardt (✉)
Institute for Disaster Management and Reconstruction, Sichuan University and Hong Kong Polytechnic University, Chengdu, China

Swiss Paraplegic Research, Nottwil, Switzerland

Department of Health Sciences and Health Policy, University of Lucerne, Lucerne, Switzerland
e-mail: reinhardt@scu.edu.cn; jan.reinhardt@paraplegie.ch

R. Escorpizo
Department of Rehabilitation and Movement Science, University of Vermont, Burlington, VT, USA
e-mail: Reuben.Escorpizo@med.uvm.edu

© Springer Nature Switzerland AG 2020
U. Bültmann, J. Siegrist (eds.), *Handbook of Disability, Work and Health*, Handbook Series in Occupational Health Sciences, https://doi.org/10.1007/978-3-030-24334-0_23

Conclusion 427
Cross-References 427
References 427

Abstract

Spinal cord injury (SCI) is a seriously disabling condition, and work participation rates among people with SCI are substantially below that of the general population. In this chapter evidence on work participation and vocational rehabilitation of people with SCI is summarized. First, the characteristics and consequences are described. These include motor and sensory impairment below the level of the SCI and possible secondary health conditions. Second, work participation rates and determinants of work are described. An overall work participation rate of 37% has been reported but with wide variation across countries. A multitude of non-modifiable determinants of work has been described, such as age, sex and ethnicity, type of SCI, and time since onset of SCI. Also, many modifiable factors influencing work have been described, such as functional ability, level of education, motivation, and the availability of workplace accommodations and vocational rehabilitation services. Third, vocational rehabilitation (VR) is described. VR should ideally start early after onset of SCI and be tailored to the individual with SCI. Evidence on specific VR interventions is sparse, but beneficial effects of individual placement and support have been reported.

Keywords

Spinal cord injuries · Vocational rehabilitation · Work disability · Employment

Introduction

This chapter describes work-related issues among people with spinal cord injury (SCI). According to a recent review of qualitative studies, work fulfills important functions for people with SCI. These include regaining a sense of being somebody who cannot be reduced to a person with disability, who is in control of life, and who has a motivation to living. Work also plays an important role in perceiving oneself as a full member of the community, somebody who is embedded in social networks, and has an impact on society. Finally, work is important for establishing and reassuring economic self-sufficiency (Ullah et al. 2018).

This chapter begins with a description of the condition and its consequences. This section is meant for people who are not familiar with SCI. After that, the evidence on work participation among people with SCI and factors associated with having work is presented. Finally, vocational rehabilitation as part of SCI rehabilitation is described, and evidence on specific interventions is discussed.

Spinal Cord Injury

Spinal cord injury (SCI) refers to a lesion or damage to the spinal cord. This damage is irreparable and hampers the transportation of sensory information to the brain, as well as motor control from the brain to the remainder of the body. Damage to the spinal cord can occur due to, for example, traffic accidents, falls, violence, spinal degeneration, infections, and benign or malignant tumors. Although the term SCI refers to traumatic etiologies only, we will follow the habit to use the term SCI irrespective of etiology and only specify this as traumatic SCI (TSCI) or non-traumatic SCI (NTSCI) if relevant.

The spinal cord is situated within the spine and consists of neurological segment levels. These neurological segments are named after the spinal roots that enter and leave the spinal column between each of the vertebral segments. Therefore, particularly the lower segment levels of the spinal cord do not correspond with the vertebral levels. The T3 through T12 cord segments are situated between T3 to T8 vertebra. The lumbar cord segments are situated at the T9 through T11 vertebrae. The sacral segments are situated from T12 to L1 vertebra. The lower end of the spinal cord or conus is situated at about the L2 vertebral level. Below L2 there are only nerve roots within the cauda equina. A lesion to the cauda equina is therefore not diagnosed as SCI.

The severity of SCI is defined by two parameters: (1) the level of the spinal cord where the lesion occurs, since a higher lesion affects more body parts than a low lesion, and (2) the degree to which this damage is incomplete or complete. A detailed examination according to the International Standards for the Neurological Classification of SCI (INSCSCI) is required to describe these characteristics (Kirshblum et al. 2011). This examination consists of testing muscle strength in key muscles and of sensory impairment in key dermatomes or skin areas.

The level of SCI is defined as the lowest unimpaired segment of the spinal cord. Since this may be different for motor and sensory muscles and different for the left and right side of the body, the neurological level of injury (NLI) is defined as the lowest (most rostral) level of these four (Kirshblum et al. 2011). The term tetraplegia refers to damage in the cervical spinal cord, thus affecting function in all body parts, whereas paraplegia refers to damage in the thoracic, lumbar, or sacral segments of the spinal cord, leaving arm/hand functioning spared.

Completeness of the lesion is expressed on the American Spinal Injury Association (ASIA) impairment scale (AIS). The grades are:

- A: No motor or sensory function is preserved below the NLI.
- B: Sensory but no motor function is preserved below the NLI.
- C: Motor function is preserved below the NLI, but more than half of the key muscles below the NLI have a muscle grade less than 3.
- D: At least half of the muscles below the NLI have a muscle grade > 3.
- E: No sensory or motor deficits (this grade is only used to track recovery in patients with previous deficits). (Kirshblum et al. 2011).

Epidemiology

Fortunately, SCI is a rare condition. The estimated global total SCI incidence is 40–80 new cases per million persons per year (Bickenbach et al. 2013). Figures on NTSCI are however largely lacking. The estimated global incidence of TSCI is 23 cases per million per year. The incidence of TSCI is highest in the United States (40–53 per million), compared to Western Europe (average 16 per million), Australia (15 per million), and 20–30 per million in other parts of the world (Lee et al. 2014; Jain et al. 2015).

The life expectancy of people with SCI is associated with the severity of the lesion and on average substantially below that of the general population. However, most people who experience SCI may expect to live for many more years. According to US figures, adults who suffer from TSCI at 40 years of age and survive their first post-injury year have a life expectancy of 36 years if their TSCI is AIS grade D and still 22 years if they have high tetraplegia (C1–C4) with AIS grade A–C (National Spinal Cord Injury Statistical Center 2018).

SCI affects people of all ages. However, the distribution of age at onset of TSCI shows peaks in young adults and elderly. The large majority of people with TSCI are male, whereas sex distribution is more even in people with NTSCI. People of lower socioeconomic status or certain ethnic minorities are overrepresented in the TSCI statistics (National Spinal Cord Injury Statistical Center 2018).

In the United States, the most frequent etiologies of TSCI in 2010–2017 were vehicle crashes (38%), falls (31%), acts of violence (primarily gunshot wounds (14%)), and sports/recreation activities (9%) (National Spinal Cord Injury Statistical Center 2018). TSCI due to violence or sports injuries occurs relatively often in young adults, road traffic accidents are the leading cause of TSCI across adulthood, and low falls are the leading cause of TSCI in the elderly. Work-related onset of TSCI is relatively high in low-income countries due to unsafe working environments, e.g., from fall from a coconut tree, mining accidents, or cervical TSCI from losing balance while carrying a heavy load on the head. The proportion of TSCI from land transport is decreasing or stable in developed but increasing in developing countries due to their transition to motorized transport, poor infrastructure, and regulatory challenges (Bickenbach et al. 2013).

In a retrospective file study of NTSCI utilizing data from nine countries, the most common etiologies of NTSCI were degeneration of the spinal column (30.8%), malignant tumors (16.2%), ischemia (10.9%), benign tumors (8.7%), and bacterial infections (7.1%) but with substantial variation across countries (New et al. 2015).

Impairments and Activity Limitations

The most visible consequence of SCI is the partial or complete paralysis of the affected body parts. Also, altered or absent sensation is present in the affected body parts, further limiting functional abilities and leading to vulnerability for skin damage. In case of complete SCI, the type and degree of activity limitations are

23 Return to Work After Spinal Cord Injury

Table 1 Expected levels of independence in daily activities related to level of motor complete SCI

Level	Functional goals
C1–C4	**Breathing, communication**: Depends on a ventilator for breathing and talking may be difficult or impossible (C1–C3). Independent communication can be accomplished by using a mouth stick and a computer for speech or typing
	Daily tasks: Mostly dependent on help from others. Assistive devices can enable independence in tasks such as turning pages and operating lights and appliances
	Mobility: Can operate an electric wheelchair by using a head control, mouth stick, or chin control
C5	**Daily tasks**: Independence with activities such as eating, brushing of teeth, and hair care after assistance in setting up specialized equipment
	Mobility: A power wheelchair with hand controls is typically used for daily activities. Driving a car may be possible with special equipment needs
C6	**Daily tasks**: Partial independence in daily tasks of bathing, personal hygiene, and dressing using specialized equipment. May be able to perform a transfer using a sliding board. May independently perform light housekeeping duties
	Mobility: Can use a manual wheelchair for daily activities but may use power wheelchair for greater ease of independence
C7	**Daily tasks**: Able to perform household duties. Need fewer adaptive aids in independent living
	Mobility: Daily use of manual wheelchair. Can transfer with greater ease
C8–T1	**Daily tasks**: Can live independently without assistive devices in bathing, dressing, bladder management, and bowel management
	Mobility: Uses manual wheelchair. Can transfer independently
T2–T12	**Mobility**: Uses manual wheelchair. A few individuals are capable of limited walking with extensive bracing
L1–S5	**Mobility**: Walking can be a viable function, with the help of specialized leg and ankle braces. Lower levels walk with greater ease with the help of assistive devices

largely determined by the level of the lesion. Dependent on the severity of the damage, much more variation is seen in people with incomplete SCI. Table 1 provides an overview of functional rehabilitation goals related to level of complete SCI.

Secondary Health Problems

SCI results in a series of direct and indirect (due to increased vulnerability) secondary health problems that may affect work capacity and quality of life. The problems that are most important in the context of work are briefly described here:

(a) Decreased pulmonary function and increased vulnerability for respiratory tract infections. SCI above T12 affects the abdominal muscles that contribute to breathing and coughing, and with increasing level of SCI, pulmonary function is increasingly affected (see also Table 1). Also, people with SCI are at increased risk of obstructed sleep apnea, leading to daytime sleepiness.

(b) Most people with SCI experience bladder dysfunction and, consequently, are at risk of incontinence, overfilling, or both. If spontaneous voiding is not possible, intermittent catheterization is usually advised. Catheterization is, however, associated with a greater risk of urinary tract infections. Bladder accidents or the fear for bladder accidents may hamper work participation.
(c) The same applies to bowel function. Bowel management may include dietary and lifestyle measures, supported by medication. Defecation may take much extra time.
(d) Spasticity, uncontrolled reflex movement of body parts, may hinder daily activities or sleep, although it is sometimes helpful, for example, in performing a transfer from wheelchair to toilet.
(e) People with SCI, in particular those with complete SCI, are at risk of pressure sores. If present, healing of such wounds requires prolonged periods of immobilization. Minimizing this risk may limit the number of hours one can sit in a wheelchair.
(f) Most people with SCI experience pain and may experience different types of pain simultaneously. Overload can lead to shoulder or wrist pain. Neuropathic pain can be present at or below the level of the lesion ("phantom pain").
(g) Autonomic dysreflexia is a potentially life-threatening complication that can occur in people with SCI above T6. It is an uncontrolled reaction of the autonomous system leading to, among others, excessively high blood pressure.
(h) Other health problems include osteoporosis with increased risk of fractures, hyper or hypothermia, deep vein thrombosis, and edema.

This long list might imply that people with SCI are unlikely to be able to work. This is however not true. But it does mean that long-term medical care and good self-management are required to keep these secondary problems as much as possible under control. It also means that work capacity may be reduced, for example, the amount of time that one can work without having a break. Also, workplace adaptations construction work to realize wheelchair accessibility (entrance, stairs, toilet, etc.) may be needed. People with tetraplegia might need a helping hand, e.g., for taking something of the shelf. Having an SCI further takes extra time and energy for self-care, transportation, and other (Van der Meer et al. 2017). This may also limit the work capacity of people with SCI.

Employment

When we speak about work participation of people with acquired disabilities, we usually differentiate between employment and return to work. Employment refers to the percentage of a population in employable age engaged in paid work. Return to work rates, in contrast, refer to the percentage engaged in paid work of a population in employable age who were engaged in paid work at the onset of their condition.

Employment is defined by the International Labor Organization as being engaged in any activity to produce goods or provide services for pay or profit, for at least 1 h during some short period of time (usually a week). This includes self-employed persons as well as those who are temporarily absent from work, e.g., on sick leave, during the reference periods. It also includes people in sheltered employment. It excludes people who produce goods or services solely for their household's or family's subsistence, volunteers, and those in unpaid internships or apprenticeships (International Labor Organization 2019).

Unfortunately, researchers rarely adhere to this international standard definition which makes comparison across studies difficult if not impossible (Bloom et al. 2019).

Employment Rates

In a systematic review of 21 studies conducted between 1992 and 2005, employment rates ranged from 22% to 55% with an aggregate estimate of 36.8% (Young and Murphy 2009). The highest employment rates were found in Europe (pooled estimate 54%), followed by Australia (about 47%), and the lowest rates were found in Asia (about 35%) and North America (about 32%). These variations suggest an impact of differential health systems performance, employment policies, and welfare regimes, although variance in definitions of employment, composition of sampled populations, and sampling frames are likely to have contributed as well.

Recent studies with systematic sampling frames from Asia and Europe confirm the above findings for these continents, e.g., reporting an employment rate of 27.5% in South Korea (Kang et al. 2014), 35% in Taiwan (Huang 2017), and a higher 53.4% rate in Switzerland (Reinhardt et al. 2016). This higher figure, however, is still 30% below the employment rate of the Swiss general population, with the greatest differences found for males with tetraplegia aged between 40 and 54 years (Reinhardt et al. 2016). Unfortunately, differences between employment rates of people with SCI and those of the general population are rarely reported in spite of this being an important measure of relative disadvantage.

Return to Work Rates

Lidal et al. (2007) carried out the only systematic review of return to work rates so far, including studies from 2000 to 2006 reports return to work rates to vary between 21% and 67%. Individual studies and the comparison between different studies suffer from similar issues as mentioned in the above section. It is also important to emphasize here that it can take a considerable time for individuals with SCI to return to work (Krause et al. 2010) and that taking up work again after injury can entail significant changes in the employment situation including reduced working hours and a shift to physically less demanding jobs (Ferdiana et al. 2014).

Determinants of Labor Market Participation and Return to Work

In a systematic review of the literature including 39 studies published between 1952 and 2014, the authors identified a large number of non-modifiable and modifiable determinants of employment outcomes after SCI (Trenaman et al. 2015).

Non-modifiable factors positively associated with post-SCI employment in a majority of studies investigating the respective factors were younger age at time of the study, younger age at injury, being male, Caucasian race, belonging to the majority ethnic group, nonviolent etiology, less severe injury, longer time since injury, and higher pre-injury education.

Modifiable determinants negatively affecting post-injury employment found in a majority of studies analyzing those factors were secondary health conditions and rehospitalizations, financial disincentives due to welfare benefits, insurance status being Medicaid or Workers' Compensation, experience of barriers related to accessibility, emotional control, perceived lack of skills, and finding work not important.

Modifiable determinants positively associated with post-injury employment reported in a majority of studies examining those determinants were access to and ability to use independent transportation, increased motor control, greater functional independence, higher neighborhood socioeconomic status, greater employment rates in the general population, social support, being married, receiving vocational rehabilitation related services, perceived discrimination, higher post-injury education, and increased motivation (Trenaman et al. 2015).

More recent research found that nonmanual high or middle level pre-injury occupations were also associated with an increased likelihood of returning to work (Ferdiana et al. 2014; Leiulfsrud et al. 2020).

Also, several studies highlighted the importance for those with pre-injury employment to have the opportunity to return to their pre-injury employer which was in particular associated with shorter time of returning to work (Krause et al. 2010; Trezzini et al. 2018; Hilton et al. 2018).

Vocational Rehabilitation in SCI

One way to mitigate the negative effects of work disability is through a comprehensive, holistic, and multidisciplinary vocational rehabilitation. Vocational rehabilitation has been defined as a "multi-professional evidence-based approach that is provided in different settings, services, and activities to working age individuals with health-related impairments, limitations, or restrictions with work functioning, and whose primary aim is to optimize work participation" (Escorpizo et al. 2011). This definition of vocational rehabilitation lays the foundation for an overarching perspective on the complexity of work as a life area and also the benefits of vocational rehabilitation using a dynamic, nonlinear, and worker-centered process that aims at enhancing assessment procedures of return to work and the consequent intervention or plan that includes work strategies to sustain work participation and capacity. As a process, vocational rehabilitation should address the complexity of work – in terms of worker interactions, workplace environment including colleagues and peers, and the work culture – all considering the biopsychosocial model (Escorpizo et al. 2015). In order to mitigate the negative consequences of work disability, we must recognize and define the contributing factors that could be assessed and intervened upon by way of a systematic process. Two major components of vocational rehabilitation include first, the valid and reliable assessment methods to properly gauge rehabilitation needs and potential of the worker, and second, to plan and implement an intervention program based on the information derived from the assessment process.

Vocational Rehabilitation as Part of SCI Rehabilitation

Vocational rehabilitation in SCI needs to cover a comprehensive view of the different aspects of functioning that is affected by such a debilitating health condition. These aspects of functioning may involve not only work life but also aspects of life that is outside work. Hence, vocational rehabilitation should not only include the physical or mental functioning of an individual in the context of work and life but also the global picture of the individual's role in the family, community, and the society.

Vocational rehabilitation in the context of SCI will need to consider multimodal approach across a continuum of care. For example, rehabilitation must start as early as possible by way of an in-depth assessment of the individual's history, pre-injury characteristics and work situation, educational experience and training, and an identification of the individual's interest to inform the selection and training for the prospective job. Vocational rehabilitation must consider the bigger picture of community reintegration by way of building social support and relationships (Gupta et al. 2019) to promote participation at the highest level. Service providers must consider multiple outcomes to gauge the success of return to work strategies such as the global indicator of quality of life, (Cotner et al. 2018a) in addition to body impairment level indicators such as muscle weakness or inability to move. A battery of existing standardized instruments or questionnaires can be used for this purpose. One such questionnaire is the Work Rehabilitation Questionnaire (WORQ) (www.myworq.org). WORQ, which was developed using the ICF Core Set for vocational rehabilitation, captures information essential in the return to work efforts such as work status, education, specific interventions or services available, previous type or nature of job and prospective job, and environmental facilitators such as support from family, employer, and vocational services. In addition to this information, WORQ also obtains measures around the individual worker's body impairment such as energy and anxiety, thinking and decision-making, pain, muscle strength, and skin impairments (e.g., pressure injuries), activity limitations such as learning and completing daily tasks, and mobility and ambulation. All these functioning aspects are particularly critical in planning return to work for people with SCI. Amidst these items, WORQ emphasizes the need for future planning given the current status of the person.

Individuals with work disability also have different trajectories or pathways to return to work (Trezzini et al. 2018; Marti et al. 2017); hence, nothing in vocational rehabilitation is "one-size-fits-all." These pathways must be taken into account so as to inform risk factors and predictors to return to work – an understanding that needs to be common across different healthcare or vocational rehabilitation service providers. Vocational rehabilitation must be tailor fit to the individual depending on their needs and potential or capacity. Factors that we know facilitate return to work for people with SCI, as described in the previous section, must be considered by case managers right from the beginning of rehabilitation, so identification and mitigation of problems can be put in place by a multidisciplinary team. Such would also allow efficient transition of care from inpatient acute setting to outpatient to community-based job training setting such as "sheltered" work setting to the open labor market.

Evidence-Based VR Interventions

There are various trends in the scientific literature that support vocational rehabilitation and the service of providing work-related support in order to facilitate return to work among individuals with SCI. The evidence supports the practice of early intervention as early as when the patient is in an inpatient rehabilitation phase (Bloom et al. 2019) versus waiting much later before concrete high-level work rehabilitation strategies can be implemented such as job planning and placement and skills training. One area of much interest is this strategy Individual Placement and Support (IPS) which has been proven to help facilitate work engagement for people with SCI (Cotner et al. 2015, 2018a; Ottomanelli et al. 2017). The challenge remains on how to keep the cost of implementing the program down while ensuring benefits and value of the program from an ecological validity perspective. Cotner et al. (2018b) identified ways and means for providers of SCI-related services that can facilitate return to work. These examples include the individual placement and support model, orientation to SCI, supported employment, job accommodations, and benefits planning. The practice of supported employment has been found to have the strongest evidence to support employment after SCI. Other vocational rehabilitation interventions found to facilitate employment include vocational counseling and vocational training. Moreover, risk factors have also been identified to either help combat the negative effects of SCI on unemployment and help mitigate the consequence of unemployment. Comorbidities such as pain and depression play a crucial role in determining work outcomes (Goetz et al. 2018; Mehta et al. 2018), hence must also be considered in the overall planning for return to work.

The Spinal Cord Injury Research Evidence (SCIRE) group based in Canada has been instrumental in laying down the foundation for work- and employment-related interventions that is reflective of current evidence and contemporary practice (https://scireproject.com/evidence/rehabilitation-evidence/work-and-employment/). Two of their works were around factors that contribute to work outcomes (Trenaman et al. 2015) and interventions that either enhance or hamper work participation (The SCIRE Research Team et al. 2014). To take into account the current state of evidence, these works have been updated in 2018 (Escorpizo et al. 2018). According to SCIRE, returned to work strategies for people with SCI can be enhanced by implementing assistive technology that would provide individual support such as assistive devices, access to transportation, social support including family, employer support, and job accommodations such as reduced work hours. There are also factors that have been found to impede work participation such as financial disincentives (receiving less benefits when working more hours), discrimination from people around, and the lack of appropriate workplace that can support and accommodate work-related needs of the worker such as limited capacity to work full time (Trenaman et al. 2015). Balancing these two sets of factors amidst the interplay between different healthcare systems and labor policies is crucial in attaining successful and sustained return to work, long-term work satisfaction, and an employment strategy that will keep people with SCI remain at work for a long period and ensure their productivity.

Conclusion

Despite the severity and multitude of consequences of SCI, many people with SCI are able to work part-time or full-time. Return to work is one of the main indicators of successful rehabilitation and community reintegration after SCI. Vocational rehabilitation is crucial to get as many as possible people with SCI back to work.

Cross-References

- ▶ Concepts of Work Ability in Rehabilitation
- ▶ Employment as a Key Rehabilitation Outcome
- ▶ Facilitating Competitive Employment for People with Disabilities
- ▶ Implementing Best Practice Models of Return to Work
- ▶ Personal and Environmental Factors Influencing Work Participation Among Individuals with Chronic Diseases
- ▶ Regulatory Contexts Affecting Work Reintegration of People with Chronic Disease and Disabilities
- ▶ Shifting the Focus from Work Reintegration to Sustainability of Employment

References

Bickenbach J, Officer A, Shakespeare T, von Groote P (eds) (2013) International perspectives on spinal cord injury. World Health Organization, Geneva

Bloom J, Dorsett P, McLennan V (2019) Investigating employment following spinal cord injury: outcomes, methods, and population demographics. Disabil Rehabil 2019:2359–2368

Cotner BA, Ottomanelli L, O'Connor DR, Njoh EN, Barnett SD, Miech EJ (2018a) Quality of life outcomes for veterans with spinal cord injury receiving individual placement and support (IPS). Top Spinal Cord Inj Rehabil 24:325–335

Cotner BA, Ottomanelli L, O'Connor DR, Trainor JK (2018b) Provider-identified barriers and facilitators to implementing a supported employment program in spinal cord injury. Disabil Rehabil 40:1273–1279

Cotner BA, Njoh EN, Trainor JK, O'Connor DR, Barnett SD, Ottomanelli L (2015) Facilitators and barriers to employment among veterans with spinal cord injury receiving 12 months of evidence-based supported employment services. Top Spinal Cord Inj Rehabil 21:20–30

Escorpizo R, Brage S, Homa D, Stucki G (eds) (2015) Handbook of vocational rehabilitation and disability evaluation: application and implementation of the ICF. Springer, Cham

Escorpizo R, Reneman MF, Ekholm J, Fritz J, Krupa T, Marnetoft SU, Maroun CE, Guzman JR, Suzuki Y, Stucki G, Chan CC (2011) A conceptual definition of vocational rehabilitation based on the ICF: building a shared global model. J Occup Rehabil 21:126–133

Escorpizo R, Smith E, Finger ME, Miller WC (2018) Work and employment following spinal cord injury. Available from: https://scireproject.com/evidence/rehabilitation-evidence/work-and-employment/. Accessed 22 July 2019

Ferdiana A, Post MW, de Groot S, Bültmann U, van der Klink JJ (2014) Predictors of return to work 5 years after discharge for wheelchair-dependent individuals with spinal cord injury. J Rehabil Med 46:984–990

Goetz LL, Ottomanelli L, Barnett SD, Sutton B, Njoh E (2018) Relationship between comorbidities and employment among veterans with spinal cord injury. Top Spinal Cord Inj Rehabil 24:44–53

Gupta S, Jaiswal A, Norman K, DePaul V (2019) Heterogeneity and its impact on rehabilitation outcomes and interventions for community reintegration in people with spinal cord injuries: an integrative review. Top Spinal Cord Inj Rehabil 25:164–185

Hilton G, Unsworth CA, Stuckey R, Murphy GC (2018) The experience of seeking, gaining and maintaining employment after traumatic spinal cord injury and the vocational pathways involved. Work 59:67–84

Huang IC (2017) Employment outcomes following spinal cord injury in Taiwan. Int J Rehabil Res 40:84–90

International Labor Organization (2019) Employment. Available from: https://www.ilo.org/global/statistics-and-databases/statistics-overview-and-topics/WCMS_470295/lang%2D%2Den/index.htm. Accessed 7 Oct 2019

Jain NB, Ayers GD, Peterson EN, Harris MB, Morse L, O'Connor KC, Garshick E (2015) Traumatic spinal cord injury in the United States, 1993–2012. JAMA 313:2236–2243

Kang EN, Shin HI, Kim HR (2014) Factors that influence employment after spinal cord injury in South Korea. Ann Rehabil Med 38:38–45

Kirshblum SC, Waring W, Biering-Sorensen F, Burns SP, Johansen M, Schmidt-Read M, Donovan W, Graves D, Jha A, Jones L, Mulcahey MJ, Krassioukov A (2011) Reference for the 2011 revision of the international standards for neurological classification of spinal cord injury. J Spinal Cord Med 34:547–554

Krause JS, Terza JV, Saunders LL, Dismuke CE (2010) Delayed entry into employment after spinal cord injury: factors related to time to first job. Spinal Cord 48:487–491

Lee BB, Cripps RA, Fitzharris M, Wing PC (2014) The global map for traumatic spinal cord injury epidemiology: update 2011, global incidence rate. Spinal Cord 52:110–116

Leiulfsrud AS, Solheim EF, Reinhardt JD, Post MWM, Horsewell J, Biering-Sørensen F, Leiulfsrud H (2020) Gender, class, employment status and social mobility following spinal cord injury in Denmark, the Netherlands, Norway and Switzerland. Spinal Cord 58:224–231

Lidal IB, Huynh TK, Biering-Sørensen F (2007) Return to work following spinal cord injury: a review. Disabil Rehabil 29:1341–1375

Marti A, Escorpizo R, Schwegler U, Staubli S, Trezzini B (2017) Employment pathways of individuals with spinal cord injury living in Switzerland: a qualitative study. Work 58:99–110

van der Meer P, Post MW, van Leeuwen CM, van Kuppevelt HJ, Smit CA, van Asbeck FW (2017) Impact of health problems secondary to SCI one and five years after first inpatient rehabilitation. Spinal Cord 55:98–104

Mehta S, Janzen S, McIntyre A, Iruthayarajah J, Loh E, Teasell R (2018) Are comorbid pain and depressive symptoms associated with rehabilitation of individuals with spinal cord injury? Top Spinal Cord Inj Rehabil 24:37–43

National Spinal Cord Injury Statistical Center (2018) Facts and figures at a glance. University of Alabama at Birmingham, Birmingham

New PW, Reeves RK, Smith É, Townson A, Eriks-Hoogland I, Gupta A, Maurizio B, Scivoletto G, Post MW (2015) International retrospective comparison of inpatient rehabilitation for patients with spinal cord dysfunction epidemiology and clinical outcomes. Arch Phys Med Rehabil 96:1080–1087

Ottomanelli L, Goetz LL, Barnett SD, Njoh E, Dixon TM, Holmes SA, LePage JP, Ota D, Sabharwal S, White KT (2017) Individual placement and support in spinal cord injury: a longitudinal observational study of employment outcomes. Arch Phys Med Rehabil 98:1567–1575

Reinhardt JD, Post MW, Fekete C, Trezzini B, Brinkhof MW, SwiSCI Study Group (2016) Labor market integration of people with disabilities: results from the Swiss spinal cord injury cohort study. PLoS One 11:e0166955

The SCIRE Research Team, Trenaman LM, Miller WC, Escorpizo R (2014) Interventions for improving employment outcomes among individuals with spinal cord injury: a systematic review. Spinal Cord 52:788–794

Trenaman L, Miller WC, Querée M, Escorpizo R (2015) Modifiable and non-modifiable factors associated with employment outcomes following spinal cord injury: a systematic review. J Spinal Cord Med 38:422–431

Trezzini B, Schwegler U, Reinhardt JD, for the SwiSCI Study Group (2018) Work and wellbeing-related consequences of different return-to-work pathways of persons with spinal cord injury living in Switzerland. Spinal Cord 56:1166–1175

Ullah MM, Fossey E, Stuckey R (2018) The meaning of work after spinal cord injury: a scoping review. Spinal Cord 56:92–105

Young AE, Murphy GC (2009) Employment status after spinal cord injury (1992–2005): a review with implications for interpretation, evaluation, further research, and clinical practice. Int J Rehabil Re 32:1–11

Coronary Heart Disease and Return to Work 24

Angelique de Rijk

Contents

Introduction	432
Outline of This Chapter	433
Risk Factors for Recurrence of a Cardiac Event and Barriers for RTW in Employees with Coronary Heart Disease	435
Cardiac Risk Factors	435
Work-Related Risk Factors: Psychosocial Risk Factors	437
Work-Related Risk Factors: Physical Risk Factors	438
Barriers to a Successful RTW	439
RTW Interventions for Employees with Coronary Heart Disease	441
Recommendations by Experts for the Support of RTW in CR	442
Conclusions	443
Cross-References	444
References	444

Abstract

After a cardiac event, up to 80% of the employees return to work within one year. Cardiac rehabilitation (CR), which focuses on the physical, psychological, and social functioning, contributes to faster return to work (RTW). Specific attention for work-related issues might improve the RTW rate. Three systematic reviews were done on: (1) risk factors in the workplace for cardiac patients; (2) factors that prolonged sickness absence in cardiac patients; and (3) the effectiveness of RTW interventions for cardiac patients. Existing guidelines, expert knowledge of representatives of 11 different health professions, and a working group of psychologists were additionally used to select risk factors and management to promote RTW in cardiac patients as part of CR. The reviews, guidelines, and expert knowledge identified four groups of risk factors for RTW: eight cardiac

A. de Rijk (✉)
Department of Social Medicine, Care and Public Health Research Institute (CAPHRI), Faculty of Health, Medicine and Life Sciences, Maastricht University, Maastricht, The Netherlands
e-mail: Angelique.derijk@maastrichtuniversity.nl

risk factors; four psychosocial job-related risk factors; six physical risk factors; and 17 psychosocial risk factors (barriers to a successful RTW). Positive effects of interventions were found for the more comprehensive interventions. Key recommendations based on scientific evidence and expert advice are targeting via a short intake that eliminates those patients that do not need RTW support; early start of (part-time) RTW during CR; tailor-made RTW support based on individual risk assessment and interventions within and outside CR that address the individual risks; and frequent communication between the CR team and the workplace (occupational physician), upon patient agreement.

Keywords

Cardiovascular disease · Coronary heart disease · Return to work · Cardiac rehabilitation · Risk factors · Assessment · Intervention · Tailoring

Introduction

Generally, 80% of employees who have been admitted at a hospital for myocardial infarction (MI), coronary artery bypass graft surgery (CABG) ("bypass"), or percutaneous coronary intervention (PCI, an intervention to treat the stenotic coronary arteries) have returned to work after one year (Perk and Alexanderson 2004; Worcester et al. 2014). This rate seems rather stable over the years and populations, but there is room for improvement. Return to work (RTW) can take place faster and become more effective when the RTW support is given earlier (Jelinek 2014) and when the RTW support takes into account patient-specific risk factors (Smedegaard et al. 2017; Reibis et al. 2019).

RTW support can be offered as part of cardiac rehabilitation (CR). CR is delivered in hospitals, in rehabilitation centers, or at local physiotherapists combined with telemonitoring at home (Kraal et al. 2017). It is offered to patients after their stay in the hospital for an acute cardiac condition such as MI, CABG, and PCI. In recent years, it is also offered to patients with more chronic conditions such as heart failure (reduced pumping function of the heart). CR has four goals: (1) physical recovery, (2) psychological recovery, (3) social recovery, and (4) lifestyle improvement. CR improves functional capacity, recovery, and psychological well-being and is cost-effective (Piepoli et al. 2010). Effectiveness lies in CR improving the physical condition, lifestyle (e.g., smoking cessation), medication adherence, and psychological well-being (Piepoli et al. 2010). The latter is of utmost importance since 75% of cardiac patients have elevated levels of depressive symptoms and/or symptoms of anxiety. About one fifth of cardiac patients suffer from depressive disorder (De Jong et al. 2004; Thombs et al. 2006). These conditions reduce the patient's health status in itself but are also risk factors for recurrent cardiovascular morbidity (disease) and mortality, and, finally, they reduce compliance with medical and lifestyle interventions. CR will thus indirectly contribute to RTW by improving physical condition, lifestyle, and psychological well-being.

CR that focuses on physical recovery has been offered to patients since the 1960s. This exercise-based CR is proven effective in reducing total and cardiovascular mortality and hospital admissions (Jolliffe et al. 2001; Piepoli et al. 2010; Heran et al. 2011). Next, CR has been extended with lifestyle interventions: quitting smoking, active lifestyle, no or moderate alcohol consumption, weight reduction, and healthy diet (reduction in saturated and trans fat, improve the consumption of n-3 fatty acids, improve consumption of fruit and vegetables, and reduce salt consumption). Often, psychological approaches are used to change unhealthy behavior into healthy behavior (Piepoli et al. 2010). CR is well implemented in the Western world although intensity varies (Piepoli et al. 2010).

However, specific attention to work-related issues or RTW is often lacking within CR (Reibis et al. 2019). In some countries, specialized occupational physicians or insurance physicians are available to support patients during their sickness absence and RTW. Only in recent years, specific interventions have been developed, but initially with little success. In their review of studies between 1982 and 2000, Perk and Alexanderson (2004) found no effects of specific RTW interventions for patients after MI, PCI, and CABG. An important aspect that was lacking in these interventions is tailoring to the specific needs of the employee with coronary heart disease, for example, reducing work demands (O'Hagan et al. 2012; Reibis et al. 2019). (Occupational) health professionals need to be aware of the possible patient-specific risk factors for delayed RTW and be able to decide on the individual patient's risk factors and on interventions to decrease or eliminate the patient's risk factors.

Outline of This Chapter

This chapter aims to familiarize the reader with the specific risk factors for RTW and possible interventions to improve the RTW of employees with coronary heart disease. This knowledge is not only important for research but also for (medical) practice, as most guidelines and directions for cardiac patients do not yet address the work situation or RTW support (cf Piepoli et al. 2016) or only offer broad directions (Reibis et al. 2019). This chapter will therefore address three topics:

1. Factors that impede RTW in employees with coronary heart disease (cardiac risk factors, psychosocial and physical work-related risk factors, and barriers to a successful RTW)
2. Interventions for employees with coronary heart disease that improve their RTW
3. Recommendations by experts for the organization of support of RTW of employees with coronary heart disease including tools (within CR)

Topics 1 and 2 are addressed via systematic reviews of the literature, except for cardiac risk factors and physical work-related risk factors, for which several guidelines already exist (see below). The searches were conducted in the context of developing a multidisciplinary guideline for CR in the Netherlands during 2008–2011 (van Stipdonk et al. 2011) and done during autumn 2010 for publications

Table 1 Search strategies and quality assessment of reviews

Stage	Review topic: 1. Psychosocial work-related risk factors	2. Barriers to a successful RTW	3. Interventions for employees with coronary heart disease that improve RTW
# hits review 2010	1220	130	664
# relevant on the basis of the title 2010	419	86	300
# relevant on the basis of the abstract 2010	380	67	216
# full articles available 2010	291	63	180
(# added on basis of references 2010)	39	14	4
# met inclusion criteria on basis of full article 2010	32	21	14
# hits review 2018	152		
# added on basis of relevance of title, abstract and full article 2018	3	14	3
Total number of articles	**35**	**35**	**17**
Quality of studies	$N = 35$: fair	$N = 35$: fair	$N = 13$: fair

in the previous 10 years (and thus not overlapping those in Perk and Alexanderson 2004) in the following databases: PsycINFO, CINAHL, and PubMed. The findings of these searches for the guideline were supplemented by a recent search of literature on RTW in patients with cardiovascular disease (2010–September 2018). The quality of individual studies was assessed (high quality, randomized controlled trial; fair quality, non-randomized trial, cohort study, and patient-control study; low quality, study with major flaws). The search strategy and quality assessment are presented in Table 1.

The conclusions of the reviews will be supplemented by three very recent reviews and recommendations on aspects of RTW of cardiac patients (Gragnano et al. 2018; O'Brien et al. 2018; Reibis et al. 2019). Moreover, the reviews will be supplemented by expert knowledge generated in the context of the guideline development described above. Experts were representatives of 12 scientific societies of professions involved in CR in the Netherlands (cardiologists, psychiatrists, psychologists, rehabilitation physicians, cardiac nurses, occupational therapists, physiotherapists, social workers, occupational physicians, occupational experts, social insurance physicians, and general practitioners). Also, representatives of the cardiac patient's association were involved. The discussions with experts covered 11 meetings over a period of 18 months and resulted in recommendations. In addition to these experts, a temporary working group of nine psychologists advised on psychological screening instruments and cutoff points to be used within CR. Thus, first risk factors for the recurrence of a cardiac event and barriers to RTW in employees with coronary heart disease will be addressed, and next evidence for RTW interventions for patients with coronary heart disease and, finally, a RTW support procedure within CR including practical tools will be presented. This chapter will be finished with conclusions for research and practice.

Risk Factors for Recurrence of a Cardiac Event and Barriers for RTW in Employees with Coronary Heart Disease

When addressing RTW in employees with coronary heart disease, it is important to distinguish between preventing a recurrent cardiac event (through managing cardiac, psychosocial, and physical work-related risk factors) and removing barriers for RTW (by managing risk factors for impaired RTW).

Cardiac Risk Factors

International and national guidelines (Bjarnason-Wehrens et al. 2004; van Dijk et al. 2006; Piepoli et al. 2010; Reibis et al. 2019) and the experts referred to above agree on eight cardiac factors that might affect work ability and/or increase the chance for recurrence of the cardiac event, possibly in interaction with certain working conditions (see Table 2). Table 2 also presents norms for when a factor is assumed to be a risk factor. First, (1) residual ischemia and (2) reduced heart function (left ventricular ejection factor <40%) are indications that working under heavy circumstances is dangerous. Next, (3) medication for the patient with coronary heart disease might have side effects that interfere with functioning at work. For example, ß-blockers reduce physical endurance and hamper performing heavy physical jobs. Stress at work can provoke (4) arrhythmia (irregular heart rate) and (5) tachycardia (too rapid heart rate), which the treating cardiologist might judge as being harmful, depending on the specific medical condition and level of stress at work. When untreated or resistant to treatment, (6) hypertension is regarded harmful above 160/100 mmHg and an extra risk for the respective patient for recurrence of a cardiac event. When the work situation demands (7) higher physical endurance than the patients has, this is again a risk for recurrence. Low physical endurance is also a risk for delayed RTW, as two recent studies showed (Salzwedel et al. 2016; Boschetto et al. 2016).

Existence of these cardiac risk factors does not imply that RTW will not be possible. However, they need to be interpreted in relation to the type of work. In practice, occupational health expertise is needed to weigh up the cardiac risk factors in relation to the exposure at work and to formulate recommendations for work adaptations or alternative work (van Dijk et al. 2006) as there is still no agreement on norms (Reibis et al. 2019).

Table 2 Cardiac risk factors that might interfere with performing work

Cardiac risk factors	Explanation including norms	References
1. Residual ischemia	Four classes of severity are distinguished by the New York Heart Association (NYHA classes) related to chest pain when climbing stairs (no pain = class I; pain after 3 stairs of 15 steps = class II; pain after 1 stair of 15 steps = class III) or even in rest (class IV) Precise exercise capacity and ischemic threshold can be established by bicycle ergometry or treadmill maximal stress test →Working conditions might provoke ischemia	Bjarnason-Wehrens et al. 2004; van Dijk et al. 2006; Piepoli et al. 2010; Boschetto et al. 2016; Salzwedel et al. 2016; Reibis et al. 2019
2. Reduced heart function (left ventricular ejection factor <40%).	→If reduced, the patient cannot perform physically heavy work	
3. Medication (particularly ß-blockers)	→Side effects might interfere with working conditions (e.g., ß-blockers reduce physical endurance)	
4. Arrhythmias (atrial or ventricular)	→ Stress or physical work demands might provoke arrhythmias	
5. Ventricular tachycardia (with strain and stress)	→ Stress might provoke ventricular tachycardia	
6. Untreated/therapy-resistant hypertension (≥160/100 mmHg)	Treatment is recommended for hypertension ≥140/90 mmHg, but some patients have low treatment adherence or their hypertension is resistant to therapy → Employees need to have a blood pressure <140/90 mmHg during rest	
7. Low physical endurance tolerance (determined by an endurance test)	Precise exercise capacity and ischemic threshold can be established by bicycle ergometry or treadmill maximal stress test →Working conditions should be below the patient's physical endurance	
8. ICD/PM implant	→ ICD/PM implant might interfere with electromagnetic exposure in the workplace	

Work-Related Risk Factors: Psychosocial Risk Factors

There is firm scientific evidence for the relationship between psychosocial work characteristics and coronary heart disease. Primarily, research regarding recurrence of coronary heart disease is relevant for defining risk factors for lack of RTW, but – as there is little research on work-related risk factors for impeded RTW – also research regarding the work-related etiology of coronary heart diseases is regarded informative (see Table 3).

Stressors at work are risk factors for RTW in persons with coronary heart disease, as they may increase the chance for recurrent cardiac events. There is moderate evidence regarding job demands and job strain (combination of high demands and low autonomy) in relation to recurrent cardiac incidence. Only for men there is enough evidence that high work demands are a strong prognostic risk factor for a recurrent cardiac event, particularly when combined with low autonomy at work. Recent research of Biering et al. (2015) demonstrated more sickness absence after PCI (percutaneous coronary intervention; see above) when having high demands and low autonomy, however, not an increased risk for cardiac events after RTW – which might be explained by changes in perceived or actual working conditions. Söderberg et al. (2015) showed that acute coronary syndrome (e.g., MI) survivors, who worked under adverse psychosocial work conditions, had lower return-to-work expectations compared to those working under better psychosocial work conditions. Salzwedel et al. (2016), however, found a higher psychosocial workload to *increase* the

Table 3 Psychosocial risk factors for (recurrent) cardiac event

Psychosocial risk factors for...	References
1. High work demands (in combination with low autonomy) for recurrent cardiac event	Belkic et al. 2004; Eaker et al. 2004; Malinauskiene et al. 2004; Riese et al. 2004; De Bacquer et al. 2005; Kivimäki et al. 2006; Kornitzer et al. 2006; Peter et al. 2006; Lallukka et al. 2006; Nomura et al. 2007; Wang et al. 2007; Eller et al. 2009; Bonde et al. 2009
2. High effort-reward imbalance for first cardiac event	Peter et al. 2002; Ala-Mursula et al. 2005; Chandola et al. 2005; van Vegchel et al. 2005; Peter et al. 2006
3. Lack of support from colleagues/supervisor for first cardiac event	Belkic et al. 2004; De Bacquer et al. 2005; Kuper et al. 2006; André-Petersson et al. 2007; Chandola et al. 2008; Eller et al. 2009
4. Other stressors at work for first cardiac event: financial setbacks, bankruptcy, not realizing a promotion, increase or decrease of responsibility, conflict, too many deadlines, too much competition at work, too much criticism of supervisor, change of workplace, and job dissatisfaction	Falger and Schouten 1992; Ferrie et al. 1995, 1998, 2002; Kivimäki et al. 2003; Theorell et al. 2003; Virtanen et al. 2003; Lee et al. 2004; Vahtera et al. 2004; Müller-Nordhorn et al. 2003; Gallo et al. 2006; Huisman et al. 2008; Väänänen et al. 2008; Eller et al. 2009; Fiabane et al. 2013

probability of RTW. Again, the results were primarily found among men, which could result from few female study participants or gender differences in RTW mechanisms. Gragnano et al. (2018), who reviewed work-related predictors for RTW in patients with cardiovascular disease published between 1994 and 2016, concluded that job strain and job control were the most important predictors of RTW, in addition to work ability.

A high effort-reward imbalance also increases the risk for a first cardiac event.

Recent research by Biering et al. (2015) among PCI patients showed that high work pace, low commitment to the workplace, low recognition (rewards), and low job control were associated with sickness absence at three months, but not after one year.

As Table 3 shows, lack of support from colleagues/supervisor is a risk factor for first cardiac events. There is evidence that other stressors at work also increase the risk for (first) cardiac events. Finally, and also shown in Table 3, there is suggestive evidence that diverse other stressors at work increase the risk for a first cardiac event.

Work-Related Risk Factors: Physical Risk Factors

For physical risk factors, guidelines already exist and no new review has been performed. These guidelines agree on four physical working environment factors that increase the risk for a cardiac event (Table 4). There is strong evidence for exposure to chemical and physical hazards and to noise. Shift work has direct negative effects on cardiovascular disease but also via a bad lifestyle. The evidence for sedentary work is weak, and often inconclusive, as studies often do not control for active lifestyle, groups are selective, and measures for sedentary work might not be valid. Findings are inconclusive for the following factors. Physically heavy work (e.g., lifting) is only regarded dangerous when performed irregularly by employees with a bad physical endurance. It is recommended that during an 8-hour working day, physical demands do not exceed 30–40% of VO2 maximal (Wiedeman et al. 1984). For working under extreme temperatures, which might trigger cardiac events,

Table 4 Physical risk factors in the working environment for cardiac events

Physical risk factor	References
1. Chemical and physical hazards, e.g., passive smoking, carbon monoxide, small particles ($\leq$2.5 μm)	Allred et al. 1989, He et al. 1999; Peters et al. 2001; Whincup et al. 2004
2. Noise ($\geq$85 dB)	Babisch et al. 2005; Willich et al. 1993
3. Shift work	Schnall et al. 2000; Knutsson 2003;
4. Sedentary work without compensating active lifestyle	van Uffelen et al. 2010
5. Physically heavy work	Wiedeman et al. 1984
6. Working under extreme temperatures	van Dijk et al. 2006; van Stipdonk et al. 2011

findings are contradictory and, according to the guideline, up to the discretion of occupational physicians (van Dijk et al. 2006).

Barriers to a Successful RTW

Many factors prolong sickness absence in cardiac patients. Four areas of psychosocial barriers to RTW can be distinguished: (1) vulnerable social-demographic status; (2) health problems and unhealthy lifestyle; (3) mental health problems; and (4) negative perceptions. In total, 17 barriers to a successful RTW are identified (see Table 5). A recent review that includes studies on factors related to RTW in

Table 5 Barriers to a successful RTW

Risk factor for RTW after cardiac event	References
Social-demographic factors	
1. Low education	Soejima et al. 1999; Söderman et al. 2003; Earle et al. 2006; Smedegaard et al. 2017; Butt et al. 2018
2. Low social support in their environment	Soejima et al. 1999; Sykes et al. 2000;
3. Female gender	Kragholm et al. 2015; Dreyer et al. 2016; Smedegaard et al. 2017; Butt et al. 2018;
4. >50 years of age	Kragholm et al. 2015; Butt et al. 2018
Health problems and unhealthy lifestyle	
5. Persistence of angina symptoms after hospitalization	Froom et al. 1999; Clarke et al. 2000; Shrey and Mital 2000; Mittag et al. 2001; Kamphuis et al. 2002; Earle et al. 2006; Samkange-Zeeb et al. 2006;
6. Cardiac health limits daily functioning	
7. Experience reduced physical activity on a daily basis	Sykes et al. 2000; Mittag et al. 2001; Slebus et al. 2007
8. Excessive alcohol use	
9. Prior cardiovascular disease symptoms	Froom et al. 1999; Clarke et al. 2000; Shrey and Mital 2000; Mittag et al. 2001; Kamphuis et al. 2002; Earle et al. 2006; Samkange-Zeeb et al. 2006; Butt et al. 2018
10. Other health problems	
Mental health problems	
11. Depressive symptoms	O'Neil et al. 2010; Ervasti et al. 2015; Haschke et al. 2012; de Jonge et al. 2014; Smedegaard et al. 2017
12. Anxiety symptoms	Gragnano et al. 2018; Reibis et al. 2019
Negative perceptions	
13. Lack of acceptance of the illness	Clarke et al. 2000; Müller-Nordhorn et al. 2003; Earle et al. 2006; Hemingway et al. 2007; Bergvik et al. 2012; Fiabane et al. 2013; Söderberg et al. 2015
14. Low recovery expectations	
15. Lack of self-confidence	
16. Low internal locus of control	
17. Lack of job satisfaction or motivation for RTW	

cardiovascular disease published between 1994 and 2016 parallels these findings (Gragnano et al. 2018).

Social-demographic factors. As Table 5 shows, cardiac patients with low education and/or low social support in their environment have increased risk not to return to their work. Several recent studies showed that women return to work less than men and, also, older cardiac patients return to work less often than younger patients.

Health problems and unhealthy lifestyle. If patients experience symptoms of angina after hospital dismissal and/or limitations in daily functioning, this hampers their RTW (see Table 5). Unhealthy lifestyle in terms of low physical activity and high alcohol consumption also hamper RTW. Patients with a history of cardiovascular disease are also hampered, as are those who have other health problems. Recently, Butt et al. (2018) found absence of major comorbidities to be associated with return to work 1 year after discharge for CABG.

Mental health problems. Depressive symptoms decrease the RTW chance considerably (the literature on anxiety is scarce but also points toward an increased risk for less RTW). Levels of depression and anxiety can be measured via assessment instruments (questionnaires). In the context of the guideline development, a systematic review and meeting with a specific working group of psychologists was organized to establish the top 3 of best assessment instruments (leaving discretion to the hospitals) with corresponding norm scores (van Engen-Verheul et al. 2012) (Table 6). Severe levels of depression and/or anxiety are an indication for a diagnostic interview to judge whether the patient fulfills the criteria for a depressive disorder or anxiety disorder or not. Low levels, though, indicate the absence of a risk factor. The HADS is widely accepted in hospitals, but psychometric qualities are low, particularly for anxiety, even though Reibis et al. (2019) recommend the HADS

Table 6 Norm scores for depression and anxiety in patients with coronary heart disease

	Depression	Anxiety
First choice	*Patient Health Questionnaire 9 items (PHQ-9)* (Spitzer et al. 1999) Severe: 10–27 Moderate: 5–9 Low: 0–4	*Generalized Anxiety Disorder 7 items (GAD-7)* (Spitzer et al. 2006) Severe: 10–27 Moderate: 5–9 Low: 0–4
Second choice	*Beck Depression Inventory (BDI)* (Beck et al. 1996) Severe: 10–63 Moderate: 5–9 Low: 0–4	*Beck Anxiety Inventory (BAI)* (Beck et al. 1988) Severe: 10–63 Moderate: 5–9 Low: 0–4
Third choice	*Hospital Anxiety and Depressions Scale – Depression (HADS-D)* (Spinhoven et al. 1997) Severe: 8–21 Moderate: 5–7 Low: 0–4	*Hospital Anxiety and Depressions Scale – Anxiety (HADS-A)* (Spinhoven et al. 1997) Severe: 8–21 Moderate: 5–7 Low: 0–4

to assess psychosocial parameters to improve RTW after an acute coronary syndrome such as MI.

Negative perceptions. As Table 5 shows, lack of acceptation of the illness, low recovery expectations, lack of self-confidence, and lower internal locus of control and motivation for RTW are all related to lower RTW rates. These negative thoughts that function as barriers to RTW might be explained by depression and/or might be rooted in adverse psychosocial working conditions. Söderberg et al. (2015) demonstrated in a cross-sectional study that such conditions are related to lower RTW expectations via fear-avoidance beliefs toward the workplace.

RTW Interventions for Employees with Coronary Heart Disease

Thirteen studies on RTW interventions for cardiac patients that met the inclusion criteria (published between January 2000 and September 2018; listed in PsycINFO, CINAHL, PubMed; evaluation study of RTW intervention in patients with a coronary heart disease) are included. Positive effects of interventions are found for ten of the interventions (Mital et al. 2000; Varvaro 1991; Higgins et al. 2001; Kutzleb and Reiner 2006; Hanssen et al. 2007; Broadbent et al. 2009; McKee 2009; Lamberti et al. 2016; Babić et al. 2015; Pirhonen et al. 2017). Generally, they are more comprehensive than the three interventions that did not yield results (Pfund 2001; Hanssen et al. 2009; Yonezawa et al. 2009). Still, the effective interventions vary largely regarding content. They include interventions focusing on reduction of barriers in terms of lifestyle, physical condition, and psychological symptoms by health education strategies; making a return-to-work plan; occupational counselling; establishing work modifications; and extensive assessment of the patient's condition in order to advise on when to return to work. Lamberti et al. (2016) and Babić et al. (2015) demonstrate that lack or delayed CR was related to reduced RTW. In checking the references of the hits, another four studies of fair quality were found that had been published before 2000 but had not been included in the review of Perk and Alexanderson (2004) (Picard et al. 1989; Haussler and Keck 1997; Dumont et al. 1999; Johnston et al. 1999). These studies present extensive and effective interventions. For example, one German intervention included a guided trajectory consisting of making up a problem analysis and a reintegration plan during rehabilitation; next a meeting with the employer regarding work modifications; and finally administrative and psychological support to safeguard RTW (Haussler and Keck 1997). The recent study by Pirhonen et al. (2017) showed positive effects of person-centered care on increased self-efficacy, but the positive effects on RTW were nonsignificant due to too short follow-up. Their intervention consists of patients and clinicians identifying and discussing problems and next considering both the outcomes of clinical tests and the practical, social, and emotional effects of their condition(s) and treatment(s) on their daily lives. A shared decision-making process informs a plan of action. O'Brien et al. (2018) showed with a meta-analysis of 18 RTW interventions for MI patients, a 3-month increase in RTW rate compared to usual care.

Recommendations by Experts for the Support of RTW in CR

On the basis of the scientific literature and expert opinion, a RTW support procedure within CR is recommended (Fig. 1). Basically, this procedure aligns with the support strategies that Reibis et al. (2019) recommend after CR.

In essence, the RTW support procedure needs to be tailored to the cardiac patient's individual risk factors and should be comprehensive enough the tackle risk factors for CVD and barriers to RTW. Further, the experts, with the occupational physicians in particular, advocate for gradual RTW during CR, so CR patients are supported by the CR team and have plenty opportunities to discuss work-related problems. Indeed, system delays decrease RTW (Laut et al. 2014). Reibis et al. (2019) also emphasize part-time, stepwise reintegration into work. However, they envision that RTW support is part of prolonged CR, rather than an integral part of CR. Because prolonged CR hardly exists across different countries (Reibis et al. 2019), it is recommended though to incorporate RTW support within regular CR.

The RTW support procedure should start with referral of the patient to CR by the treating cardiologist. To target the RTW support and align with other services, first, whether the patient has a work-related problem and is in need of RTW support needs to be checked and, if so, the risk factors from Tables 2, 3, 4, and 5 be assessed (the CR-WORK checklist with questions to support targeting during the intake for CR is available with the author upon request). In line with this, Reibis et al. (2019) also recommend risk stratification and making up a work-related diagnosis.

This assessment requires a trained nurse or reintegration professional. On the basis of risks for hampered RTW, interventions within and outside the CR/hospital

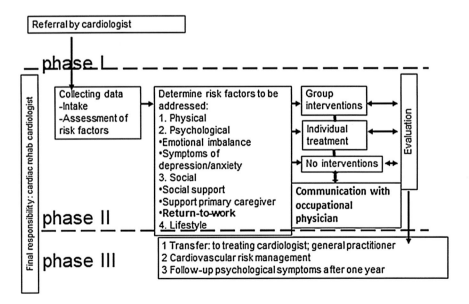

Fig. 1 RTW support procedure within CR

setting need to be selected and be prioritized together with the patient (the CR matrix with RTW interventions and referral options within and outside the hospital is available with the author upon request). In line with privacy laws, it is of utmost importance that healthcare workers do not contact the employer directly but communicate via the occupational physician and patient. This is to avoid (1) that employers receive medical, and thus private, information and (2) bypassing a possible occupational physician who – if available in a country's system – has a key role in translating medical status into work opportunities. Further and in line with the law on exchange of medical information, patients need to agree with the cardiologist on sending medical information to his or her occupational physician (if available). Lack of clarity regarding legislation and roles might lead to a reserved attitude regarding RTW support of cardiac patients.

During the support procedure, all CR professionals should monitor the patient's (steps toward) gradual RTW and the bottlenecks experienced by (in)formal talks with the patient, discuss the monitoring results in interdisciplinary meetings, and take adequate action if needed. Finally, the intervention results need to be evaluated. Within a CR setting, this is after 2–3 months. If the results are satisfying for the patient and professionals, the patient is transferred to guidance by the treating physician.

As part of the guideline project, we did a pilot study on using the CR-WORK checklist in one hospital during 2 weeks. Generally, the healthcare workers acknowledged two types of patients: those who feel pressed by the return to their work and those who hesitated to return to work and searched for ways to legitimize the delay of their RTW. The healthcare workers preferred a checklist format that fits their work routines. Also, the healthcare workers needed more knowledge about interventions to manage the risk factors and a standardized "tick-box format" letter to communicate with the patients' occupational physician.

Conclusions

There is evidence that specific support for RTW within CR improves the RTW rate, but interventions vary widely and are not integrated well in CR nor address the various types of risks. In this chapter, it is proposed to target the cardiac patients in need of RTW support, to screen them for risk factors, and to select interventions that fit with the individual risk factors, which are delivered both within and outside CR.

The review results have led to a guideline for RTW within CR in the Netherlands (van Stipdonk et al. 2011) and have implications for CR in other countries. In many countries, occupational physicians are not available or do not have tasks regarding RTW guidance. Even though in the Netherlands, occupational physicians have a key role in RTW guidance, they are not available to an increasing number of patients at working age (e.g., the self-employed, those working for temporary agencies, etc.). Bridging hospital treatment (rehabilitation) with workplace requirements is thus a bottleneck in all countries. CR is of utmost importance to support cardiac patients in their RTW (Piepoli et al. 2010; Reibis et al. 2019). It can be concluded that RTW guidance should be part of CR in order not to delay RTW unnecessarily and offer the patient tailor-made support. Standardized checklists such as the CR-WORK checklist, valid psychological questionnaires, and the CR matrix with RTW interventions offer healthcare workers more grip on an important aspect of CR that they might be insecure about. Reintegration agencies outside hospitals can also use the information in this chapter to develop their interventions. Next, the effectiveness of the new checklist and the intervention recommendations need to be studied in studies of high quality.

Cross-References

▶ Employment as a Key Rehabilitation Outcome
▶ IGLOO: A Framework for Return to Work Among Workers with Mental Health Problems
▶ Implementing Best Practice Models of Return to Work
▶ Occupational Determinants of Cardiovascular Disorders Including Stroke
▶ Promoting Workplace Mental Wellbeing

References

Ala-Mursula L, Vahtera J, Linna A, Pentti J, Kivimäki M (2005) Employee worktime control moderates the effects of job strain and effort-reward imbalance on sickness absence: the 10-town study. J Epidemiol Community Health 59:851–857

Allred EN, Bleecker ER, Chaitman BR, Dahms TE, Gottlieb SO, Hackney JD, Hayes D, Pagano M, Selvester RH, Walden SM (1989) Acute effects of carbon monoxide exposure on individuals with coronary artery disease. Res Rep Health Eff Inst 25:1–79

André-Petersson L, Engström G, Hedblad B, Janzon L, Rosvall M (2007) Social support at work and the risk of myocardial infarction and stroke in women and men. Soc Sci Med 64:830–834

Babić Z, Pavlov M, Oštrić M, Milošević M, Misigoj Duraković M, Pintarić H (2015) Re-initiating professional working activity after myocardial infarction in primary percutaneous coronary intervention networks era. Int J Occup Med Environ Health 28:999–1010

Babisch W, Beule B, Schust M, Kersten N, Ising H (2005) Traffic noise and risk of myocardial infarction. Epidemiology 16:33–40

Beck AT, Epstein N, Brown G, Steer RA (1988) An inventory for measuring clinical anxiety: psychometric properties. J Consult Clin Psychol 56:893–897

Beck AT, Steer RA, Ball R, Ranieri WF (1996) Comparison of Beck Depression Inventories-I and -II in psychiatric outpatients. J Pers Assess 67:588–597

Belkic KL, Landsbergis PA, Schnall PL, Baker D (2004) Is job strain a major source of cardiovascular disease risk? Scand J Work Environ Health 30:85–128

Bergvik S, Sørlie T, Wynn R (2012) Coronary patients who returned to work had stronger internal locus of control beliefs than those who did not return to work. Br J Health Psychol 17(5):96–608

Biering K, Lund T, Andersen JH, Hjollund NH (2015) Effect of psychosocial work environment on sickness absence among patients treated for ischemic heart disease. J Occup Rehabil 25:776–782

Bjarnason-Wehrens B, Mayer-Berger W, Meister ER, Baum K, Hambrecht R, Gielen S (2004) German Federation for Cardiovasular Prevention and Rehabilitation. Recommendations for resistance exercise in cardiac rehabilitation. Eur J Cardiovasc Prev Rehabil 11:352–361

Bonde JP, Munch-Hansen T, Agerbo E, Suadicani P, Wieclaw J, Westergaard-Nielsen N (2009) Job strain and ischemic heart disease: a prospective study using a new approach for exposure assessment. J Occup Environ Med 51:732–738

Boschetto P, Vaccari A, Groccia R, Casimirri E, Stendardo M, Maietti E, Volpato S, Sarcone M, Fucili A (2016) Forced expiratory volume in one second: predicting return to work within 3 months after chronic heart failure diagnosis. Int J Cardiol 203:798–799

Broadbent E, Ellis CJ, Thomas J, Gamble G, Petrie KJ (2009) Further development of an illness perception intervention for myocardial infarction patients: a randomized controlled trial. J Psychosom Res 67:17–23

Butt JH, Rørth R, Kragholm K, Kristensen SL, Torp-Pedersen C, Gislason GH, Køber L, Fosbøl EL (2018) Return to the workforce following coronary artery bypass grafting: a Danish nationwide cohort study. Int J Cardiol 251:15–21

Chandola T, Siegrist J, Marmot M (2005) Do changes in effort-reward imbalance at work contribute to an explanation of the social gradient in angina? Occup Environ Med 62:223–230

Chandola T, Britton A, Brunner E, Hemingway H, Malik M, Kumari M, Badrick E, Kivimäki M, Marmot M (2008) Work stress and coronary heart disease: what are the mechanisms? Eur Heart J 29:640–648

Clarke SP, Frasure-Smith N, Lespérance F, Bourassa MG (2000) Psychosocial factors as predictors of functional status at 1 year in patients with left ventricular dysfunction. Res Nurs Health 23:290–300

De Bacquer D, Pelfrene E, Clays E, Mak R, Moreau M, De Smet P, Kornitzer M, De Backer G (2005) Perceived job stress and incidence of coronary events: 3-year follow-up of the Belgian Job Stress Project cohort. Am J Epidemiol 161:434–441

de Jong MJ, Chung ML, Roser LP, Jensen LA, Kelso LA, Dracup K, McKinley S, Yamasaki K, Kim CJ, Riegel B, Ball C (2004) A five-country comparison of anxiety early after acute myocardial infarction. Eur J Cardiovasc Nurs 3:129–134

de Jonge P, Zuidersma M, Bültmann U (2014) The presence of a depressive episode predicts lower return to work rate after myocardial infarction. Gen Hosp Psychiatry 36:363–367

Dreyer RP, Xu X, Zhang W, Du X, Strait KM, Bierlein M, Bucholz EM, Geda M, Fox J, D'Onofrio G, Lichtman JH, Bueno H, Spertus JA, Krumholz HM (2016) Return to work after acute myocardial infarction: comparison between young women and men. Circ Cardiovasc Qual Outcomes 9:S45–S52

Dumont S, Jobin J, Deshaies G, Trudel L, Chantale M (1999) Rehabilitation and the socio-occupational reintegration of workers who have had a myocardial infarct: a pilot study. Can J Cardiol 15:453–461

Eaker ED, Sullivan LM, Kelly-Hayes M, D'Agostino RB Sr, Benjamin EJ (2004) Does job strain increase the risk for coronary heart disease or death in men and women? The Framingham offspring study. Am J Epidemiol 159:950–958

Earle A, Ayanian JZ, Heymann J (2006) Work resumption after newly diagnosed coronary heart disease: findings on the importance of paid leave. J Women's Health 15:430–441

Eller NH, Netterstrøm B, Gyntelberg F, Kristensen TS, Nielsen F, Steptoe A, Theorell T (2009) Work-related psychosocial factors and the development of ischemic heart disease: a systematic review. Cardiol Rev 17:83–97

Ervasti J, Vahtera J, Pentti J, Oksanen T, Ahola K, Kivekäs T, Kivimäki M, Virtanen M (2015) Return to work after depression-related absence by employees with and without other health conditions: a cohort study. Psychosom Med 77:126–135

Falger PR, Schouten EG (1992) Exhaustion, psychological stressors in the work environment, and acute myocardial infarction in adult men. J Psychosom Res 36:777–786

Ferrie JE, Shipley MJ, Marmot MG, Stansfeld S, Smith GD (1995) Health effects of anticipation of job change and non-employment: longitudinal data from the Whitehall II study. BMJ 311:1264–1269

Ferrie JE, Shipley MJ, Marmot MG, Stansfeld SA, Smith GD (1998) An uncertain future: the health effects of threats to employment security in white-collar men and women. Am J Public Health 88:1030–1036

Ferrie JE, Shipley MJ, Smith GD, Stansfeld SA, Marmot MG (2002) Change in health inequalities among British civil servants: the Whitehall II study. J Epidemiol Community Health 56:922–926

Fiabane E, Argentero P, Calsamiglia G, Candura SM, Giorgi I, Scafa F, Rugulies R (2013) Does job satisfaction predict early return to work after coronary angioplasty or cardiac surgery? Int Arch Occup Environ Health 86:561–569

Froom P, Cohen C, Rashcupkin J, Kristal-Boneh E, Melamed S, Benbassat J, Ribak J (1999) Referral to occupational medicine clinics and resumption of employment after myocardial infarction. J Occup Environ Med 41:943–947

Gallo WT, Teng HM, Falba TA, Kasl SV, Krumholz HM, Bradley EH (2006) The impact of late career job loss on myocardial infarction and stroke: a 10 year follow up using the health and retirement survey. Occup Environ Med 63:683–687

Gragnano A, Negrini A, Miglioretti M, Corbiere M (2018) Common psychosocial factors predicting return to work after common mental disorders, cardiovascular diseases, and cancers: a review of reviews supporting a cross-disease approach. J Occup Rehabil 28:215–231

Hanssen TA, Nordrehaug JE, Eide GE, Hanestad BR (2007) Improving outcomes after myocardial infarction: a randomized controlled trial evaluating effects of a telephone follow-up intervention. Eur J Cardiovasc Prev Rehabil 14:429–437

Hanssen TA, Nordrehaug JE, Eide GE, Hanestad BR (2009) Does a telephone follow-up intervention for patients discharged with acute myocardial infarction have long-term effects on health-related quality of life? A randomised controlled trial. J Clin Nursing 18:1334–1345

Haschke A, Hutter N, Baumeister H (2012) Indirect costs in patients with coronary artery disease and mental disorders: a systematic review and meta-analysis. Int J Occup Med Environ Health 25:319–329

Haussler B, Keck M (1997) Improvement in occupational rehabilitation of myocardial infarct patients – results of a model study in Rhineland-Pfalz. Rehabilitation 36:106–110

He J, Vupputuri S, Allen K, Prerost MR, Hughes J, Whelton PK (1999) Passive smoking and the risk of coronary heart disease – a meta-analysis of epidemiologic studies. New Engl J Med 25:920–926

Hemingway H, Vahtera J, Virtanen M, Pentti J, Kivimäki M (2007) Outcome of stable angina in a working population: the burden of sickness absence. Eur J Cardiovasc Prev Rehabil 14:373–379

Heran BS, Chen JM, Ebrahim S, Moxham T, Oldridge N, Rees K, Thompson DR, Taylor RS (2011) Exercise-based cardiac rehabilitation for coronary heart disease. Cochrane Database Syst Rev CD001800

Higgins HC, Hayes RL, McKenna KT (2001) Rehabilitation outcomes following percutaneous coronary interventions (PCI). Patient Educ Couns 43:219–230

Huisman M, Van Lenthe F, Avendano M, Mackenbach J (2008) The contribution of job characteristics to socioeconomic inequalities in incidence of myocardial infarction. Soc Sci Med 66:2240–2252

Jelinek M (2014) Resumption of work after acute coronary syndrome or coronary artery bypass surgery. Heart Lung Circ 23:1094

Johnston M, Foulkes J, Johnston DW, Pollard B, Gudmundsdottir H (1999) Impact on patients and partners of inpatient and extended cardiac counseling and rehabilitation: a controlled trial. Psychosom Med 61:225–233

Jolliffe JA, Rees K, Taylor RS, Thompson D, Oldridge N, Ebrahim S (2001) Exercise-based rehabilitation for coronary heart disease. Cochrane Database Syst Rev CD001800

Kamphuis M, Ottenkamp J, Vliegen HW, Vogels T, Zwinderman KH, Kamphuis RP, Verloove-Vanhorick SP (2002) Health related quality of life and health status in adult survivors with previously operated complex congenital heart disease. Heart 87:356–362

Kivimäki M, Vahtera J, Elovainio M, Pentti J, Virtanen M (2003) Human costs of organizational downsizing: comparing health trends between leavers and stayers. Am J Community Psychol 32:57–67

Kivimäki M, Virtanen M, Elovainio M, Kouvonen A, Väänänen A, Vahtera J (2006) Work stress in the etiology of coronary heart disease-a meta-analysis. Scand J Work Environ Health 32:431–442

Knutsson A (2003) Health disorders of shift workers. Occup Med 53:103–108

Kornitzer M, Desmet P, Sans S, Dramaix M, Boulenguez C, DeBacker G, Ferrario M, Houtman I, Isacsson SO, Ostergren PO, Peres I (2006) Job stress and major coronary events: results from the Job Stress, Absenteeism and Coronary Heart Disease in Europe study. Eur J Cardiovasc Prev Rehabil 13:695–704

Kraal JJ, Van den Akker-Van Marle ME, Abut-Hanna A, Stut W, Peek N, Kemps HMC (2017) Clinical and cost-effectiveness of home-based cardiac rehabilitation compared to conventional, centre-based cardiac rehabilitation: results of the FIT@Home study. Eur J Prev Cardiol 24:1260–1273

Kragholm K, Wissenberg M, Mortensen RN, Fonager K, Jensen SE, Rajan S, Lippert FK, Christensen EF, Hansen PA, Lang-Jensen T, Hendriksen OM, Kober L, Gislason G, Torp-Pedersen C, Rasmussen BS (2015) Return to work in out-of-hospital cardiac arrest survivors: a nationwide register-based follow-up study. Circulation 131:1682–1690

Kuper H, Adami HO, Theorell T, Weiderpass E (2006) Psychosocial determinants of coronary heart disease in middle-aged women: a prospective study in Sweden. Am J Epidemiol 164:349–457

Kutzleb J, Reiner D (2006) The impact of nurse-directed patient education on quality of life and functional capacity in people with heart failure. J Am Acad Nurse Pract 18:116–123

Lallukka T, Martikainen P, Reunanen A, Roos E, Sarlio-Lähteenkorva S, Lahelma E (2006) Associations between working conditions and angina pectoris symptoms among employed women. Psychosom Med 8:348–354

Lamberti M, Ratti G, Gerardi D, Capogrosso C, Ricciardi G, Fulgione C, Latte S, Tammaro P, Covino G, Nienhaus A, Grazillo EM, Mallardo M, Capogrosso P (2016) Work-related outcome after acute coronary syndrome: implications of complex cardiac rehabilitation in occupational medicine. Int J Occup Med Environ Health 29:649–657

Laut KG, Hjort J, Engstrøm T, Jensen LO, Tilsted Hansen HH, Jensen JS, Pedersen F, Jørgensen E, Holmvang L, Pedersen AB, Christensen EF, Lippert F, Lang-Jensen T, Jans H, Hansen PA, Trautner S, Kristensen SD, Lassen JF, Lash TL, Clemmensen P, Terkelsen CJ (2014) Impact of health care system delay in patients with ST-elevation myocardial infarction on return to labor market and work retirement. Am J Cardiol 114:1810–1816

Lee S, Colditz GA, Berkman LF, Kawachi I (2004) Prospective study of job insecurity and coronary heart disease in US women. Ann Epidemiol 14:24–30

Malinauskiene V, Theorell T, Grazuleviciene R, Malinauskas R, Azaraviciene A (2004) Low job control and myocardial infarction risk in the occupational categories of Kaunas men, Lithuania. J Epidemiol Community Health 58:131–135

McKee G (2009) Are there meaningful longitudinal changes in health related quality of life-SF36, in cardiac rehabilitation patients? Eur J Cardiovasc Nurs 8:40–47

Mital A, Shrey DE, Govindaraju M, Broderick TM, Colon-Brown K, Gustin BW (2000) Accelerating the return to work (RTW) chances of coronary heart disease (CHD) patients: part 1 – development and validation of a training programme. Disabil Rehabil 22:604–620

Mittag O, Kolenda KD, Nordman KJ, Bernien J, Maurischat C (2001) Return to work after myocardial infarction/coronary artery bypass grafting: patients' and physicians' initial viewpoints and outcome 12 months later. Soc Sci Med 52:1441–1450

Müller-Nordhorn J, Gehring J, Kulig M, Binting S, Klein G, Gohlke H, Völler H, Bestehorn K, Krobot KJ, Willich SN (2003) Return to work after cardiologic rehabilitation. Sozial- und Praventivmedizin 48:370–378

Nomura K, Nakao M, Sato M, Ishikawa H, Yano E (2007) The association of the reporting of somatic symptoms with job stress and active coping among Japanese white-collar workers. J Occup Health 49:370–375

O'Brien L, Wallace S, Romero L (2018) Effect of psychosocial and vocational interventions on return-to-work rates post-acute myocardial infarction: a systematic review. J Cardiopulm Rehabil Prev 38:215–223

O'Hagan FT, Coutu MF, Thomas SG, Mertens D (2012) Work reintegration and cardiovascular disease: medical and rehabilitation influences. J Occup Rehabil 22:270–281

O'Neil A, Sanderson K, Oldenburg B (2010) Depression as a predictor of work resumption following myocardial infarction (MI): a review of recent research evidence. Health Qual Life Outcomes 8:95

Perk J, Alexanderson K (2004) Sick leave due to coronary artery disease or stroke. Scand J Public Health 32(63S):181–206

Peter R, Siegrist J, Hallqvist J, Reuterwall C, Theorell T (2002) Psychosocial work environment and myocardial infarction: improving risk estimation by combining two complementary job stress models in the SHEEP Study. J Epidemiol Community Health 56:294–300

Peter R, Hammarström A, Hallqvist J, Siegrist J, Theorell T, SHEEP Study Group (2006) Does occupational gender segregation influence the association of effort-reward imbalance with myocardial infarction in the SHEEP study? Int J Behav Med 13:34–43

Peters A, Dockery DW, Muller JE, Mittleman MA (2001) Increased particulate air pollution and the triggering of myocardial infarction. Circulation 103:2810–2815

Pfund A (2001) Coronary intervention and occupational rehabilitation – a prospective, randomized intervention study. Z Kardiol 90:655–660

Picard MH, Dennis C, Schwartz RG, Ahn DK, Kraemer HC, Berger WE III, Blumberg R, Heller R, Lew H, DeBusk RF (1989) Cost-benefit analysis of early return to work after uncomplicated acute myocardial infarction. Am J Cardiol 63:1308–1314

Piepoli MF, Corra U, Benzer W, Bjarnason-Wehrens B, Dendale P, Gaita D, McGee H, Mendes M, Niebauer J, Zwisler AD, Schmid JP (2010) Seconday prevention through cardiac rehabilitation: from knowledge to implementation. A position paper from the Cardiac Rehabilitation Section of the European Association of Cardiovascular Prevention and Rehabilitation. Eur J Cardiovasc Prev Rehabil 17:1–17

Piepoli MF, Hoes AW, Agewall S, Albus C, Brotons C, Catapano AL, Cooney MT, Corra U, Cosyns B, Deaton C, Graham I, Hall MS, Hobbs FDR, Løchen M-L, Löllgren H, Marques-Vidal P, Perk J, Prescott E, Redon J, Richter DJ, Sattar N, Smulders Y, Tiberi M, van der Worp BH, van Dis I, Verschuren M (2016) European guidelines on cardiovascular disease prevention in clinical practice: The Sixth Joint Task Force of the European Society of Cardiology and Other Societies on Cardiovascular Disease Prevention in Clinical Practice (constituted by representatives of 10 societies and by invited experts) Developed with the special contribution of the European Association for Cardiovascular Prevention & Rehabilitation (EACPR). Eur Heart J 37:2315–2381

Pirhonen L, Olofsson EH, Fors A, Ekman I, Bolin K (2017) Effects of person-centred care on health outcomes-A randomized controlled trial in patients with acute coronary syndrome. Health Policy 121:169–179

Reibis R, Salzwedel A, Abreu A, Corra U, Davos C, Doehner W, Doherty P, Frederix I, Hansen D, Iliou M, Vigorito C, Völler H (2019) The importance of return to work: How to achieve optimal reintegration in ACS patients. Eur J Prev Cardiol 26:1358–1369

Riese H, Van Doornen LJ, Houtman IL, De Geus EJ (2004) Job strain in relation to ambulatory blood pressure, heart rate, and heart rate variability among female nurses. Scand J Work Environ Health 30:477–485

Salzwedel A, Reibis R, Wegscheider K, Eichler S, Buhlert H, Kaminski S, Völler H (2016) Cardiopulmonary exercise testing is predictive of return to work in cardiac patients after multicomponent rehabilitation. Clin Res Cardiol 105:257–267

Samkange-Zeeb F, Altenhöner T, Berg G, Schott T (2006) Predicting non-return to work in patients attending cardiac rehabilitation. Int J Rehabil Res 29:43–49

Schnall P, Belkić K, Landsbergis P, Baker D (2000) Why the workplace and cardiovascular disease? Occup Med 15:1–6

Shrey DE, Mital A (2000) Accelerating the return to work (RTW) chances of coronary heart disease (CHD) patients: part 2 – development and validation of a vocational rehabilitation programme. Disabil Rehabil 22:621–626

Slebus FG, Kuijer PP, Willems HJ, Sluiter JK, Frings-Dresen MH (2007) Prognostic factors for work ability in sicklisted employees with chronic diseases. Occup Environ Med 64:814–819

Smedegaard L, Numé AK, Charlot M, Kragholm K, Gislason G, Hansen PR (2017) Return to work and risk of subsequent detachment from employment after myocardial infarction: insights from Danish nationwide registries. J Am Heart Assoc 10:e006486

Söderberg M, Rosengren A, Gustavsson S, Schiöler L, Härenstam A, Torén K (2015) Psychosocial job conditions, fear avoidance beliefs and expected return to work following acute coronary syndrome: a cross-sectional study of fear-avoidance as a potential mediator. BMC Public Health 15:1263

Söderman E, Lisspers J, Sundin O (2003) Depression as a predictor of return to work in patients with coronary artery disease. Soc Sci Med 56:193–202

Soejima Y, Steptoe A, Nozoe SI, Tei C (1999) Psychosocial and clinical factors predicting resumption of work following acute myocardial infarction in Japanese men. Int J Cardiol 72:39–47

Spinhoven P, Ormel J, Sloekers PP, Kempen GI, Speckens AE, Van Hemert AM (1997) A validation study of the Hospital Anxiety and Depression Scale (HADS) in different groups of Dutch subjects. Psychol Med 27:363–370

Spitzer RL, Kroenke K, Williams JB (1999) Validation and utility of a self-report version of PRIME-MD: the PHQ primary care study. JAMA 282:1737–1744

Spitzer RL, Kroenke K, Williams JB, Lowe B (2006) A brief measure for assessing generalized anxiety disorder. The GAD-7. Arch Intern Med 166:1092–1097

Sykes DH, Hanley M, Boyle DM, Higginson JDS (2000) Work strain and the post-discharge adjustment of patients following a heart attack. Psychol Health 15:609–623

Theorell T, Oxenstierna G, Westerlund H, Ferrie J, Hagberg J, Alfredsson L (2003) Downsizing of staff is associated with lowered medically certified sick leave in female employees. Occup Environ Med 60:E9

Thombs BD, Bass EB, Ford DE, Stewart KJ, Tsilidis KK, Patel U, Fauerbach JA, Bush DE, Ziegelstein RC (2006) Prevalence of depression in survivors of acute myocardial infarction. J Gen Intern Med 21:30–38

Väänänen A, Koskinen A, Joensuu M, Kivimäki M, Vahtera J, Kouvonen A, Jäppinen P (2008) Lack of predictability at work and risk of acute myocardial infarction: an 18-year prospective study of industrial employees. Am J Public Health 98:2264–2271

Vahtera J, Kivimäki M, Pentti J, Linna A, Virtanen M, Virtanen P, Ferrie JE (2004) Organisational downsizing, sickness absence, and mortality: 10-town prospective cohort study. BMJ 328:555

van Dijk JL, Bekedam MA, Brouwer W, Buijvoets M, Gielen CMJ, Jambroes G, Robeer GG, Smeenk D, Willems MLN (2006) Achtergronddocument bij de richtlijn ischemische hartziekten. Handelen van de bedrijfsarts bij werknemers met ischemische hartziekten. NVAB Kwaliteitsbureau, Utrecht

van Engen-Verheul MM, de Rijk AE, Peek N (eds) (2012) Beslisboom Poliklinische Indicatiestelling Hartrevalidatie 2012. Nederlandse Vereniging voor Cardiologie, Utrecht

van Stipdonk T, Kuijpers P, de Rijk A, van Dijk J, projectgroep PAAHR (2011) Intervenies gericht op sociale doelen. In: Revalidatiecommissie NVVC/NHS en projectgroep PAAHR (ed) Multi-disciplinaire Richtlijn Hartrevalidatie 2011. Nederlandse Vereniging Voor Cardiologie, Utrecht

van Uffelen JG, Wong J, Chau JY, van der Ploeg HP, Riphagen I, Gilson ND, Burton NW, Healy GN, Thorp AA, Clark BK, Gardiner PA (2010) Occupational sitting and health risks: a systematic review. Am J Prev Med 39:379–388

van Vegchel N, De Jonge J, Bosma H, Schaufeli W (2005) Reviewing the effort-reward imbalance model: drawing up the balance of 45 empirical studies. Soc Sci Med 60:1117–1131

Varvaro FF (1991) Women with coronary heart disease: an application of Roy's Adaptation Model. Cardiovasc Nurs 27:31–35

Virtanen M, Kivimäki M, Elovainio M, Vahtera J, Ferrie JE (2003) From insecure to secure employment: changes in work, health, health related behaviours, and sickness absence. Occup Environ Med 60:948–953

Wang HX, Leineweber C, Kirkeeide R, Svane B, Schenck-Gustafsson K, Theorell T, Orth-Gomér K (2007) Psychosocial stress and atherosclerosis: family and work stress accelerate progression of coronary disease in women. The Stockholm Female Coronary Angiography Study. J Intern Med 26:245–254

Whincup PH, Gilg JA, Emberson JR, Jarvis MJ, Feyerabend C, Bryant A, Walker M, Cook DG (2004) Passive smoking and risk of coronary heart disease and stroke: prospective study with cotinine measurement. BMJ 329:200–205

Wiedeman HP, Gee JB, Balmes JR, Loke J (1984) Exercise testing in occupational lung disease. Clin Chest Med 5:157–171

Willich S, Lewis M, Lowel H (1993) Physical exertion as a trigger of acute myocardial infarction. N Engl J Med 329:1684–1690

Worcester MU, Elliott PC, Turner A, Pereira JJ, Murphy BM, Le Grande MR, Middleton KL, Navaratnam HS, Nguyen JK, Newman RW, Tatoulis J (2014) Resumption of work after acute coronary syndrome or coronary artery bypass graft surgery. Heart Lung Circ 23:444–453

Yonezawa R, Masuda T, Matsunaga A, Takahashi Y, Saitoh M, Ishii A, Kutsuna T, Matsumoto T, Yamamoto K, Aiba N, Hara M (2009) Effects of phase II cardiac rehabilitation on job stress and health-related quality of life after return to work in middle-aged patients with acute myocardial infarction. Int Heart J 50:279–290

Return to Work After Stroke

25

Akizumi Tsutsumi

Contents

Introduction	452
Current RTW Rate	453
Prognostic Factors for RTW	453
Recurrent Stroke	454
Functional Disability	454
Higher Brain Function	454
Post-stroke Fatigue and Depression	455
Demographic and Socioeconomic Factors (Social Determinants)	455
Psychosocial Factors	456
Current States of Interventions	456
Pharmacological Interventions	456
Rehabilitation	456
Cognitive Behavioral Therapy	457
Work- and Employment-Related Interventions	457
Supervisor Training	458
Social Systems (Case Examples)	458
Remaining Challenges	460
Intervention on Psychosocial Factors	460
Management of Workers with Disabilities	460
Fitness for Work and Workplace Accommodation	461
Social Systems	462
Conclusions	462
Cross-References	463
References	463

A. Tsutsumi (✉)
Department of Public Health, Kitasato University School of Medicine, Sagamihara, Japan
e-mail: akizumi@kitasato-u.ac.jp

© Springer Nature Switzerland AG 2020
U. Bültmann, J. Siegrist (eds.), *Handbook of Disability, Work and Health*, Handbook Series in Occupational Health Sciences, https://doi.org/10.1007/978-3-030-24334-0_25

Abstract

Stroke is recognized as the single largest cause of severe disability worldwide. The cost of stroke is greater for young people because of a greater loss in productivity. Return to work (RTW) following stroke represents a major psychosocial complication. Approximately 40%–55% of patients with stroke need active rehabilitation, and 60% of stroke survivors need job modification after stroke. Factors associated with RTW include functional recovery, higher brain dysfunction, post-stroke fatigue and depression, socioeconomic status, employer flexibility, social benefits, and support from family or coworkers. Although rehabilitation techniques have been improved and some rehabilitation programs have been shown to be effective, there is a paucity of studies on vocational outcomes after stroke. RTW after stroke is a challenge for younger stroke survivors as well as for the older working population in general and people with disabilities who want to work. The system of RTW for workers with disabilities, such as disease treatment (including rehabilitation), workplace accommodation, and cooperation and coordination among stakeholders, should be consolidated. Overcoming the challenges of RTW after stroke is a key milestone for harmonizing work and disease treatment.

Keywords

Fitness for work · Functional disability · Harmonizing work and disease treatment · Higher brain dysfunction · Psychosocial work environment · Rehabilitation · Social determinants · Workplace accommodation

Introduction

Stroke is recognized as the single largest cause of severe disability worldwide (Arauz 2013) and is a leading cause of mortality, accounting for 11.8% of total deaths worldwide (Centers for Disease Control and Prevention (CDC) 2009). In the USA, stroke accounts for about 1 in every 20 deaths and has serious consequences for healthcare expenditure (Mozaffarian et al. 2016). Direct medical expenditure for stroke was around $71.6 billion in 2012, with this expenditure estimated to be $184.1 billion in 2030 (Ovbiagele et al. 2013). Approximately 60% of economic loss due to stroke is indirect loss associated with lost productivity (Taylor et al. 1996). Aging populations and prolonged stroke survival mean that the prevalence of stroke survivors among the working-age population is expected to increase in the near future (Arauz 2013).

Stroke in young patients is a major socioeconomic issue, as survivors have a longer time to live with any resulting physical impairments. Approximately 20% of stroke survivors in industrial nations are of working age or younger (Luengo-Fernandez et al. 2009). Young stroke patients face difficulty in return to work (RTW) (Teasell et al. 2000), and stroke in young people costs a greater deal of money than stroke in older people in terms of loss in productivity (Jacobs et al. 2002). Vocational needs for RTW after stroke are often neglected during medical rehabilitation. Returns on investment in vocational rehabilitation were reported to be far from idealistic when RTW was set as the primary outcome; that is, many stroke survivors who received vocational rehabilitation ended up on a disability pension allowance (Treger et al. 2007).

This chapter aims to clarify the major challenges and rehabilitation approaches with regard to RTW after stroke, by reviewing the current RTW rate, the relevant prognostic factors for RTW, and the current states of interventions and social systems.

Current RTW Rate

It is difficult to estimate true RTW rates after stroke because previous studies in this area differ in aspects such as study populations, definitions and types of stroke studied, definitions of work, study designs and methodologies, and company healthcare systems.

Daniel et al. (2009) reviewed 70 studies that reported data on RTW after stroke and found that the proportion of RTW ranged from 0% to 100% (average 44%). However, most studies reported RTW as a proxy for recovery or measure of rehabilitation outcomes (Daniel et al. 2009). Another review summarized 24 studies on RTW after ischemic stroke and reported RTW rates of 9%–91% (Wozniak and Kittner 2002). The cumulative full RTW rate appears to be improving each year. For example, a cohort study from Denmark showed that the odds for return to gainful occupation 2 years after stroke increased from 54% in 1996 to 72% in 2006 (Hannerz et al. 2012b).

For a more accurate estimation of RTW rate, Wozniak and Kittner (2002) argued for the necessity of time-to-event (life table or survival) analysis; however, there have been few studies on the time course of RTW after stroke. Recently, Endo et al. (2016) reported RTW in 382 Japanese stroke survivors using an objective measurement of sickness absence based on data from the occupational health register (clinically certified sickness absence using physicians' certificates). The cumulative RTW rate was 15.1% at 60 days post-stroke, 33.6% at 120 days post-stroke, 43.5% at 180 days post-stroke, and 62.4% at 365 days post-stroke (Endo et al. 2016).

Prognostic Factors for RTW

Functional ability is one of the most robust predictors of RTW. However, functional ability alone is not an indication of RTW after stroke. Stroke survivors who have high function scores should still be assessed for workability and assisted with the RTW process where possible. Glozier et al. (2008) noted that potentially treatable psychiatric morbidity and physical disability are determinants of RTW after stroke.

Appropriate management of both emotional and physical sequelae therefore appears necessary to optimize recovery and RTW in younger adults after stroke (Glozier et al. 2008).

Recurrent Stroke

Based on a previous estimation on stroke prognosis, the proportion of the target population that need active rehabilitation, after excluding the deceased and those that reach functional independence (recovery without disability), is approximately 40%–55% of patients with stroke (Macdonell and Dewey 2001). Recurrent stroke is a key factor that inhibits rehabilitation and is associated with increased difficulty in RTW. Even in the chronic phase, there is a strong association between recurrent stroke and prognosis. The cumulative risk of suffering stroke recurrence is estimated at 30% by 5 years. This risk is highest soon after the first stroke (13% by 1 year), with the average annual risk about 4% after the first year. The risk of stroke recurrence did not appear to be related to age or pathological type of stroke (Burn et al. 1994).

Functional Disability

An individual's functional disability (e.g., hemiplegia) at 5 to 10 years may be determined by 1 year after stroke onset. Newman observed that little neurological improvement occurred after the 14th week, the average interval from onset to 80% final recovery was 6 weeks, and functional recovery closely followed neurological recovery (Newman 1972). Functional recovery after stroke reaches a plateau by 6 months after disease onset. Actual accumulation of RTW indicates that RTW rarely starts during or immediately after this 6-month period. It has been suggested that factors other than functional recovery (e.g., provision of vocationally directed rehabilitation) are associated with RTW, such as higher brain dysfunction, mental dysfunction, employer flexibility, social benefits, and support from family or coworkers (Alaszewski et al. 2007).

Higher Brain Function

Higher brain function is related to social dysfunction after stroke in patients who return to work. Among stroke survivors with mild physical impairment, those with dysfunctions in attention, memory, and intelligence had a significantly lower likelihood of an early RTW (Tanaka et al. 2011). However, few studies have examined strong predicting factors in terms of RTW prognosis among stroke survivors with impairment of higher brain function.

Kauranen et al. (2013) showed that the cognitive severity of stroke in the first weeks after stroke predicted an inability to RTW 6 months after a stroke. Deficits evaluated as cognitive functions included executive functions (a set of processes concerned with managing oneself and one's resources to achieve a goal), psychomotor speed, episodic memory, working memory, language, visuospatial and constructional skills, and motor skills. Similarly, subtle cognitive deficits in survivors of cerebellar stroke adversely affected RTW, including impairments in working memory, mental speed and flexibility, and visuospatial ability (Malm et al. 1998).

Post-stroke Fatigue and Depression

Post-stroke fatigue is considered one of the greatest impairment-related barriers to RTW and tends to persist as a relevant impediment over time (Hartke and Trierweiler 2015). Evidence suggests that people who complain of fatigue at the time of hospital discharge rarely return to work. The prevalence of post-stroke fatigue has been reported to range from 30% to 68% (De Groot et al. 2003). In young adults, post-stroke fatigue has a pronounced negative influence on functional outcomes (Maaijwee et al. 2015).

Depression is also common among patients with stroke. A systematic review of observational studies revealed that a pooled estimate of 33% (95% confidence interval [CI] 29%–36%) of all stroke survivors experienced depression (Hackett and Pickles 2014). Post-stroke depression is considered a factor that may hinder RTW after stroke, although not all studies support this concept.

Demographic and Socioeconomic Factors (Social Determinants)

Older age seems to increase the difficulty of RTW (Howard et al. 1985; Wozniak et al. 1999), although socioeconomic factors such as retirement may confound this association. Female sex was also reported to be a negative predictor of RTW (Saeki and Toyonaga 2010; Wozniak et al. 1999).

Higher socioeconomic status appears to be related to successful RTW. High educational attainment (Bergmann et al. 1991; Neau et al. 1998) and increased total household income (Wozniak et al. 1999) were positively associated with RTW. One study showed that with a few exceptions, white-collar workers tended to RTW more often than blue-collar workers (Treger et al. 2007). Stroke survivors in professional-managerial positions were also more likely to RTW than farm or blue-collar workers (Bergmann et al. 1991; Howard et al. 1985; Neau et al. 1998).

A prospective analysis based on nationwide data on enterprise size from Statistics Denmark merged with data from the Danish occupational hospitalization register revealed a statistically significant positive association between enterprise size and an increase in the estimated odds of RTW (Hannerz et al. 2012a). Provision of occupational health services largely depends on enterprise size, and occupational health activities are often insufficient, especially in small-sized businesses. Larger companies were also reported to be more positive in their attitude toward hiring persons with disabilities (Rimmerman 1998). In contrast, smaller companies are less likely to have flexible working systems, sufficient paid sick leave systems, or RTW systems.

Psychosocial Factors

Perceived stress or worry about RTW (e.g., expectation for a successful RTW and adjusting to performing job tasks with new limitations) is considered the greatest impediment to RTW. Attitudes of coworkers and flexibility in work schedules are the most helpful for the RTW process (Hartke and Trierweiler 2015). Social support at work, particularly emotional support, may be a strong promoter of RTW (Glass et al. 1993). In particular, good supervisor support facilitates RTW, as the employer's attitude toward disabilities is influential (Treger et al. 2007).

Work stress measured by the relevant occupational stress models, such as the job demand-control model (Karasek and Theorell 1990) and the effort-reward imbalance model (Siegrist 1996), was associated with an increased relative risk of recurrent coronary heart diseases events by 65% (Li et al. 2015). However, evidence is lacking on prognostic factors for RTW after stroke explored by using these occupational stress models.

Current States of Interventions

Pharmacological Interventions

The greatest risk factor for stroke recurrence is hypertension. Active treatment of high blood pressure reduced the risk of stroke among both hypertensive and non-hypertensive individuals with a history of stroke or transient ischemic attack (relative risk reduction 28%) (PROGRESS Collaborative Group 2001). A subtype analysis revealed that the relative risk for any stroke during follow-up was reduced by 26% (95% CI 12–38) among patients whose baseline cerebrovascular event was an ischemic stroke and by 49% (95% CI 18–68) among those whose baseline event was an intracerebral hemorrhage (Chapman et al. 2004).

A systematic review including 16 trials (1655 participants at entry) revealed beneficial effects of pharmacotherapy in terms of complete remission of depression and a reduction in scores on depression rating scales after stroke. However, there was also evidence of an increase in adverse events. In the natural history of post-stroke depression, there were self-limited cases in most studies after several months. It has also been reported that few stroke patients receive effective management for their depression (Hackett et al. 2005).

Rehabilitation

There is robust evidence showing stroke rehabilitation in diverse settings provides beneficial effects for improving patients' functional status, survival, cardiovascular disease risk profiles, quality of life, and reduction of recurrent stroke risk and psychological disorders (Winstein et al. 2016). Of those stroke survivors who received vocational rehabilitation counseling, two times as many reported a RTW

1 year after their stroke than survivors that did not receive counseling (Sinclair et al. 2014).

To establish recommendations for the practice of rehabilitation for cognitive disability after traumatic brain injury and stroke, the Cognitive Rehabilitation Task Force evaluated 370 cognitive rehabilitation interventions published from 1971 to 2008 based on 3 consecutive systematic reviews (see Cicerone et al. (2011) for the latest review). They provided evidence for the comparative effectiveness of cognitive rehabilitation, including support for visuospatial rehabilitation after right hemisphere stroke, and interventions for aphasia and apraxia after left hemisphere stroke. A number of recommended practice standards reflect the lateralized nature of cognitive dysfunction that is characteristic of stroke. For example, after right hemisphere stroke, visuospatial rehabilitation that includes visual scanning training for left visual neglect is recommended. Cognitive-linguistic interventions for aphasia and gestural strategy training for apraxia are recommended after left hemisphere stroke. Computer-based training programs may be considered as an adjunct to clinician-guided treatment for the remediation of attention deficits after stroke, although the level of recommendation was low; however, such programs may help to increase working memory capacity (Westerberg et al. 2007).

Cognitive Behavioral Therapy

Cognitive behavioral therapy may be used for stress control in patients post-stroke. The effectiveness of cognitive remediation and cognitive behavioral psychotherapy was tested for participants with persisting complaints after mild or moderate traumatic brain injury. Cognitive remediation consisted of direct attention training along with training in use of a memory notebook and problem-solving strategies. Cognitive behavioral therapy was used to increase coping behaviors and reduce stress. Participants demonstrated improved performance on a measure of complex attention and reduced emotional distress compared with a control group (Tiersky et al. 2005). Cognitive training has also been applied to treat post-stroke fatigue. A program combining cognitive treatment to reduce fatigue and graded activity training tested with patients with post-stroke fatigue reported positive short- and long-term effects in terms of fatigue complaints and improved fitness (Zedlitz et al. 2011).

Work- and Employment-Related Interventions

Adaptation of the working environment for patients with stroke that have disabilities is essential to support their RTW. A study of rehabilitation patients reported that over 90% of patients after stroke had been transferred to a job suited for people with disabilities or their workplace had been restructured (Bergmann et al. 1991). A US survey revealed that nearly 60% of stroke survivors who had held full-time jobs before their stroke acknowledged that their jobs required modification because of stroke-related changes in their abilities (Black-Schaffer and Osberg 1990). Many studies have shown that over 70% of stroke survivors resumed full-time employment (Bergmann et al. 1991; Neau et al. 1998; Wozniak et al. 1999). However, some studies showed that these rates lowered to around 50% and that 22% of patients had to RTW half time or less (Black-Schaffer and Osberg 1990). The proportions of those that needed adjustment in their occupation, working hours, or type of employment were lower among young patients with stroke compared with older patients (23% and 26%, respectively) (Neau et al. 1998). In addition, many patients needed accommodating or workplace restructuring according to special needs after stroke.

A workplace intervention comprising workability assessments and workplace visits was effective in facilitating RTW for stroke survivors (Ntsiea et al. 2015), with stroke survivors who received individualized RTW programs being three times as likely to return to work than survivors who received usual care. The program was tailored according to the functional ability and workplace challenges of each stroke survivor and was administered by a physiotherapist and an occupational therapist. The program comprised (1) assessment to identify potential problems in the fit between work and stroke survivors' skills, including psychosocial work environment (Karasek and Theorell 1990); (2) separate interviews with the stroke survivor and employer to establish perceived barriers and enablers of RTW; and (3) a work visit for the stroke survivor to demonstrate what they do at work and identify what they could still do safely and what they could not do. Where possible, a plan for reasonable accommodation was discussed with a social worker/psychologist/speech therapist as necessary. Both workplace accommodation (change of job description and work adaptations) and vocational rehabilitation programs were provided. Most stroke survivors in the intervention group had work adaptations and job description changes following communication and contact between employers and therapists.

Supervisor Training

A trial was conducted to determine the competencies supervisors need to facilitate a worker's RTW following absence due to a mental health condition or a musculoskeletal disorder (Johnston et al. 2015). RTW competencies were allocated to nine clusters of related items (Table 1). Nearly all respondents (who represented a variety of rehabilitation professionals and jurisdictions) agreed that supervisors should receive training to achieve competencies for supporting RTW. Although developed for mental health conditions or musculoskeletal disorders, these competencies are applicable for RTW following many other disabilities or injuries, including stroke.

Social Systems (Case Examples)

The "fit note system" may be applicable to facilitate cooperation among stakeholders. In the UK, general practitioners (i.e., attending physicians) assess the fitness of workers on leave due to health problems and use a "Statement of Fitness for

Table 1 Essential competency clusters for supervisors who manage return to work (Johnston et al. 2015)

Enabling behaviors and personal attributes
Knowing return-to-work systems, processes, and procedures
Understanding and giving support to the injured worker
Communicating effectively with the injured worker
Liaising with key stakeholders (other than the injured worker)
Accessing knowledge and support for themselves
Developing, establishing, and monitoring the RTW plan
Managing the impact of the RTW on teams and coworkers
Managing impact of RTW programs on organizational effectiveness

Work" (fit note). This system allows physicians to provide advice on the types of assistance required of an employer. A fit note is not a conventional medical certificate that indicates the need for a leave of absence, but rather focuses on the conditions required for a worker to RTW. Therefore, it is effective in preventing the prolongation of leave of absence by altering workplace perceptions and behaviors regarding leave of absence and RTW. In the UK, fit notes are commonly used for illnesses and injuries to encourage the employer and patient to come to an agreement regarding working conditions by considering the patient's condition and helping them RTW. Fit notes are forms on which an attending physician checks either "not fit for work" or "you may be fit for work if you take into account the following advice" and provides details on the minimum required clinical considerations. Fit notes currently used in the UK include four check boxes that indicate detailed instructions to be followed in cases where a worker may be fit to return to work: "a phased return to work," "altered hours," "amended duties," and "workplace adaptations." There is also a blank space in which a physician can write their opinion. In such cases, a physician must consider work conditions at the individual's workplace. However, as a physician cannot be expected to have specialized knowledge about an individual's workplace and occupational health and safety issues, the physician's advice forms the basis for discussing these issues. The role of determining the actual extent of feasible compliance with this advice is the responsibility of the patient (worker) and their employer. Fit notes that are currently used generally allow a physician to state their opinion regarding a patient's recuperation, work restrictions, and taking a leave of absence based on clinical findings related to the patient (worker). Fit notes are used by physicians to provide advice from a medical perspective that is useful in promoting the continuation of work while considering workplace conditions. The fit note system has undergone provisional adoption in countries outside the UK.

On February 23, 2016, the Japan Ministry of Health, Labour and Welfare released *Guidelines for Supporting the Ability to Work at Workplaces while Undergoing Treatment*, which describe workplace initiatives designed to ensure that consideration is given to appropriate workplace conditions and the treatment of workers suffering from cancer, stroke, and other illnesses so that they can continue working while undergoing treatment. The recommendations in that report include the following: (1) workers request employer support (the attending physician submits a written opinion regarding items that require consideration); (2) the employer considers the opinions of occupational physicians and others regarding required measures and considerations; and (3) the employer determines and implements workplace measures (the creation of a "Support Plan" is recommended). Although these recommendations relate to cases of cancer or stroke, forms used to provide information on employment with attending physicians, as well as those used when attending physicians are asked to provide an opinion, are similar to those used in the UK fit note system. A problem hindering cooperation between employers and attending physicians is that they use different language (i.e., technical terms). It has also been noted that patients may need psychological assistance because of various difficulties they experience, such as economic stress due to job loss. To improve communication between stakeholders, training of coordinators to assist patients has started.

Remaining Challenges

Intervention on Psychosocial Factors

Many factors that are known to influence vocational outcomes after other illnesses have not been examined in terms of stroke (Wozniak and Kittner 2002). Psychosocial job characteristics are such factors, and factors conceptualized by the relevant occupational stress models (Karasek and Theorell 1990; Siegrist 1996) can be utilized for the theory-based interventions (Tsutsumi and Kawakami 2004). Actually, evaluation of psychosocial job characteristics was effectively utilized for individualized RTW programs for stroke survivors (Ntsiea et al. 2015). Low workplace social support and low levels of job control were associated with colleagues' negative perceptions of individuals with a psychiatric disorder returning to work (Eguchi et al. 2017). Improving psychosocial job characteristics may lead to successful RTW for stroke survivors through changing colleagues' negative perceptions. Further studies are necessary to investigate the impact of psychosocial job characteristics on RTW after stroke.

High levels of social support were associated with faster and more extensive recovery of functional status (Glass et al. 1993) and health-related quality of life after stroke (King 1996). However, evidence of a direct association between social support and RTW is lacking. Interventions to improve social support at work should be tested in the near future.

Management of Workers with Disabilities

There are insufficient studies that have evaluated any therapy for depression after stroke. Intervention studies are limited, and knowledge about effective management has important gaps. In addition, there is no robust evidence about how to treat patients with mild to moderate depression after stroke and a paucity of evidence on how to manage people with suspected depression in whom mood cannot be formally assessed because of aphasia (Hackett et al. 2014).

In terms of higher brain function, job modification through occupational management is required to maximize the performance of patients with stroke to compensate for their disabilities (Tanaka et al. 2011). Although some evidence-based practical recommendations have been established, there remain challenges to improve their working capacity (Cicerone et al. 2011). For example, benefits from targeting visual attention deficits skills are limited, and there is need for specific, functional skill training to improve driving ability after stroke (Mazer et al. 2003). It is also acknowledged that additional research is needed to investigate patient characteristics that influence treatment effectiveness (Cicerone et al. 2011).

There is limited evidence to suggest stroke patients may benefit from specific executive function training and learn compensatory strategies to reduce the consequences of executive impairments. Although it is estimated that around 75% of stroke survivors will experience executive dysfunction, high-quality evidence that supports generalized conclusions about the effect of cognitive rehabilitation on executive function or other secondary outcome measures is insufficient (Chung et al. 2013).

Fitness for Work and Workplace Accommodation

A recent systematic review targeting diverse disability groups found moderate evidence on the effectiveness of some workplace accommodations (vocational counseling and guidance, education and self-advocacy, help of others, changes in work schedules, work organization, and special transportation) to promote employability among persons with physical disabilities and reduce costs (Nevala et al. 2015). In particular, evidence on the effectiveness of liaison, education, work aids, or work techniques coordinated by case managers was low. The review suggested the necessity of more high-quality studies and identified self-advocacy, support from the employer and community, amount of training and counseling, and flexibility of work schedules and work organization as key facilitators and barriers of employment (Nevala et al. 2015).

Employers and line managers are pivotal in RTW after stroke. A qualitative study conducted in the UK provided insights from the employer perspective to promote RTW after stroke (Coole et al. 2013). The researchers gathered data using semi-structured interviews with employer stakeholders, including small business owners, line managers, human resources, and occupational health staff. The analyses revealed employers' concerns about the RTW of stroke survivors and the necessity of the individual's (stroke survivors) personal motivation to RTW. Those that had received support from a healthcare professional with knowledge of both vocational rehabilitation and stroke appeared to benefit. Because stakeholders' understanding relevant to RTW after stroke improved with the help of healthcare professionals (occupational health staff, rehabilitation team, and clinicians), promoting communication among professionals and stakeholders is essential.

Cooperation between the physician in charge and occupational health staff (occupational physicians) appeared to contribute to RTW (Tanaka et al. 2011). To facilitate cooperation with occupational physicians, it may be necessary to obtain information about the patient's medical and psychosocial background early in the disease onset. This would support provision of appropriate advice regarding RTW, such as relocation of the patient and workplace arrangements based on their medical condition.

Social Systems

Although there is evidence demonstrating stroke rehabilitation is offered in diverse settings (e.g., outpatient, in-hospital, and post-acute care settings), opportunities to reach stroke survivors have been missed (Ayala et al. 2018). It has also been suggested that vocational rehabilitation services are under-used (Hartke and Trierweiler 2015).

Interventions from a broad public health perspective are needed to reduce socioeconomic disparities in RTW. Rehabilitation opportunities do not reach some populations because of sex, race, and level of education (Ayala et al. 2018). People working for themselves or for small-sized enterprises are also less likely to have access to occupational health services. Health insurance coverage is needed that includes stroke rehabilitation, education for stroke survivors on rehabilitation opportunities, and healthcare professionals to guide referral to appropriate opportunities at hospital discharge (Ayala et al. 2018). Cooperation among employers (occupational health professionals) and attending physicians should be systematically facilitated. Economic support may be necessary for small-sized companies to establish RTW support systems for workers with disabilities, such as flexible working systems or paid sick leave systems. Other than occupational health service issues, factors limiting RTW after stroke include constructional and transportation problems that restrict social activities of impaired persons and stigma and prejudice regarding the workability of stroke survivors (Treger et al. 2007).

Conclusions

It is expected that people who return to work after stroke have better quality of life compared with those who do not (Ntsiea et al. 2015). It has become increasingly important to evaluate the social prognosis (i.e., health-related quality of life) of stroke survivors, because patients with stroke are getting older and the severity of disease is becoming worse. Although rehabilitation techniques have been improved and the effectiveness of some rehabilitation programs has been shown (Cicerone et al. 2011), investigations on vocational outcomes after stroke have been limited. Study outcomes should include sustained RTW. To achieve sustained RTW, worker-based vocational rehabilitation and creating supportive work environment are needed (Dekkers-Sanchez et al. 2011). To improve the RTW rate after stroke, it is also necessary to overcome identified evidence gaps.

Harmonizing work and disease treatment is an emerging topic. RTW after stroke is a challenge for younger stroke survivors, as well as for the older working population in general and people with disabilities who want to work. The whole RTW system for workers with disabilities, such as disease treatment (including rehabilitation), workplace accommodation, and cooperation among stakeholders and coordination of these factors, should be consolidated. Overcoming the challenges of RTW after stroke is a key milestone for harmonizing work and disease treatment.

Cross-References

▶ Coronary Heart Disease and Return to Work
▶ Implementing Best Practice Models of Return to Work
▶ Policies of Reducing the Burden of Occupational Hazards and Disability Pensions

Acknowledgments This work was supported by Ministry of Health, Labour and Welfare (Industrial Disease Clinical Research Grants: Grant Number 170401 and 180701-1). We also thank Audrey Holmes, MA, from Edanz Group (www.edanzediting.com/ac) for editing a draft of this manuscript.

References

Alaszewski A, Alaszewski H, Potter J, Penhale B (2007) Working after a stroke: survivors' experiences and perceptions of barriers to and facilitators of the return to paid employment. Disabil Rehabil 29(24):1858–1869. https://doi.org/10.1080/09638280601143356

Arauz A (2013) Return to work after stroke: the role of cognitive deficits. J Neurol Neurosurg Psychiatry 84(3):240. https://doi.org/10.1136/jnnp-2012-303328

Ayala C, Fang i, Luncheon C, King SC, Chang T, Ritchey M, Loustalot F (2018) Use of outpatient rehabilitation among adult stroke survivors—20 states and the District of Columbia, 2013, and four states, 2015. MMWR Morb Mortal Wkly Rep 67:575–578. https://doi.org/10.15585/mmwr.mm6720a2

Bergmann H, von Kuthmann M, Ungern-Sternberg A, Weimann VG (1991) Medical educational and functional determinants of employment after stroke. J Neural Transm Suppl 33:157–161

Black-Schaffer RM, Osberg JS (1990) Return to work after stroke: development of a predictive model. Arch Phys Med Rehabil 71(5):285–290

Burn J, Dennis M, Bamford J, Sandercock P, Wade D, Warlow C (1994) Long-term risk of recurrent stroke after a first-ever stroke. The Oxfordshire community stroke project. Stroke 25(2):333–337

Centers for Disease Control and Prevention (CDC) (2009) Prevalence and most common causes of disability among adults–United States, 2005. MMWR Morb Mortal Wkly Rep 58(16):421–426

Chapman N, Huxley R, Anderson C, Bousser MG, Chalmers J, Colman S, Davis S, Donnan G, MacMahon S, Neal B, Warlow C, Woodward M (2004) Effects of a perindopril-based blood pressure-lowering regimen on the risk of recurrent stroke according to stroke subtype and medical history: the PROGRESS trial. Stroke 35(1):116–121. https://doi.org/10.1161/01. Str.0000106480.76217.6f

Chung CS, Pollock A, Campbell T, Durward BR, Hagen S (2013) Cognitive rehabilitation for executive dysfunction in adults with stroke or other adult non-progressive acquired brain damage, CD008391. Cochrane Database Syst Rev 2013(4). https://doi.org/10.1002/14651858. CD008391.pub2

Cicerone KD, Langenbahn DM, Braden C, Malec JF, Kalmar K, Fraas M, Felicetti T, Laatsch L, Harley JP, Bergquist T, Azulay J, Cantor J, Ashman T (2011) Evidence-based cognitive rehabilitation: updated review of the literature from 2003 through 2008. Arch Phys Med Rehabil 92(4):519–530. https://doi.org/10.1016/j.apmr.2010.11.015

Coole C, Radford K, Grant M, Terry J (2013) Returning to work after stroke: perspectives of employer stakeholders, a qualitative study. J Occup Rehabil 23(3):406–418

Daniel K, Wolfe CD, Busch MA, McKevitt C (2009) What are the social consequences of stroke for working-aged adults? Syst Rev Stroke 40(6):e431–e440. https://doi.org/10.1161/strokeaha.108.534487

De Groot MH, Phillips SJ, Eskes GA (2003) Fatigue associated with stroke and other neurologic conditions: implications for stroke rehabilitation. Arch Phys Med Rehabil 84(11):1714–1720

Dekkers-Sanchez PM, Wind H, Sluiter JK, Hw Frings-Dresen MH (2011) What promotes sustained return to work of employees on long-term sick leave? Perspectives of vocational rehabilitation professionals. Scand J Work Environ Health 37(6):481–493. https://doi.org/10.5271/sjweh.3173

Eguchi H, Wada K, Higuchi Y, Smith DR (2017) Psychosocial factors and colleagues' perceptions of return-to-work opportunities for workers with a psychiatric disorder: a Japanese population-based study. Environ Health Prev Med 22(1):23

Endo M, Sairenchi T, Kojimahara N, Haruyama Y, Sato Y, Kato R, Yamaguchi N (2016) Sickness absence and return to work among Japanese stroke survivors: a 365-day cohort study. BMJ Open 6(1):e009682

Glass TA, Matchar DB, Belyea M, Feussner JR (1993) Impact of social support on outcome in first stroke. Stroke 24(1):64–70

Glozier N, Hackett ML, Parag V, Anderson CS (2008) The influence of psychiatric morbidity on return to paid work after stroke in younger adults: the Auckland regional community stroke (ARCOS) study, 2002 to 2003. Stroke 39(5):1526–1532. https://doi.org/10.1161/strokeaha.107.503219

Hackett ML, Pickles K (2014) Part I: frequency of depression after stroke: an updated systematic review and meta-analysis of observational studies. Int J Stroke 9(8):1017–1025. https://doi.org/10.1111/ijs.12357

Hackett ML, Yapa C, Parag V, Anderson CS (2005) Frequency of depression after stroke: a systematic review of observational studies. Stroke 36(6):1330–1340. https://doi.org/10.1161/01.Str.0000165928.19135.35

Hackett ML, Kohler S, O'Brien JT, Mead GE (2014) Neuropsychiatric outcomes of stroke. Lancet Neurol 13(5):525–534. https://doi.org/10.1016/s1474-4422(14)70016-x

Hannerz H, Ferm L, Poulsen OM, Pedersen BH, Andersen LL (2012a) Enterprise size and return to work after stroke. J Occup Rehabil 22(4):456–461. https://doi.org/10.1007/s10926-012-9367-z

Hannerz H, Mortensen OS, Poulsen OM, Humle F, Pedersen BH, Andersen LL (2012b) Time trend analysis of return to work after stroke in Denmark 1996–2006. Int J Occup Med Environ Health 25(2):200–204. https://doi.org/10.2478/s13382-012-0017-7

Hartke RJ, Trierweiler R (2015) Survey of survivors' perspective on return to work after stroke. Top Stroke Rehabil 22(5):326–334. https://doi.org/10.1179/1074935714z.0000000044

Howard G, Till JS, Toole JF, Matthews C, Truscott BL (1985) Factors influencing return to work following cerebral infarction. JAMA 253(2):226–232

Jacobs BS, Boden-Albala B, Lin IF, Sacco RL (2002) Stroke in the young in the northern Manhattan stroke study. Stroke 33(12):2789–2793

Johnston V, Way K, Long MH, Wyatt M, Gibson L, Shaw WS (2015) Supervisor competencies for supporting return to work: a mixed-methods study. J Occup Rehabil 25(1):3–17. https://doi.org/10.1007/s10926-014-9511-z

Karasek R, Theorell T (1990) Healthy work: stress, productivity, and the reconstruction of working life. Basic Books, New York

Kauranen T, Turunen K, Laari S, Mustanoja S, Baumann P, Poutiainen E (2013) The severity of cognitive deficits predicts return to work after a first-ever ischaemic stroke. J Neurol Neurosurg Psychiatry 84(3):316–321. https://doi.org/10.1136/jnnp-2012-302629

King RB (1996) Quality of life after stroke. Stroke 27(9):1467–1472

Li J, Zhang M, Loerbroks A, Angerer P, Siegrist J (2015) Work stress and the risk of recurrent coronary heart disease events: a systematic review and meta-analysis. Int J Occup Med Environ Health 28(1):8–19. https://doi.org/10.2478/s13382-014-0303-7

Luengo-Fernandez R, Gray AM, Rothwell PM (2009) Costs of stroke using patient-level data: a critical review of the literature. Stroke 40(2):e18–e23. https://doi.org/10.1161/strokeaha.108.529776

Maaijwee NA, Arntz RM, Rutten-Jacobs LC, Schaapsmeerders P, Schoonderwaldt HC, van Dijk EJ, de Leeuw FE (2015) Post-stroke fatigue and its association with poor functional outcome after stroke in young adults. J Neurol Neurosurg Psychiatry 86(10):1120–1126. https://doi.org/10.1136/jnnp-2014-308784

Macdonell RA, Dewey HM (2001) Neurological disability and neurological rehabilitation. Med J Aust 174(12):653–658

Malm J, Kristensen B, Karlsson T, Carlberg B, Fagerlund M, Olsson T (1998) Cognitive impairment in young adults with infratentorial infarcts. Neurology 51(2):433–440

Mazer BL, Sofer S, Korner-Bitensky N, Gelinas I, Hanley J, Wood-Dauphinee S (2003) Effectiveness of a visual attention retraining program on the driving performance of clients with stroke. Arch Phys Med Rehabil 84(4):541–550. https://doi.org/10.1053/apmr.2003.50085

Mozaffarian D, Benjamin EJ, Go AS, Arnett DK, Blaha MJ, Cushman M, Das SR, de Ferranti S, Despres JP, Fullerton HJ, Howard VJ, Huffman MD, Isasi CR, Jimenez MC, Judd SE, Kissela BM, Lichtman JH, Lisabeth LD, Liu S, Mackey RH, Magid DJ, McGuire DK, Mohler ER, Moy CS, Muntner P, Mussolino ME, Nasir K, Neumar RW, Nichol G, Palaniappan L, Pandey DK, Reeves MJ, Rodriguez CJ, Rosamond W, Sorlie PD, Stein J, Towfighi A, Turan TN, Virani SS, Woo D, Yeh RW, Turner MB (2016) Heart disease and stroke Statistics-2016 update: a report from the American Heart Association. Circulation 133(4):e38–e360. https://doi.org/10.1161/cir.0000000000000350

Neau JP, Ingrand P, Mouille-Brachet C, Rosier MP, Couderq C, Alvarez A, Gil R (1998) Functional recovery and social outcome after cerebral infarction in young adults. Cerebrovasc Dis 8(5):296–302. https://doi.org/10.1159/000015869

Nevala N, Pehkonen I, Koskela I, Ruusuvuori J, Anttila H (2015) Workplace accommodation among persons with disabilities: a systematic review of its effectiveness and barriers or facilitators. J Occup Rehabil 25(2):432–448

Newman M (1972) The process of recovery after hemiplegia. Stroke 3(6):702–710

Ntsiea MV, Van Aswegen H, Lord S, Olorunju SS (2015) The effect of a workplace intervention programme on return to work after stroke: a randomised controlled trial. Clin Rehabil 29(7):663–673. https://doi.org/10.1177/0269215514554241

Ovbiagele B, Goldstein LB, Higashida RT, Howard VJ, Johnston SC, Khavjou OA, Lackland DT, Lichtman JH, Mohl S, Sacco RL, Saver JL, Trogdon JG (2013) Forecasting the future of stroke in the United States: a policy statement from the American Heart Association and American Stroke Association. Stroke 44(8):2361–2375. https://doi.org/10.1161/STR.0b013e31829734f2

PROGRESS Collaborative Group (2001) Randomised trial of a perindopril-based blood-pressure-lowering regimen among 6,105 individuals with previous stroke or transient ischaemic attack. Lancet 358(9287):1033–1041. https://doi.org/10.1016/s0140-6736(01)06178-5

Rimmerman A (1998) Factors relating to attitudes of Israeli corporate executives toward the employability of persons with intellectual disability. J Intellect Develop Disabil 23(3):245–254. https://doi.org/10.1080/13668259800033731

Saeki S, Toyonaga T (2010) Determinants of early return to work after first stroke in Japan. J Rehabil Med 42(3):254–258. https://doi.org/10.2340/16501977-0503

Siegrist J (1996) Adverse health effects of high-effort/low-reward conditions. J Occup Health Psychol 1(1):27–41

Sinclair E, Radford K, Grant M, Terry J (2014) Developing stroke-specific vocational rehabilitation: a soft systems analysis of current service provision. Disabil Rehabil 36(5):409–417

Tanaka H, Toyonaga T, Hashimoto H (2011) Functional and occupational characteristics associated with very early return to work after stroke in Japan. Arch Phys Med Rehabil 92(5):743–748. https://doi.org/10.1016/j.apmr.2010.12.009

Taylor TN, Davis PH, Torner JC, Holmes J, Meyer JW, Jacobson MF (1996) Lifetime cost of stroke in the United States. Stroke 27(9):1459–1466

Teasell RW, McRae MP, Finestone HM (2000) Social issues in the rehabilitation of younger stroke patients. Arch Phys Med Rehabil 81(2):205–209

Tiersky LA, Anselmi V, Johnston MV, Kurtyka J, Roosen E, Schwartz T, Deluca J (2005) A trial of neuropsychologic rehabilitation in mild-spectrum traumatic brain injury. Arch Phys Med Rehabil 86(8):1565–1574. https://doi.org/10.1016/j.apmr.2005.03.013

Treger I, Shames J, Giaquinto S, Ring H (2007) Return to work in stroke patients. Disabil Rehabil 29(17):1397–1403. https://doi.org/10.1080/09638280701314923

Tsutsumi A, Kawakami N (2004) A review of empirical studies on the model of effort-reward imbalance at work: reducing occupational stress by implementing a new theory. Soc Sci Med 59(11):2335–2359

Westerberg H, Jacobaeus H, Hirvikoski T, Clevberger P, Ostensson ML, Bartfai A, Klingberg T (2007) Computerized working memory training after stroke–a pilot study. Brain Inj 21(1):21–29. https://doi.org/10.1080/02699050601148726

Winstein CJ, Stein J, Arena R, Bates B, Cherney LR, Cramer SC, Deruyter F, Eng JJ, Fisher B, Harvey RL, Lang CE, MacKay-Lyons M, Ottenbacher KJ, Pugh S, Reeves MJ, Richards LG, Stiers W, Zorowitz RD (2016) Guidelines for adult stroke rehabilitation and recovery: a guideline for healthcare professionals from the American Heart Association/American Stroke Association. Stroke 47(6):e98–e169. https://doi.org/10.1161/str.0000000000000098

Wozniak MA, Kittner SJ (2002) Return to work after ischemic stroke: a methodological review. Neuroepidemiology 21(4):159–166. https://doi.org/10.1159/000059516

Wozniak MA, Kittner SJ, Price TR, Hebel JR, Sloan MA, Gardner JF (1999) Stroke location is not associated with return to work after first ischemic stroke. Stroke 30(12):2568–2573

Zedlitz AM, Fasotti L, Geurts AC (2011) Post-stroke fatigue: a treatment protocol that is being evaluated. Clin Rehabil 25(6):487–500. https://doi.org/10.1177/0269215510391285

Common Mental Disorders and Work

Barriers and Opportunities

26

Silje Endresen Reme

Contents

Introduction	468
Consequences of Exclusion from the Labor Market	468
Positive Health Effects of Work	470
Negative Health Effects of Work	471
Barriers and Opportunities of RTW in Common Mental Disorders	471
Individual Perspective	471
Healthcare Perspective	474
Workplace Perspective	475
Compensation System and Societal Perspective	476
Summary and Concluding Remarks	477
Cross-References	478
References	478

Abstract

Common mental disorders, such as anxiety and depression, are responsible for a significant loss of capacity for work. Exclusion from the labor market can *in and of itself* lead to severe health consequences.

Keywords

Common mental disorders · Work disability · Workplace inclusion · Return to work

---

S. E. Reme (✉)
University of Oslo, Oslo, Norway
e-mail: s.e.reme@psykologi.uio.no

© Springer Nature Switzerland AG 2020
U. Bültmann, J. Siegrist (eds.), *Handbook of Disability, Work and Health*, Handbook Series in Occupational Health Sciences, https://doi.org/10.1007/978-3-030-24334-0_26

Introduction

Common mental disorders (CMDs), which primarily refer to affective disorders such as anxiety and depression, are responsible for a significant loss of capacity for work. This includes not only a reduced productivity at work but also high rates of sickness absence, disability, and unemployment (Ahola et al. 2011; OECD 2012). In particular, mental illness causes many young people to leave the labor market, or never really enter it, through early exits out into disability benefit. Across the OECD countries, between one-third and one-half of all new disability benefit claims are for reasons of mental ill-health, and among young adults, that proportion goes up to over 70% (OECD 2012). Anxiety and depression are the most common diagnoses.

CMDs are highly prevalent (Stansfeld et al. 2011) and may affect up to 50% percent of the general population in a lifetime perspective (Kessler et al. 2012). However, despite no clear increase in prevalence rates of affective disorders (Kessler et al. 2005; Spiers et al. 2011; Wittchen et al. 2011), sickness absence with mental disorders as a primary diagnosis has increased markedly over the past decade and now accounts for more incapacity benefit claims than any other disorders (Cattrell et al. 2011; OECD 2013). Longer duration of sickness absence reduces the chances of return to work (RTW) – the longer a person is off work due to sickness absence, the smaller are the chances of that person to ever RTW (Blank et al. 2008; Waddell et al. 2007). A crucial challenge is therefore to disrupt the process of prolonged sickness absence before it progresses into permanent disability (Henderson et al. 2005).

In this chapter we will take a closer look at barriers and opportunities for work in people with common mental disorders. Consequences of *not working* will be explored, as well as benefits involved in *staying at/returning to work*, provided that the workplace is a good place to be and not contaminated by hazardous risk factors. Significant barriers and opportunities of RTW from various perspectives will be presented, including the individual, healthcare, workplace, and societal perspective. Work (dis)ability is a complex phenomenon involving not only processes within the individual worker but also all the various contexts that the individual is a part of (Loisel and Anema 2014). Complex problems call for integrated and interdisciplinary solutions; thus, work (dis)ability needs to be investigated and discussed in light of this complexity (see Fig. 1).

Consequences of Exclusion from the Labor Market

Common mental disorders are a frequent reason for exclusion from the labor market, but exclusion from the labor market can *in and of itself* lead to severe health consequences. On average, those who are involuntarily out of work have higher levels of psychological distress than those who have work. The consequences of being involuntary out of work are also not only mental but general health consequences, such as functional disorders and mortality. Unemployment is, for instance, prospectively associated with poor cardiovascular health and a threefold higher risk

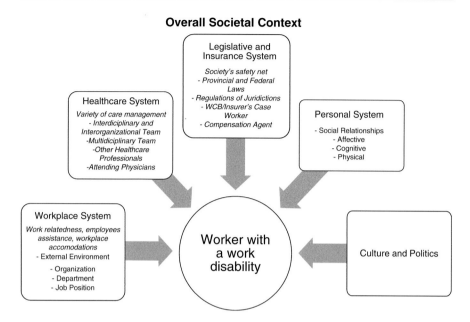

Fig. 1 An integrated work disability model based on Loisel and Anema 2014

of all-cause mortality (Meneton et al. 2015). Unemployment has also been found to more than double the risk of limiting illness (e.g., musculoskeletal complaints, anxiety/depression, high blood pressure) and also to reduce the chances of recovery once an illness has occurred (Bartley et al. 2004). A rigorous and systematic review of the unemployment literature correspondingly supports a causal association between unemployment and mortality (Roelfs et al. 2011).

A common objection to the alleged causal association between unemployment and mortality is that pre-existing health conditions confound the relationship. In other words, a poorer health is the common factor predicting both unemployment and negative health outcomes (e.g., mortality). However, in this thorough study, pre-existing health problems accounted for only a small portion of the association between unemployment and mortality (Roelfs et al. 2011). Thus, pre-existing health conditions do *not* seem to be the common cause of both unemployment and mortality. Instead, unemployment was associated with a substantially increased risk of death among broad segments of the population. The risk was higher earlier in the career compared to later, it was considerably higher in men than in women, and it was not substantially influenced by differences in national welfare and healthcare systems (Roelfs et al. 2011).

Other studies have looked more closely at various causes of death, with substantial evidence demonstrating that suicide rates are considerably higher in unemployed (Milner et al. 2013). There also seems to be a dose-response relationship – a longer duration of the unemployment period is associated with a greater risk of suicide and suicide attempt.

Positive Health Effects of Work

The abovementioned consequences of being out of work seem to imply that *returning to work* could be therapeutic, and maybe even a cure, for people with mental illness. Being employed seems to be a very efficient way to stay healthy. However, the fact that unemployment leads to negative health consequences does not necessarily imply that returning to work reverses the negative consequences caused by being out of work. The positive health effects observed in those who work could simply be a result of selection effects rather than a causal effect of work. The question of whether social factors are a cause or consequence of disease and illness is often framed in the context of the debate over the *social selection hypothesis* versus the *social causation hypothesis* (Adda et al. 2003; Bartley 1988; Ross and Mirowsky 1995).

The social causation hypothesis suggests that employment leads to health benefits, while the social selection hypothesis proposes that health is a necessary condition for employment. Although some support has been found in favor of the selection effect (i.e., healthy workers being more likely to be employed in the first place), a systematic review was able to document stronger support in favor of the social causation hypothesis (i.e., that work leads to good health) (Rueda et al. 2012). In the review, most of the longitudinal studies found a positive association between returning to work and health outcomes in a variety of populations, at different times, and in different settings. For instance:

- In one study reemployment reversed the negative effect of unemployment on mental health (Ginexi et al. 2000).
- In another study, the high prevalence of heavy drinking among the unemployed was mostly explained by unemployment preceding heavy drinking rather than alcohol abuse causing unemployment (Claussen 1999).
- In yet another study, participants who returned to work reported less psychological distress than did those who remained unemployed, while participants who were unable to find employment reported no change in distress over time (Vuori and Vesalainen 1999).

An earlier meta-analysis of 16 longitudinal studies found similar effects; job loss and unemployment were associated with increased mental distress, while reemployment reversed the negative effects of unemployment on mental health (Murphy and Athanasou 1999). However, these authors wanted to go even further and looked at the *size* of these effects. They did this by dividing the studies into two categories: (1) studies looking at the effects of *gaining* employment and (2) studies looking at the effects of *losing* employment. In their analyses they found a moderate effect size for the first category (0.54) and a small effect size for the second category (0.36). This implies that a move from unemployment to employment is associated with improvements to mental well-being that are of such size that they imply practical significance (Murphy and Athanasou 1999).

Nevertheless, there have also been solid documentation in support of the social selection hypothesis (Rueda et al. 2012). For instance:

- In one study, no support was found for an increase in psychological distress over time for those who were continuously unemployed (Breslin and Mustard 2003).
- In another study, a tendency of improved psychological health was found in participants who were continuously unemployed, suggesting that an adaptation to unemployment sets in after a certain amount of time (Schaufeli and VanYperen 1992).
- In yet another study, a considerable long-term selection of the physically unhealthy into unemployment was found – the mental health of the observed participants in the study had deteriorated even before the unemployment started (Stauder 2018).

Despite stronger support in favor of the social causation hypothesis, the overall conclusion supported by most studies involves seeing these processes as both significant and mutually reinforcing (Rueda et al. 2012).

Negative Health Effects of Work

There is thus good evidence to support the therapeutic effects of work on our health and well-being, but work is not always health promoting. In some cases, the situation and conditions at the workplace can be directly harmful for the mental health of the individual worker (Harvey et al. 2017). Comprehensive summaries of the literature have identified three overlapping clusters of workplace risk factors: (1) imbalanced job design, (2) occupational uncertainty, and (3) a lack of value and respect within the workplace (Harvey et al. 2017). *Imbalanced job design* relates to various work stress models and includes workplace factors such as job demands, job control, effort-reward imbalance, and occupational social support. *Occupational uncertainty* also includes job control but additionally incorporates procedural justice, organizational change, job insecurity, and temporary employment status. *Lack of value and respect within the workplace* includes several of the factors mentioned in the previous clusters (e.g., effort-reward imbalance, procedural justice, temporary employment status) but additionally includes relational justice and workplace conflict/bullying (Fig. 2).

Work can thus make us ill. However, provided that the abovementioned factors are not too dominating in the workplace, the arrow will most often point in the other direction, namely, from work to positive (mental) health consequences for the individual worker, as outlined in the previous paragraph.

Barriers and Opportunities of RTW in Common Mental Disorders

Individual Perspective

Several individual factors can act as barriers of RTW for people with common mental disorders. A history of either common mental disorders or absenteeism predicts sickness absence, while other individual predictors of sickness absence

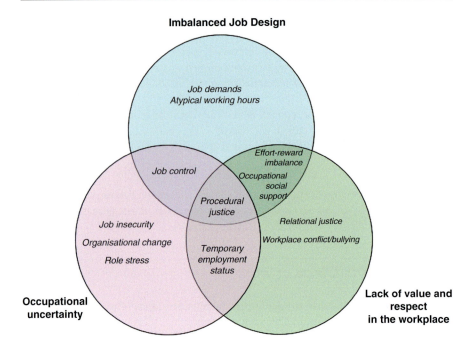

Fig. 2 Unifying model of workplace risk factors

are higher symptom severity, comorbidity and a low perceived general health (de Vries et al. 2018). More stable demographic factors, such as lower educational level, higher age, and female gender, are also significant predictors of sickness absence (Lagerveld et al. 2010) but usually receive less attention since they are less modifiable by nature (Cornelius et al. 2011). Still, lower educational level seems to be a consistent barrier of RTW (Cornelius et al. 2011), while high socioeconomic status has been found to be associated with faster RTW across various conditions, including in common mental disorders (Gragnano et al. 2018). The evidence on socioeconomic position as predictor of RTW is, however, somewhat inconsistent. This could be related to the complex interplay between different structural factors. To exemplify, in a large Finnish study, high occupational position was associated with quicker RTW (Ervasti et al. 2017), whereas in a Canadian study, the association was reversed (Ebrahim et al. 2013). The very different social security policies in Finland and Canada are likely to have influenced these contrasting results and again speak to the importance of considering the various contexts surrounding the disabled worker and the complex interplay between them which will have an impact on the outcome for the individual worker (see more below under "Compensation System and Societal Perspective").

When searching for significant factors acting as barriers and opportunities for work, the *absence* of significant associations may be as interesting as the *presence* of associations. One interesting association that is often absent is the association between symptom severity (in depressed workers) and work participation in prospective studies (Lagerveld et al. 2010). Common sense would imply that the more severe symptoms, the more unfavorable employment outcomes. But that does not always seem to be the case. There is no one-to-one relationship between disorder, symptom levels, and work participation (Henderson et al. 2005). Symptom reduction and RTW seem to be somewhat separate processes. That is probably also why the level of integrated work focus in the mental health treatment is so important for successful RTW, as we will see in the next section ("Healthcare Perspective").

Nevertheless, characteristics of the mental disorders are not irrelevant factors in the RTW process. Strong associations have, for instance, been found between a long duration of depression and more severe types of depressive disorders and disability (Lagerveld et al. 2010). Lifestyle factors have also been documented, including weight (underweight as well as overweight), being a smoker, and being drug dependent (Blank et al. 2008).

A few studies have looked at personality factors in relation to various work-related outcomes and find that higher neuroticism is related to more limitations in work functioning (Lagerveld et al. 2010). On the more positive side, moderate-quality evidence suggest that higher conscientiousness is associated with quicker RTW (Ervasti et al. 2017) and can thus act as a facilitator in the RTW process. It is very plausible that other personality traits may influence the RTW process and outcomes as well, but in this particular area, more high-quality studies are needed as there is a scarcity of studies of mental health and RTW that also include personality assessments.

An interesting factor that consistently and precisely predicts RTW outcomes is individuals' own beliefs about possibilities for work participation, in other words, their RTW expectations (Cornelius et al. 2011). These expectations have not only been found to predict work-related outcomes in people with common mental disorders but also to predict RTW across several conditions (Ebrahim et al. 2015; Mondloch et al. 2001). The most common theoretical framework applied to understand the role of these predictive expectations is Bandura's concept of self-efficacy (Bandura 1977). Self-efficacy has been described as "the belief in ones' abilities to organize and execute the courses of actions required to produce given attainments" (p. 3) (Bandura 1997). RTW expectations are thus essentially beliefs about and expectations of RTW. According to Bandura, the main influential source of self-efficacy is direct enactment, which implies that RTW expectations could be shaped by previous work-related experiences, but vicarious learning, verbal persuasion, and social support could also contribute to the formation of self-efficacy. It has been suggested that both intrapersonal factors, interpersonal factors, and system-level factors influence the formation of RTW expectations (Ebrahim et al. 2015).

Workers' own expectations of RTW are in many sense the "canary in the coal mine," providing a warning of what lies ahead. They could, of course, just represent a precise evaluation of reality, and thus not have any direct potential of change in itself, but there are several indications pointing in other directions. RTW expectations have, for instance, been found to be a better predictor of RTW than symptom severity in common mental disorders (Lovvik et al. 2014), and various studies across different patient populations indicate that recovery expectations are amendable to change and that this change acts as a mediator of the effect (e.g., Goldin et al. 2012; Kadden and Litt 2011; Montgomery et al. 2010; Turner et al. 2007).

Healthcare Perspective

RTW interventions provided by the healthcare system show mixed results. While some interventions, such as work-focused cognitive behavioral therapy, has been shown to be quite effective in both reducing symptoms and increasing RTW in patients with CMDs (Kroger et al. 2015; Lagerveld et al. 2012; Reme et al. 2015), other RTW interventions have been shown to instead delay RTW (Erik et al. 2013; Martin et al. 2013). These paradoxical effects may be explained by the content and focus of the various interventions.

In general, most RTW interventions include one or more of the following four elements: (1) organizational change, which often includes enhanced collaboration or integration between central stakeholders; (2) graded RTW as a therapeutic means; (3) therapeutic elements, often involving some sort of therapy, or support through conversation with a healthcare provider; and (4) contact with the workplace. In a recent systematic review, these components were considered when reviewing the evidence for RTW interventions in people with mental health disorders, mostly studies that targeted common mental disorders (Mikkelsen and Rosholm 2018). They found strong evidence for interventions that included contact with the workplace and for including more than one of the four elements mentioned above. They also found moderate evidence for including graded RTW, which by definition also involves contact with the workplace. This particular element, contact with the workplace, therefore appears to be of particular importance for a successful RTW process, as well as including more than one component in the intervention (Mikkelsen and Rosholm 2018). Again, this speaks to the multidimensional nature of work disability and the corresponding need to consider this complexity when intervening (Loisel and Anema 2014).

Along those same lines, another important aspect that often separates more effective from less effective RTW interventions in the healthcare setting is to what degree they include and integrate an explicit focus on RTW. Even though common sense implies that a reduction in symptoms would automatically lead to RTW, this is not necessarily how it works in reality (see, for instance, Ejeby et al. 2014). As previously discussed, there is no one-to-one relationship between symptom reduction and RTW. It appears as if *work* needs to be explicitly included in the intervention in order to increase the odds of an actual RTW. Still, the majority of psychological interventions aiming to increase RTW do not include an explicit focus on RTW in their interventions. This was demonstrated in a recent meta-analysis of psychological RTW interventions in common mental disorders. The results of the meta-analysis showed a small but significant effect in favor of the psychological treatments, but most of the included studies did not specifically address RTW in their interventions (Finnes et al. 2018). There is as such a potential of increasing the effect sizes in the future, by adopting and integrating an explicit RTW focus in healthcare interventions for disabled workers.

RTW interventions with negative results serve as an example of how healthcare intervention may in itself act as a barrier for RTW. Despite the very best intentions, it can actually make the situation worse for the patient by delaying RTW. In the two examples cited above, the authors conclude with program failure in both cases (Martin et al. 2013; Noordik et al. 2013). The authors should be applauded for publishing these important studies to help us understand more about what works and what does not work. One hypothesis to draw from these studies could be that the ignorance of the complex interplay between the various contexts of the individual worker is (partly) responsible for the negative results. In the study by Noordik et al., for instance, an exposure-based RTW program delayed RTW in workers on sick leave due to common mental disorders. However, neither the work conditions nor the self-efficacy of the individual worker was considered before exposing participants to the various work situations, which could have contributed to the negative results.

Workplace Perspective

High job demands/strain and low job control are all predictors of sickness absence in workers with common mental disorders (de Vries et al. 2018), and although it could be argued that these are more individual rather than workplace factors, they are still closely linked to the workplace and work tasks. Especially when high perceived job demands are combined with low control, and when high-strain jobs are combined with low support, the risk of sickness absence is high.

Organizational justice is another factor related to sickness absence. We recognize this factor from the paragraph on bad work conditions, where it was stated that a perception of low organizational justice increases the risk of mental health consequences. Here we show that it also increases the risk of sickness absence, as do reorganizational stress and threat of unemployment (Blank et al. 2008). Not surprisingly, many of the same factors at the workplace that predict poor mental health also predict sick leave and thus act as barriers of RTW.

A previous history of sick leave or mental disorders was mentioned as predictor of future work disability in the section describing the individual perspective. Similarly, a previous history of low level of functioning at work is associated with work disability in the future (Lagerveld et al. 2010).

On the more positive side, contact between supervisor and other professionals besides the occupational physician is associated with shorter time to RTW in depressed workers (Lagerveld et al. 2010). Correspondingly, communication between key stakeholders is also important in non-depressed workers, particularly between the supervisor and the employee, which has been associated with a shortened time to full RTW (Cornelius et al. 2011). An interesting finding when it comes to communication between the supervisor and the disabled worker is that this could be both an opportunity *and* a barrier for faster RTW. In general, workplace support plays an important role in disability management and enhances RTW. However, some studies indicate that this effect of support is only beneficial in those with low depression scores, while in workers with more severe conditions, perceived support could actually be a barrier and delay RTW (Cornelius et al. 2011). A possible explanation for this apparently paradoxical finding could be a small but important nuance in the nature of support – validation (empathy-based support) vs solicitousness (sympathy-based support). While the former support involves empathic responses that validate the experience yet encourage coping behaviors, the latter provides support as well as helping behaviors that might have an unintended detrimental effect in encouraging illness behavior.

The third detrimental workplace factor mentioned in the previous paragraph involves a lack of value and respect. Not surprisingly, this factor is also an important barrier for work in many workers with (or without) common mental disorders. Workplace bullying appears to be a particular toxic factor, which has been associated with sickness absence in studies from both the USA (Asfaw et al. 2014) and Europe (Niedhammer et al. 2013). In a large, prospective study among healthcare workers, it was found that exposure to bullying resulted in a 26% higher risk of sickness absence (Kivimaki et al. 2000), and there also seems to be a dose-response relationship – more frequent exposure leads to worse RTW outcomes (Ortega et al. 2011).

Compensation System and Societal Perspective

Few studies have investigated how structural factors at the societal level can act as barriers or opportunities for work. Although the impact of the large societal context has been emphasized (e.g., in several OECD reports), few studies have investigated this directly. One recent attempt, however, is worth mentioning. In a Finnish study, a natural experiment was used to investigate legislative changes and the effect it had on RTW and work participation (Halonen et al. 2016). The legislative changes involved (1) obligating the employer to notify the occupational health service provider whenever a worker had been on sick leave for more than 30 days, (2) including suggestions for work modification and rehabilitation in the sick note, and (3) requiring an assessment by an occupational physician of remaining work ability and possibilities to continue working after 90 days of sick leave. These legislative changes did in fact show some effects in terms of enhancing sustainable RTW. The effects were mainly seen in the short term, however, and diluted over time. The impact of these changes in the long run is therefore questionable.

The large differences in sickness absence rates between countries, for instance, in OECD countries, have to a large extent been attributed to the different compensation systems as well as other social and cultural differences. To exemplify, the most comprehensive compensation system is found in Norway, where workers on sick leave receive 100% coverage for lost income from day 1 up to 52 weeks, after which long-term benefits set in that provide approximately 66% of the former income. In the national statistics, there is correspondingly seen an enormous rise in recovery rates just prior to 1 year when the compensation drops from 100% to 66% (Markussen et al. 2011), implying the influence of these structural factors.

Structural factors at the societal level could thus act as both barriers and opportunities for work in disabled workers with common mental disorders. For some, a generous and comprehensive welfare system could become a "welfare trap" (OECD 2013), keeping them away from work for unnecessary long periods of time, while for others it could act as a health-promoting safety net, providing them with a sense of security and assurance that allows them to focus their energy and efforts on RTW. Legislative changes could similarly contribute to both hamper and facilitate a fast and sustainable RTW, but the scarcity of studies from this perspective calls for more research and careful conclusions.

Summary and Concluding Remarks

In this chapter, we have seen that a large proportion of sickness absence across Europe and elsewhere are caused by common mental disorders such as depression and anxiety. This represents an enormous challenge not only from the societal perspective but also from the individual perspective. Being involuntarily excluded from the labor market is associated with severe negative health consequences, within both somatic and mental health domains. RTW, on the other hand, is associated with positive health consequences and could in fact reverse the negative consequences of work exclusion, that is, of course, provided that the workplace is a good enough place to be and not intoxicated by detrimental factors characterized by imbalance, uncertainty, or lack of value and respect. Several barriers and opportunities for work exist and could operate on different levels and in different contexts. Processes within, and in the near vicinity of the individual, are naturally influencers of the RTW process, with the most important being a history of either sick leave or common mental disorders, comorbidity, low education, high age, and negative RTW expectations. The healthcare system and interventions can also play a crucial role, for good or bad, in the RTW process of the individual worker. Symptom reduction is important, but no guarantee of RTW, and some interventions can even lead to negative results and delay RTW. Healthcare interventions with an explicit focus on work appear to be crucial, as well as multicomponent interventions that include contact with the workplace. The workplace in itself is an important context to consider, which can contribute both positively and negatively in the RTW process. High job demands/strain and low job control are for many workers barriers of RTW. Still, it is important to also remember that a job with high decision latitude can largely neutralize the risk of high job demands. Uncertainty and lack of value and respect in the workplace are also important factors in the RTW process, with workplace bullying being particularly harmful for the individual and his/her prognosis of RTW. The larger societal context the individual is a part of will also have a substantial impact on the opportunities and barriers for work, particularly the compensation system. Legislative changes or larger structural interventions to improve opportunities for work in workers with common mental disorders are, however, gravely understudied and to a large degree unknown.

Cross-References

▶ Facilitating Competitive Employment for People with Disabilities
▶ IGLOO: A Framework for Return to Work Among Workers with Mental Health Problems
▶ Occupational Determinants of Affective Disorders
▶ Work-Related Burden of Absenteeism, Presenteeism, and Disability: An Epidemiologic and Economic Perspective

References

Adda J, Chandola T, Marmot M (2003) Socio-economic status and health: causality and pathways. J Econ 112:57–63. https://doi.org/10.1016/S0304-4076(02)00146-X

Ahola K, Virtanen M, Honkonen T et al (2011) Common mental disorders and subsequent work disability: a population-based Health 2000 Study. J Affect Disord 134:365–372. https://doi.org/10.1016/j.jad.2011.05.028

Asfaw AG, Chang CC, Ray TK (2014) Workplace mistreatment and sickness absenteeism from work: results from the 2010 National Health Interview survey. Am J Ind Med 57:202–213. https://doi.org/10.1002/ajim.22273

Bandura A (1977) Self-efficacy: toward a unifying theory of behavioral change. Psychol Rev 84:191

Bandura A (1997) Self-efficacy: the exercise of control. WH Freeman, New York

Bartley M (1988) Unemployment and health: selection or causation – a false antithesis? Sociol Health Illn 10:41–67. https://doi.org/10.1111/1467-9566.ep11340114

Bartley M, Sacker A, Clarke P (2004) Employment status, employment conditions, and limiting illness: prospective evidence from the British household panel survey 1991–2001. J Epidemiol Community Health 58:501–506. https://doi.org/10.1136/jech.2003.009878

Blank L, Peters J, Pickvance S et al (2008) A systematic review of the factors which predict return to work for people suffering episodes of poor mental health. J Occup Rehabil 18:27–34. https://doi.org/10.1007/s10926-008-9121-8

Breslin FC, Mustard C (2003) Factors influencing the impact of unemployment on mental health among young and older adults in a longitudinal, population-based survey. Scand J Work Environ Health 29:5–14

Cattrell A, Harris EC, Palmer KT et al (2011) Regional trends in awards of incapacity benefit by cause. Occup Med (Lond) 61:148–151. https://doi.org/10.1093/occmed/kqr008

Claussen B (1999) Alcohol disorders and re-employment in a 5-year follow-up of long-term unemployed. Addiction 94:133–138

Cornelius LR, van der Klink JJ, Groothoff JW et al (2011) Prognostic factors of long term disability due to mental disorders: a systematic review. J Occup Rehabil 21:259–274. https://doi.org/10.1007/s10926-010-9261-5

de Vries H, Fishta A, Weikert B et al (2018) Determinants of sickness absence and return to work among employees with common mental disorders: a scoping review. J Occup Rehabil 28:393–417. https://doi.org/10.1007/s10926-017-9730-1

Ebrahim S, Guyatt GH, Walter SD et al (2013) Association of psychotherapy with disability benefit claim closure among patients disabled due to depression. PLoS One 8:e67162. https://doi.org/10.1371/journal.pone.0067162

Ebrahim S, Malachowski C, Kamal El Din M et al (2015) Measures of patients' expectations about recovery: a systematic review. J Occup Rehabil 25:240–255. https://doi.org/10.1007/s10926-014-9535-4

Ejeby K, Savitskij R, Ost LG et al (2014) Symptom reduction due to psychosocial interventions is not accompanied by a reduction in sick leave: results from a randomized controlled trial in primary care. Scand J Prim Health Care 32:67–72. https://doi.org/10.3109/02813432.2014.909163

Erik N, van der Klink JJ, Geskus RB et al (2013) Effectiveness of an exposure-based return-to-work program for workers on sick leave due to common mental disorders: a cluster-randomized controlled trial. Scand J Work Environ Health 39:144–154. https://doi.org/10.5271/sjweh.3320

Ervasti J, Joensuu M, Pentti J et al (2017) Prognostic factors for return to work after depression-related work disability: a systematic review and meta-analysis. J Psychiatr Res 95:28–36. https://doi.org/10.1016/j.jpsychires.2017.07.024

Finnes A, Enebrink P, Ghaderi A et al (2018) Psychological treatments for return to work in individuals on sickness absence due to common mental disorders or musculoskeletal disorders: a systematic review and meta-analysis of randomized-controlled trials. Int Arch Occup Environ Health. https://doi.org/10.1007/s00420-018-1380-x

Ginexi EM, Howe GW, Caplan RD (2000) Depression and control beliefs in relation to reemployment: what are the directions of effect? J Occup Health Psychol 5:323–336

Goldin PR, Ziv M, Jazaieri H et al (2012) Cognitive reappraisal self-efficacy mediates the effects of individual cognitive-behavioral therapy for social anxiety disorder. J Consult Clin Psychol 80:1034–1040. https://doi.org/10.1037/a0028555

Gragnano A, Negrini A, Miglioretti M et al (2018) Common psychosocial factors predicting return to work after common mental disorders, cardiovascular diseases, and cancers: a review of reviews supporting a cross-disease approach. J Occup Rehabil 28:215–231. https://doi.org/10.1007/s10926-017-9714-1

Halonen JI, Solovieva S, Pentti J et al (2016) Effectiveness of legislative changes obligating notification of prolonged sickness absence and assessment of remaining work ability on return to work and work participation: a natural experiment in Finland. Occup Environ Med 73:42–50. https://doi.org/10.1136/oemed-2015-103131

Harvey SB, Modini M, Joyce S et al (2017) Can work make you mentally ill? A systematic meta-review of work-related risk factors for common mental health problems. Occup Environ Med 74:301–310. https://doi.org/10.1136/oemed-2016-104015

Henderson M, Glozier N, Holland Elliott K (2005) Long term sickness absence. BMJ 330:802–803. https://doi.org/10.1136/bmj.330.7495.802

Kadden RM, Litt MD (2011) The role of self-efficacy in the treatment of substance use disorders. Addict Behav 36:1120–1126. https://doi.org/10.1016/j.addbeh.2011.07.032

Kessler RC, Demler O, Frank RG et al (2005) Prevalence and treatment of mental disorders, 1990 to 2003. N Engl J Med 352:2515–2523. https://doi.org/10.1056/NEJMsa043266

Kessler RC, Petukhova M, Sampson NA et al (2012) Twelve-month and lifetime prevalence and lifetime morbid risk of anxiety and mood disorders in the United States. Int J Methods Psychiatr Res 21:169–184. https://doi.org/10.1002/mpr.1359

Kivimaki M, Elovainio M, Vahtera J (2000) Workplace bullying and sickness absence in hospital staff. Occup Environ Med 57:656–660

Kroger C, Bode K, Wunsch EM et al (2015) Work-related treatment for major depressive disorder and incapacity to work: preliminary findings of a controlled, matched study. J Occup Health Psychol 20:248–258. https://doi.org/10.1037/a0038341

Lagerveld SE, Bultmann U, Franche RL et al (2010) Factors associated with work participation and work functioning in depressed workers: a systematic review. J Occup Rehabil 20:275–292. https://doi.org/10.1007/s10926-009-9224-x

Lagerveld SE, Blonk RW, Brenninkmeijer V et al (2012) Work-focused treatment of common mental disorders and return to work: a comparative outcome study. J Occup Health Psychol 17:220–234. https://doi.org/10.1037/a0027049

Loisel P, Anema JR (2014) Handbook of work disability. Prevention and management. Springer, New York

Lovvik C, Shaw W, Overland S et al (2014) Expectations and illness perceptions as predictors of benefit recipiency among workers with common mental disorders: secondary analysis from a randomised controlled trial. BMJ Open 4:e004321. https://doi.org/10.1136/bmjopen-2013-004321

Markussen S, Roed K, Rogeberg OJ et al (2011) The anatomy of absenteeism. J Health Econ 30:277–292. https://doi.org/10.1016/j.jhealeco.2010.12.003

Martin MH, Nielsen MB, Madsen IE et al (2013) Effectiveness of a coordinated and tailored return-to-work intervention for sickness absence beneficiaries with mental health problems. J Occup Rehabil 23:621–630. https://doi.org/10.1007/s10926-013-9421-5

Meneton P, Kesse-Guyot E, Mejean C et al (2015) Unemployment is associated with high cardiovascular event rate and increased all-cause mortality in middle-aged socially privileged individuals. Int Arch Occup Environ Health 88:707–716. https://doi.org/10.1007/s00420-014-0997-7

Mikkelsen MB, Rosholm M (2018) Systematic review and meta-analysis of interventions aimed at enhancing return to work for sick-listed workers with common mental disorders, stress-related disorders, somatoform disorders and personality disorders. Occup Environ Med 75:675–686. https://doi.org/10.1136/oemed-2018-105073

Milner A, Page A, LaMontagne AD (2013) Long-term unemployment and suicide: a systematic review and meta-analysis. PLoS One 8:e51333. https://doi.org/10.1371/journal.pone.0051333

Mondloch MV, Cole DC, Frank JW (2001) Does how you do depend on how you think you'll do? A systematic review of the evidence for a relation between patients' recovery expectations and health outcomes. CMAJ 165:174–179

Montgomery GH, Hallquist MN, Schnur JB et al (2010) Mediators of a brief hypnosis intervention to control side effects in breast surgery patients: response expectancies and emotional distress. J Consult Clin Psychol 78:80–88. https://doi.org/10.1037/a0017392

Murphy GC, Athanasou JA (1999) The effect of unemployment on mental health. J Occup Organ Psychol 72:83–99. https://doi.org/10.1348/096317999166518

Niedhammer I, Chastang JF, Sultan-Taieb H et al (2013) Psychosocial work factors and sickness absence in 31 countries in Europe. Eur J Pub Health 23:622–629. https://doi.org/10.1093/eurpub/cks124

Noordik E, van der Klink JJ, Geskus RB et al (2013) Effectiveness of an exposure-based return-to-work program for workers on sick leave due to common mental disorders: a cluster-randomized controlled trial. Scand J Work Environ Health 39:144–154. https://doi.org/10.5271/sjweh.3320

OECD (2012) Sick on the job? Myths and realities about mental health and work. OECD, Paris

OECD (2013) Mental health and work: Norway. OECD, Paris

Ortega A, Christensen KB, Hogh A et al (2011) One-year prospective study on the effect of workplace bullying on long-term sickness absence. J Nurs Manag 19:752–759. https://doi.org/10.1111/j.1365-2834.2010.01179.x

Reme SE, Grasdal AL, Lovvik C et al (2015) Work-focused cognitive-behavioural therapy and individual job support to increase work participation in common mental disorders: a randomised controlled multicentre trial. Occup Environ Med 72:745–752. https://doi.org/10.1136/oemed-2014-102700

Roelfs DJ, Shor E, Davidson KW et al (2011) Losing life and livelihood: a systematic review and meta-analysis of unemployment and all-cause mortality. Soc Sci Med 72:840–854. https://doi.org/10.1016/j.socscimed.2011.01.005

Ross CE, Mirowsky J (1995) Does employment affect health? J Health Soc Behav 36:230–243

Rueda S, Chambers L, Wilson M et al (2012) Association of returning to work with better health in working-aged adults: a systematic review. Am J Public Health 102:541–556. https://doi.org/10.2105/AJPH.2011.300401

Schaufeli WB, VanYperen NW (1992) Unemployment and psychological distress among graduates: a longitudinal study. J Occup Organ Psychol 65:291–305. https://doi.org/10.1111/j.2044-8325.1992.tb00506.x

Spiers N, Bebbington P, McManus S et al (2011) Age and birth cohort differences in the prevalence of common mental disorder in England: National Psychiatric Morbidity Surveys 1993–2007. Br J Psychiatry 198:479–484. https://doi.org/10.1192/bjp.bp.110.084269

Stansfeld SA, Fuhrer R, Head J (2011) Impact of common mental disorders on sickness absence in an occupational cohort study. Occup Environ Med 68:408–413. https://doi.org/10.1136/oem.2010.056994

Stauder J (2018) Unemployment, unemployment duration, and health: selection or causation? Eur J Health Econ. https://doi.org/10.1007/s10198-018-0982-2

Turner JA, Holtzman S, Mancl L (2007) Mediators, moderators, and predictors of therapeutic change in cognitive-behavioral therapy for chronic pain. Pain 127:276–286. https://doi.org/10.1016/j.pain.2006.09.005

Vuori J, Vesalainen J (1999) Labour market interventions as predictors of re-employment, job seeking activity and psychological distress among the unemployed. J Occup Organ Psychol 72:523–538. https://doi.org/10.1348/096317999166824

Waddell G, Burton K, Aylward M (2007) Work and common health problems. J Insur Med 39:109–120

Wittchen HU, Jacobi F, Rehm J et al (2011) The size and burden of mental disorders and other disorders of the brain in Europe 2010. Eur Neuropsychopharmacol 21:655–679. https://doi.org/10.1016/j.euroneuro.2011.07.018

Work-Related Interventions to Reduce Work Disability Related to Musculoskeletal Disorders

27

Dwayne Van Eerd and Peter Smith

Contents

Introduction	484
Burden of MSD	484
Factors Associated with MSD	485
What Is the Evidence for Workplace Interventions to Reduce Disability Related to MSD?	486
The Scientific Evidence	486
The Seven Principles of Return to Work	487
The Evidence Since the Seven Principles	488
Does More Recent Research Evidence Support the Seven Principles?	492
Emerging Topics in MSD and Work Disability	494
Sex and Gender	494
Sitting and Standing	495
Aging	496
Conclusion	498
Cross-References	499
References	499

Abstract

Musculoskeletal disorders (MSD) cause considerable disability and lost productivity in many economic sectors worldwide. In fact, the most common MSD (low back pain and neck pain) rank as the first and fourth highest disability causes among noncommunicable diseases globally. Research has shown there is a strong link between work factors and MSD. The goal of this chapter is to provide an overview of work-related interventions designed to reduce the work disability burden resulting from MSD. The chapter also covers some emerging topics relevant to conducting research on MSD and work disability. The research findings described in this overview suggest that seven return-to-work principles

D. Van Eerd (✉) · P. Smith
Institute for Work and Health, Toronto, ON, Canada
e-mail: dvaneerd@iwh.on.ca; PSmith@iwh.on.ca

© Springer Nature Switzerland AG 2020
U. Bültmann, J. Siegrist (eds.), *Handbook of Disability, Work and Health*, Handbook Series in Occupational Health Sciences, https://doi.org/10.1007/978-3-030-24334-0_27

created over a decade ago continue to be supported by the scientific literature. In particular there is consistent support for employers providing work accommodations and communication between healthcare providers and the workplace. However, there are more high-quality studies required as the available evidence regarding interventions to reduce the work disability caused by MSD is not strong. Emerging topics related to sex and gender, sitting and standing, and aging are important to MSD and work disability. The existing research evidence on these topics is equivocal; however, it is clear that workplaces must consider them in RTW and accommodation practices. More high-quality research, while challenging to conduct, would be beneficial contributing to positive workplace results.

Keywords

Musculoskeletal disorders, Return to work · Work disability · Interventions · Prognosis · Sex and gender · Aging

Introduction

Burden of MSD

Musculoskeletal disorders (MSD) cause substantial disability and lost productivity in many economic sectors worldwide (Hoy et al. 2014; Smith et al. 2014a; Tornqvist et al. 2009; Vos et al. 2012). MSD are defined as painful disorders of muscles, tendons, joints, and nerves which can affect all body parts, although the neck and lower back are the most common areas (Hagberg et al. 1995; Schneider and Irastorza 2010; Silverstein and Evanoff 2011). Symptoms reported for MSD include pain, burning, or numbness/tingling which can be mild or become quite severe especially if not treated (Silverstein and Evanoff 2011). In 2010, low back pain was ranked the 6th leading contributor to global disease burden (years lost from premature mortality or years lived in ill health), up from 11th in 1990 (Buchbinder et al. 2013). In 2017, low back pain was in the top three causes of disability for both sexes (GBD 2017 Disease and Injury Incidence and Prevalence Collaborators 2018). The increase in ranking for MSD, like low back pain, is cause for great concern particularly for the workplace as the most common MSD (neck pain and back pain) affect those typically in their formative and peak income earning years (Briggs et al. 2018).

Buchbinder et al. (2013) notes that low back pain is the leading cause of disability among noncommunicable diseases in both developed and developing countries and consistently ranks in the top three causes globally. In the Global Burden of Disease 2010 study, low back pain (LBP) ranked the highest in terms of disability, while neck pain (NP) ranked the fourth highest for disability (Briggs et al. 2018; Haldeman et al. 2018). Duffield et al. (2017) found MSD are pervasive in multimorbidity. The role of MSD in multimorbidity suggests a potentially larger impact on work disability as working population age. For example, a Canadian study observed that the impacts of back pain when co-occurring with arthritis on labor-market participation were greater (super-additive) than the impacts of either of these factors in isolation (Smith et al. 2014a).

Overall work-related MSD account for 29% of all US workplace injuries (Silverstein and Evanoff 2011). In Canada, MSD account for between 40 and 60% of lost-time claims since 2000 (Workers Compensation Board of Manitoba 2014; Workplace Safety and Insurance Board 2013; WorkSafeBC 2013; Workers' Compensation Board of Nova Scotia 2013). In addition, in Canada and the United States (US), MSD are the leading causes of disabling work-related injuries. In Europe, MSD are considered to be an increasing and significant health problem, making up to approximately 39% of occupational diseases (Schneider and Irastorza 2010).

Furthermore, it has been estimated that work-related MSD costs are between 0.5% and 2% of the EU's gross national product (GNP) (Schneider and Irastorza 2010). Direct compensation costs for MSD are estimated to be between $13 and $20 billion dollars annually in the United States, and on average they result in a median of 9 days off work (Silverstein and Evanoff 2011). In summary, MSD are prevalent and costly in developed and developing countries (Hurwitz et al. 2018) demanding focused prevention and rehabilitation campaigns. Briggs and Dreinhofer (2017) also support the view that the rising burden of MSD requires effective rehabilitation strategies. Briefly, in a recent call to action called "Rehabilitation 2030," Briggs and Dreinhofer (2017) note that increasing disability rates such as that related to MSD requires careful planning to improve and maintain access to quality rehabilitation for the future. They point out that to address the rising burden, changes will likely be required at multiple levels (including health governance, policy, and how individuals access and participate in care) across jurisdictions. Briggs and Dreinhofer (2017) point out that MSD impact on functional health such as mobility, participation, financial security, as well as mental well-being and therefore emphasize the importance of improved rehabilitation for these conditions globally.

Factors Associated with MSD

Studies examining global burden of MSD consistently note the link between work factors and MSD, particularly neck and back pain (Buchbinder et al. 2013; Hoy et al. 2014; Johnson et al. 2018). High-quality epidemiological investigations have identified a broad range of physical, psychological, psychosocial, and organizational risk factors for MSD (Hagberg et al. 1995; National Research Council 2001; Silverstein and Evanoff 2011; Wells et al. 2004). Commonly reported risk factors include mechanical factors (force, posture, repetition, duration), work organizational factors (worker perceptions of demand, control, and co-worker and supervisor support; psychosocial factors), as well as individual factors (such as health and health habits (smoking, drinking, fitness), rest, and recovery) (Hagberg et al. 1995; Wells et al. 2004). Therefore, there is relatively little debate among the scientific community regarding the work-relatedness of MSD. While there continue to be prevalence studies published, largely the research focus has moved from establishing cause to prevention and treatment effectiveness studies (Silverstein and Evanoff 2011). However, there is more high-quality research on well-implemented interventions needed in these areas (Kristensen 2005; Neumann et al. 2010).

The goal of this chapter is to summarize research evidence on workplace-based interventions that can reduce the burden of MSD. We also provide a few thoughts on areas for future research/emerging topics, in areas of how work impacts MSD and how MSD impact work.

What Is the Evidence for Workplace Interventions to Reduce Disability Related to MSD?

The Scientific Evidence

Early descriptions of evidence-based practice noted the importance of referring to the best available scientific evidence in decision-making (Sackett et al. 1996). The suggestion of a hierarchy of evidence stems from these early evidence-based practice descriptions and spawned several versions of the evidence pyramid (Alper and Haynes 2016; McMaster University 2016; Murad et al. 2016). While there are a number of different ways to represent the pyramid, they all convey that there is a hierarchy and moving up the pyramid results in better evidence with which to make decisions. Figure 1 depicts our version of the hierarchy showing the superiority of filtered information and like many other pyramids, shows systematic reviews at the top.

Systematic reviews refer to studies which appraise and summarize the results of primary research from the scientific literature on a specific research topic or question

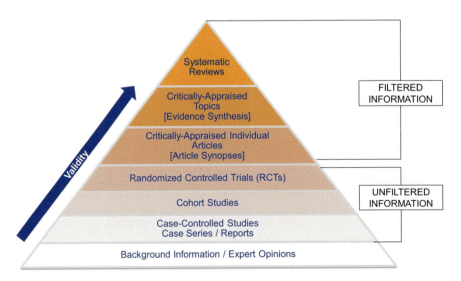

Fig. 1 An evidence pyramid

(Irvin et al. 2010). A systematic review focuses on reducing bias by using replicable, scientific, and transparent methods. A key aspect of what makes the systematic review a higher level of evidence is the critical appraisal of study quality in the synthesis. Therefore, the results of a systematic review are ideal to inform decision-makers including clinicians, occupational health practitioners, researchers, consumers, and policy makers by providing an up-to-date summary of the current evidence on a topic.

In the following section, we summarize some systematic reviews of the scientific literature covering a range of workplace-based interventions.

The Seven Principles of Return to Work

Just a little over a decade ago, two reviews were published describing the workplace-based return-to-work (RTW) interventions for MSD (Franche et al. 2005; MacEachen et al. 2006). The review by Franche et al. (2005) examined peer-reviewed quantitative studies of workplace-based RTW interventions for workers with MSD and other pain-related conditions. Using a rigorous review process, the authors considered over 4000 references and found 10 relevant articles of sufficient quality. The review focused on RTW interventions that could be employed in workplaces: early contact with the worker by the workplace, work accommodation offers, contact between healthcare provider and the workplace, ergonomic work site visits, staff replacements, and RTW coordination.

The synthesis of the best available research evidence suggested there was strong evidence that (1) a work accommodation offer and (2) contact by a healthcare provider with the workplace significantly reduces work disability duration. There was a moderate level of evidence that (1) early contact with the worker, (2) ergonomic work site visits, and (3) interventions which include the presence of a RTW coordinator significantly reduce work disability duration. There was insufficient evidence to support the effectiveness of supernumerary replacements impact on work disability duration.

In an accompanying review of the qualitative literature, MacEachen et al. (2006) examined the processes and practices of RTW for workers with MSD and pain-related conditions. Qualitative research can address the gap related to RTW process and practice in workplaces by providing the viewpoint of those involved.

MacEachen and colleagues found 13 qualitative studies of sufficient quality from the same 4000 plus articles described in Franche et al. (2005). Conducting a meta-ethnographic synthesis of these relevant studies, the authors report eight key concepts: role of goodwill; relations between workers and systems; contact between worker and workplace after injury and prior to RTW; employer contact with physicians; modified work; union role; supervisor role; and organizational environment. In all concepts there are potential positive or negative consequences, for example, the role of the supervisor could facilitate or be a barrier to RTW outcomes. From these eight concepts, the authors put forward three overarching findings: (1) RTW processes have great scope and complexity, involving the interaction between many different individuals and systems; (2) goodwill and trust are central to RTW given the complexity and number of potential individuals involved; therefore, (3) social and communication barriers are key concerns to be addressed in the RTW process.

The findings from these two reviews were used to create a practical RTW tool: Seven Principles for Successful Return to Work (Institute for Work and Health 2008).

1. The workplace has a strong commitment to health and safety, which is demonstrated by the behaviors of the workplace parties.
2. The employer makes an offer of modified work (also known as work accommodation) to injured/ill workers so they can return early and safely to work activities suitable to their abilities.
3. RTW planners ensure that the plan supports the returning worker without disadvantaging co-workers and supervisors.
4. Supervisors are trained in work disability prevention and included in RTW planning.
5. The employer makes early and considerate contact with injured/ill workers.
6. Someone has the responsibility to coordinate RTW.
7. Employers and healthcare providers communicate with each other about the workplace demands as needed, and with the worker's consent.

The seven principles were based on the best available research evidence and have become one of the most popular tools for download on the IWH website (Institute for Work and Health 2017).

The Evidence Since the Seven Principles

There have been a number of reviews of the research evidence completed since the creation of the seven principle tool (Institute for Work and Health 2008). The remainder of this section compares recent review findings to the seven principles – indicating whether the reviews support or not the individual principles. The reviews considered here were found using the literature search strategy from Cullen et al. (2018), selecting only recent systematic literature reviews (from 2008 to 2018). We also ran a search in Medline for systematic reviews on the topic of MSD and RTW for the years 2008 to 2018. Additional reviews and some supporting studies were found in the reference lists of the included literature reviews from the original search yield. We note this is not a systematic review approach but a narrative review.

We chose reviews that synthesized evidence on work-related prognostic factors as well as those focused on work disability outcomes (primarily RTW) and considered workplace-based interventions for MSD. Our summary of the reviews is presented with brief details of the review findings. Following this we provide our assessment of whether the findings supported the seven principles (see list above).

Prognostic Factors Evidence

There have been quite a number of reviews in the past decade examining prognostic factors related to MSD and RTW (e.g., Campbell et al. 2013; Verkerk et al. 2012). We also found a review of reviews by Cancelliere et al. (2016) which considers and synthesizes the evidence from systematic reviews. A review of already-filtered evidence moves us up to the peak of the evidence pyramid. Importantly the review covers a variety of health conditions and not solely MSD. However, of the 56 reviews they examined, 35 included MSD, therefore we were easily able to extract the findings related to MSD.

The factors associated with positive RTW outcomes for MSD included higher self-efficacy/optimistic perceptions and expectations, stakeholder participation in the RTW process, work modification/accommodation, and RTW coordination. Interventions involving a workplace component were associated with positive RTW outcomes. These interventions included multidisciplinary, education, psychological, and outpatient interventions/comprehensive treatment. In addition, interventions that included exercise and early contact with the worker by the workplace (i.e., within the first 3 months following onset of work disability) were linked to positive RTW outcomes.

Factors associated with negative RTW outcomes for MSD included older age, higher pain or disability, and higher physical work demands. Also receiving higher compensation (e.g., higher weekly wage compensation rates from workers' compensation due to occupational back injuries) was commonly associated with negative RTW outcomes.

The authors report factors not associated with RTW outcomes for MSD were having anxiety or stress, smoking, and level of work satisfaction showed no association with RTW outcomes. There were a number of additional factors where the authors note there is insufficient or conflicting evidence of association such as the type of occupation and vocational rehabilitation programs.

Cancelliere and colleagues (2016) compared their findings to the seven principles (Institute for Work & Health 2008) and concluded their synthesis results generally supported the principles. They point out they did not find studies to support principles three and four but note these principles made sense regardless. They, however, suggested adding a "principle" based on their findings. They called the additional principle – "the worker has access to multidisciplinary resources (including clinical interventions for the management of pain, disability, depression and poor expectations for recovery), where necessary, working in combination with the other stakeholders."

Intervention Evidence

Participatory ergonomics (PE) interventions are a popular method of reducing risk factors for musculoskeletal and traumatic injuries in workplaces and can be used for RTW (Loisel et al. 2001; Van Eerd et al. 2016). Rivilis et al. (2008) conducted a systematic review of the literature on the effectiveness of PE as a workplace intervention to improve health outcomes. PE interventions strive to improve workplace conditions through participation, communication, and group problem-solving.

Twelve articles were relevant and considered to have sufficient methodological quality to contribute to the evidence synthesis. These studies came from various jurisdictions and industries and addressed two broad categories of health outcomes related to work disability: MSD injury records or claims and MSD lost workdays/sick leave. Using a best-evidence synthesis approach encompassing methodological quality, quantity of studies, and consistency, the review team found limited evidence that PE can improve MSD claims and lost days of work. Subsequent PE studies most often focused on the prevention of MSD rather than preventing work disability. This is the most current synthesis of the literature that we are aware of as the review has not been updated.

In a Cochrane review of workplace interventions for neck pain, Aas et al. (2011) found ten randomized controlled trial (RCT) studies from various jurisdictions. The included studies evaluated a variety of interventions either single component or multicomponent that included modified work, participatory ergonomic, ergonomic workplace visits, return-to-work interventions, or multidisciplinary ergonomic interventions. The review considered outcomes related to pain and work disability. The authors concluded there was moderate quality evidence from one study that a multicomponent intervention reduced sickness absence. The multicomponent intervention in the study was a PE approach conducted in Finland.

Carroll et al. (2010) conducted a review of workplace involvement in interventions to improve RTW with back pain. Key elements of the interventions described in the studies of this review were related to communication or coordination with the workplace. Interventions included work modification meetings among occupational health practitioners, employees, and employers with a PE approach as well as interventions focused on exercise therapy at the workplace. The review considered a variety of study designs in studies from a variety of jurisdictions. They found ten articles of sufficient quality and found early intervention was effective as were interventions where employees, health practitioners, and employers worked together to implement workplace modifications.

A review of community and workplace interventions by Palmer et al. (2012) found 42 relevant studies with interventions of exercise therapy, behavioral change techniques, workplace adaptations, and provision of additional services. The review included RCT and cohort designs in studies from a variety of jurisdictions. The outcomes of interest for this review were sickness absence, MSD-related job loss, and RTW. Workplace interventions were evaluated in 17 of the 42 studies and typically included workplace adaptations. Overall, the authors found most interventions were effective at reducing sickness absence, but the effects were rather small. However, the authors note interventions involving workplace adaptations/assessments were somewhat more beneficial in reducing days lost than the others in the review.

Gensby et al. (2014) conducted a Campbell review exploring workplace disability management programs (WPDM). Gensby et al. consider a broad range of study designs, and studies were conducted in a variety of jurisdictions. The findings are from 12 studies covering 10 different WPDM of which 8 programs focused on MSD. The authors concluded there was insufficient evidence about the effectiveness of employer WPDM program for RTW. A unique aspect of the Gensby review was the description of the common program policies and practices. The authors found a total of 15 policies and practices and found evidence to support 10 used most frequently: (1) RTW policies guiding program management and procedures, (2) offer of suitable work accommodation, (3) onsite physical rehabilitation services, (4) workplace assessment with job analysis, (5) tailored job modification, (6) corporate located RTW coordinators/disability case managers, (7) internal disability claim information system, (8) early contact and intervention, (9) involvement of joint labor-management committee, and (10) active employee participation.

van Vilsteren et al. (2015) conducted a Cochrane review and found 14 RCT studies conducted in various jurisdictions that evaluated workplace interventions to prevent work disability. Eight of the studies included workers with MSD. In a subgroup analysis focused on MSD studies, the authors found workplace MSD interventions reduced time to RTW more than usual care. The MSD interventions reviewed tended to include modified work/accommodations, contact with health professionals, and some type of case management. Williams-Whitt et al. (2016) considered the findings and studies from the van Vilsteren review (2015) along with gray literature and a stakeholder panel. The authors support the key findings from the systematic review but suggest more emphasis should be placed on organizational factors in workplace interventions. A key aspect of the recommendations is to provide managers and supervisors with training and ensure they are fully involved along with employees in the RTW process.

Vargas-Prada et al. (2016) reviewed studies that examined effectiveness of very early (<15 days) workplace-based RTW interventions on sickness absence. Despite a rather inclusive literature search strategy, only four RCT articles (describing three studies) were considered relevant and of at least moderate quality. Two of the included studies considered MSD, both conducted in European countries. One intervention was a guideline-based care with workplace involvement including counselling, work modifications/accommodations, and case management. The other intervention was an early part-time (P/T) sick leave for workers with MSD where daily work-time was reduced to approximately 50%. The authors conclude there is a lack of evidence from the literature to support the effectiveness of early RTW interventions. It is important to note that Vargas-Prada et al. only included two studies examining MSD in their review based on a somewhat arbitrary definition of "very early."

Vogel et al. (2017) recently completed a Cochrane review of RTW coordination interventions to improve RTW outcomes. They found 14 RCT studies from various jurisdictions, with 12 including workers with MSD. Importantly the review only considered public or private insurers offered (or contracted) return-to-work coordination programs and excluded employer programs. The interventions were varied, and all started within 6 months of the worker inclusion. The interventions also varied with respect to the contact with the workplace, with only eight studies describing involvement of the workplace in the intervention. The overall findings of the review were that RTW coordination programs offered (or contracted by) public or private insurers were not more effective than usual care for work disability outcomes.

Cullen et al. (2018) recently completed a systematic review examining the effectiveness of workplace-based RTW and work disability management interventions for workers with MSD and pain-related conditions as well as mental health conditions. The search found 36 medium- and high-quality studies from a variety of jurisdictions. Of these, 14 studies examined MSD or pain-related conditions. The review found a strong level of evidence of a positive effect for comprehensive multi-domain interventions to reduce lost time related to MSD from four high- and ten medium-quality studies. They also found moderate evidence that graded activity programs have a positive effect on reducing lost time, work modification interventions (accommodations) had a positive effect on reducing lost time, and multi-domain interventions had a positive effect on work functioning after RTW. Overall the authors suggest interventions with multiple components aimed at service coordination, work modification, and improving worker health for reducing lost time associated with MSD.

Does More Recent Research Evidence Support the Seven Principles?

The review of systematic reviews on the topic of MSD and work disability in this chapter is neither exhaustive nor systematic. We have provided some details about how we searched for the various reviews but note it was not a comprehensive search strategy. Our intent was to provide an overview of the current evidence on workplace-based interventions and their impact on work disability outcomes. We compare our overview results to the seven principles of return to work as they are popular and practical. However, they were derived from two systematic reviews completed over a decade ago (Franche et al. 2005; MacEachen et al. 2006). Therefore, we considered reviews from 2008 and on and used the information presented in the reviews about the interventions and level of evidence to make a judgment about whether any of the seven principles were supported or not. We appreciate the potential bias in these judgments and wish to be transparent here, so the reader can proceed accordingly.

Generally, our overview suggests the recent evidence about MSD and work disability continues to support the seven principles (see Table 1). However, the support is not universal as we found some reviews that did not support any principles (Vargas-Prada et al. 2016; Vogel et al. 2017). Not all principles are supported equally, although there was no expectation the included systematic reviews would have provided evidence on all principles. The most often supported principles are two (employer makes an offer of modified work) and seven (employers and healthcare providers communicate with each other). The support for principles two and seven may be related to current work disability practices across jurisdictions where these elements are included in research because they are required by the workplace or system. Alternatively, they may be the easiest aspects to include in practices and policies and therefore are available in interventions in research studies. We found there was support for each of the seven principles from at least three systematic reviews (see Table 1).

Table 1 Support (+)/nonsupport (−) of seven principles according to recent systematic reviews

Principle	Cancelliere et al. (2016)[a]	Rivilis et al. (2008)	Aas (2011)	Carroll et al. (2010)	Palmer (2012)	Gensby et al. (2014)	van Vilsteren et al. (2015)[b]	Vargas-Prada et al. (2016)	Vogel et al. (2017)	Cullen et al. (2018)
1. The workplace has a strong commitment to health and safety, which is demonstrated by the behaviors of the workplace parties	+	+				+				
2. The employer makes an offer of modified work (also known as work accommodation) to injured/ill workers so they can return early and safely to work activities suitable to their abilities	+	+	+	+	+	+	+	−		+
3. RTW planners ensure that the plan supports the returning worker without disadvantaging co-workers and supervisors						+	+			+
4. Supervisors are trained in work disability prevention and included in RTW planning			+			+	+			
5. The employer makes early and considerate contact with injured/ill workers	+			+		+		−	−	+
6. Someone has the responsibility to coordinate RTW	+		+			+				+
7. Employers and healthcare providers communicate with each other about the workplace demands as needed, and with the worker's consent	+	+	+	+		+	+			+

[a] review of reviews
[b] including findings of Williams-Whitt et al. (2016)

Cancelliere et al. (2016) suggested adding an eighth principle to address review findings that multicomponent interventions tended to be more effective than single-component interventions. In our overview it seems multicomponent interventions better encompass or address a number of the existing seven principles. Whether or not this should be added to the principles is beyond the scope of this chapter, but with more research it is possible the principles could be expanded to include the multi-component concept.

Emerging Topics in MSD and Work Disability

Before concluding this chapter, we would like to focus on some specific emerging issues in the area of MSD as they relate to work. These are (a) the need for better integrating concepts of sex (biological differences between men and women) and gender (social differences between men and women) into understanding the risk factors and work consequences of MSD conditions; (b) the available evidence on sitting and standing at work as they relate to MSD conditions; and (c) the role of the aging of the labor market in MSD incidence and the effects on work.

Sex and Gender

The labor market in many countries remains highly segregated for men and women. For example, in Canada between 1987 and 2015, the proportion of the employed labor force that is female increased from 45% to 49%, with an absolute increase in the labor force of 1.8 million men and 2.7 million women. Despite these increases the 12 most gender-segregated occupations, which represent 40% of all labor force participants, have remained unchanged (Smith presented at Women, work and health: precarious and invisible labour. Women's College Hospital: women's Xchange, November 25th, 2016. Women's College Hospital, Toronto). Previous work in Quebec suggests more than half of all workers would have to change jobs in order for men and women to be distributed equally across employment categories (Armstrong and Messing 2014). Despite these changes in labor market participation and the consistent finding of male/female differences in RTW outcomes, very little research has specifically examined potential gender/sex differences in either the risk factors that lead to musculoskeletal injuries or the differences in the impact of modifiable workplace and individual factors on RTW outcomes.

A 2010 systematic review on disability following a work-related musculoskeletal injury could only identify 32 articles (7%), from an original sample of 475 articles, which specifically explored gender differences (rather than adjusting for gender in analyses) (Cote and Coutu 2010). This review identified some key areas of relevance to better understanding gender differences in work disability following musculoskeletal injury. Women are more likely than men to suffer from work-related injuries and illnesses with a complex etiology and fewer visible manifestations. These characteristics may result in more strained relationships between women and their physicians and their workplace (both supervisors and co-workers) in the RTW process, leading to increased feelings of distrust and longer absence durations.

The different family and societal roles of men and women (men as a breadwinner and women as the person who is pivotal to the family structure and function) may impact the RTW process differently for men and women. One specific area where these impacts may be felt is in relation to gender differences in non-work roles and subsequent levels of domestic strain. Women returning to work after injury are more likely than men to be engaged in dual roles, balancing family responsibilities with rehabilitation priorities (Cote and Coutu 2010). While a previous review concluded there was moderate evidence of no effect of having dependent children and strong evidence of no effect of marital status on RTW (Laisne et al. 2012), these findings were from studies where gender had been adjusted for, not examined specifically. When examined in stratified models, the effect of dependent children on having time to relax and exercise differs for men and women, with dependent children having a negative effect on relaxation and exercise time among women, but no effect among men (Strazdins and Bammer 2004). In turn, less time to relax and exercise has been associated with greater symptoms of musculoskeletal pain among both genders (Strazdins and Bammer 2004).

There is also a reasonably large body of literature that documents increased pain sensitivity among women compared to men (Fillingham et al. 1999; Frot et al. 2004). These gender/sex differences in pain are potentially due to both biological and social differences between men and women (Cote 2012). It is therefore important to better understand not only the factors related to differences in pain among men and women but also to understand the relative contribution that differences in pain have to subsequent differences in absence from work. There are also biological factors such as smaller body size and muscle fiber composition that may lead to women being more likely to suffer upper body musculoskeletal injuries than men (Cote 2012). It is therefore important to better understand the role that part of body plays in gender/sex differences in RTW outcome for particular types of conditions.

Sitting and Standing

The last decade has seen increasing interest in the impacts of sedentary sitting time at work and its impact on a variety of health outcomes (Buckley et al. 2015). While a 2003 publication from the World Health Organization identifies prolonged sitting as a posture that might be a risk factor for musculoskeletal disorders (World Health Organisation 2003), the risks associated with prolonged sitting time at work likely depend on what sitting time is replaced with and the way this is done. Specifically, much of the work to reduce sitting time at work has involved the introduction of sit/stand workstations; however, it is possible replacing sitting with standing could exacerbate, rather than reduce, MSD symptoms (Antle et al. 2013; Callaghan et al. 2015; Coenen et al. 2017), as well as potentially leading to higher risks of other cardiovascular conditions (Smith et al. 2018).

The recent research literature on the optimal combinations or sitting and standing at work, as they relate to muscular discomfort is mixed. A multicomponent intervention involving a height-adjustable workstation and activity prompts, along with pain self-management, demonstrated a reduction in pain over a 6-month period (Barone Gibbs et al. 2018), although it was not possible to separate the effects of increases in standing from pain management. Conversely, a study examining the impacts of a 2-h standing task demonstrated increased discomfort in all body areas, as well as reducing mental state (Baker et al. 2018). Another study demonstrated while standing for 1 h resulted in greater motion (potentially associated with reduced MSD burden) compared to sitting, it was also associated with the higher discomfort (Le and Marras 2016). A Finnish intervention study demonstrated standing, compared to sitting over a 3-month period, resulted in decreased musculoskeletal pain in the neck and shoulders, but increased pain in the legs and feet, with no differences observed in mental alertness between groups (Makkonen et al. 2017). Finally, a study among blue-collar workers in Denmark demonstrated prolonged sitting, among workers who normally stand, was associated with a more favorable course of low back pain over a 1-year period (Korshoj et al. 2018). While mixed, the take-home message from the above studies may be that providing opportunities to move or change positions is most beneficial for workers, in relation to reducing musculoskeletal symptoms, as workers who sit for prolonged periods may find relief in opportunities to stand and move, while workers who stand for prolonged periods will find relief in opportunities to sit. Further, it is likely there is not one prescribed pattern of sitting, standing, and moving that will work for all workers (Holtermann et al. 2018). It is possible that advances in technology might enable workers to more easily track there standing, sitting, and moving patterns throughout the day, as well as levels of musculoskeletal discomfort, allowing for specific prompts to be developed over time over optimal sit/stand/move combinations that suit them.

Aging

The global population is aging with a projection that one in five people will be over the age of 60 by 2050 (UN 2012). For example, the Canadian population aged 65 and over is expected to double over the next 25 years (Statistics Canada 2010). The Canadian workforce is also aging with a large proportion of workers (42.4%) in the 45 to 64 age group in 2011 (Human Resources and Skills Development Canada 2011), and the average age of labor market participant predicted to continue to rise until 2031 (Martel et al. 2012).

There are studies that have explored the link between MSD (e.g., Whalin et al. 2013; Monteiro et al. 2009) and aging; however, the nature of the association remains unclear. Smith et al. (2014b) showed older workers did not have higher rates of MSD despite having longer durations of disability. Smith et al. (2013) also found no association between age and the probability of a lost time claim for musculoskeletal conditions, with the risk of injury peaking among workers

35–44 years of age, among both men and women. Guest et al. (2014) showed older workers did not sustain more injuries than younger workers in construction jobs. Pransky et al. (2005) suggests older workers recover from injury more quickly than younger workers. An analysis on the interplay between physical demands and age for MSD requiring 10 or more days off work revealed the relationship between occupational demands and risk of injury was highest among workers 25–45 years of age, flattening slightly among workers 45 and older (Smith and Berecki-Gisolf 2014). Barros et al. (2015) also found older workers do not consider physical demands as a reason for earlier exit from their jobs.

A challenge in the area of age and work is how to best measure the concept of aging. Aging has been defined as "changes that occur in biological, psychological and social functioning throughout time" (Settersten and Mayer 1997). Often, researchers focus on chronological age as part of their analytical models examining aging, but they are not explicit about what chronological age represents, or the conceptual diversity in meanings of age (Settersten and Mayer 1997). Over two decades ago, Sterns and Doverspike (1989) proposed five approaches to define older age that are relevant to understanding the relationship between age and work outcomes. These are (1) chronological/legal age; (2) functional age (which reflects performance-based measures and is influenced by health and chronic conditions); (3) psychosocial age (reflecting perceptions from the individual or others, about their age relative to personal or social standards); (4) organizational age (reflecting the time an individual has spent in the labor market, in their workplace, or in their current occupations); and (5) life stage age (which reflects where an individual perceives themselves to be, in relation to their life course). While these dimensions are related, they also likely capture unique aspects of the aging process. For example, studies focusing on RTW and healthcare following a work-related MSD injury suggest that preexisting chronic conditions (a measure of functional age) only explain a small proportion of age differences in these two outcomes, leaving a substantial proportion of age differences in each outcome unexplained (Smith et al. 2014b, c). Given each of the dimensions of age may have a role to play in relation to the impacts of MSD conditions on work outcomes, future research should attempt to better measure each of these dimensions and determine their relative impacts. Importantly, some of these dimensions of age are potentially modifiable, unlike chronological age.

An aging population and workforce is a reality. The link between aging and MSD is not clear, and specific research related to strategies to reduce MSD suggests age is but one of many factors to address. Workplace policies supporting accommodation and development may be the most useful to address MSD in older workers as they can lead to innovative interventions and programs such as participatory and problem-solving approaches (Koolhaas et al. 2015; Van Eerd et al. 2016), ergonomics (Gonzalez and Morer 2016; Stedmon et al. 2012), and health promotion approaches (Hughes et al. 2011; Pitt-Catsouphes et al. 2015). More research regarding MSD and aging is required so workplaces/employers can better develop policies and practices regarding older workers. Specific research on fatigue and recovery (Bos et al. 2013; Clendon and Walker 2016; Riethmeister et al. 2016) should be a priority. Current research suggests supporting healthy aging will be beneficial for productivity as well as society. The World Health Organization (WHO) *World Report on Ageing and Health* defines healthy aging as "the process of developing and maintaining the functional ability that enables well-being in older age" (World Health Organization 2015). The WHO report provides strategies for creating age-friendly environments that we propose can be adapted and applied to workplaces to reduce the burden of MSD: (i) *combating ageism*, (ii) *enabling autonomy*, and (iii) *supporting healthy aging in policy*.

Conclusion

This chapter has provided an overview of evidence and emerging topics related to MSD and work disability. The burden of MSD is great across industrial sectors in both developed and developing economies. While there have been many studies and reviews devoted to this topic, there remain challenges. Our overview encompassed a wide variety of workplace-based interventions and considered the evidence from systematic reviews. Yet there is no strong scientific evidence for any single intervention. And while this is no excuse for inaction on the part of workplaces or work disability professionals, it is disconcerting. In fact, it is important to point out the lack of scientific evidence is not necessarily a reflection of the quality of the interventions studied. It is primarily a problem with the amount and quality of the research carried out to evaluate the interventions. Consequently, systematic reviews to date have not been able to provide strong guidance for practice.

However, the seven "principles" of successful return to work (Institute for Work and Health 2008) do provide some guidance to reduce work disability. A particular strength of the seven principles is they were constructed using evidence from systematic reviews of the quantitative and qualitative literature. While these reviews are over a decade old now, our overview of recent systematic reviews suggest the principles are generally supported. Despite the support we suggest more research is required. We anticipate that practitioners have created (and continue to create) workplace-based interventions to reduce work disability using practice evidence (their training, expertise, and experience). However, challenges of conducting well-designed, rigorous evaluations of these interventions have been a barrier to building the strong scientific evidence necessary to guide practice. Studies that evaluate weak or poorly implemented interventions do a disservice to the scientific literature by suggesting interventions which are not effective. When, in fact, they may be effective if implemented properly (Kristensen 2005). Kristensen (2005) has referred to this as program failure versus theory failure.

Emerging topics important to MSD and work disability will continue to provide challenges to the conduct of high-quality research. However, the burden of MSD is high, and what is needed are creative researchers and willing workplaces working together to conduct evaluations with the level of rigor required to provide sufficient levels of evidence of effectiveness.

Cross-References

▶ Concepts of Work Ability in Rehabilitation
▶ Employment as a Key Rehabilitation Outcome
▶ Implementing Best Practice Models of Return to Work

References

Aas RW, Tuntland H, Holte KA et al (2011) Workplace interventions for neck pain in workers. Cochrane Database Syst Rev (4):CD008160
Alper BS, Haynes RB (2016) EBHC pyramid 5.0 for accessing preappraised evidence and guidance. Evid Based Med 21(4):123–125. https://doi.org/10.1136/ebmed-2016-110447
Antle DM, Vezina N, Messing K et al (2013) Development of discomfort and vascular and muscular changes during a prolonged standing task. Occup Ergon 11(1):21–33
Armstrong P, Messing K (2014) Taking gender into account in occupational health research: continuing tensions. Policy Pract Health Saf 14:3–16
Baker RP, Coenen E, Howie J et al (2018) A detailed description of the short-term musculoskeletal and cognitive effects of prolonged standing for office computer work. Ergonomics 61:877–890
Barone Gibbs B, Hergenroeder AL, Perdomo SJ et al (2018) Reducing sedentary behavior to decrease chronic low back pain: the stand back randomised trial. J Occup Environ Med 75:321–327
Barros C, Carnide F, Cunha L et al (2015) Will I be able to do my work at 60? An analysis of working conditions that hinder active ageing. Work 51(3):579–590
Bos JT, Donders NCGM, Schouteten RLJ et al (2013) Age as a moderator in the relationship between work-related characteristics, job dissatisfaction and need for recovery. Ergonomics 56(6):992–1005
Briggs AM, Dreinhofer KE (2017) Rehabilitation 2030: a call to action relevant to improving musculoskeletal health care globally. J Orthop Sports Phys Ther 47(5):297–300. https://doi.org/10.2519/jospt.2017.0105
Briggs AM, Woolf AD, Dreinhöfer K et al (2018) Reducing the global burden of musculoskeletal conditions. Bull World Health Organ 96(5):366–368. https://doi.org/10.2471/BLT.17.204891
Buchbinder R, Blyth FM, March LM et al (2013) Placing the global burden of low back pain in context. Best Pract Res Clin Rheumatol 27(5):575–589. https://doi.org/10.1016/j.berh.2013.10.007
Buckley JP, Hedge A, Yates T et al (2015) The sedentary office: an expert statement on the growing case for change towards better health and productivity. Br J Sports Med 49(21):1357–1362
Callaghan JP, De Carvalho D, Gallagher K et al (2015) Is standing the solution to sedentary office work. Ergon Des 23(3):20–24
Campbell P, Wynne-Jones G, Muller S et al (2013) The influence of employment social support for risk and prognosis in nonspecific back pain: a systematic review and critical synthesis. Int Arch Occup Environ Health 86(2):119–137
Cancelliere C, Donovan J, Stochkendahl MJ et al (2016) Factors affecting return to work after injury or illness: best evidence synthesis of systematic reviews. Chiropr Man Ther 24(1):32
Carroll C, Rick J, Pilgrim H et al (2010) Workplace involvement improves return to work rates among employees with back pain on long-term sick leave: a systematic review of the effectiveness and cost-effectiveness of interventions. Disabil Rehabil 32(8):607–621
Clendon J, Walker L (2016) The juxtaposition of ageing and nursing: the challenges and enablers of continuing to work in the latter stages of a nursing career. J Adv Nurs 72(5):1065–1074. https://doi.org/10.1111/jan.12896
Coenen P, Willenberg L, Parry S et al (2017) Associations of occupational standing with musculoskeletal symptoms: a systematic review with meta-analysis. Br J Sports Med 52(3):176–183

Cote JN (2012) A critical review on physical factors and functional characteristics that may explain a sex/gender difference in work-related neck/shoulder disorders. Ergonomics 55:173–182

Cote D, Coutu MF (2010) A critical review of gender issues in understanding prolonged disability related to musculoskeletal pain: how are they relevant to rehabilitation? Disabil Rehabil 32:87–102

Cullen KL, Irvin E, Collie A et al (2018) Effectiveness of workplace interventions in return-to-work for musculoskeletal, pain-related and mental health conditions: an update of the evidence and messages for practitioners. J Occup Rehabil 28(1):1–15

Duffield SJ, Ellis BM, Goodson N et al (2017) The contribution of musculoskeletal disorders in multimorbidity: implications for practice and policy. Best Pract Res Clin Rheumatol 31(2):129–144. https://doi.org/10.1016/j.berh.2017.09.004

Fillingham RB, Edwards RR, Powell T (1999) The relationship of sex and clinical pain to experimental pain responses. Pain 83:419–425

Franche RL, Cullen K, Clarke J et al (2005) Workplace-based return-to-work interventions: a systematic review of the quantitative literature. J Occup Rehabil 15(4):607–631

Frot M, Feine JS, Buchnell MC (2004) Sex differences in pain perception and anxiety. A psychophysical study with topical capsaicin. Pain 108:230–246

GBD 2017 Disease and Injury Incidence and Prevalence Collaborators (2018) Global, regional, and national incidence, prevalence, and years lived with disability for 354 diseases and injuries for 195 countries and territories, 1990–2017: a systematic analysis for the Global Burden of Disease Study 2017. Lancet 392:1789–1858

Gensby U, Labriola M, Irvin E et al (2014) A classification of components of workplace disability management programs: results from a systematic review. J Occup Rehabil 24(2):220–241. https://doi.org/10.1007/s10926-013-9437-x

Gonzalez I, Morer P (2016) Ergonomics for the inclusion of older workers in the knowledge workforce and a guidance tool for designers. Appl Ergon 53(Pt A):131–142

Guest M, Boggess MM, Viljoen DA et al (2014) Age-related injury and compensation claim rates in heavy industry. Occup Med 64(2):95–103

Hagberg M, Silverstein B, Wells R et al (1995) Work related musculoskeletal disorders (WMSDs): a reference book for prevention. Taylor & Francis, London

Haldeman S, Nordin M, Chou R et al (2018) The Global Spine Care Initiative: World Spine Care executive summary on reducing spine-related disability in low- and middle-income communities. Eur Spine J 27(Suppl 6):776–785. https://doi.org/10.1007/s00586-018-5722-x

Holtermann A, Mathiassen SE, Straker L (2018) Promoting health and physical capacity during productive work: the Goldilocks Principle. Scand J Work Environ Health 45:90. https://doi.org/10.5271/sjweh.3754

Hoy D, Geere JA, Davatchi F et al (2014) A time for action: opportunities for preventing the growing burden and disability from musculoskeletal conditions in low- and middle-income countries. Best Pract Res Clin Rheumatol 28(3):377–393. https://doi.org/10.1016/j.berh.2014.07.006

Hughes SL, Seymour RB, Campbell RT et al (2011) Comparison of two health-promotion programs for older workers. Am J Public Health 101(5):883–890. https://doi.org/10.2105/AJPH.2010.300082

Human Resources & Skills Development Canada (2011) National occupational classification career handbook. Government of Canada, Ottawa

Hurwitz EL, Randhawa K, Torres P et al (2018) The Global Spine Care Initiative: a systematic review of individual and community-based burden of spinal disorders in rural populations in low- and middle-income communities. Eur Spine J 27(Suppl 6):802–815. https://doi.org/10.1007/s00586-017-5393-z

Institute for Work & Health (2008) Seven 'principles' for successful return to work. Institute for Work & Health, Toronto

Institute for Work & Health (2017) Seven "principles" used in return-to-work policies and practices. IWH case impact study. Available via https://www.iwh.on.ca/impact-case-studies/seven-principles-guidelines-used-in-return-to-work-policies-and-practices. Accessed 10 Oct 2018

Irvin E, Van Eerd D, Amick BC et al (2010) Introduction to special section: systematic reviews for prevention and management of musculoskeletal disorders. J Occup Rehabil 20(2):123–126

Johnson CD, Haldeman S, Chou R et al (2018) The Global Spine Care Initiative: model of care and implementation. Eur Spine J 27(Suppl 6):925–945. https://doi.org/10.1007/s00586-018-5720-z

Koolhaas W, Groothoff JW, de Boer MR et al (2015) Effectiveness of a problem-solving based intervention to prolong the working life of ageing workers. BMC Public Health 15:76. https://doi.org/10.1186/s12889-015-1410-5

Korshoj M, Jorgensen MB, Hallman DM et al (2018) Prolonged sitting at work is associated with a favorable time course of low-back pain among blue-collar workers: a prospective study in the DPhacto cohort. Scand J Work Environ Health 44:530–538

Kristensen TS (2005) Intervention studies in occupational epidemiology. Occup Environ Med 62:205–210

Laisne F, Lecomte C, Corbiere M (2012) Biopsychosocial predictors of prognosis in musculoskeletal disorders: a systematic review of the literature. Disabil Rehabil 34:355–382

Le P, Marras WS (2016) Evaluating the low back biomechanics of three different office workstations: seated, standing, and perching. Appl Ergon 56:170–178

Loisel P, Gosselin L, Durand P et al (2001) Implementation of a participatory ergonomics program in the rehabilitation of workers suffering from subacute back pain. Appl Ergon 32(1):53–60

MacEachen E, Clarke J, Franche RL et al (2006) Systematic review of the qualitative literature on return to work after injury. Scand J Work Environ Health 32:257–269

Makkonen M, Silvennoinen M, Nousiainen T (2017) To sit or to stand, that is the question: examining the effects of work posture change on the well-being at work of software professionals. Int J Networking Virtual Organ 17:371–391

Martel L, Malenfant EC, Morency JD et al (2012) Projected trends to 2031 for the Canadian labour force. Statistics Canada, Ottawa. Available via: http://www.statcan.gc.ca/pub/11-010-x/2011008/part-partie3-eng.htm. Accessed 22 Nov 2018

McMaster University (2016) Resources for evidence-based practice: the 6S pyramid. http://hsl.mcmaster.libguides.com/ebm. Accessed 10 Oct 2018

Monteiro MS, Alexandre NMC, Ilmarinen J et al (2009) Work ability and musculoskeletal disorders among workers from a public health institution. Int J Occup Saf Ergon 15(3):319–324

Murad MH, Asi N, Alsawas M et al (2016) New evidence pyramid. Evid Based Med 21(4):125–127

National Research Council (2001) Musculoskeletal disorders in the workplace: low back and upper extremities. National Academic Press, Washington, DC

Neumann WP, Eklund J, Hansson B et al (2010) Effect assessment in work environment interventions: a methodological reflection. Ergonomics 53(1):130–137. https://doi.org/10.1080/00140130903349914

Palmer KT, Harris EC, Linaker C (2012) Effectiveness of community- and workplace-based interventions to manage musculoskeletal-related sickness absence and job loss: a systematic review. Rheumatology (Oxford) 51(2):230–242

Pitt-Catsouphes M, James JB, Matz-Costa C (2015) Workplace-based health and wellness programs: the intersection of aging, work, and health. Gerontologist 55(2):262–270. https://doi.org/10.1093/geront/gnu114

Pransky GS, Benjamin KL, Savageau JA et al (2005) Outcomes in work-related injuries: a comparison of older and younger workers. Am J Ind Med 47(2):104–112

Riethmeister V, Brouwer S, van der Klink J et al (2016) Work, eat and sleep: towards a healthy ageing at work program offshore. BMC Public Health 16(1):134

Rivilis I, Van Eerd D, Cullen K et al (2008) Effectiveness of participatory ergonomic interventions on health outcomes: a systematic review. Appl Ergon 39(3):342–358

Sackett DL, Rosenberg WM, Gray JA et al (1996) Evidence based medicine: what it is and what it isn't. BMJ 312(7023):71

Schneider E, Irastorza X (2010) OSH in figures: work-related musculoskeletal disorders in the EU – facts and figures. European Agency for Safety and Health at Work (EU-OSHA), Luxembourg

Settersten RA, Mayer KU (1997) The measurement of age, age structuring, and the life course. Annu Rev Sociol 23:233–261

Silverstein B, Evanoff B (2011) Musculoskeletal disorders. In: Levy BS, Wegman DH, Baron SL et al (eds) Occupational and environmental health: recognizing and preventing disease and injury. Oxford University Press, New York, pp 335–365

Smith PM, Berecki-Gisolf J (2014) Age, occupational demands and the risk of serious work injury. Occup Med 64(8):571–576. https://doi.org/10.1093/occmed/kqu125

Smith PM, Bielecky A, Mustard CA et al (2013) The relationship between age and work injury in British Columbia: examining differences across time and nature of injury. J Occup Health 55(2):98–107

Smith P, Chen C, Mustard C et al (2014a) Examining the relationship between chronic conditions, multi-morbidity and labour market participation in Canada: 2000 to 2005. Ageing Soc 34(10):1730–1748

Smith P, Bielecky A, Ibrahim S et al (2014b) Impact of pre-existing chronic conditions on age differences in sickness absence after a musculoskeletal work injury: a path analysis approach. Scand J Work Environ Health 40(2):167–175. https://doi.org/10.5271/sjweh.3397

Smith P, Bielecky A, Ibrahim S et al (2014c) How much do pre-existing chronic conditions contribute to age differences in health care expenditures following a work-related musculoskeletal injury? Med Care 52:71–77

Smith P, Ma H, Gilbert-Ouimet M et al (2018) The relationship between occupational standing and sitting and incident heart disease over a 12-year period in Ontario, Canada. Am J Epidemiol 187(1):27–33

Statistics Canada (2010) Estimates of population, by age group and sex for July 1, Canada, provinces and territories, annual (CANSIM Table 051-0001). Statistics Canada, Ottawa

Stedmon AW, Howells H, Wilson JR et al (2012) Ergonomics/human factors needs of an ageing workforce in the manufacturing sector. Health Promot Perspect 2(2):112–125

Sterns HL, Doverspike D (1989) Aging and the retraining and learning process in organisations. In: Goldstein I, Katze R (eds) Training and development in work organizations. Jossey-Bass, San Francisco, pp 299–332

Strazdins L, Bammer G (2004) Women, work and musculoskeletal health. Soc Sci Med 58:997–1005

Tornqvist EW, Hagberg M, Hagman M et al (2009) The influence of working conditions and individual factors on the incidence of neck and upper limb symptoms among professional computer users. Int Arch Occup Environ Health 82(6):689–702

UN (2012) Ageing in the twenty-first century: a celebration and a challenge. United Nations Population Fund (UNFPA)/HelpAge International, New York/London

Van Eerd D, Cole DC, Steenstra IA (2016) Chapter 16: participatory ergonomics for return to work. In: Schultz IZ, Gatchel RJ (eds) Handbook of return to work: from research to practice. Springer, New York, pp 289–305

van Vilsteren M, van Oostrom SH, de Vet HC et al (2015) Workplace interventions to prevent work disability in workers on sick leave. Cochrane Database Syst Rev (10):CD006955

Vargas-Prada S, Demou E, Lalloo D et al (2016) Effectiveness of very early workplace interventions to reduce sickness absence: a systematic review of the literature and meta-analysis. Scand J Work Environ Health 42(4):261–272

Verkerk K, Luijsterburg PA, Miedema HS et al (2012) Prognostic factors for recovery in chronic nonspecific low back pain: a systematic review. Phys Ther 92(9):1093–1108

Vogel N, Schandelmaier S, Zumbrunn T et al (2017) Return-to-work coordination programmes for improving return to work in workers on sick leave. Cochrane Database Syst Rev (3):CD011618

Vos T, Flaxman AD, Naghavi M et al (2012) Years lived with disability (YLDs) for 1160 sequelae of 289 diseases and injuries 1990-2010: a systematic analysis for the Global Burden of Disease Study 2010. Lancet 380(9859):2163–2196

Wells R, Van Eerd D, Hagg G (2004) Mechanical exposure concepts using force as the agent. Scand J Work Environ Health 30(3):179–190

Whalin C, Ekberg K, Persson J et al (2013) Evaluation of self-reported work ability and usefulness of interventions among sick-listed patients. J Occup Rehabil 23(1):32–43

Williams-Whitt K, Bültmann U, Amick B 3rd et al (2016) Workplace interventions to prevent disability from both the scientific and practice perspectives: a comparison of scientific literature, grey literature and stakeholder observations. J Occup Rehabil 26(4):417–433

Workers Compensation Board of Manitoba (2014) Manitoba workplace injury and illness statistics 2000–2013. Workers Compensation Board of Manitoba, Winnipeg. Available from http://www.wcb.mb.ca/sites/default/files/resources/annualInjurystats2000_2013%20v3.1.pdf

Workers Compensation Board of Nova Scotia (2013) Workers' Compensation Board of Nova Scotia 2013 Annual Report. Workers' Compensation Board of Nova Scotia, Halifax

Workplace Safety and Insurance Board (WSIB) (2013) By the numbers: 2013 WSIB statistical report (schedule 1). Workplace Safety and Insurance Board (WSIB), Toronto

WorkSafeBC (2013) WorkSafeBC 2013 statistics. Vancouver: WorkSafeBC

World Health Organisation (2003) Preventing musculoskeletal disorders in the workplace. In: Protecting workers' health series. World Health Organisation, Geneva

World Health Organization (2015) World report on ageing and health WHO press. World Health Organization, Geneva

Addictive Disorders: Problems and Interventions at Workplace

28

Clemens Veltrup and Ulrich John

Contents

Introduction	506
Diagnosis and Detection	506
Diagnosis	506
Detection	507
Epidemiology	509
Epidemiologic Data	509
Risk Factors	510
Interventions	511
Workplace Interventions	511
Other Interventions with Relevance for Working Life	515
Conclusions	520
Cross-References	520
References	521

Abstract

Addictive disorders may cause severe problems at work. Among them, alcohol intoxication and alcohol dependence are the most important ones. Organizational, social, and individual risk factors may contribute to addictive disorders. The consequences of harmful substance use for work are mental and physical in kind, but substance misuse may also contribute to job loss. Workplace interventions may help to cope with addictive behavior. They include (1) psychosocial interventions concerning substance use problems, (2) substance-use related brief interventions, (3) peer-supported interventions, (4) web-based interventions, (5) mandatory screening, and (6) general health promotion programs. Acute

C. Veltrup
Fachklinik Freudenholm Ruhleben, Ploen, Germany
e-mail: veltrup.clemens@fachklinik-freudenholm-ruhleben.de

U. John (✉)
University Medicine Greifswald, Institute of Community Medicine, Greifswald, Germany
e-mail: ulrich.john@med.uni-greifswald.de

© Springer Nature Switzerland AG 2020
U. Bültmann, J. Siegrist (eds.), *Handbook of Disability, Work and Health*, Handbook Series in Occupational Health Sciences, https://doi.org/10.1007/978-3-030-24334-0_28

and postacute treatment programs support individuals in regaining the ability to work or to find a new job.

> **Keywords**
>
> Addictive disorders · Risk · Work · Rehabilitation

Introduction

Work environments may add to the protection of employees against addictive disorders and may help to cope with problems of addiction. But working life may also bear risks of addictive disorders. These include loss of productivity, disciplinary problems, accidents, and criminal behavior at the workplace (Anderson 2012).

According to Marlatt and Witkiewitz (2010), more than 70% of current illicit drug users and heavy drinkers belong to the workforce. However, addictive behavior increases the risk of unemployment. Data from Germany revealed that 45.4% of the patients suffering from alcohol dependency and 77.1% of the drug-dependent patients in rehabilitation programs were unemployed (Fachverband Sucht 2017). In this chapter, we explain the diagnosis and detection of substance use disorders and present epidemiological data as well as risk factors that explain the development of such disorders. Furthermore, we introduce interventions in work environments and other interventions that seem to be relevant for working life and may help people to become or stay sober. This contribution is limited to alcohol and drugs and does not include nicotine consumption.

Diagnosis and Detection

Diagnosis

Addictive disorders include problematic substance use and nonsubstance addictive disorders such as gaming disorders. Problematic substance use includes at-risk use and substance use disorders (SUD). Substances are alcohol, nicotine, and other psychotropic drugs such as cannabis, cocaine, or opiates. These substances have in common that they may change the mood of the consumer. Alcohol at-risk drinking is defined as consuming alcohol in such a quantity, frequency, and binging that an increased risk of disease, social, psychological, or other consequences may arise. Recent research has shown that even amounts of drinking less than 12 g pure alcohol per day among women and less than 24 g pure alcohol per day among men may add to developing severe diseases such as cancer. One conclusion is that abstaining from alcohol is the best way to prevent oneself from cancer compared to any alcohol consumption (Scoccianti et al. 2015). Guidelines for low risk drinking differ by country. According to other substances such as nicotine or drugs, any consumption may be a risk of health.

Impaired Control	Use of the substance for longer periods of time than intended or using larger amounts than intended
	Wanting to reduce use, yet being unsuccessful doing so
	Spending time getting or using the drug or recovering from its use
	Craving for the substance
Social Impairment	Continued use of the substance despite problems with work, school or family/social obligations
	Continuing to use despite having interpersonal or social problems because of the substance use
	Important and meaningful social and recreational activities may be given up or reduced because of substance use
Risky Use	Repeated use of the substances in physically dangerous situations
	Continuing to use substance despite being aware it is causing or worsening physical and psychological problems
Pharmacological Indicators	Development of tolerance
	Development of withdrawal symptoms

Fig. 1 Criteria for substance use disorders (DSM-V; American Psychiatric Association 2013)

SUD are classified according to two classification systems, the International Classification of Diseases and Related Health Problems in its current version ICD-10 (World Health Organization 1992), its upcoming version ICD-11 (World Health Organization 2016), and the Diagnostic and Statistical Manual of the American Psychiatric Association (DSM-5; American Psychiatric Association 2013). The ICD-10 includes acute intoxication, harmful use, dependence, and withdrawal state as the central mental and behavioral disorders due to psychoactive substance use. The ICD-11 includes diagnostic criteria due to substance use or addictive behaviors: intoxication, single episode of harmful substance use, harmful patterns of substance use, dependence, and withdrawal. Hazardous use increases the risk of harmful consequences for the user. ICD 11 differentiates degrees of, while according to ICD-10 harmful use is causing damage to physical or mental health. For the diagnosis of dependence, three out of six criteria must have been fulfilled in the last 12 months: (a) craving, (b) difficulties in controlling substance use behavior, (c) physiological withdrawal state (d) evidence of tolerance, (e) increasing neglect of pleasures or interests because of psychoactive substance use, (f) persisting substance use despite clear evidence of harmful consequences. According to DSM-5, substance use disorders are categorized into mild, moderate, and severe. Two or three among 11 symptoms indicate a mild, four or five symptoms moderate, and six or more symptoms severe substance use disorder. The criteria belong to four problem areas: impaired control, social impairment, risky substance use, and pharmacological indicators (Fig. 1).

Detection

Typical symptoms of addictive disorders at work include absenteeism, work performance, behavior change, and signs of intoxication (Soyka 2017) (Fig. 2).

One promising way to detect SUD is to use systematic screening. Screening questionnaires provide information on the existence and severity of any substance

Absenteeism	Increasing frequency of single days not at work
	Absenteeism during work-time
	Notificaton of sickness by significant others
	Arriving too late at work
	Retroactively application for vacation
Performance	Instable working results
	Attention deficits
	Loss of concentration
	Unreliability
Behavior Change	Severe mood changes
	Inadequate irritated, nervous, sociable
	Aggressive behavior,
	Submissive behavior
	Neglect of personal hygiene
Signs of intoxication	Foetor and attempt to hide foetor
	Slurred speech
	Change of pupils (narrowed or expanded)
Withdrawal symptoms	Nausea
	Hands shaking
	Sweat outbreak
	Reddened face
	Attempt to hide signs of withdrawal
Consequences	Loss of driving license for more than three months
	Liabilities

Fig. 2 Work-related symptoms of problematic substance use

problem as well as on the necessity of treatment. The questionnaires may be filled in by the individual without assistance. The Alcohol Use Disorder Identification Test (AUDIT, Reinert and Allen 2007) includes 10 items. It informs on current quantity and frequency of alcohol drinking, on binge drinking, and on typical consequences of increased alcohol drinking. The Cannabis Use Disorder Identification Test (Adamson and Sellman 2003) works in a similar manner. One limitation of these self-statement instruments is that they are open to reporting bias. This raises the question whether laboratory parameters measured in blood samples or other body fluids might overcome the limitation.

Hermansson et al. (2000) examined a sample of workers in the transport sector of Sweden over 16 months. They asked employees who used the routine health service in a company to answer the AUDIT. In addition, blood samples were taken to provide alcohol-related laboratory parameters: carbohydrate-deficient transferrin (CDT) and gamma-glutamyl-transferase (GGT). Among the 570 study participants, 105 (18.4%) screened positive according to AUDIT or CDT, or both. If GGT was added, the proportion of positive screening results was 22.0%. Laboratory parameters may detect employees with SUD in addition to self-statement instruments and may inform about probable SUD as it is known that individuals tend to underreport alcohol consumption. However, laboratory parameters have their own limitations such as being cost intensive and time consuming. Above that, if screening information is needed for further counseling, it is not of primary interest whether the information disclosed by the individual is valid or not. Instead, the self-statements are used to get into contact for the purpose of counseling. For counseling it is crucial what the individual is open to present.

Epidemiology

Epidemiologic Data

According to survey data from European countries, 3.4% of the adult population suffered from an alcohol dependence in the last 12 months (Wittchen et al. 2011).

Alcohol use disorders hold rank three on the "Disability Adjusted Life Year" (DALY) rate per 10,000 persons. The rate is 17.2 for women and 82.8 for men (Wittchen et al. 2011). In Germany more than 70,000 persons die per year because of alcohol-related disorders (John and Hanke 2002). This adds to the loss of about 900,000 life years and 285,000 years of employment. Rehm et al. (2009) pointed out that alcohol-related disorders are the most important cause for DALies among men. The typical diseases for men and women are neuropsychiatric disorders, alcohol-induced accidents or injuries, and cardiovascular diseases (Rehm et al. 2006, 2009). The peak age of alcohol-related death is in the age of peak performance at work, particularly the age between 45 and 64 years (Rehm et al. 2006).

Alcohol consumption, intoxication, and dependence in the workforce are more prevalent than use, intoxication, or dependence of any illicit drugs (Frone 2013). Occupations with the highest alcohol-related death rates were found to be bar staff, seafarers, and publicans and people who work in catering, entertainment and construction industries or in the medical field (Anderson 2012; Hemmingsson et al. 1997). While male medical practitioners were among the occupations with the highest alcohol-related mortality in the England and Wales in the 1960s to 1980s, they were among the occupations with the lowest alcohol-related mortality in 2001 to 2005 (Romeri et al. 2007). Ennenbach and Soyka (2007) showed that 26% of the employees of a medical rehabilitation center disclosed problematic alcohol consumption levels according to the AUDIT. Rosta (2008) examined a sample of German physicians working in hospitals. Among the physicians who consumed alcohol during the past year, there were 9.5% abstainers. Binge drinking (five or more drinks per occasion) once a month was reported by 10.7%; 2.7% did so weekly, and 0.1% daily or almost daily.

Data from a telephone survey of a random sample of 2805 employed adults in the United States of America revealed that workplace alcohol use and impairment directly affected 15% of the workforce (19.2 million workers). An estimated 1.8% (2.3 million workers) drank alcohol before work, and 7.1% (8.9 million workers) drank during the workday (Frone 2006). Frone (2013) points out that more than 90% of the workforce did not drink any alcohol before or during the workday. However, about 5% of workers may have an alcohol use disorder (during the last 12 months). About 2% of the workforce in the United States reported illicit drug use or impairment at work one or more days per week. Illicit drug use disorders, mainly marihuana use disorders, were found in 2.5%.

Alcohol problems may cause absenteeism (not coming to work) due to hangovers or disease following from alcohol consumption (Bacharach et al. 2010).

Further studies show that social norms concerning substance use at the workplace combined with other work-related factors such as job stress or work group cohesion may add to the consumption of psychoactive substances (Bennett et al. 2004). Problem drinkers seem to be more likely to be aware of the availability of alcohol than those who drink at lower risk (Berger 2009). In a study of 6000 workers of one plant, those who estimated that co-workers consumed alcohol frequently and in high amounts also reported more drinking themselves than workers who believed that their co-workers drank infrequently. The perception of alcohol consumption of co-workers turned out to be a strong correlate of workplace drinking (Ames and Grube 1999).

Three groups of workers turned out to be more likely than others to abuse substances or to be dependent of these: young men and women in high-risk occupations and young men in low-risk occupations. They represent around 5% of the overall workforce (Frone 2013). But selection processes should be considered in regards of these findings. Workers at higher age might have lost their workplace, suffered from severe disease, or even might have lost their lives due to substance use. Addictive behavior increases the risk of job loss, whereas job loss may add to worsen addictive behavior.

Three work place characteristics might add to substance use at work places: (1) the availability of psychotropic substances at work, (2) social norms that favor or tolerate substance use and the compliance to these norms at the work place, and (3) tolerance of psychoactive substance use during working time by colleagues and supervisors (Anderson 2012).

The consequences of substance use for work-related issues may be: (1) substance related mental and physical abnormalities which reduce the working capacity, i.e., poor attendance, poor work performance, and job injuries (Frone 2013), and (2) severe consequences because of substance misuse or abuse. Furthermore, working under the influence of a substance (intoxication) adds to impairment which is relevant for work safety, as Rummel et al. (2004) showed for alcohol (Fig. 3).

Risk Factors

The bio-psychosocial model of addiction demonstrates the complexity and the interdependence between different factors for the development of an addiction. No single factor may explain addiction (John 2015), rather many aspects act together. Bode et al. (2017) distinguish between organizational, social, and individual risk factors for the development of mental disorders. Organizational risks include qualitative or quantitative over- or under-demands, physically heavy work, multitasking, or low responsibility. Social risk factors include social conflicts in the workplace ("bullying"), conflicts with customers, and high emotional demands. Individual risk factors include professional gratification crises (Siegrist 1996), a level of expenditure of the

Blood alcohol concentration (Promille)	Consequences in Work
> 0.2	Disturbances of equilibrium system
> 0.3	Attention disorder, reduction of concentration, ability to perceive moving objects disturbed
> 0.4	Prolongation of reaction time
> 0.5	Increase of risk-taking behavior, misjudgement of speed, reduction of hearing performance
> 0.8	Increase of disinhibition and of limitation of perception, reduction of visual field, reduction of control of movement, increase of reaction time
> 1.0	Severe symptoms concerning attention disorder, misjudgement, reduction of oral and visual perception, reduction of reaction time
> 2.0	Blackout
> 3.0	Severe intoxication, coma

Fig. 3 Consequences of alcohol intoxication for work (according to Rummel et al. 2004)

employee that does not lead to sufficient approval. Also, low self-efficacy, the expectation of the employee to succeed in fulfilling job demands, may increase the risk of a mental disorder. The risk factors become significant if inadequate compensatory components and lack of protective factors disable the employee to reach own goals.

Psychological and social conditions may add to problematic substance use. In a sample of US workers (N = 2790), work overload and job insecurity were found to be associated with alcohol and illicit drug use among employees before, during, and after work (Frone 2008). But also social conflicts or the use of alcohol for the improvement of social relationships among employees may induce problematic consumption of alcohol. Psychological problems at work such as burnout may also add to substance use. Honkonen et al. (2006) among 3276 employees (1637 women and 1639 men aged 30–64 years) of a general population sample found that the prevalence of current alcohol dependence was associated with burnout both among men and women.

There is large evidence for work stress and addictive behavior being correlates (Frone 1999; Cooper et al. 1990). Quantitative and qualitative demands may lead to job dissatisfaction or feelings of job insecurity but also to problems of combining work and family roles.

Interventions

Workplace Interventions

Workplaces are a suited setting for the prevention of SUD. Co-workers, supervisors, or employers may notice early signs of SUD and motivate the employee to request treatment or counseling for addictive behavior (Roman and Blum 2002). Intervention programs either focus on addressing behavior change directly or apply via change of environments or rules (Veltrup 2011). Different workplace interventions exist: first, psychosocial interventions concerning substance use problems, second, substance use related brief interventions, third, peer supported interventions for substance abusers, fourth, web-based interventions for workers with a problematic substance use, fifth, mandatory screening, and sixth, general health promotion programs including substance-related modules.

A systematic review of workplace interventions for alcohol-related problems (Webb et al. 2009) found 10 intervention studies: 5 psychosocial interventions, 4 brief intervention (mail, feedback) studies, and one peer support program.

Psychosocial interventions include psychosocial skills training (team building, stress management), brief intervention with feedback to self-reports of drinking, lifestyle factors and general health checks (e.g., smoking, diet, weight, blood pressure), and alcohol education via Internet. The counseling-based interventions either had no (Hermansson et al. 1998) or small effects (Bennett et al. 2004). In one study employees were randomly assigned to either (1) an 8h training for psychosocial skills ("Team Awareness" program), (2) an informational training (4 h), or no intervention (Bennett et al. 2004). The "Team Awareness" program illustrated how to deal with problems, and participants learned alternative ways to improve social relationships instead of drinking alcohol. The employees received information about the guidelines on how to deal with alcohol at work, about an employee assistance program, and drug testing. Both intervention groups reported reduced problem drinking, whereas the control group did not show any changes in problem drinking.

The "Team Awareness" program was adapted to the use with young restaurant workers, and a modified intervention ("Team Resilience") was offered in three 2h sessions (Bennett et al. 2010). Participants learned how to stimulate social support, personal confidence, coping, and stress management. A first study among 124 workers aged 16 to 34 years found increased awareness of alcohol and other drug risks, increased help seeking, and increased personal resilience. The second study was a randomized controlled trial including 235 employees of 28 stores from a restaurant chain. The employees in these stores reported larger decreases in heavy drinking and workrelated problems with alcohol than workers in control stores who did not receive the intervention (Broome and Bennett 2011).

Another psychosocial intervention study (Hermansson et al. 2010) found that out of 990 employees from a transport company (68% men) who volunteered for an alcohol screening, 194 (20%) had positive results of the AUDIT (Babor et al. 1989) or CDT testing. Among them, 158 subjects attended a follow-up session after 12 months. The positive screening results had been decreased. At baseline, 51% were positive according to the AUDIT and 58% according to CDT, at follow-up 23% by the AUDIT and 34% by CDT. These reductions were statistically significant, and they were independent of whether the individuals had taken part in a brief intervention or comprehensive intervention or whether they were in the control group. There may have been an effect of the alcohol screening.

Cook et al. (2003, 2004) evaluated health promotion programs with or without substance abuse prevention. In a first study (Cook et al. 2003) they showed that workers of an insurance company who participated in stress management sessions decreased their alcohol consumption. In a second study (Cook et al. 2004)

374 construction workers participated in a health promotion program with substance abuse prevention. The data revealed that the intervention group increased their intention to reduce alcohol drinking.

Because of the high proportion of problematic alcohol drinking among the employees of a medical rehabilitation center (Ennenbach and Soyka 2007), a prevention program was established that showed to be effective (Ennenbach et al. 2009).

The brief intervention studies (Anderson and Larimer 2002; Richmond et al. 2000; Matano et al. 2007; Walters and Woodall 2003) showed a small positive effect on the drinking behavior according to Webb et al. (2009). Anderson and Larimer (2002) used a sample of 155 employees of a food and retail service company who were randomly assigned to either a nontreatment control group or a brief alcohol abuse prevention program featuring personal feedback, alcohol education, and training of skills (e.g., refusing alcohol). Female problem drinkers who had received the intervention were more likely than females in the control group to reduce alcohol-related negative consequences at 6 month follow-up. Another brief intervention was conducted among 48 employees at a manufacturing company (Walters and Woodall 2003). Alcohol consumers received mailed feedback on their drinking. The participants significantly decreased their alcohol consumption after having received the feedback. Other data of a brief intervention ("Workscreen") among 1206 post office employees in Sydney, Australia, revealed that women in the intervention group significantly reduced their number of alcoholic drinks during the 10month followup time, however men did not (Richmond et al. 2000).

One study used trends of injuries as an outcome measure to describe the influence of peer-focused substance abuse program in the transportation industry. The program focused on changing workplace attitudes towards on-the-job substance use in addition to training workers to recognize colleagues who have a problem and intervene among them. There was an estimated US $ 1850 reduction of the employer's injury costs per employee, corresponding to a benefit–cost ratio of 26:1.

Several web-based interventions focus on alcohol use (Balhara and Verma 2014). Doumas and Hannah (2008) evaluated the efficacy of a webbased personalized feedback program delivered at workplace to 124 adults aged 18–24 years. Participants were randomly assigned to either receive webbased feedback, webbased feedback plus a 15min motivational interviewing session, or to a control group without intervention. Participants who had received an intervention reported significantly less alcohol consumption than those in the control group at the 30 days followup. Participants who had been classified as high risk drinkers (binge drinking once or more often during the previous 2 weeks at the initial assessment) reported the largest decreases in drinking between initial assessment and the 30days followup assessment. No differences were found between the two intervention groups, indicating that the addition of a 15min motivational interviewing session did not increase the efficacy of the webbased feedback program.

The U.S. Department of Defense evaluated a webbased alcohol intervention ("Drinker's Check-Up") using a sample of 3070 individuals from military staff. Follow-up information was provided by 1072 participants 1 month and by 532 participants 6 months after baseline. At 1-month follow-up significant reductions of the mean number of drinks consumed per occasion, of frequent heavy episodic drinking, and of peak blood alcohol concentration were found. The reductions in alcohol use were still present 6 months after baseline (Pemberton et al. 2011).

In a study of Billings et al. (2008), 309 workers from a technology firm were randomly assigned to either a web-based intervention program on stress and mood management or to a waitlist control condition. After 3 months, in contrast to control subjects, intervention program participants reported reductions in drug and alcohol use to manage stress. Another positive intervention result is reported by Hester et al. (2009). They recruited alcohol-dependent workers through advertisement and randomly assigned the study participants to different Internetbased programs. All participants significantly reduced their drinking as well as alcohol-related problems.

One simple intervention approach is to advise car drivers to use drug and alcohol testing before driving a car in work settings. This might help to reduce accidents. The evidence in this field is still insufficient (Cashman et al. 2009).

Action to reduce alcohol consumption may be embedded in more general health promotion programs. Such programs focus on lifestyle changes including health behavior change rather than specific disease. Such programs have shown higher acceptance, higher participation, and higher success than programs that are more punitive in character (Sieck and Heirich 2010). However, the evidence for the impact of health promotion programs in work environments is limited. Kuoppala et al. (2008) identified 46 studies. The findings suggest that workplace health promotion could improve work ability but does not decrease sickness absence, and overall, no impact on mental or physical well-being could be shown. Exercise programs were effective in increasing well-being, but education and psychological methods were not. Only few effects on presenteeism were found in workplace health promotion programs using different intervention approaches (Cancelliere et al. 2011).

The findings so far suggest that the reductions in alcohol consumption found in single studies seem promising to further reduce alcohol and other substance use problems at the workplace. This is in accordance with recommendations of Anderson (2012). In addition to initiatives that promote well-being at work, including management and leadership styles, increasing alcohol-free workplaces may help to reduce substance use problems in the work field (Anderson 2012). There should also be regular proof of staying free from alcohol, drugs, sedatives, and other psychotropic substances. Companies should have a detailed agreement about how to deal with employees who suffer from SUD. Such action may be expected to result in reductions of alcohol-related workplace accidents and injuries, as well as in an increase of a culture of more healthy relationships. Three target groups should be in the focus according to Anderson (2012): those working in the retail alcohol trade, blue collar workers in the construction industry, seafarers, and dockers. Particularly young men suffer from unemployment and risk drinking. The middle-aged workers and employees have the highest rates of alcohol-related disability.

Other Interventions with Relevance for Working Life

One focus of interventions should be to motivate employees to reduce substance use and cope with SUD by utilizing adequate treatment. Contracts between the management and the work council help to convince laborers with substance use problems to request support. The agreement should include different options to change and stepped care. Stepped care delivers brief intervention at low cost such as one web-based intervention first. Only in case of insufficient success more intervention is provided. It follows a psychosocial approach and includes counseling and brief interventions to motivate the individual to change behavior as well as different employment-related measures. A warning of job loss should be included. The employee who takes part in treatment is offered the opportunity to return to work. The intervention process begins when a worker or employee arrives intoxicated on her/his workplace or is in conflict with the rules of the company concerning substance use. The principle of "constructive pressure" is generally applied, providing a system of assistance and employment. It should exist with written rules and be transparent to every worker in the company. In most cases, the supervisor approaches the employee if she/he suspects signs of SUD. The employee will be recommended to seek treatment from a family doctor or an outpatient addiction counseling center and, if necessary, is also requested to consult the company physician or company addiction nurse. In case of another conspicuousness, the Human Resources Department as well as the Employee Representatives will be asked to take part in the interview and a request to seek treatment will be accompanied by a reminder or warning. If the employee does not comply with the urgent recommendation and is intoxicated again or shows clear withdrawal symptoms at the workplace, a dismissal can also be issued. In Germany, the national guideline for alcohol use disorders in working life (Mann et al. 2015) includes a 3-step approach: (1) brief intervention, (2) acute treatment (detoxification treatment), and (3) postacute treatment to overcome SUD. These approaches also are successful in case of other problematic substance use.

Brief Interventions

Brief interventions may be provided by psychologists, physicians, social workers, or psychotherapists. Available data suggest that brief interventions are effective in reducing alcohol consumption both in men and women (Kaner et al. 2018). Evidence-based strategies include interventions based on motivational interviewing (MI) (Miller and Rollnick 2012). Brief intervention is based on six elements (Miller and Sanchez 1994): provide Feedback on personal risks, emphasize the importance of taking personal Responsibility for changing one's behavior, give Advice to change, provide a Menu of options for change, support with Empathy, and increase Self-efficacy to make such a change successful (FRAMES). Core techniques of MI are: Open questions, Affirmation, Reflective listening, and Summarizing (OARS). Clients become able to decide for themselves and to solve their conflict between urges for the substance on the one hand side and aversion against it on the other hand side. MI is evidence-based and has been shown to be effective in helping people to change their behavior. Brief intervention has been proven to be effective particularly in medical settings (Babor et al. 2007; Kaner et al. 2018). It helps to easily support patients in medical practices, general or psychiatric hospitals to look for adequate help (John et al. 2003). It is helpful to use screening instruments for entering change talk according to problematic substance use.

Acute Treatment

Among patients with mental health disorders related to problematic substance use (excluding tobacco), there are five times more unemployed than employed, and unemployed people spend more days staying inpatient in hospitals than employed (Zoike and König 2006). Unemployment seems to add to risky patterns of alcohol consumption (Dee 2001).

In German treatment programs for dependent patients in psychiatric hospitals 92,575 were treated in addiction psychiatric competence centers in the year 2016 (Destatis 2016). In contrast, 322,608 patients, including 234,785 men, were treated in general or psychiatric hospitals because of alcohol problems in the year 2016 (Destatis 2016). In many cases, alcohol-attributable disease other than alcohol dependence was treated.

As part of the withdrawal treatment in addition to the medical treatment of intoxication and withdrawal symptoms, psycho- and socio-therapeutic intervention elements are provided to promote readiness and ability to change. This includes the motivation to use further (postacute) interventions, such as medical rehabilitation or participation in self-help groups. Withdrawal treatment may support the acceptance of further help. In order to improve health care utilization, it is possible to begin postacute inpatient rehabilitation directly after acute treatment.

Postacute Treatment

Postacute treatments can be further inpatient or outpatient psychiatric and psycho-therapeutic treatment, addiction treatment, and in addition participation in self-help groups. In Germany, medical rehabilitation is provided for addicted patients in a routine program. Its purpose is to restore the patient's ability to work. The inpatient treatments last up to 15 weeks for alcohol dependence and up to 6 months for drug dependence. The outpatient medical rehabilitation includes a treatment period of 12 to 18 months with single and group therapy sessions. In addition, special rehabilitation programs combine outpatient and inpatient treatment phases. In Germany, almost 48,000 patients took part in these programs in 2016 (Die Drogenbeauftragte der Bundesrepublik Deutschland 2018) (Table 1).

The German Council of Addiction annually publishes the data of the users of medical rehabilitation (alcohol, medical drugs, illegal drugs) in different settings. Socio-demographic data are shown in Table 2 (Fachverband Sucht 2017).

The programs include single and group psychotherapeutic components for staying abstinent. In inpatient rehabilitation, evidence-based treatment modules have been developed. They include precise instructions on modules in which the

Table 1 Postacute treatment (medical rehabilitation) in Germany (2016)

	Inpatient rehabilitation program	Outpatient rehabilitation program
Alcohol dependence	28,252	10,438
Prescription drug dependence	649	151
Other drug dependence	15,402	2583

Table 2 Sociodemographic data of patients in rehabilitation in 2016 (Fachverband Sucht 2017)

	Men	Women	Age	Living with partner	Partnership	Own dwelling
Inpatient rehabilitation alcohol, prescription drugs N = 15,479	70.7%	29.3%	M = 46.1 SD = 11.6	23.6%	43.3%	86.3%
Inpatient rehabilitation illegal drugs N = 3411	79.1%	20.9%	M = 30.4 SD = 7.9	4.7%	32.0%	56.6%
Outpatient rehabilitation alcohol, all drugs N = 302	66.6%	33.4%	M = 47.0 SD = 11.2	32.6%	60.3%	–
Day hospital rehabilitation alcohol, all drugs N = 480	35.0%	65.0%	M = 45.4 SD = 10.1	26.2%	56.7%	–

M = mean; SD = standard deviation

patients have to take part. The treatment includes addiction-therapeutic elements, social work, interventions for the family, and measures to promote health (nutritional counseling, tobacco smoking cessation, exercise and sports therapy, training of occupational skills). Work-related interventions are of central importance. They are utilized by unemployed patients to a greater extent than by patients still in the workforce. Since 2013, many treatment facilities have made additional efforts to promote return to work, as it has been shown that a job may help to stay abstinent (Fachverband Sucht 2017).

The work-related program includes intra- and extramural trainings during inpatient rehabilitation and specific occupational and work-related groups as well as treatment options to promote social skills and stress management, topics that are of particular relevance for employment. The programs for employed persons are often similar to the first five sessions in the "return-to work" module by Lagerveld and Blonk (2017). It has shown to accelerate vocational reintegration (Dalgaard et al. 2017). Recordings of occupational biography and developing plans to return to work are part of this program.

In Table 3 the results of the medical rehabilitation concerning ability to work are shown. Most of the inpatient rehabilitees are able to work (without any health restrictions) directly after treatment. More than 75% have the capacity to work in

Table 3 Ability to work and capacity to work at discharge from medical rehabilitation (Fachverband Sucht 2017)

	Ability to work	Capacity to work in the former job	General capacity to work
Inpatient rehabilitation alcohol, prescription drugs	N = 13,587 69.6%	N = 13,424 76.7%	N = 13,387 82.5%
Inpatient rehabilitation illegal drugs	N = 3023 89.4%	N = 3009 89.3%	N = 3009 93.6%
Outpatient rehabilitation alcohol, all drugs	–	–	–
Day hospital rehabilitation alcohol, all drugs	–	–	N = 471 93.4%

Table 4 Change of employment during medical rehabilitation (Fachverband Sucht 2017)

	Work contract at admission	Work contract at discharge
Inpatient rehabilitation alcohol, prescription drugs	N = 15,098 38.3%	N = 15,042 37.0%
Inpatient rehabilitation illegal drugs	N = 3323 16.3%	N = 3275 13.6%
Outpatient rehabilitation alcohol, drugs	N = 299 67.6%	N = 295 68.1%
Day hospital rehabilitation alcohol, drugs	N = 465 49.9%	N = 463 50.1%

their former job for more than 6 h a day. General capacity to work means that the rehabilitees are able to work longer than 6 h a day (regardless of their former job).

Table 4 shows employment before and after medical rehabilitation. The proportion of unemployed patients is higher in inpatient than in outpatient treatment. Part of the inpatient rehabilitees with drug use disorders loses their job during treatment.

In medical addiction rehabilitation, annual follow-up postal surveys are conducted among former patients using questionnaires. The following data are from patients who terminated their rehabilitation in 2015 (Bachmeier et al. 2018; Fischer et al. 2018; Schneider et al. 2018; Lange et al. 2018). Rates of all former patients who sent their filled in questionnaires back (response rates) were between 33.9% and 66.9% depending on the setting (see Table 5). The rates of former patients with continuous abstinence since rehabilitation refer to the total number of rehabilitation patients and not just responders.

The importance of working life is demonstrated by abstinence among employed versus nonemployed patients of the inpatient rehabilitation program. During treatment the rate of patients who had a work contract increased from 46.6% at admission to 51.1% at discharge (Bachmeier et al. 2018). The follow-up survey data revealed that among employed patients, 46.9% of the responders remained abstinent 12 months after treatment discharge. Among patients who had been unemployed

Table 5 Abstinence in the first 12 months after medical rehabilitation (Fachverband Sucht 2017)

	Continuous abstinence (12 months)
Inpatient rehabilitation: Alcohol, medical drugs N = 10,230, response rate: 52.0%	2989 (29.2%)
Inpatient rehabilitation: Illegal drugs N = 1453, response rate: 33.9%	232 (16.0%)
Outpatient rehabilitation: Alcohol, medical drugs, illegal drugs N = 302, response rate: 66.9%	144 (47.7%)
Day hospital rehabilitation: Alcohol, medical drugs, illegal drugs N = 225, response rate: 55.1%	76 (33.8%)

at admission into rehabilitation, 30.8% of the responders, significantly less, remained abstinent 12 months after discharge (Bachmeier et al. 2018). The continuation of work after inpatient rehabilitation was associated with abstinence.

Among unemployed persons who found a job in the first year after treatment, 78.3% were abstinent for 12 months or sober after relapse for more than 30 days compared to 64.3% who remained unemployed (Bachmeier et al. 2018).

For addicts with special risks (high relapse risk according to the estimation of therapists, homelessness, unemployment) adaptation treatment, an additional rehabilitation module of 3 to 4 months duration may be provided after inpatient medical rehabilitation. Among 1265 participants in adaption treatment in the year 2016, 80.7% were men and 85.5% were unemployed. Unemployment had lasted 1 year or less in 15.2% of the unemployed, 1–3 years in 21.4%, 3–5 years in 17.1%, and six or more years before rehabilitation in 19.4%. The mean age of the unemployed patients was 36.9 years.

The rehabilitation follow-up data (Fabricius et al. 2018) show that 19.9% (n = 118) of the sample (N = 592) said that they were alcohol abstinent. Among the 194 rehabilitees who provided data at the beginning of the adaptation and the completion of the 12-month follow-up survey, the employment rate increased from 9.4% to 40.1%. This suggests that adaption treatment might be the only element in medical rehabilitation which helps patients to get a work contract after postacute treatment.

A program for coping with joblessness as a major problem for addicts has been used as a module in the community reinforcement program (CRA) since years: The "Job-Finding Club" (Azrin and Besalel 1980a, 1980b) is a psychosocial intervention conducted in a group. The techniques include mutual assistance among job-seekers, a "buddy" system, and family support. The program includes the training of practices such as searching want-ads, role-playing, phoning, motivating the job-seeker, constructing a résumé, and contacting friends. The program has been evaluated in a matched-control design. Within 2 months, 90% of the 60 job-seekers who had received counseling obtained employment, whereas only 55% of the job-seekers who had not received counseling obtained employment. The average starting salary

Group meetings	2 to 8 clients
	First two sessions: 3 hours each
	Subsequent sessions: 1 to 2 hours each
Elements and Strategies	Buddy system
	Building motivation and self-efficacy
	Strengthen family support
	"Job search as a full-time job " – Continuous job searching
	Widening variety of positions considered
	Advice for dress and hygiene
	Strategies for obtaining jobs
Methods	Discussion
	Role plays
	Training

Fig. 4 Elements of the Job-Finding Club (according to Azrin and Besalel 1980a, 1980b)

was about 30% higher for the counseled than for the noncounseled job-seekers. This program may be integrated into outpatient rehabilitation treatments for improving the likelihood to get a job and to improve social participation according the International Classification of International Classification of Functioning, Disability and Health (ICF, World Health Organization 2001) (Fig. 4).

Conclusions

A significant proportion of the workforce suffers from problematic substance use. Diagnostic tools to identify workers with SUD and effective psychosocial interventions to cope with problematic substance exist. Several small studies showed promising results concerning intervention effectiveness. However, systematic studies that include a variety of work settings are missing. In addition to single behavior change interventions, clear rules in work settings according to psychoactive substances help to reduce alcohol and drug consumption and related disorders at the workplace. Such rules should include regular proof of staying free of alcohol and drugs. Detailed regulations how to deal with employees who suffer from SUD should exist. Treatment of addicted persons is rather successful when focusing on the maintenance of abstinence. Adaption treatment may help to induce reemployment.

Cross-References

- ▶ Employment as a Key Rehabilitation Outcome
- ▶ Facilitating Competitive Employment for People with Disabilities
- ▶ Promoting Workplace Mental Wellbeing

References

Adamson SJ, Sellman JD (2003) A prototype screening instrument for cannabis use disorder: the Cannabis Use Disorders Identification Test (CUDIT) in an alcohol-dependent clinical sample. Drug Alcohol Rev 22:309–315

American Psychiatric Association (2013) Diagnostic and statistical manual of mental disorders, 5th edn. American Psychiatric Association, Arlington

Ames GM, Grube JW (1999) Alcohol availability and workplace drinking: mixed method analyses. J Stud Alcohol 60(3):383–393

Anderson P (2012) Alcohol and the workplace. Department of Health, Government of Catalonia, Barcelona

Anderson BK, Larimer ME (2002) Problem drinking and the workplace: an individualized approach to prevention. Psychol Addict Behav 16:243–251

Azrin NH, Besalel V (1980a) Job club counselor's manual: a beahvioral approach to vocational counselling. University Press, Baltimore

Azrin NH, Besalel VA (1980b) A job Club counselors manual: a behavioral approach to vocational counseling. Pro-Ed Publisher, Austin

Babor TF, de la Fuente JR, Saunders J, Grant M (1989) The alcohol use disorders identification test: guidelines for use in primary health care. World Health Organization, Genf

Babor TF, McRee BG, Kassebaum PA, Grimaldi PL, Ahmed K, Bray J (2007) Screening, brief intervention, and referral to treatment (SBIRT): toward a public health approach to the management of substance abuse. Subst Abus 28:7–30

Bacharach SB, Bamberger P, Biron M (2010) Alcohol consumption and workplace absenteeism: the moderating effect of social support. J Appl Psychol 95:334–348

Bachmeier R, Bick-Dresen S, Dreckmann I, Feindel H, Kemmann D, Kersting S, Kreutler A, Lange N, Medenwaldt J, Mielke D, Missel P, Premper V, Regenbrecht G, Sagel A, Schneider B, Strie M, Teigeler H, Weissinger V (2018) Effektivität der stationären Suchtrehabilitation – FVS-Katamnese des Entlassjahrgangs 2015 von Fachkliniken für Alkohol- und Medikamentenabhängige [Effectiveness of inpatient addiction rehabilitation – FVS catamnesis of the discharge year 2015 of specialist clinics for alcohol and drug addicts]. Sucht aktuell 1:49–65

Balhara YPS, Verma R (2014) A review of web based interventions focusing on alcohol use. Ann Med Health Sci Res 4:472–480

Bennett BJ, Patterson CR, Reynolds GS, Wiitala WL, Lehman WEK (2004) Team awareness, problem drinking, and drinking climate: workplace social health promotion in a policy context. Am J Health Promot 19:103–113

Bennett JB, Aden CA, Broome K, Mitchell K, Rigdon WD (2010) Team resilience for young restaurant workers: research-to-practice adaptation and assessment. J Occup Health Psychol 15:223–236

Berger LK (2009) Employee drinking practices and their relationships to workplace alcohol social control and social availability. J Work Behav Health 24:367–382

Billings DW, Cook RF, Hendrickson A, Dove DC (2008) A web-based approach to managing stress and mood disorders in the workforce. J Occup Environ Med 5:960–968

Bode K, Maurer F, Kröger C (2017) Arbeitswelt und psychische Störungen. Fortschritte der Psychotherapie. Band 66 [Work and mental disorders. Advances in psychotherapy. Volume 66]. Hogrefe, Göttingen

Broome KM, Bennett JB (2011) Reducing heavy alcohol consumption in young restaurant workers. J Stud Alcohol Drugs 72:117–124

Cancelliere C, Cassidy JD, Ammendolia C, Cote P (2011) Are workplace health promotion programs effective at improving presenteeism in workers? A systematic review and best evidence synthesis of the literature. BMC Public Health 11:395

Cashman CM, Ruotsalainen JH, Greiner BA, Beirne PV, Verbeek JH (2009) Alcohol and drug screening of occupational drivers for preventing injury. Cochrane Database Syst Rev 2

Cook RF, Back AS, Trudeau JV, McPherson T (2003) Integrating substance abuse prevention into health promotion programs in the workplace: a social cognitive intervention targeting the mainstream user. In: Bennett JB, Lehman WEK (eds) Preventing workplace substance abuse. American Psychological Association, Washington, DC, pp 97–133

Cook RF, Hersch RK, Back AS, McPherson TL (2004) The prevention of substance abuse among construction workers: a field test of a social- cognitive program. J Prim Prev 25:337–357

Cooper ML, Russel M, Frone MR (1990) Work stress and alcohol effects: a test of stress-induced drinking. J Health Soc Behav 31:260–276

Dalgaard VL, Aschbacher K, Andersen JH, Glasscock DJ, Willert MV, Carstensen O, Biering K (2017) Return to work after work-related stress: a randomized controlled trial of a work-focused cognitive behavioral intervention. Scand J Work Environ Health 43:436–446

Dee TS (2001) Alcohol abuse and economic conditions: evidence from repeated cross-sections of individueal-level data. Health Econ 10:257–270

Destatis (2016) Statistisches Bundesamt [Federal Statistical Office]. Internet https://www.destatis.de/DE

Die Drogenbeauftragte der Bundesrepublik Deutschland (2018) Drogen- und Suchtbericht 2018 [Drug and addiction report 2018]

Doumas DM, Hannah E (2008) Preventing high-risk drinking in youth in the workplace: a web-based normative feedback program. J Subst Abus Treat 34:263–271

Ennenbach M, Soyka M (2007) Suchtprävention im Betrieb. Identifikation von pathogenem Alkoholkonsum -Ergebnisse einer Mitarbeiterbefragung an einer Rehabilitationsklinik [On-the-job addiction prevention during operation. Identification of pathogenic alcohol consumption – results of an employee survey at a rehabilitation clinic]. Nervenarzt 78:530–535

Ennenbach M, Gass B, Reinecker H, Soyka M (2009) Zur Wirksamkeit betrieblicher Suchtprävention -Ergebnisse einer empirischen Untersuchung [The effectiveness of on-the-job addiction prevention – results of an empirical study]. Nervenarzt 80:3051–3314

Fabricius B, Teigeler H, Bick-Dresen S, Doris Braun D, Burger H, Danninger A, Donczewski I, Häberlein G, Kallina U, Liebrich M, Missel P, Müller V, Nels-Lindemann C, Reger F, Urban K, Wulf F, Bachmeier R, Medenwaldt J, Reichinger I, Sagel WV (2018) Effektivität der Adaptionsphase – FVS-Katamnese des Entlassjahrgangs 2015 [Effectiveness of the adaptation phase – FVS catamnesis of the discharge year 2015]. Sucht aktuell 1:66–76

Fachverband Sucht (2017) Basisdokumentation 2016. Reihe: Qualitätsförderung in der Entwöhnungsbehandlung. Band 24 [Basic documentation 2016. Series: quality promotion in the postacute addiction treatment. Volume 24]. Bonn

Fischer F, Kemmann D, Domma-Reichart J, Heinrich J, Post Y, Schulze M, Susemihl I, Tuchtenhagen F, Missel P, Weissinger V (2018) Effektivität der stationären abstinenzorientierten Drogenrehabilitation. FVS- Katamnese des Entlassjahrgangs 2015 von Fachkliniken für Drogenrehabilitation [Effectiveness of inpatient abstinence-oriented drug rehabilitation. FVS catamnesis of the discharge year 2015 from clinics for drug rehabilitation]. Sucht aktuell 1:77–86

Frone MR (1999) Work stress and alcohol use. Alcohol Res Health 23:284–291

Frone MR (2006) Prevalence and distribution of alcohol use and impairment in the workplace: a U.S. national survey. J Stud Alcohol 67:147–156

Frone MR (2008) Are work stressors related to employee substance use? The importance of temporal context in assessments of alcohol and illicit drug use. J Appl Psychol 93:199–206

Frone MR (2013) Alcohol and illicit drug use in the workforce and workplace. US: American Psychological Association, Washington, DC

Hemmingsson T, Lundberg I, Romelsjö A, Alfredsson L (1997) Alcoholism in social classes and occupations in Sweden. Int J Epidemiol 26:584–591

Hermansson U, Knutsson A, Rönnberg S, Brandt L (1998) Feasibility of brief intervention in the workplace for the detection and treatment of excessive alcohol consumption. Int J Occup Environ Health 4:71–78

Hermansson U, Helander A, Huss A, Brandt L, Rönnberg S (2000) The Alcohol Use Disorders Identification Test (AUDIT) and carbohydrate-deficient transferrin (CDT) in a routine workplace health examination. Alcohol Clin Exp Res 24:180–187

Hermansson U, Helander A, Brandt L, Huss A, Rönnberg S (2010) Screening and brief intervention for risky alcohol consumption in the workplace: results of a 1-year randomized controlled study. Alcohol Alcohol 4:252–257

Hester RK, Delaney HD, Campbell W, Handmaker N (2009) A web application for moderation training: initial results of a randomized clinical trial. J Subst Abus Treat 37:266–276

Honkonen T, Ahola K, Pertovaara M, Isometsä E, Kalimo R, Nykyri E, Aromaa A, Lönnqvist J (2006) The association between burnout and physical illness in the general population–results from the Finnish Health 2000 Study. J Psychosom Res 61:59–66

John U (2015) Addictions: general considerations. In: Wright JD (ed) International encyclopedia of the social and behavioral sciences, vol 1. Elsevier, Oxford, pp 97–102

John U, Hanke M (2002) Tobacco smoking- and alcohol drinking-attributable cancer mortality in Germany. Eur J Cancer Prev 11:11–17

John U, Veltrup C, Driessen M, Wetterling T (2003) Motivational intervention: an individual counselling vs a group treatment approach for alcohol-dependent in-patients. Alcohol Alcohol 38:263–269

Kaner EF, Beyer FR, Muirhead C, Campbell F, Pienaar ED, Bertholet N, Daeppen JB, Saunders JB, Burnand B (2018) Effectiveness of brief alcohol interventions in primary care populations. Cochrane Database Syst Rev 2:CD004148. https://doi.org/10.1002/14651858.CD004148.pub4

Kuoppala J, Lamminpää A, Husman P (2008) Work health promotion, job well-being, and sickness absences-a systematic review and meta-analysis. J Occup Environ Med 50:1216–1227

Lagerveld S, Blonk R (2017) Therapiemodul – return to work bei psychischen Erkrankungen (KBT-A). Ein ergänzendes Therapiemodul [Therapy module – return to work in case of mental illness (GIBT-DA). A complementary therapy module]. In: Kahl KG, Winter L (eds) Arbeitsplatzbezogene Psychotherapie. Intervention, Prävention und Rehabilitation [Workplace psychotherapy. Intervention, prevention and rehabilitation]. Kohlhammer, Stuttgart, pp 221–243

Lange N, Neeb K, Parusel F, Missel P, Bachmeier R, Brenner R, Fölsing S, Funke W, Herder F, Kersting S, Klein T, Kramer D, Löhnert B, Malz D, Medenwaldt J, Bick-Dresen S, Sagel A, Schneider B, Steffen D, Verstege R, Weissinger V (2018) Effektivität der ambulanten Suchtrehabilitation – FVS-Katamnese des Entlassjahrgangs 2015 von Ambulanzen für Alkohol- und Medikamentenabhängige [Effectiveness of outpatient addiction rehabilitation – FVS catamnesis of the discharge year 2015 of ambulances for alcohol and drug addicts]. Sucht aktuell 1:87–94

Mann K, Hoch E, Batra A (eds) (2015) S3-Leitlinie: Screening, Diagnose und Behandlung alkoholbezogener Störungen [S3 guideline: screening, diagnosis and treatment of alcohol-related disorders]. Springer, Heidelberg

Marlatt GA, Witkiewitz K (2010) Update on harm-reduction policy and intervention research. Annu Rev Clin Psychol 6:591–560

Matano RA, Koopman C, Wanat SF, Winzelberg AJ, Whitsell SD, Westrup D, Futa K, Clayton JB, Mussman L, Taylor CB (2007) A pilot study of an interactive web site in the workplace for reducing alcohol consumption. J Subst Abus Treat 32:71–80

Miller WR, Rollnick S (2012) Motivational interviewing. Helping people change, 3rd edn. Guilford Press, New York

Miller WR, Sanchez VC (1994) Motivating young adults for treatment and lifestyle change. In: Howard G (ed) Issues in alcohol use and misuse in young adults. University of Notre Dame Press, Notre Dame

Pemberton MR, Williams J, Herman-Stahl M, Calvin SL, Bradshaw MR, Bray RM, Ridenhour JL, Cook R, Hersch RK, Hester RK, Mitchell GM (2011) Evaluation of two web-based alcohol interventions in the U.S.military. J Stud Alcohol Drugs 72:480–489

Rehm J, Taylor B, Room R (2006) Global burden of disease from alcohol, illicit drugs and tobacco. Drug Alcohol Rev 25:503–513

Rehm J, Mathers C, Popova S, Thavorncharoensap M, Teerawattananon Y, Patra J (2009) Global burden of disease and injury and economic cost attributable to alcohol use and alcohol-use disorders. Lancet 373(9682):2223–2233

Reinert DF, Allen JP (2007) The alcohol use disorders identification test: an update of research findings. Alcohol Clin Exp Res 31:185–199

Richmond RL, Klein L, Heather N, Wodak A (2000) Evaluation of a workplace brief intervention for excessive alcohol consumption: the workscreen project. Prev Med 30:51–63

Roman M, Blum TC (2002) The workplace and alcohol problem prevention. Alcohol Res Health 26:49–57

Romeri E, Baker A, Griffiths C (2007) Alcohol-related deaths by occupation, England and Wales, 2001-05. Health Stat Q 35:6–12

Rosta J (2008) Hazardous alcohol use among hospital doctors in Germany. Alcohol Alcoholism 43:198–203

Rummel M, Rainer L, Fuchs R (2004) Alkohol im Unternehmen. Praxis der Personalpsychologie [Alcohol in the company. Practice of personal psychology]. Hogrefe, Göttingen

Schneider B, Mielke D, Bachmeier R, Bick-Dresen S, Deichler ML, Forschner L, Missel P, Sagel A, Weissinger V (2018) Effektivität der Ganztägig Ambulanten Suchtrehabilitation – Fachverband Sucht – Katamnese des Entlassjahrganges 2015 aus Einrichtungen Alkohol- und Medikamentenabhängiger [Effectiveness of the all-day outpatient addiction rehabilitation – Fachverband Sucht- Catamnese of the discharge year 2015 from institutions for alcohol and drug dependents]. Sucht aktuell 1:95–105

Scoccianti C, Cecchini M, Anderson AS, Berrino F, Boutron-Ruault MC, Espina C, Key TJ, Leitzmann M, Norat T, Powers H, Wiseman M, Romieu I (2015) European code against cancer 4th edition: alcohol drinking and cancer. Cancer Epidemiol 39(Suppl 1):67–74

Sieck M, Heirich M (2010) Focusing attention on substance abuse in the workplace: a comparison of three workplace interventions. J Work Behav Health 25:72–87

Siegrist J (1996) Soziale Krisen und Gesundheit [Social crises and health]. Hogrefe, Göttingen

Soyka M (2017) Die Rolle von Alkohol in der Arbeitswelt [The role of alcohol in the workplace]. In: Kahl KG, Winter L (eds) Arbeitsplatzbezogene Psychotherapie. Intervention, Prävention und Rehabilitation [Workplace psychotherapy. Intervention, prevention and rehabilitation]. Kohlhammer, Stuttgart, pp 44–50

Veltrup C (2011) Vom konstruktiven Druck zum effektiven Vorgehen: Paradigmenwechsel in der betrieblichen Suchtprävention [From constructive pressure to effective action: paradigm shift in company addiction prevention]. In: Breitstadt R, Müller U (eds) Herr und Frau "Co" wollen nicht mehr. Beiträge für eine betriebliche Drogenpolitik [Mr. and Mrs. "Co" do not want anymore. Contributions to an operational drug policy]. Shaker, Aachen, pp 79–86

Walters ST, Woodall WG (2003) Mailed feedback reduces consumption among moderate drinkers who are employed. Prev Sci 4:287–294

Webb G, Shakeshaft A, Sanson-Fisher R, Havard A (2009) A systematic review of work place interventions for alcohol-related problems. Addiction 104:365–377

Wittchen HU, Jacobi F, Rehm J, Gustavsson A, Svensson M, Jonsson B, Olesen J, Allgulander C, Alonso J, Faravelli C, Fratiglioni L, Jennum P, Lieb R, Maercker A, van Os J, Preisig M, Salvador-Carulla L, Simon R, Steinhausen HC (2011) The size and burden of mental disorders and other disorders of the brain in Europe 2010. Eur Neuropsychopharmacol 21:655–679

World Health Organisation (1992) ICD-10 classification of mental and behavioural disorders: clinical descriptions and diagnostic guidelines, Geneva

World Health Organisation (2001) International classification of functioning, disability and health (ICF), Geneva

World Health Organisation (2016) International statistical classification of diseases and related health problems (the) ICD-10. 5th, Geneva

Zoike E, König C (2006) Suchterkrankungen und Psychische Störungen – wen trifft's? Widerspiegelungen in Leistungsdaten der BKK [Addictions and mental disorders – who is affected? Reflections in performance data of the BKK]. Sucht aktuell:36–42

Factors of Competitive Employment for People with Severe Mental Illness, from Acquisition to Tenure

29

Marc Corbière, Élyse Charette-Dussault, and Patrizia Villotti

Contents

Introduction	526
Policies and Legal Framework (Europe, North America, Australia)	528
Environmental Factors to Predict the Work Integration of People with SMI	530
Related to Disability Benefits	530
Related to Stigma and Social Support	531
Related to Vocational Services and Employment Specialists Competencies	533
Related to the Workplace: Work Accommodations and Natural Supports	534
Individual Factors to Predict the Work Integration of People with SMI	534
Demographic Factors	534
Related to Illness: Psychiatric and Physical Conditions	536
Related to Experience and Skills	538
Related to Self and Motivational Factors	541
Discussion	543
Cross-References	545
References	545

M. Corbière (✉)
Department of Education, Career Counselling, Université du Québec à Montréal (UQAM), Montréal, QC, Canada

Centre de Recherche de l'Institut Universitaire en Santé Mentale de Montréal (CR-IUSMM), Research Chair in Mental and Work, Foundation of IUSMM, Montréal, QC, Canada
e-mail: Corbiere.marc@uqam.ca

É. Charette-Dussault
Department of Psychology, Université du Québec à Montréal, Montréal, QC, Canada
e-mail: charette-dussault.elyse@courrier.uqam.ca

P. Villotti
Department of Education, Career Counselling, Université du Québec à Montréal (UQAM), Montréal, QC, Canada
e-mail: villotti.patrizia@uqam.ca

© Springer Nature Switzerland AG 2020
U. Bültmann, J. Siegrist (eds.), *Handbook of Disability, Work and Health*, Handbook Series in Occupational Health Sciences, https://doi.org/10.1007/978-3-030-24334-0_29

Abstract

People with severe mental illness (SMI) face numerous obstacles in order to obtain and sustain employment in the regular labor market. Yet, work represents the cornerstone of recovery. Although supported employment programs are recognized as evidence-based practices to help people with SMI in their work integration, the literature highlights a ceiling effect for job acquisition (approximately 60% of participants registered in supported employment programs) and brief job tenure for most, regardless of the length of study follow-ups (short or longer) and the number of jobs obtained. This chapter reviews individual and environmental factors of employment outcomes – job acquisition and job tenure – by considering reviews, trials, and studies conducted in the domain. The goal of this chapter is also to introduce the systems, policies, and strategies implemented in different countries to facilitate the work integration of people with disabilities, particularly people with SMI. Finally, a short discussion will highlight strengths and limitations identified by researchers and health professionals regarding the work integration of people with SMI, and will mention emerging ideas and eventual recommendations on this research topic.

Keywords

Severe mental illness · Job acquisition · Job tenure · Individual factors · Environmental factors · Review

Introduction

People with severe mental illness (SMI) are often stigmatized and marginalized, and a substantial proportion of them remain, accordingly, unemployed (Taskila et al. 2014; Bejerholm et al. 2015; Hampson et al. 2016). Helping clients to obtain competitive employment is coherent with the recovery movement. In fact, work represents the cornerstone of recovery since it emphasizes the possibility of rebuilding one's life after the onset of mental illness (Corbière and Lecomte 2009). Many advantages and life improvements are associated with employment and are highlighted in the scientific literature as follows (Becker et al. 2007; Mueser and McGurk 2014; Netto et al. 2016; Pachoud 2017): (1) Work is a major determinant of social inclusion and plays a critical role in the life and recovery of people with mental disorders; (2) Work implies managing time in a way that is more like the dominant lifestyle, allowing persons to develop a greater sense of social inclusion; (3) Work establishes a routine, helps to develop communication skills, and to pay the bills; (4) By dealing with job demands and overcoming obstacles, the person gains self-efficacy, develops a sense of control over his/her life, and reaches self-actualization; (5) Work also gives the person the opportunity to be recognized for his/her skills, capacities, and contribution to collective work, which forms a pillar of self-esteem; (6) Work offers the opportunity for social recognition, which results in a sense of social inclusion and belonging to a community; (7) By meeting people outside the family circle, work provides the person with the means to develop friendships and to break the vicious cycle of isolation; (8) Through their work, people with SMI develop a professional identity that helps them to dissociate themselves from the stigmatized identity of a "mentally ill person." Even though employment is often associated with several benefits, employment rates for people with SMI are lower than for people with other disabilities, and the majority of the former want to penetrate the regular labor market (Schindler 2014).

People with SMI face numerous obstacles to getting and sustaining employment. Supported employment programs (and augmented supported employment programs) are recognized in the literature as evidence-based practices to promote the work integration of people with SMI in the open market (Hoffmann et al. 2014). Despite this, success in job acquisition remains limited, with a review of 20 randomized controlled trials indicating a median rate of 60% (Drake and Bond 2014) of people with SMI being successful in getting a job. Another study conducted by Johannesen et al. (2007) reported a drop out rate of 40–50% by individuals with SMI prior to obtaining employment, even with the assistance of supported employment programs. Even when people with SMI are successful in obtaining competitive employment, studies published in the last three decades indicate that most of the jobs obtained are part-time. Furthermore, job tenure for people with a SMI is often brief, with studies showing that nearly half of all clients leave or lose their supported employment positions within 6–8 months (Xie et al. 1997; Resnick and Bond 2001; Becker et al. 2007; Bond et al. 2013; Corbière et al. 2014; Glynn et al. 2017). More recently, Suijkerbuijk et al. (2017) added further details in their Cochrane review: the duration of job tenure can vary, on average, 13 weeks or 33 weeks, respectively, according to short- (≤ 1 year) and long-term (>1 year) follow-ups of trials. Moreover, even though studies on job tenure of people with SMI consist of long-term follow-ups (from 3 to 12 years), samples are usually very small, around 50 persons, preventing us from drawing clear conclusions (Salyers et al. 2004; Hoffmann et al. 2014). Furthermore, reasons for job terminations are often unsatisfactory, and people with SMI quit without other plans for employment (Johannesen et al. 2007). Studies over time report that close to two-thirds of the job termination decisions were voluntary, made by the employee with a SMI (Wong et al. 2004; Lanctôt et al. 2013), due to external and uncontrollable causes (e.g., work conditions, schedule, symptoms).

This evidence shows that: (1) most people with SMI struggle to obtain work and maintain employment in the regular labor market, even when they are registered in supported employment programs and (2) many individuals who obtain a job quit their job after a few weeks, often without plans for the next job. Consequently, it is important to identify factors that contribute to job acquisition and tenure in people with SMI. In the scientific literature, several initiatives have attempted to disentangle the factors associated with work integration for people with SMI, often by exploring a specific category of factors related to job acquisition and job tenure, together or separately (Bassett et al. 2001; McGurk and Mueser 2004; Wewiorski and Fabian 2004; McGurk et al. 2005; Razzano et al. 2005; Corbière et al. 2006; Burke-Miller et al. 2006; Catty et al. 2008; Tsang et al. 2010; Campbell et al. 2010; Williams et al. 2016; Charette-Dussault and Corbière 2019). Among the most reviewed categories of factors are those related to individual characteristics, such as demographic (e.g., age), cognitive (e.g., work memory), clinical (e.g., symptoms), psychosocial (e.g., self-esteem), and those related to the environment, such as service features (e.g., employment specialist skills) and workplace (e.g., work accommodations). These categories of factors may be more or less relevant, depending on the targeted outcomes, job acquisition (e.g., motivation to work), or job tenure (e.g., work accommodations).

This chapter reviews individual and environmental factors of employment outcomes – job acquisition and job tenure – by considering reviews, trials, and studies conducted in the domain. Before describing the categories of individual and environmental factors, for which several subcategories exist, we will first introduce the systems, policies, and strategies implemented in different countries to facilitate the work integration of people with disabilities, particularly people with SMI. Finally, a short discussion will allow us to summarize and discuss the results by highlighting strengths and limitations identified by researchers and health professionals, and to suggest future avenues of research.

Policies and Legal Framework (Europe, North America, Australia)

Because of its societal, economic, and health-related relevance, employment for disabled people is regulated by most Western countries. Although these policies and systems often do not specifically target people with SMI, they do provide overarching frameworks that help this population to obtain and sustain employment. Severe mental disorders are defined by three indicators (Corbière et al. 2013): (1) difficulties interfering with or limiting the person's functioning in one or more areas of life activity; (2) persistence of mental health problems over time (e.g., frequency and intensity of use of psychiatric services); and (3) the predominant psychiatric diagnoses are schizophrenia, schizoaffective disorders, bipolar disorders, and major depression. Due to their health condition and important restrictions on their participation in society, people with SMI are often considered disabled individuals and, thus, eligible for support in employment.

In the following paragraphs, we provide a general overview of policies and system strategies developed in Europe, North America, and Australia to secure employment for people with SMI. Policies are defined as mandatory and non-mandatory legislative frameworks (e.g., law) that guide the work (re)integration process at the local, regional, national, or international level. System strategies are defined as actions of support, programs, or incentives (e.g., disability pension) supporting unemployed and inactive individuals to obtain or return to paid employment, to remain at work or, more generally, to support and facilitate the work participation of vulnerable persons (Scaratti et al. 2018).

Most countries in Europe, North America, and Australia have policies or legislative frameworks against discrimination and provide support to persons with disabilities. Despite different political and legislative histories, most European Countries ratified the U.N. Convention on the Rights of Persons with Disabilities (UNCRPD 2006). These countries committed themselves to fighting discrimination against people with disabilities (Article 4), ensuring they have the right to work and are provided with reasonable accommodations at work, as well as promoting job retention and return-to-work programs (Article 27). Canadian legislation prohibits discrimination in employment based on disability at both the federal and provincial levels (The U.N. Convention on the Rights of Persons with Disability was ratified in 2010). Human rights and protection against discrimination in the area of employment are also guaranteed by Federal acts and programs, such as the Canadian Human Rights Act (1985), and the Employment Equity Act (1995). These acts state that employers have a duty to accommodate employees, to achieve workplace equity and to create opportunities for individuals with disabilities by removing barriers to employment. In the United States, the Americans with Disabilities Act (ADA 1990) protects the fundamental civil rights of people with disabilities. Inspired by anti-discrimination policy, this act posits for all individuals with mental and/or physical disabilities equal opportunities and full integration into the workplace. Under the provisions of the ADA, employers must adopt unbiased hiring and promotion criteria, and make reasonable accommodations for the known limitations of disabled individuals, unless this will cause undue hardship. In the United States, the Rehabilitation Act of 1973 requires federal employers to hire and retain individuals with disabilities, with the goal of 7% of all employees being persons with disabilities. Australia ratified the U.N. Convention in 2008 and committed to ensure that people with a disability have the same rights, choices, and opportunities as other Australians, including the right to a meaningful job. Discrimination is prohibited by the Disability Discrimination Act of 1992, which deals with all areas of work including recruitment, employment promotion, dismissal, and access to premises. The 1986 Disability Services Act provides a coordinated approach to assist people with disabilities gain and maintain employment. It is a legislative and funding framework for a range of disability services, most significantly, employment services.

The system strategies used by European countries differ based on how much emphasis is put on support, incentives, or obligations to promote the integration of disabled individuals in the open labor market. In general, they adopt either passive measures to support people with disabilities (cash benefits, disability pensions) or active measures (active labor market policies) to promote employment of people with disabilities, or a combination of the two.

Passive measures are generally provided through different types of programs, such as universal programs, contributory programs, and noncontributory programs. The active measures usually offered by European countries include guidance and counselling, training, education, and job placement. Support in employment is offered in the open labor market through social enterprises or social cooperatives as well as through sheltered work. Supported employment programs are widely implemented in Canada to help people with disabilities obtain competitive employment with the help of an employment specialist. The general tendency in the United

States is to try to integrate disabled individuals into the workplace through supported and competitive initiatives, such as supported employment programs, rather than through sheltered work (considered as obsolete). Several social security incentives are available to encourage those receiving disability benefits to work. These incentives include medical coverage for people who work, continued payment under a vocational rehabilitation program and reimbursement for impairment-related work expenses. Taxation measures are also used to integrate disabled individuals into the workplace, such as tax deductions and tax credits to help employers to adapt their work environment. In Australia, the Disability Services Act (1986) provides a coordinated approach to assisting people with disabilities to gain and maintain employment within the framework of several disability services, most significantly, employment services. Currently, the National Disability Strategy is the main guide for improving outcomes for people with disabilities in Australia in the years 2010–2020. Although analyzing the policies, systems, and strategies implemented in several countries to facilitate the work integration of people with SMI allows us to better understand the context of work integration, many studies, reviews, and meta-analyses have been conducted to document the factors related to work integration, particularly obtaining and maintaining competitive employment. The results of these studies will be presented in the next section.

Environmental Factors to Predict the Work Integration of People with SMI

Related to Disability Benefits

Disability Benefits
Although disability benefits provide financial stability for people with SMI, they can also represent an important barrier to employment. People receiving disability benefits may be afraid of losing the stability associated with these payments. It is not uncommon for jobs held by people with SMI to be entry positions with salaries at minimum wage and with few social benefits (Bond and Drake 2008). The prospect of being in an even more precarious financial situation by integrating a job can discourage them from even trying. In fact, people receiving disability benefits who integrate vocational programs tend to be less active in their job searches or leave the program faster than those without this support (Bond et al. 1995). For instance, in Sweden, Bejerholm et al. (2015) observed that Individual Placement and Support (IPS) participants left the IPS program because they risked losing their welfare benefits if they continued with IPS. They noticed that the welfare services regulations in Sweden restricted effectiveness of IPS (Bejerholm et al. 2015). Bond et al. (2007) explored the effects of the status of disability benefits on the acquisition and maintenance of employment among participants in four independent randomized controlled trials (IPS program versus regular employment services) in the United

States. Participants were divided into four groups according to their disability benefits: Supplemental Security Income (SSI), Social Security Disability Insurance (SSDI), dually eligible beneficiaries and nonbeneficiaries. Job acquisition did not differ significantly among beneficiary groups in the IPS programs. However, the difference was significant when the job was obtained through a regular employment program, with nonbeneficiaries having a higher rate of job acquisition than those with one of the types of disability benefits. According to these authors, the fact that benefit counselling is part of the IPS program can explain the difference between the programs (Bond et al. 2007). Furthermore, it is noteworthy that the majority of those integrating or reentering the labor market choose a part-time job that does not allow them enough income to leave disability benefits (Drake et al. 2013a). Yet, the total loss of benefits has been referred to as "falling off a cliff" (Bond et al. 2007). One of the solutions proposed is to act quickly after the onset of mental health disorders to promote a rapid reintegration to work and thus limit the duration of the receipt of disability benefits (Bond and Drake 2008). This solution seems adequate since it has been found that beneficiaries seem to have more opportunities to enter competitive employment if they receive benefits for a shorter period of time (Metcalfe et al. 2016).

Related to Stigma and Social Support

Stigma and Disclosure

The stigma associated with mental illness is considered to be a major obstacle to social participation for this population (Hampson et al. 2016). The misconceptions and stereotypes associated with mental illness, such as violent tendencies or unpredictable behaviors, lead to discrimination in several settings, including employment (Corrigan et al. 2009). Employers tend to perceive individuals with mental illnesses as aggressive, dangerous, unpredictable, unintelligent, unreasonable, unreliable, lacking self-control and frightening, and, as a result, question their work performance, quality of work, work attendance and tenure, and need for excessive and expensive accommodations (Russinova et al. 2011). Although this stigma has been reported by both people with SMI and health and vocational professionals as an important obstacle to employment acquisition (Boycott et al. 2015; Netto et al. 2016), it is difficult to measure its actual effects. To do so, in a field experiment, Hipes et al. (2016) responded to 635 job offers with fictive applications indicating either a mental health problem or a physical health problem to explain an absence of a few months from the labor market. They found significant discrimination against the applicant with mental illness history (15% were called back by the employer) compared to applicants with physical illness history (22% were called back). It is not surprising that people with SMI are reluctant to disclose their mental health disorder in the application process for a job.

According to Waghorn and Spowart (2010), a structured and pragmatic preparation of this disclosure can facilitate job acquisition. They proposed a tool, the formal plan to manage personal information (PMPI), which helps the participant to define employment goals, personal strengths and skills, sensitive information (i.e., diagnosis, medication and side effects), possible work limitations, terms used to describe these work limitations in a formal and informal context, and accommodations and support needed to adequately perform the job. McGahey et al. (2016) found that a group of people who completed the PMPI were significantly more likely to be employed 6 weeks after baseline than the group that chose not to disclose any information about their mental illness.

Social Support

The financial and emotional support provided by relatives can influence the job search process or the motivation to integrate or reintegrate the labor market for people with SMI. In Corbière et al. (2011), feeling supported and encouraged, specifically in relation to work, was related to job acquisition only indirectly, but directly to greater motivation to find a job, perception of fewer obstacles to job acquisition, better career search self-efficacy, and the use of more active strategies to find employment. In another study, rejection attitudes of relatives were linked to lower chances of gaining competitive employment (Mueser et al. 2001). In the same way, in an ethnographical study, Alverson et al. (2006) observed that the most active participants in job searches were those who said they had support from their relatives or who were responsible for supporting their family. However, the support of relatives is not always positive. In Corbière et al. (2005), the people who thought they could always count on their family in case of need were the ones who worked fewer hours per week. In the same way, being satisfied with one's situation, social and intimate relationships also limit motivation and effort dedicated to acquiring a job (Catty et al. 2008).

Clinician Support (or Expectations)

Without having been tested quantitatively, the support provided by mental health professionals is frequently reported by people with SMI as being a facilitating factor in their efforts to acquire a job (Marwaha and Johnson 2005; Netto et al. 2016). Just like mainstream society and relatives, mental health clinicians may have different perceptions of the signification and prognostic of mental health diseases. Professionals with a more traditional approach to rehabilitation may focus primarily on reducing symptoms and may not consider it worthwhile or realistic to aim for the integration of a competitive job if some symptoms are still present (Slade 2009). These professionals tend not to refer customers to employment services and their discourse can be perceived as discouraging by people with a SMI (Marwaha and Johnson 2005; Taskila et al. 2014). Conversely, professionals with a recovery-oriented approach through the integration of meaningful life projects for the individual with SMI, such as acquiring and maintaining a competitive job, will be more likely to support the person with SMI in their employment endeavors. According to several authors, the ability of the professional to develop and support the hope of the person related to his/her projects and goals is an important factor in recovery (Slade 2009).

Related to Vocational Services and Employment Specialists Competencies

Access and Quality of Services

Despite the proven superiority of IPS programs, an overwhelming majority of people with SMI do not have access to these services. According to US survey data from 2001 to 2012, only 2% of that population has access to supported employment programs (Bruns et al. 2016). Several obstacles to the implementation of employability programs have been identified but the most important one is related to the funding of these programs (Drake et al. 2016). Also, among the programs that have been implemented, there can be significant variability in the employment integration rate (Drake et al. 2006). One of the reasons for this variability is the degree of fidelity of these programs to the model – the highest level of fidelity leads to better acquisition rates for clients with SMI participating in these programs (Bond et al. 2012).

Employment Specialist Competencies

In addition to this inter-program variability, it appears that the employment rates vary from one employment counselor to another within the same program (Drake et al. 2006). To better understand these variations, authors focused on the skills of employment specialists and the link between them and the acquisition and maintenance of a job by their clients, but the results are still scarce. In the supported employment program model, working directly in the community is considered the core task of the employment specialist (Whitley et al. 2010). It has been demonstrated that clients who had the benefit of employment development from their employment specialists are up to five times more likely to enter a job than those who did not (Leff et al. 2005). According to Catty et al.'s study (2008), the relationship with the employment specialist helped clients to obtain competitive employment but did not affect their ability to maintain their employment. In addition, the quality of the relationships established by the employment specialist with potential employers and supervisors also facilitates their clients entering a competitive job (Corbière et al. 2017).

Working Alliance

The working alliance is the quality of the collaborative relationship created between the client and the professional and includes a shared vision of the goals and tasks to be accomplished (Bordin 1979). This alliance is considered one of the essential ingredients of psychotherapy and counselling, and its role in mental health recovery is increasingly recognized (Anthony and Mizock 2014). Although there is little research on the contribution of the working alliance on employment related outcomes, the current data indicate its importance. In two studies, the working alliance as perceived by the job seeker and by the employment specialist – including the agreement between both parties on the goals, the tasks required to reach the goals, and the bond developed – was a significant predictor of job acquisition (Catty et al. 2008; Corbière et al. 2017). This working alliance depends, in part, on the employment specialist's skills and characteristics (Drake and Bond 2014), as well as the client's characteristics, such as severity of symptoms, social functioning, and insight, that can also predict the development of the working alliance in a psychiatric treatment context (Barrowclough et al. 2010).

Related to the Workplace: Work Accommodations and Natural Supports

When natural supports are not put in place by health professionals, employment specialists, or other key persons in the workplace, employers as well as employees with a work disability should be supported to ensure that work accommodations are provided when the demand is reasonable and the accommodations feasible (MacDonald-Wilson et al. 2002). Reasonable accommodations are defined as workplace adjustments that do not slow down the productivity of the enterprise, cause undue hardship, or generate excessive costs (McDowell and Fossey 2015). Work accommodations as well as natural supports in the workplace for helping people with SMI are recognized as key elements for maintaining employment (e.g., Williams et al. 2016). However, few studies have investigated the relationship between work accommodations and job tenure (Corbière et al. 2014). Using the Work Accommodation and Natural Support Scale (WANSS), Corbière et al. (2014) showed that the "Supervisor and coworker supports" dimension was associated with reduced risk of losing the job, after controlling for all other relevant covariates (e.g., disclosure of the mental condition). Two items of this dimension were more important for predicting job tenure: *Are you receiving rewards or recognition from your supervisor and/or coworkers?* and *Are you able to exchange work tasks with others?* This dimension can be seen as a facilitator of work tenure of people with SMI but could also be considered as a protective factor against potential relapses (Corbière et al. 2014). In the same vein, the integrative review of Williams et al. (2016), based on studies from 1993 to 2013 focusing on job tenure of people with SMI, showed the importance of good interactions between the worker and supervisor, the satisfaction of the supervisor-worker relationship and supportive co-workers as critical factors improving job tenure.

Individual Factors to Predict the Work Integration of People with SMI

Demographic Factors

Many studies have looked at sociodemographic variables such as gender, age, ethnicity, and marital status, and their effects on job acquisition and tenure for people with SMI, but the results are either inconclusive or contradictory from study to study. Age and its impact on employment is a good example of a factor whose results are incongruent across studies. Although younger age predicted better competitive job acquisition in several studies (Mueser et al. 2001; Burke-Miller et al. 2006; Drake et al. 2013b; McGahey et al. 2016; Metcalfe et al. 2018), it was nonsignificant in other studies (Catty et al. 2008; Campbell et al. 2010; Fortin et al. 2017). It has been proposed that age can hide other factors that may better explain the acquisition of a job. For example, older people may have a longer history of SMI and may have experienced more job failures or have more symptoms or side effects related to their medication (Twamley et al. 2008).

In studying the effects of gender, neither interest and effort made toward employment (Mueser et al. 2001) nor rate of competitive employment acquisition differed between men and women (Drake et al. 2013b; Mueser et al. 2001; Leff et al. 2005; Burke-Miller et al. 2006; Twamley et al. 2008; Catty et al. 2008; Butler et al. 2010; Campbell et al. 2010; Metcalfe et al. 2016; Llerena et al. 2017; Fortin et al. 2017). However, in a study conducted in Hong Kong among participants of a supported employment program for people with SMI, significantly more men than women obtained a competitive job at the follow-up (6 months after entering the program). The authors explained these results by specifying that jobs with more physical demands were the most rapidly available on the job market and, thus, considered more suitable for men (Wong et al. 2004). Also, the number of hours worked per week was significantly lower for women than for men in two studies (Burke-Miller et al. 2006). Burke-Miller et al. (2006) argue that this difference can be explained by the fact that women may be less available because of the care devoted to children or other family members.

Similarly, in a large majority of studies, there was no difference between ethnic groups in the acquisition of competitive employment (Leff et al. 2005; Twamley et al. 2008; Catty et al. 2008; Butler et al. 2010; Campbell et al. 2010; Drake et al. 2013b; Llerena et al. 2017). Despite this, four studies found that being part of a visible ethnic minority (versus being Caucasian) decreased the likelihood of competitive employment acquisition (Wewiorski and Fabian 2004; Cook 2006; Butler et al. 2010). These results may reflect discrimination in hiring affected minorities for competitive jobs. Conversely, in two studies conducted in the United States (Burke-Miller et al. 2006; Metcalfe et al. 2016), Hispanic participants were more likely to gain competitive employment than the other participants. In the same way, in an ethnographic study of job search behaviors of people with SMI, Puerto Rican participants, in contrast to Euro and Afro-American participants, showed greater involvement and mobilization in their job search (Alverson et al. 2006). These differences were explained by a different cultural perception of the implications of mental illness. In fact, Euro-American and, to a lesser extent, Afro-American more often reported a perception that their mental illness was debilitating and an impediment to work, compared to Puerto Ricans, who rarely reported that view.

Age-, gender-, and ethnicity-related difficulties or discrimination are experienced by all job seekers whether or not they are diagnosed with SMI. These factors can become an additional obstacle for people with SMI and, therefore, require more steps or support to facilitate their integration into the regular job market. Age, sex, and ethnicity are not considered critical factors of job tenure (Xie et al. 1997).

Related to Illness: Psychiatric and Physical Conditions

Psychiatric Diagnosis

In the literature, the effects of the mental health diagnosis on employment acquisition and tenure are also inconclusive. The majority of studies do not report that the diagnosis has a significant impact on the acquisition and tenure of a competitive job (Twamley et al. 2008; Drake et al. 2013b). In a meta-analysis conducted by Wewiorski and Fabian in 2004, people with a schizophrenia diagnosis were significantly less likely to be employed following diverse vocational rehabilitation programs (Wewiorski and Fabian 2004). The effect sizes were, however, very small. Another meta-analysis by Campbell et al. in 2010, specifically comparing groups of persons attending IPS programs versus prevocational programs, found the diagnosis of schizophrenia to be an obstacle to job acquisition, uniquely for the participants in the prevocational group (Campbell et al. 2010). In Razzano et al. (2005), participants in supported employment programs who reported a diagnosis on the schizophrenia spectrum had fewer opportunities to work more than 40 h in a month compared to participants with another diagnosis (i.e., major depression, bipolar disorder), even after controlling for symptoms and level of social functioning. No differences were reported regarding job acquisition.

Psychiatric Symptoms

Some authors have proposed that the severity of symptoms was a better predictor of job acquisition than the specific mental illness diagnosis (Bond et al. 2012). Despite this presumption, the results of studies carried out so far do not affirm that the severity of the symptoms predict the acquisition of a competitive job for this population. Actually, general indexes of symptom scales are never significant, whether the questionnaire is self-reported, like the Brief Symptoms Inventory (BSI) (Corbière et al. 2011, 2017; Waynor et al. 2016), or completed by a professional, like the Brief Psychiatric Rating Scale (BPRS) (Mueser et al. 1997, 2001; Campbell et al. 2010), or the Positive and Negative Symptoms Scale (PANSS) (Leff et al. 2005; Razzano et al. 2005; Twamley et al. 2008; Catty et al. 2008; Puig et al. 2016). Some authors have obtained more significant results by studying the positive and negative symptoms separately. In doing so, negative symptoms appear more often as predictors of job acquisition while positive symptoms appear to be nonsignificantly related to this outcome (Tsang et al. 2010; Drake et al. 2013b), except for one case where higher positive symptoms were related to less chance to acquire competitive employment (Razzano et al. 2005).

Other authors have sought to further understand which specific symptoms may explain greater difficulty in acquiring a job, with interesting results. Mueser et al. (2001) examined the effects of different negative symptoms on the job acquisition of 528 patients with schizophrenia spectrum using a three-factor model of the Scale for the Assessment of Negative Symptoms (SANS). Of these factors, they found that only inattention-alogia and social amotivation were predictors of competitive employment but not diminished expression. In 2017, Llerena et al. (2017) used the same scale but with a two-factor model, experiential and expressive symptoms, to study their ability to predict competitive employment among people with schizophrenia spectrum diagnosis. The first factor, experiential symptoms, combining avolition, anhedonia, and asociality, was predictive of competitive employment while the second one, expressive factors that combine blunting affect and alogia, was not. Beyond the presence of symptoms (i.e., general, specific, positive, negative) in their 12-year follow-up study, Becker et al. (2007) showed that the successful management of psychiatric symptoms associated with the deployment of appropriate coping skills played an important role in finding and maintaining long-term work.

Cognitive Deficits
One of the most commonly reported barriers to various vocational outcomes is cognitive deficits associated with mental health illnesses (Tsang et al. 2010). However, when the outcome is specifically the acquisition of competitive employment, composite score results from a neurocognition battery covering various cognitive dimensions, such as attention, working memory, information processing speed, and executive functions, indicated that these dimensions are not significant predictors (Llerena et al. 2017). Other authors have studied the different dimensions separately or have targeted a specific dimension of neurocognition to explain the acquisition of a competitive job. Two studies demonstrated that better speed of information processing significantly favors job acquisition (Metcalfe et al. 2016; Corbière et al. 2017). However, in another study, neither the information processing speed nor the other cognitive domains evaluated, namely, verbal learning and memory, attention and working memory, visual organization, verbal comprehension, and social cognition, were significant predictors of that outcome (Allott et al. 2013). Other researchers postulate that it is not the cognitive skills at baseline that are important to consider but those at follow-up (McGurk and Mueser 2006). In agreement with this hypothesis, Puig et al. (2016) found that participants in a supported employment program supplemented by compensatory cognitive training were more likely to enter a competitive job if they experienced an improvement in their attention and vigilance between baseline and the 12 weeks of cognitive training. Moreover, it is becoming increasingly clear that the employment programs that incorporate cognitive training are even more efficient than IPS programs only when it comes to the competitive job acquisition rate (Suijkerbuijk et al. 2017). In their meta-analysis on augmented supported employment programs (SE programs + cognitive remediation) including 12 trials, Sauvé et al. (2018) demonstrated that this combination of services was not a significant predictor of job tenure. Beyond highlighting the limitations of studies retained in the meta-analysis, the authors suggested targeting the need for cognitive remediation for doing specific work tasks in their clients' ongoing employment, eventually improving their job tenure.

Comorbidities (Physical Disease or Condition, Substance Abuse, Personality Disorder)
Researchers were also interested in dual and concomitant disorders that could become barriers to gaining competitive employment for people with SMI. Abuse of drugs and alcohol is frequent among people with SMI but the effect of these

co-occurring disorders on employment acquisition is not clear. In one study, people with SMI who had drug or alcohol addiction were reported as being 50% less likely to gain employment than those without the addiction (Razzano et al. 2005). In other studies, the addiction was not a significant predictor at all (Campbell et al. 2010; Corbière et al. 2017). However, having physical health problems or physical or cognitive co-occurring disabilities were repeatedly associated with more difficulty in getting a job (Razzano et al. 2005; Metcalfe et al. 2018). Another concomitant disorder that can influence obtaining or maintaining employment is having a personality disorder or specific personality traits. In attempting to disentangle the impacts of these variables on work outcomes, Fortin et al. (2017) showed that prior employment, personality problems, and negative symptoms were significantly related to acquisition of competitive employment and to delays in acquisition, whereas the conscientiousness personality trait was predictive of job tenure. All of these conditions are obstacles to employment on their own, and it is therefore not surprising that they can make it more difficult for people with mental health problems to access employment and maintain competitive employment. As suggested by Fortin et al. (2017), it would be relevant to develop a person-environment fit model, considering the person's characteristics, as well as job preference and work interests, to find congruent jobs and thus maintain employment longer (see the section entitled job skills and job match).

Medication (Compliance, Side Effects)

Although adherence to medication is perceived as an important factor in the acquisition and maintenance of employment, medication side effects are also perceived as significant potential barriers (Taskila et al. 2014). For example, pharmacological treatments can cause drowsiness, sluggishness, shakiness, and other disturbed movement patterns; moreover, side effects such as weight gain (Lieberman et al. 2005) can compromise self-esteem and confidence, and this may negatively impact work participation. Studies evaluating the effect of medication on the acquisition of a job, however, report no significant effect of the type of medication (Mueser et al. 2001) or self-reported adherence to this medication (Razzano et al. 2005).

Related to Experience and Skills

Level of Education

Despite some studies linking a low level of education to lower job acquisition (Mueser et al. 2001; Burke-Miller et al. 2006), most studies conclude that this factor is not a significant obstacle (Catty et al. 2008; Campbell et al. 2010; Metcalfe et al. 2016; Fortin et al. 2017; Corbière et al. 2017). However, it is noteworthy that the level of education of people with SMI is significantly lower than the general population (Bond and Drake 2008). Indeed, the experience of SMI typically begins during adolescence and young adulthood, disrupting education, career planning, and work experiences. The typical onset age of psychotic disorders is from 10 to 30 years, which usually coincides with formal education and work training. This is a critical time-period for developing a work identity, gaining experiences, relationships, and completing education and training associated with adult work. As a consequence, the jobs most often acquired by participants are also entry-level jobs that do not require specialized training, such as service or clerical jobs (Mueser et al. 2004). There is little research on people with SMI and higher levels of education. In Wong et al.'s study (2004), higher-more educated people had greater difficulty getting a job. These authors hypothesized that it is more difficult to acquire a job for people with higher qualifications because of stronger competition for more specialized jobs compared to entry-level positions. It has also been hypothesized that people with higher levels of education and well-established careers before the development of mental health problems have specific challenges when returning to work, for example, the need to reassess one's expectations and to grieve the previous employment (Becker and Drake 2003).

Work History
In contrast to education level, employment history is much more often reported as a significant predictor of competitive job acquisition. In the majority of studies incorporating this factor, having held a job in the past year (Mueser et al. 2001; Fortin et al. 2017), the last 2 years (Metcalfe et al. 2016), or the last 5 years (Burke-Miller et al. 2006; Catty et al. 2008; Campbell et al. 2010) facilitates work integration. These results can also be more nuanced. For example, in a study conducted by Fortin et al. (2017), having job experience in the previous year facilitated the acquisition of another job, whereas job experience from more than 1 year before the start of the program (up to 5 years back) was not of benefit. To summarize these results, a longer period of work inactivity appears to be a significant obstacle to the acquisition of a competitive job (Corbière et al. 2011, 2017).

In their study on factors predicting job tenure conducted more than 20 years ago, Xie et al. (1997) reported work history as the only significant variable, resulting in a 2% drop in the risk of job termination of people with a SMI for each month of paid work. In 2008, work history remained a significant factor of work-related outcomes: people with SMI who had worked for at least 1 month in the previous 5 years were more than twice as likely to enter competitive employment as those who had not, and these workers also obtained their first job more quickly and were more likely to work for more hours (Catty et al. 2008). The authors stressed the nature of the work history factor since it is statistical per se (number of months, or years), not *a highly clinically meaningful factor* and can, consequently, hide unmeasured variables such as self-esteem, work motivation, social skills, and social functioning (Campbell et al. 2010). Or it can indirectly predict work outcomes via work centrality, work motivation, and job search behaviors (Corbière et al. 2017).

Skills, Competencies (Work-Related, Job Search-Related)
According to (Fortin et al. 2017), to have recent work experience is a significant facilitator for acquiring a competitive job. People with little or no employment experience may not be aware of which types of jobs may match their abilities and which methods or steps they could take to find these jobs. This lack of knowledge

about job search skills is reported in several qualitative studies to be a significant barrier as perceived by people with SMI (Netto et al. 2016; Hanisch et al. 2017). In addition, unlike those with little or no work experience, recent job-seekers can rely on generic work-related skills, such as punctuality, hygiene, and valued attitudes in the workplace, or more specific skills, such as the use of information technology. It may then be easier to assert these skills to potential employers. However, programs that develop work-related skills prior to supported employment programs do not improve the chances of entering a competitive job (Bond et al. 1995).

Job Match

Successful job tenure results are often perceived by researchers as a good person-environment fit and optimal supports (Glynn et al. 2016). Yet, the job match is of central importance in the job acquisition process as well; indeed, a specific work activity of the employment specialist working in the community is to develop employment, which means establishing links through direct and indirect contact with potential employers that match the objectives of the participants. The notion of job match, often defined as the degree to which a given job matches the interests, values, and competencies of the client, has received little attention in the psychiatry research literature, while a good job match can impact work satisfaction, work performance, and, ultimately, job tenure (Kukla and Bond 2012).

Some authors have examined the similarity between a client's job preferences, based on type of job (occupational types) and expressed before obtaining employment, and the actual job attained, usually using a score calculated with codes from the Dictionary of Occupational Titles. The results indicated longer job tenures for good matches, approximately twice as many weeks in these jobs as people who were in jobs that did not match their baseline preferences (Mueser et al. 2001). However, these results were not replicated by Bond et al. (2013), who criticized the limitation of the first digit of the Dot code as a crude measure. Kukla and Bond (2012) used a more precise tool to evaluate job match, including interest/enjoyment, perceived competencies, and meaningfulness. The total score and the subscale interest/enjoyment correlated significantly with months worked in the first job obtained. Contrary to their hypotheses, no significant association was found between the perceived competency and meaningfulness subscales and job tenure. In contrast with Bégin and Corbière's study (2012) based on the theory of Holland, particularly regarding job match competencies, the results indicated that the more congruent the job match between the person and the attained job, the lower the likelihood of losing employment, controlling for covariates such as gender, age, education, work history, psychiatric diagnosis, severity of symptoms, and disability benefits. Even if these results seem inconclusive, the objective of helping clients obtain personally meaningful and rewarding jobs remains a top priority, reflecting one of the main principles of supported employment programs (Bond et al. 2013).

Social Skills, Social Adjustment, and Social Functioning

Although social skills are perceived as important for job acquisition by people with SMI, few quantitative studies have focused specifically on this factor (Hanisch et al.

2017). Two studies used self-reported measures of social adjustment to determine its contribution in predicting job acquisition. First, Mueser et al. (2001), using the Social Adjustment Scale (SAS), found that patients who reported better adjustment in their social leisure activities were also more likely to acquire employment. These authors proposed that the motivation to relate to people is the common factor explaining both the best adjustment in social leisure activities and the acquisition of a job. Conversely, Catty et al. (2008) and Corbière et al. (2017) found no significant relationship between the level of social functioning – using the Groningen Social Disabilities Schedule (GSDS) and the Multnomah Community Ability Scale (MCAS), respectively – and the acquisition of a job. However, the Global Assessment of Functioning (GAF) could predict job tenure when assessed at baseline (Evensen et al. 2017). Finally, Allott et al. (2013) were interested in social cognition, specifically in abilities related to theory of mind and the recognition of emotions, and their connection to the acquisition of competitive employment. The results obtained were, however, not significant.

Related to Self and Motivational Factors

Self-Stigma, Self-Esteem, Self-Confidence, and Self-Efficacy

As we have seen above, social stigma is a major obstacle to obtaining competitive employment. Moreover, stigma is not just an external factor, and individuals with SMI who agree with the stereotypes conveyed by society and apply them to their own situation experience profound negative consequences (Corrigan et al. 2009). This internalized stigma, or self-stigma, tinges the image that individuals have of themselves and their abilities, leading to a decrease in their self-esteem and sense of self-efficacy (Lysaker et al. 2007). In the research conducted to date, the findings on the relationship between general self-esteem and job acquisition are, nevertheless, contradictory. In fact, one study concluded that the link between level of self-esteem and baseline change in self-esteem of people with SMI during their supported employment program was strongly associated with employment status at 2-year follow-up (Evensen et al. 2017), while two studies found no significant relationship between self-esteem at baseline and job acquisition at 6- and 18-month follow-up (Catty et al. 2008; Corbière et al. 2011). Corbière et al.'s study (2017) used a specific measure of self-esteem as a worker instead of a general self-esteem measure and found that the scores obtained by people with SMI were significantly related to job acquisition.

Also, although overall self-esteem is not clearly and repeatedly associated with the acquisition of a competitive job, it is related to other factors more directly linked to the chances of acquiring a competitive job, such as self-efficacy (Corbière et al. 2011). Self-efficacy, in this context, corresponds to the belief that the person has the ability to put in place the active behaviors needed to gain a competitive job. Again, the results measuring the effects of self-efficacy on job acquisition are inconclusive. Indeed, two studies reported nonsignificant effects (Corbière et al. 2011; Waynor et al. 2016). Based on the theories above, it is highly likely that good self-esteem and self-efficacy are important factors, but they are not sufficient to gain employment. The longer job tenures of people with SMI in Evensen et al.' study (2017) coincided with higher scores on self-esteem at baseline and positive changes across time.

Perceived Barriers

Another important factor in addition to self-perception is the number of perceived barriers to employment. Two studies have found that a greater number of perceived barriers is linked to a lower chance of acquiring a job (Johannesen et al. 2007; Corbière et al. 2017). In another study, however, a higher number of barriers to employment was not found to be directly related to more chances of employment acquisition but was found to negatively impact self-esteem, self-efficacy, and work-related motivation (Corbière et al. 2011). A key goal of supported employment programs is to help clients overcome the barriers they meet while searching for a job. In a study conducted by Johannesen et al. (2009), participants enrolled in a vocational rehabilitation program whose number of perceived barriers to employment had decreased during the intervention were found to be less likely to acquire a job than those whose number of perceived obstacles remained stable. It is possible that the support received from the employment specialist does not reduce the number of obstacles perceived, but, rather, increases the feeling of being able to overcome them. It was according to this hypothesis that Corbière et al. (2004) developed the Barriers to Employment and Coping Efficacy Scale (BECES) that assesses not only the perceived barriers to get a job for the person with SMI but also the feeling of being able to overcome each of them. Once employed, participants who had significant and positive changes in barriers related to illness worked nearly twice as many weeks (34 weeks on average) as those who provided stable barrier ratings (19 weeks on average). Interestingly, this effect highlights the importance of the management of illness in the workplace as mentioned above (Johannesen et al. 2009).

Motivation, Commitment to Work, and Behavioral Motivation

Several studies have investigated the link between motivation to work and acquisition of a job. In one study conducted with participants with a diagnosis in the schizophrenia spectrum (Mueser et al. 2001), those who expressed their desire to work at the beginning of the study were more likely to have had a job at the follow-up. Motivation can be more directly measured using validated and reliable tools like the Motivation to Find a Job Scale (Villotti et al. 2015). In two studies that used this scale as a measure of motivation, one found motivation had a significant effect on the acquisition of a job (Corbière et al. 2017), while the effect was not significant in the other study (Fortin et al. 2017). In general, motivation alone is not sufficient to guarantee the acquisition of a job; although they may show motivation to find a competitive job, not all participants will be equally active in the process of achieving this goal. Regardless of their expressed interest in work, some individuals are more passive and do not translate this interest into active behaviors or efforts toward their goal (Mueser et al. 2001; Alverson et al. 2006). Mueser et al. (2001) used the term "behavioral motivation" to differentiate the expressed motivation from the demonstrated one. In the same vein, Corbière et al. (2011) found that people who were most motivated to work were also those who used the most preparatory strategies and job search strategies. Motivation is a complex process due to the neurological and cognitive processes involved. According to both the theory of planned behavior and the self-efficacy theory, to act toward a goal, the person must think that the goal is valuable, attainable, and that he/she has the control and capacity to attain that goal.

Discussion

Having a competitive job represents the common means of achieving adequate economic resources essential for people to fully participate in society; it is perhaps the most consistent and profound way in which individuals interface with their social, economic, and political context (Blustein 2008). Unfortunately, the employment situation for people with SMI remains difficult, perpetrated by multiple interacting factors that systematically disadvantage mentally ill individuals in securing and maintaining employment.

This chapter reviews individual and environmental factors related to the work integration of people with SMI. While predictors of job acquisition and tenure in people with SMI enrolled in supported employment programs have been of considerable interest in recent decades, studies have yielded inconsistent findings regarding individual and environmental factors to explain the work integration of people with SMI. In the following paragraphs, we make emerging statements and eventual recommendations on this research topic.

First, several studies focused on individual factors, particularly those related to demographics (age, gender, etc.), to explain the work integration of people with SMI. Since the start of this millennium and because of inconsistent findings with these demographic factors, researchers addressed this issue by further investigating modifiable factors (versus non-modifiable). In this vein, some researchers have evaluated clinical and cognitive factors by polishing their evaluation and developing new interventions such as cognitive remediation programs (e.g., McGurk et al. 2005), also called *augmented* supported employment when combined with supported employment programs. Other authors focused on self-related factors (e.g., self-efficacy, self-esteem, work motivation).

Although relevant, these targeted factors focused on the individual characteristics of people with SMI. Furthermore, rare are the studies including these factors in a theoretical framework to better understand their direct and indirect links to predict job acquisition or job tenure. Understanding the direct and indirect relationships between these factors can support the work of employment specialists, providing better interventions for the work integration of people with SMI. We strongly recommend that future research include theories to support comprehension of the work integration and work-related outcomes.

Second, even though researchers argued, two decades ago, for assessments of the work environment, little research has been conducted in this area. The same is true for the evaluation of stakeholders involved in the work integration of people with SMI. Work accommodation is recognized as a crucial element requiring interactions and communication between stakeholders to help people with SMI keep employment. The implementation of work accommodations is a social process in which employment specialists must examine existing social interactions and supports in the workplace. As suggested by Williams et al. (2016), considering different perspectives as well as actions and perceptions could expand our current knowledge of the conditions facilitating sustainable work. Consequently, research efforts should focus on investigating the feasibility and effectiveness of measures implying several stakeholders (e.g., immediate supervisor, employment specialist) to overcome employment obstacles.

Third, from a temporal contiguity perspective, we have little information about the effect of the rehabilitation process on targeted variables, particularly psychosocial variables (e.g., professional identity, recovery). As Johannesen et al. (2009) mentioned, it seems plausible that initial barrier levels should be most predictive of early steps in the job process (job attainment), while subsequent changes in those barriers, reflecting rehabilitation progress over time, should be most predictive of later steps in the process (keeping the job). Further investigations are needed to establish the actual benefits of work integration on self-perceptions within a longitudinal design as well as their potential fluctuations with time. Thus, two important questions could be addressed: whether self-perceptions change during the rehabilitation process and whether these changes significantly predict work outcomes, job acquisition, and job tenure.

Fourth, competitive job acquisition has been defined as community jobs that pay at least minimum wage that any person can apply for, including full-time and part-time jobs (Becker et al. 2007). The details of this definition can vary subtly from a study to another, making generalization of results across studies quite complex. In their 2017 Cochrane review, Suijkerbuijk et al. (2017) identified this important limitation since job acquisition can sometimes be defined by the period of time in competitive employment (calculated in days or months) or a minimum number of hours worked per week.

The results for evaluation of job tenure are even more inconsistent. For example, outcomes such as the time worked (e.g., hours, days), number of days between the first day worked and the date of termination from the job, weeks on the longest-held competitive job, and total number of weeks worked on competitive jobs during the follow-up are all used to evaluate job tenure. Other authors suggest not assessing job tenure in a specific job but rather steady employment over the long term (Bond and Kukla 2011), i.e., the continuity of work participation (Williams et al. 2016).

In brief, the lack of a standardized definition of competitive employment, job acquisition, and job tenure for people with SMI may explain the inconsistencies between categories of factors (e.g., demographics, self-related, work environment) and work outcomes (Evensen et al. 2017). Consequently, we recommend using a clear definition and operationalization of work outcome in evaluation studies.

Fifth, given that we are most interested in enhancing recovery outcomes for people with SMI in the long term, rather than merely in the short term, more studies on maintaining competitive employment are needed to get a better understanding of whether the costs and effort are worthwhile in the long term for both the individual and society. Moreover, in a multilevel evaluation, authors should consider the social security system (e.g., pension disability), mental health and vocational services (e.g., access to supported employment programs), training of employment specialists, as well as work values and expectations for people with SMI (societal values) in their own country to describe the big picture of work integration of people with SMI.

To conclude, the myriad of factors expected to open the doors to the world of work for people with SMI, such as systems and politics strategies, legislation and pension benefits in support of disabled persons, advancement in treatment efficacy, and development of vocational services and programs, alongside the desire and ability of individuals to work productively, have not had the anticipated impact. As a result, job acquisition and job tenure remain a major challenge for this population. Consequently, considerable work remains to address the challenge of mental health disability in the workplace. Only by integrating the efforts of researchers, policy-makers, healthcare practitioners, employers, and persons with mental health disabilities can the challenge of mental disability in the workplace be addressed.

Cross-References

▶ Facilitating Competitive Employment for People with Disabilities
▶ IGLOO: A Framework for Return to Work Among Workers with Mental Health Problems
▶ Occupational Determinants of Cognitive Decline and Dementia
▶ Reducing Inequalities in Employment of People with Disabilities

References

Allott KA, Cotton SM, Chinnery GL et al (2013) The relative contribution of neurocognition and social cognition to 6-month vocational outcomes following individual placement and support in first-episode psychosis. Schizophr Res 150:136–143. https://doi.org/10.1016/j.schres.2013.07.047

Alverson H, Carpenter E, Drake RE (2006) An ethnographic study of job seeking among people with severe mental illness. Psychiatr Rehabil J 30:15–22. https://doi.org/10.2975/30.2006.15.22

Anthony WA, Mizock L (2014) Evidence-based processes in an era of recovery: implications for rehabilitation counseling and research. Rehabil Couns Bull 57:219–227. https://doi.org/10.1177/0034355213507979

Barrowclough C, Meier P, Beardmore R, Emsley R (2010) Predicting therapeutic alliance in clients with psychosis and substance misuse. J Nerv Ment Dis 198:373–377. https://doi.org/10.1097/NMD.0b013e3181da4d4e

Bassett J, Lloyd C, Bassett H (2001) Work issues for young people with psychosis: barriers to employment. Br J Occup Ther 64:66–72. https://doi.org/10.1177/030802260106400203

Becker DR, Drake RE (2003) Highly trained individuals and work. In: A working life for people with severe mental illness. Oxford University Press, New York

Becker DR, Whitley R, Bailey EL, Drake RE (2007) Long-term employment trajectories among participants with severe mental illness in supported employment. Psychiatr Serv 58:922–928. https://doi.org/10.1176/appi.ps.58.7.922

Bégin É, Corbière M (2012) Les compétences perçues de la personne ayant un trouble mental grave: un facteur significatif de maintien en emploi. Can J Commun Ment Health 31:35–50. https://doi.org/10.7870/cjcmh-2012-0012

Bejerholm U, Areberg C, Hofgren C et al (2015) Individual placement and support in Sweden – a randomized controlled trial. Nord J Psychiatry 69:57–66. https://doi.org/10.3109/08039488.2014.929739

Blustein DL (2008) The role of work in psychological health and well-being: a conceptual, historical, and public policy perspective. Am Psychol 63:228–240. https://doi.org/10.1037/0003-066X.63.4.228

Bond GR, Drake RE (2008) Predictors of competitive employment among patients with schizophrenia. Curr Opin Psychiatry 21:362–369

Bond GR, Kukla M (2011) Is job tenure brief in individual placement and support (IPS) employment programs? Psychiatr Serv 62:950–953

Bond GR, Xie H, Drake RE (2007) Can SSDI and SSI beneficiaries with mental illness benefit from evidence-based supported employment? Psychiatr Serv 58:1412–1420. https://doi.org/10.1176/appi.ps.58.11.1412

Bond GR, Dietzen LL, McGrew JH, Miller LD (1995) Accelerating entry into supported employment for persons with severe psychiatric disabilities. Rehabil Psychol 40:75–94. https://doi.org/10.1037/0090-5550.40.2.75

Bond GR, Peterson AE, Becker DR, Drake RE (2012) Validation of the revised individual placement and support fidelity scale (IPS-25). Psychiatr Serv (Washington, DC) 63:758–763. https://doi.org/10.1176/appi.ps.201100476

Bond GR, Campbell K, Becker DR (2013) A test of the occupational matching hypothesis for rehabilitation clients with severe mental illness. J Occup Rehabil 23:261–269. https://doi.org/10.1007/s10926-012-9388-7

Bordin ES (1979) The generalizability of the psychoanalytic concept of the working alliance. Psychother Theory Res Pract 16:252–260. https://doi.org/10.1037/h0085885

Boycott N, Akhtar A, Schneider J (2015) "Work is good for me": views of mental health service users seeking work during the UK recession, a qualitative analysis. J Ment Health (Abingdon) 24:93–97. https://doi.org/10.3109/09638237.2015.1019044

Bruns EJ, Kerns SEU, Pullmann MD et al (2016) Research, data, and evidence-based treatment use in state Behavioral health systems, 2001–2012. Psychiatr Serv (Washington, DC) 67:496–503. https://doi.org/10.1176/appi.ps.201500014

Burke-Miller JK, Cook JA, Grey DD et al (2006) Demographic characteristics and employment among people with severe mental illness in a multisite study. Community Ment Health J 42:143–159. https://doi.org/10.1007/s10597-005-9017-4

Butler G, Howard L, Choi S, Thornicroft G (2010) Characteristics of people with severe mental illness who obtain employment | the psychiatrist | Cambridge Core. Psychiatrist 34:47–50. https://doi.org/10.1192/pb.bp.108.021683

Campbell K, Bond GR, Drake RE et al (2010) Client predictors of employment outcomes in high-fidelity supported employment: a regression analysis. J Nerv Ment Dis 198:556–563. https://doi.org/10.1097/NMD.0b013e3181ea1e53

Canadian Human Rights Act, R.S.C., 1985, c. H-6 Stat. (1985)

Catty J, Lissouba P, White S et al (2008) Predictors of employment for people with severe mental illness: results of an international six-Centre randomised controlled trial. Br J Psychiatry 192:224. https://doi.org/10.1192/bjp.bp.107.041475

Charette-Dussault É, Corbière M (2019) An integrative review of the barriers to job acquisition for people with severe mental illnesses. J Nerv Ment Dis 207:523–537. https://doi.org/10.1097/NMD.0000000000001013

Cook JA (2006) Employment barriers for persons with psychiatric disabilities: update of a report for the President's commission. Psychiatr Serv (Washington, DC) 57:1391–1405. https://doi.org/10.1176/ps.2006.57.10.1391

Corbière M, Lecomte T (2009) Vocational services offered to people with severe mental illness. J Ment Health 18:38–50. https://doi.org/10.1080/09638230701677779

Corbière M, Mercier C, Lesage A (2004) Perceptions of barriers to employment, coping efficacy, and career search efficacy in people with mental illness. J Career Assess. https://doi.org/10.1177/1069072704267738

Corbière M, Mercier C, Lesage A, Villeneuve K (2005) L'Insertion au travail de personnes souffrant d'une maladie mentale: analyse des caractéristiques de la personne [Professional integration of individuals with a mental illness: an analysis of individual characteristics]. Can J Psychiatry Rev Can Psychiatr 50:722–733. https://doi.org/10.1177/070674370505001112

Corbière M, Lesage A, Villeneuve K, Mercier C (2006) Le maintien en emploi de personnes souffrant d'une maladie mentale. Santé Ment. Au Qué 31:215–235. https://doi.org/10.7202/014813ar

Corbière M, Zaniboni S, Lecomte T et al (2011) Job acquisition for people with severe mental illness enrolled in supported employment programs: a theoretically grounded empirical study. J Occup Rehabil 21:342–354. https://doi.org/10.1007/s10926-011-9315-3

Corbière M, Negrini A, Dewa CS (2013) Mental health problems and mental disorders: linked determinants to work participation and work functioning. In: Loisel P, Anema H et al (eds) Handbook of work disability. Springer, New York, pp 267–288

Corbière M, Villotti P, Lecomte T, Bond G, Lesage A, Goldner E (2014) Work accommodations and natural supports for maintaining employment. Psychiatr Rehabil J 37(2):90–98. https://doi.org/10.1037/prj0000033

Corbière M, Lecomte T, Reinharz D et al (2017) Predictors of acquisition of competitive employment for people enrolled in supported employment programs. J Nerv Ment Dis 205:275–282. https://doi.org/10.1097/NMD.0000000000000612

Corrigan PW, Larson JE, Rüsch N (2009) Self-stigma and the "why try" effect: impact on life goals and evidence-based practices. World Psychiatry 8:75–81

Disability Discrimination Act of 1992. Retrieved from http://www9.austlii.edu.au/cgi-bin/viewdb/au/legis/cth/consol_act/dda1992264/

Disability Services Act 1986, Act no. 129 (1986)

Drake RE, Bond GR (2014) Introduction to the special issue on individual placement and support. Psychiatr Rehabil J 37:76–78. https://doi.org/10.1037/prj0000083

Drake RE, Bond GR, Rapp C (2006) Explaining the variance within supported employment programs: comment on "what predicts supported employment outcomes?". Community Ment Health J 42:315–318. https://doi.org/10.1007/s10597-006-9038-7

Drake RE, Frey W, Bond GR et al (2013a) Assisting social security disability insurance beneficiaries with schizophrenia, bipolar disorder, or major depression in returning to work. Am J Psychiatry 170:1433–1441. https://doi.org/10.1176/appi.ajp.2013.13020214

Drake RE, Xie H, Bond GR et al (2013b) Early psychosis and employment. Schizophr Res 146:111–117. https://doi.org/10.1016/j.schres.2013.02.012

Drake RE, Bond GR, Goldman HH et al (2016) Individual placement and support services boost employment for people with serious mental illnesses, but funding is lacking. Health Aff 35:1098–1105. https://doi.org/10.1377/hlthaff.2016.0001

Employment Equity Act, S.C. 1995, c. 44 Stat. (1995)

Evensen S, Ueland T, Lystad JU et al (2017) Employment outcome and predictors of competitive employment at 2-year follow-up of a vocational rehabilitation programme for individuals with schizophrenia in a high-income welfare society. Nord J Psychiatry 71:180–187. https://doi.org/10.1080/08039488.2016.1247195

Fortin G, Lecomte T, Corbière M (2017) Does personality influence job acquisition and tenure in people with severe mental illness enrolled in supported employment programs? J Ment Health 26:248–256. https://doi.org/10.1080/09638237.2016.1276534

Glynn SM, Marder SR, Noordsy DL et al (2017) An RCT evaluating the effects of skills training and medication type on work outcomes among patients with schizophrenia. Psychiatr Serv (Washington, DC) 68:271–277. https://doi.org/10.1176/appi.ps.201500171

Glynn SM, Marder SR, Noordsy DL, O'Keefe C, Becker DR, Drake RE, Sugar CA (2016) An RCT evaluating the effects of skills training and medication type on work outcomes among patients with schizophrenia. Psychiatr Serv 68:271–277. https://doi.org/10.1176/appi.ps.201500171

Hampson M, Hicks R, Watt B (2016) Understanding the employment barriers and support needs of people living with psychosis. Qual Rep 21:870–886

Hanisch S, Wrynne C, Weigl M (2017) Perceived and actual barriers to work for people with mental illness. J Vocat Rehabil 46:19–30. https://doi.org/10.3233/JVR-160839

Hipes C, Lucas J, Phelan JC, White RC (2016) The stigma of mental illness in the labor market. Soc Sci Res 56:16–25. https://doi.org/10.1016/j.ssresearch.2015.12.001

Hoffmann H, Jäckel D, Glauser S et al (2014) Long-term effectiveness of supported employment: 5-year follow-up of a randomized controlled trial. Am J Psychiatry 171:1183–1190. https://doi.org/10.1176/appi.ajp.2014.13070857

Johannesen JK, McGrew JH, Griss ME, Born D (2007) Perception of illness as a barrier to work in consumers of supported employment services. J Vocat Rehabil 27:39–47

Johannesen JK, McGrew JH, Griss ME, Born DL (2009) Change in self-perceived barriers to employment as a predictor of vocational rehabilitation outcome. Am J Psychiatr Rehabil 12:295–316. https://doi.org/10.1080/15487760903248358

Kukla M, Bond GR (2012) Job match and job tenure in persons with severe mental illness. J Rehabil 78:11–15

Lanctôt N, Bergeron-Brossard P, Sanquirgo N, Corbière M (2013) Causal attributions of job loss among people with psychiatric disabilities. Psychiatr Rehabil J 36:146–152. https://doi.org/10.1037/prj0000002

Leff HS, Cook JA, Gold PB et al (2005) Effects of job development and job support on competitive employment of persons with severe mental illness. Psychiatr Serv (Washington, DC) 56:1237–1244. https://doi.org/10.1176/appi.ps.56.10.1237

Lieberman JA, Stroup TS, McEvoy JP et al (2005) Effectiveness of antipsychotic drugs in patients with chronic schizophrenia. N Engl J Med 353:1209–1223. https://doi.org/10.1056/NEJMoa051688

Llerena K, Reddy LF, Kern RS (2017) The role of experiential and expressive negative symptoms on job obtainment and work outcome in individuals with schizophrenia. Schizophr Res. https://doi.org/10.1016/j.schres.2017.06.001

Lysaker PH, Roe D, Yanos PT (2007) Toward understanding the insight paradox: internalized stigma moderates the association between insight and social functioning, hope, and self-esteem among people with schizophrenia spectrum disorders. Schizophr Bull 33:192–199. https://doi.org/10.1093/schbul/sbl016

MacDonald-Wilson KL, Rogers ES, Massaro JM et al (2002) An investigation of reasonable workplace accommodations for people with psychiatric disabilities: quantitative findings from a multi-site study. Community Ment Health J 38:35–50. https://doi.org/10.1023/A:1013955830779

Marwaha S, Johnson S (2005) Views and experiences of employment among people with psychosis: a qualitative descriptive study. Int J Soc Psychiatry 51:302–316. https://doi.org/10.1177/0020764005057386

McDowell C, Fossey E (2015) Workplace accommodations for people with mental illness: a scoping review. J Occup Rehabil 25:197–206. https://doi.org/10.1007/s10926-014-9512-y

McGahey E, Waghorn G, Lloyd C et al (2016) Formal plan for self-disclosure enhances supported employment outcomes among young people with severe mental illness. Early Interv Psychiatry 10:178–185. https://doi.org/10.1111/eip.12196

McGurk SR, Mueser KT (2004) Cognitive functioning, symptoms, and work in supported employment: a review and heuristic model. Schizophr Res 70:147–173. https://doi.org/10.1016/j.schres.2004.01.009

McGurk SR, Mueser KT (2006) Cognitive and clinical predictors of work outcomes in clients with schizophrenia receiving supported employment services: 4-year follow-up. Admin Pol Ment Health 33:598–606. https://doi.org/10.1007/s10488-006-0070-2

McGurk SR, Mueser KT, Pascaris A (2005) Cognitive training and supported employment for persons with severe mental illness: one-year results from a randomized controlled trial. Schizophr Bull 31:898–909. https://doi.org/10.1093/schbul/sbi037

Metcalfe JD, Drake RE, Bond GR (2016) Predicting employment in the mental health treatment study: do client factors matter? Admin Pol Ment Health. https://doi.org/10.1007/s10488-016-0774-x

Metcalfe JD, Drake RE, Bond GR (2018) Economic, labor, and regulatory moderators of the effect of individual placement and support among people with severe mental illness: a systematic review and meta-analysis. Schizophr Bull 44:22–31. https://doi.org/10.1093/schbul/sbx132

Mueser KT, McGurk SR (2014) Supported employment for persons with serious mental illness: current status and future directions. L'Encéphale 40:S45–S56. https://doi.org/10.1016/j.encep.2014.04.008

Mueser KT, Salyers MP, Mueser PR (2001) A prospective analysis of work in schizophrenia. Schizophr Bull 27:281–296

Mueser KT, Becker DR, Torrey WC, et al (1997) Work and nonvocational domains of functioning in persons with severe mental illness: A longitudinal analysis. J Nerv Ment Dis 185:419–26. https://doi.org/10.1097/00005053-199707000-00001

Mueser KT, Clark RE, Haines M et al (2004) The Hartford study of supported employment for persons with severe mental illness. J Consult Clin Psychol 72:479–490. https://doi.org/10.1037/0022-006X.72.3.479

National Disability Strategy (2010–2020). Retrieved from https://www.dss.gov.au/our-responsibilities/disability-and-carers/publications-articles/policy-research/national-disability-strategy-2010-2020

Netto JA, Yeung P, Cocks E, McNamara B (2016) Facilitators and barriers to employment for people with mental illness: a qualitative study. J Vocat Rehabil 44:61–72. https://doi.org/10.3233/JVR-150780

Pachoud B (2017) Activité professionnelle et processus de rétablissement [Employment and recovery process]. Santé Ment Au Qué 42:57–70. https://doi.org/10.7202/1041914ar

Puig O, Thomas KR, Twamley EW (2016) Age and improved attention predict work attainment in combined compensatory cognitive training and supported employment for people with severe mental illness. J Nerv Ment Dis 204:869–872. https://doi.org/10.1097/NMD.0000000000000604

Razzano LA, Cook JA, Burke-Miller JK et al (2005) Clinical factors associated with employment among people with severe mental illness: findings from the employment intervention demonstration program. J Nerv Ment Dis 193:705–713

Resnick SG, Bond GR (2001) The Indiana job satisfaction scale: job satisfaction in vocational rehabilitation for people with severe mental illness. Psychiatr Rehabil J 25:12–19. https://doi.org/10.1037/h0095055

Russinova Z, Griffin S, Bloch P et al (2011) Workplace prejudice and discrimination toward individuals with mental illnesses. J Vocat Rehabil 35:227–241

Salyers MP, Becker DR, Drake RE et al (2004) A ten-year follow-up of a supported employment program. Psychiatr Serv (Washington, DC) 55:302–308. https://doi.org/10.1176/appi.ps.55.3.302

Sauvé G, Lepage M, Corbière M (2018) Impacts de la combinaison de programmes de soutien à l'emploi et de remédiation cognitive sur le maintien en emploi de personnes souffrant de schizophrénie: une méta-analyse. Ann Méd-Psychol Rev Psychiatr. https://doi.org/10.1016/j.amp.2018.01.015

Scaratti C, Leonardi M, Silvaggi F et al (2018) Mapping European welfare models: state of the art of strategies for professional integration and reintegration of persons with chronic diseases. Int J Environ Res Public Health 15. https://doi.org/10.3390/ijerph15040781

Schindler VP (2014) Community engagement: outcomes for occupational therapy students, faculty and clients. Occup Ther Int 21:71–80. https://doi.org/10.1002/oti.1364

Slade M (2009) Personal recovery and mental illness: a guide for mental health professionals. Cambridge University Press, New York

Suijkerbuijk YB, Schaafsma FG, van Mechelen JC et al (2017) Interventions for obtaining and maintaining employment in adults with severe mental illness, a network meta-analysis. Cochrane Database Syst Rev 9:CD011867. https://doi.org/10.1002/14651858.CD011867.pub2

Taskila T, Steadman K, Gulliford J et al (2014) Working with schizophrenia: experts' views on barriers and pathways to employment and job retention. J Vocat Rehabil 41:29–44. https://doi.org/10.3233/JVR-140696

The Americans with Disabilities Act, 42 U.S.C. 12101 et seq. Stat. (1990)

The Rehabilitation Act of 1973, Pub. L. 93-112 Stat. (1973)

Tsang HWH, Leung AY, Chung RCK et al (2010) Review on vocational predictors: a systematic review of predictors of vocational outcomes among individuals with schizophrenia: an update since 1998. Aust N Z J Psychiatry 44:495–504. https://doi.org/10.3109/00048671003785716

Twamley EW, Narvaez JM, Becker DR et al (2008) Supported employment for middle-aged and older people with schizophrenia. Am J Psychiatr Rehabil 11:76–89. https://doi.org/10.1080/15487760701853326

United Nations (UN) (2006) Convention on the rights of persons with disabilities. https://www.un.org/development/desa/disabilities/convention-on-the-rights-of-persons-with-disabilities/convention-on-the-rights-of-persons-with-disabilities-2.html

Villotti P, Corbière M, Zaniboni S et al (2015) Evaluating the motivation to obtain and sustain employment in people with psychiatric disabilities. Psicol Soc 10:57–70. https://doi.org/10.1482/79437

Waghorn G, Spowart CE (2010) Managing personal information in supported employment for people with mental illness. In: Vocational rehabilitation and mental health. Wiley Blackwell, Oxford, UK, pp 201–210

Waynor WR, Gill KJ, Gao N (2016) The role of work related self-efficacy in supported employment for people living with serious mental illnesses. Psychiatr Rehabil J 39:62–67. https://doi.org/10.1037/prj0000156

Wewiorski NJ, Fabian ES (2004) Association between demographic and diagnostic factors and employment outcomes for people with psychiatric disabilities: a synthesis of recent research. Ment Health Serv Res 6:9–21

Whitley R, Kostick KM, Bush PW (2010) Desirable characteristics and competencies of supported employment specialists: an empirically-grounded framework. Admin Pol Ment Health 37:509–519. https://doi.org/10.1007/s10488-010-0297-9

Williams AE, Fossey E, Corbière M et al (2016) Work participation for people with severe mental illnesses: an integrative review of factors impacting job tenure. Aust Occup Ther J 63:65–85. https://doi.org/10.1111/1440-1630.12237

Wong KK, Chiu L, Tang S et al (2004) A supported employment program for people with mental illness in Hong Kong. Am J Psychiatr Rehabil. https://doi.org/10.1080/15487760490465004

Xie H, Dain BJ, Becker DR, Drake RE (1997) Job tenure among persons with severe mental illness. Rehabil Couns Bull 40:230–239

Concepts of Work Ability in Rehabilitation 30

Kari-Pekka Martimo and Esa-Pekka Takala

Contents

Introduction	552
Medical Concept of Work Ability	553
Balance Concept of Work Ability	554
Psychosocial Concepts of Work Ability	555
Biopsychosocial Concepts of Work Ability	557
The Integrated "Individual in the Work Community" Concept	560
The Employability Concept of Work Ability	562
Work Ability as a Social Construct of Various Systems	563
Emerging Concepts of Work Ability and Rehabilitation	564
Managing the Process of Rehabilitation	565
Cross-References	567
References	567

Abstract

How work ability is understood has an influence on what kinds of rehabilitation activities are implemented and which aspects of the activity are emphasized. This chapter presents eight concepts of work (dis)ability based on scientific literature. In the medical concept, work disability is related to the health status impaired by medical condition, and therefore rehabilitation is focused on restoring health with medical care. The balance concept emphasizes the role of rehabilitation in correcting the imbalance between the individual's functional capacity and the demands at work. Psychosocial concepts explain work ability with psychological and psychosocial theories, which are applied in rehabilitation and supporting return to work. Biopsychosocial concepts consider dynamic interactions of body,

K.-P. Martimo (✉)
Ilmarinen Mutual Pension Insurance Company, Helsinki, Finland
e-mail: kari-pekka.martimo@ilmarinen.fi

E.-P. Takala
Finnish Institute of Occupational Health, Helsinki, Finland
e-mail: Esa-Pekka.Takala@ttl.fi

mind, and environment, which all influence the results of rehabilitation. In the integrated "individual in the work community" concept, work ability is defined as the individual's performance at work, and work ability is best restored by developing work. The employability concept of work ability includes all actions that help the person to get work, retain employment, and advance in the employment. Work ability can also be understood as a social construct resulting from negotiations on the different levels of society. Emerging integrative concepts emphasize the processes of individual and contextual factors that define the person's capability to work. In rehabilitation, a comprehensive concept of work ability should be preferred and shared by all stakeholders to develop optimal rehabilitation processes aiming at the common goal.

Keywords

Work ability · Disability · Rehabilitation · ICF · Work Ability House · Employability · Return to work

Introduction

Rehabilitation is an active, time-limited collaboration where a person with disability together with professionals and other relevant stakeholders produces sustained reductions in the impact of disease and disability on daily life. Interventions focus on the individual, on the physical or social environment, or on a combination of these (Royal College of Physicians 2010). In this chapter the main emphasis is on work-related rehabilitation, i.e., in those aspects of both medical and vocational rehabilitation that aim to enable a disabled person to secure, retain, and advance in suitable employment and thereby to further such person's integration or reintegration into society (ILO 1983).

Vocational rehabilitation has been defined as a multidisciplinary evidence-based approach that is provided in different settings, services, and activities to working-age individuals with health-related impairments, limitations, or restrictions with work functioning, and the primary aim is to optimize work participation (Escorpizo et al. 2011b).

Work ability and work disability are the key concepts in the rehabilitation of working-age people. How these concepts are understood has an influence on rehabilitation, i.e., what kinds of work ability promotion and restoration activities are implemented and which aspects of the activity are emphasized. The understanding and expectations of the rehabilitee and the rehabilitation provider have an influence on the concepts and priorities of the rehabilitation process. The way they think can restrict attention to factors that are not important for the rehabilitation result and leave less room for factors that are vital for a successful rehabilitation process.

This chapter is based on a review by Järvikoski, Takala, Juvonen-Posti, and Härkäpää who published a review in Finnish on the concepts of work ability in

Table 1 Research traditions behind some concepts of work ability. (Modified from Järvikoski et al. 2018; Schultz et al. 2007); *RTW* return to work

Concept	Research traditions	Main determinants of RTW
Medical	Medicine	Medically verifiable injury
Psychosocial	Health and rehabilitation psychology	Psychosocial factors: beliefs, ideas, experiences, and expectations about RTW
Forensic	Medicine, psychology	Secondary gain, benefits, and losses
Ecological, based on research on work life and employment	Sociology, anthropology, social, organizational, and occupational health psychology	Proactive system-based policies and practices promoting RTW
Economic	Health economics	Financial incentives embedded in the macro system
Biopsychosocial	Multi- and transdisciplinary	Interaction of medical, psychosocial, and systemic factors on RTW

research and rehabilitation (Järvikoski et al. 2018). They describe research traditions behind some of the concepts of work ability (Table 1), while other concepts are combinations or applications of previously published concepts or theories. The aim is to describe the characteristics of each construct and to make a preliminary conclusion on what kinds of aspects are emphasized in rehabilitation when each of these viewpoints is followed.

Medical Concept of Work Ability

A disease or an injury has a central role in social insurance when assessing work disability. A medical condition is regarded as objectively assessable and independent of the individual's own aims and intentions. Medical methods are assumed to show objective findings, and the idea is to distinguish "real" work disability from untrue or pretended and to separate those who genuinely cannot work from those who for some reason do not want to work. The medical concept of work ability argues that without a medical condition an individual has full work ability, and all deviations from this are due to malingering. An individual may not be eligible for disability benefits if she/he has symptoms or functional limitations but no objective findings.

The traditional medical work ability concept can be divided into two parts. In the *injury-based concept*, the restoration of work ability and rehabilitation are considered to require rigorous medical examination to verify the causes of the injury, followed by treatment of the disease and injury. By means of the medical treatment, the main problems related to work ability can be solved. The application of this concept is supported by the fact that most new episodes of work disability (sickness absences) are short, and return to work (RTW) takes place without additional rehabilitation actions. Moreover, the diagnosis of some severe diseases alone can be considered to suffice as a proof of work disability.

In the *functional capacity-based concept*, work ability is primarily or exclusively assessed according to physical and mental functional capacity. Medical rehabilitation is focused on reducing the physical and mental impairments caused by disease/injury, as well as improving functional capacity through various exercises. As an example, in Great Britain, the work capability assessment method was developed to be used in assessing the person's eligibility for the Employment and Support Allowance. The basic principles of this method have been criticized (Baumberg et al. 2015), because it is a standardized test battery that does not include any assessment of work or work environment, nor any assessment of how the person copes with the demands at work.

The logical consequence of the medical concept is to cure the disease or injury and thereby restore functional ability and, consequently, work ability. The challenge is, however, that not all medical conditions are curable. The two main diagnostic groups related to work disability are mental and musculoskeletal disorders. Typical of these diagnoses is that they have recurrences or often become chronic. In addition, medical management of these conditions may be time-consuming. If, at the same time, also related work disability and absence from work prolong, RTW becomes more complicated. This linear concept assumes that a disease or an injury is associated with functional limitations and work disability. Most people, however, continue working in full capacity despite their medical conditions.

From the rehabilitation point of view, the functional capacity-based concept includes the use of interventions aiming at improving the individual's physical and mental capacity to restore work ability. The maintenance of physical capacity has also played a crucial role in many rehabilitation programs aiming at RTW. However, the evidence shows that the results of rehabilitation based on this concept are worse the longer the absence from work has lasted before the rehabilitation started. Consequently, rehabilitation is recommended before the absence from work is prolonged, applying a concept that is more comprehensive than the medical concept (Stay at Work and Return to Work Process Improvement Committee 2006).

Balance Concept of Work Ability

The most common methods to determine work ability are based on the individual's ability to continue working in the present job, given the characteristics of the job along with the employee's personal resources. Work disability is understood as a situation where the individual is no longer capable of performing at work because of workload or requirements at work. Additionally, work ability has been described as a result of the interaction between the individual and his/her work reflecting the balance between the individual's resources and the physical, mental, and social demands at work (Ilmarinen 2001).

Work ability has also been defined as the compatibility of physical, mental, social, environmental, and organizational requirements at work and the individual's capabilities (Fadyl et al. 2010). Therefore, the assessment of work ability must include many aspects: capacity to perform physically heavy work, ability to cope with cognitive and communicative tasks, as well as skills to act appropriately in the social context and environment of work (Turner-Stokes et al. 2014).

The balance concept of work ability emphasizes the fact that work disability caused by a disease or related functional impairment depends on work tasks and the work environment. The narrowest interpretation of the balance concept is based on the "workload-work strain" model, where workload leads to work strain, but the work strain is also modified by the personal characteristics (Ilmarinen et al. 2008). Additionally, it has been emphasized that work disability is always affected by work and the norms in work life. Therefore, the actions taken in the workplaces and, more generally, in work life constitute an important part of the solutions to work disability.

In rehabilitation, the balance between an individual and work can be restored by strengthening the individual's resources and/or by changing work or the work environment. If needed, the imbalance can be solved by finding new and more suitable work or retraining the individual to a new job with more compatible demands and exposures. The concept, however, does not consider the rehabilitee as an active player with his/her own aims and plans, nor does it pay attention to the divergent interests of the various parties in the rehabilitation network, or the collaboration needed to negotiate these differences.

The other aspect questioning the balance concept of work ability is the fact that changes at the workplace challenge the achieved balance. In addition, despite the apparent balance assessed by experts, sometimes RTW is not sustainable and remains unsuccessful.

Psychosocial Concepts of Work Ability

Psychosocial concepts are based on the need to find answers to questions, why a disease or an injury explains work disability so poorly, and how we can explain the delay in RTW even if the individual's functional capacity seems to be restored. In these cases, the individual's perceptions become crucial in relation to work ability, as well as all factors that have an impact on the individual's perception on the possibilities to continue at work and in work life in general. Psychosocial factors are usually categorized into employee-related individual factors and factors related to workplace or the context. It is important to differentiate psychosocial factors from mental problems, which both can be related to work disability (Sullivan et al. 2005).

According to the psychosocial theories, the core factors related to RTW are individual experiences, perceptions, beliefs, attitudes, coping mechanisms, and expectations concerning RTW. Especially the readiness to RTW and the decisions related to RTW have been studied (Franche and Krause 2002; Schultz et al. 2007; Young et al. 2005). Workplace-related factors include psychosocial stress factors, work climate, rewarding practices (e.g., effort-reward imbalance), perceived fairness, and supervisor support (Kivimäki et al. 2007).

In vocational rehabilitation, the psychosocial concepts emphasize the importance of the individual's perception of readiness, expectations related to RTW, problem-solving skills, and resource building, as well as various interventions related to work and the workplace. These approaches have increased the likelihood of RTW among, e.g., individuals with musculoskeletal disorders (e.g., Sullivan et al. 2005).

Studies applying the psychosocial concept have focused primarily on questions related to staying at work and RTW. The crucial question is which factors explain RTW or disability retirement when impairments caused by disease seem not to explain them? The situation has been explored using various processes and phase concepts, as well as using variables describing the psychological status of the rehabilitee or the psychosocial characteristics of the work environment.

The RTW process has been analyzed using the phase concepts of work disability and transtheoretical stages of change concept by Prochaska and DiClemente (Franche and Krause 2002). They assume that the longer work disability or the absence from work lasts, the stronger are the psychosocial factors prolonging the work disability. In their model, RTW advances from precontemplation to contemplation, preparation for change, active change, and finally maintenance of change through four psychosocial dimensions related to change. The psychosocial dimensions are ability to decide (factors promoting and hindering change), self-efficacy, processes preparing for change (perceptions and functional), and commitment to change (motivation), which requires, e.g., trust.

The factors related to health care, the insurance system, the work life, and the workplace are pertinent in the different stages of decision-making, action, and commitment. Decisions are based on, e.g., knowledge and personal expectations concerning the impact that the job might have on disease and symptoms, how permanent the possible job could be, how the employer and the colleagues react to RTW, as well as the possibly needed adjustments at work and in work conditions. The attitudes of various stakeholders and their willingness to collaborate have an influence on the individual process, and therefore, efforts must be made to influence them.

RTW has also been described as development process with several stages: being off-work, reentry, maintenance, and advancement (Young et al. 2005) (Fig. 1). RTW happens either to the previous job or a new job. The question is about making necessary adjustments in the present job to achieve a suitable job or exploring new alternatives. Various stakeholders decide whether work performance is acceptable or how it could be improved or how new achievable goals are set. At the maintenance stage, the individual's integration to the organizational culture is assessed, and new goals are set of advancing in employment, maintaining the present situation, or leaving the labor force. In the fourth, advancement stage, the question is about maintaining the good performance, formulating the plans to advance at work, and finding suitable opportunities. The RTW process can proceed systematically from one stage to another, but sometimes the individual must return to an earlier stage.

Besen et al. (2015) analyzed the relevance of individual psychosocial factors on successful RTW applying the stage concept of RTW, the concept of fear avoidance from pain research, and the theory of planned behavior. They studied two mechanisms that both influence the result of RTW attempts. One mechanism works through avoiding fears related to pain and activity restrictions: strong fears weaken positive

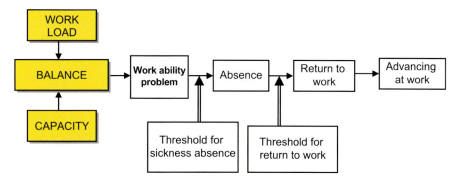

Fig. 1 Process of sickness absence and RTW. (Adapted from European Foundation for the Improvement of Living and Working Conditions 1997)

expectations concerning RTW, which in turn reduce the possibilities to successful RTW. The other mechanism works through the expectations of the employee in relation to the support offered by the workplace. The employees' perception of the support from the workplace showed to be related to the level of confidence they have concerning RTW (measured by return-to-work self-efficacy scale).

Biopsychosocial Concepts of Work Ability

Biopsychosocial and multidimensional concepts are comprehensive and interactive models that consider functional capacity and work ability as results of an interaction between individual physical, mental, and social factors and various environmental factors. In this category, two different frameworks have been widely used. The first is the International Classification of Functioning, Disability and Health (ICF framework) developed by the WHO (2001) (Fig. 2), emphasizing the interaction between the individual and environmental factors in the development and management of problems related to health and functional capacity. The second framework is the Work Ability House (Fig. 3) developed at the Finnish Institute of Occupational Health (FIOH) (Ilmarinen et al. 2008).

The ICF describes human functional capacity and functioning at three different levels: (1) body functions and structures, (2) activities and performing various tasks, and (3) participation in communities and society, as well as involvement in life situations. Functional capacity is based on the interaction between the health condition and individual as well as environmental factors, but, at the same time, the individual with his/her actions has an influence on himself/herself, the health condition, and the environment. Work performance is one dimension in the area of actions and participation. Originally, this framework does not pay any special attention to work ability, work, or the work environment. Later modifications, however, have emphasized aspects related to work ability and vocational rehabilitation.

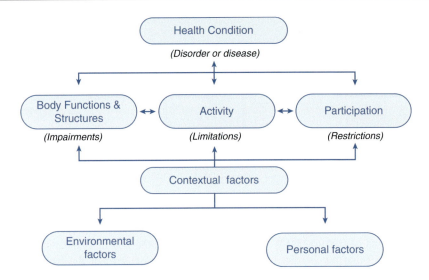

Fig. 2 ICF framework (WHO 2001)

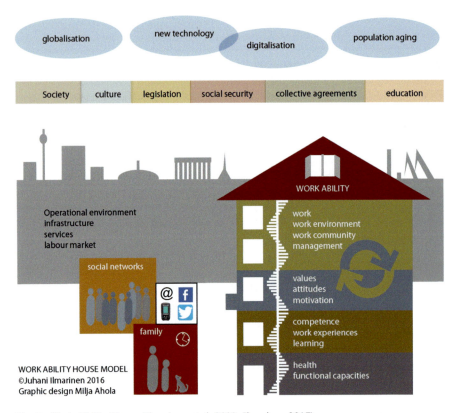

Fig. 3 Work Ability House (Ilmarinen et al. 2008; Ilmarinen 2017)

The Work Ability House illustrates work ability as a roof and related factors as four floors of the house supporting the roof. The three lower floors comprise of health and functional capacities, professional competence, as well as values and attitudes. The fourth floor describes work and includes work conditions, contents, and demands, in addition to colleagues and work organization with supervisor and management policies. The close environment outside work includes not only family but also supporting services at work, like occupational health services. The society comprises the macro environment of work ability. The Work Ability House does not consider the relationships between the various factors.

This Work Ability House has been crucial for the introduction and implementation of the concept of work disability prevention in the Finnish workplaces. It has increased interest and created a shared language between workplaces and their occupational health services. In practice, this shared language has helped stakeholders consider not only individual health but also work-related factors as targets for collaborative interventions. In addition to the cost-saving potential for employers of preventing sickness absence and disability pensions, the work ability concept emphasizes the possibility to promote employee commitment by improving health and safety at work.

The employee's ability to work is affected by macro level environmental characteristics, such as legislation, technological and economic situation, and the labor market. Factors related to work and the work environment include job contract, social relationships at work, contents of the work tasks, and working conditions in general, which all have an impact on the physical and mental strain at work. Factors at the meso level are primarily related to the workplace and its policies. The micro level includes factors related to the employee's specific work and work tasks. Work ability is constructed as the interaction between workload and the individual's resources. Education, work experience, motivation, and self-efficacy are important individual factors influencing their sources (Heerkens et al. 2004).

During the last decade, the ICF framework has been used extensively in the context of medical and multidisciplinary rehabilitation. The applicability of ICF in assessing work ability has been studied especially in insurance medicine. The problems in work ability assessments are related to the lack of standards and poor transparency of the processes and assessment results (Schwegler et al. 2012). In many countries, the eligibility to disability benefits requires similar elements, like verification of diminished health and functional capacity and need for application to rehabilitation. However, interviews with insurance physicians from various countries showed that these eligibility criteria are perceived and executed differently despite the shared ICF framework. Therefore, the assessment of work ability requires more elements than what is included in the ICF (de Boer et al. 2008).

As a response, EUMASS (European Union of Medicine in Assurance and Social Security) produced an ICF Core Set, which seems to be applicable for the assessment of work ability (Anner et al. 2013) when additionally taking the work-related experiences of the individual into consideration. The ICF framework helps to assess the health and functional capacity of the individual, but not the characteristics of work. Neither does the ICF include critical components of the assessment of work ability, e.g., time perspective or the causal relationship between health and functional capacity.

A systematic review (Escorpizo et al. 2011a) shows that the vocational rehabilitation literature includes many different measurements and variables related to the areas of activities and participation. The area of bodily functions has been widely used in vocational rehabilitation concerning mental disorders. An obvious blind spot in vocational rehabilitation research has been the area of environmental factors which were underrepresented when taking their importance into consideration.

An ICF Core Set for vocational rehabilitation has been defined to describe central factors relevant for the vocational rehabilitation (Finger et al. 2012). The comprehensive version includes the following parts belonging to various areas in the ICF framework:

- Activities and participation (40 categories, e.g., making decisions; moving around; vocational training; acquiring, keeping, and terminating a job)
- Environmental factors (33 categories, e.g., products and technology for employment; transportation services, systems, and policies; education and training services, systems, and policies; labor and employment services, systems, and policies)
- Body functions (17 categories, e.g., intellectual functions; memory functions; muscle endurance functions).

In the shorter version, the corresponding numbers of categories are six, four, and three, respectively (Finger et al. 2012).

The Integrated "Individual in the Work Community" Concept

This concept derives from the proposition that individual work ability is promoted primarily as part of the overall development of the organization and with the management of diversity and well-being at the workplace. Therefore, work ability promotion and rehabilitation are integral parts of general practices related to management, planning, and development of work processes and work organization, as well as to human resource policies and personnel training (Kristman et al. 2017). The aim is to define a set of work tasks for each employee, so that the individual can use his/her abilities as effectively and well-balanced as possible to reach the basic goals of the organization. In case work ability is assessed, it is based on work ability observed at work and as part of all activities of the work organization. An assessment of the employee's personal work ability unrelated to work tasks, or individual rehabilitation supporting functional capacity in general, is not valid to the workplace operations.

To demonstrate the individual in the work community, Fig. 4 shows the activity system, originally by Bryant and colleagues, defined by Leontiev and later redefined by Engeström (1987). In this framework the employee aims to reach a target (outcome) with his/her work by using the (concrete or tacit) instruments in relation

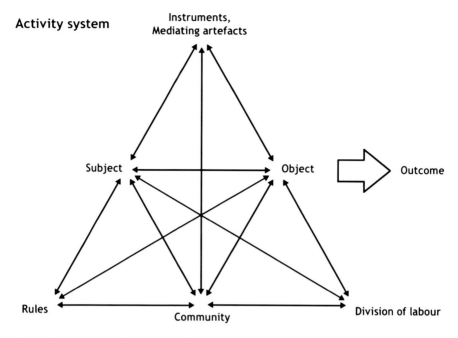

Fig. 4 Activity system (Engeström 1987)

to the object. The employee is not alone in his/her activities, but the work community works in the same direction with the same aim. This collaboration is guided by rules and the set division of labor. The activity system shows how individual performance is dependent on appropriate tools (instruments) in relation to the desired outcome when taking the needs of an employee with disability into consideration. The rules guiding collaboration can either support work performance or restrict necessary adjustments at work required to support an employee with disability. In addition, the supportive role of colleagues is dependent on the division of labor and how this division can be accommodated.

According to the integrated "individual in the work community" concept, work ability is constructed in the constant change of work and work organization, which creates both risks and opportunities to work ability. Individual work ability should be assessed as part of activities of the entire workplace. Interventions improving an individual's work ability are related to improving the performance of the entire workplace. Rehabilitation can be directed to work and/or individual characteristics. The main emphasis of rehabilitation is not directed toward maintenance or improvement of the individual's work ability but in planning and organizing work at the workplace, so that everything works as good as possible, and the skills capacity as well as physical and psychosocial capacity of all employees is in optimal use. According to this concept, work ability assessment is more relevant in real-life situations, where the individual is part of the organization, and health is only one part of the whole picture, and not very interesting as such.

The Employability Concept of Work Ability

According to the employability concept, work ability consists primarily of the ability and possibility to be employed, maintain employment, and advance at work. Therefore, work ability is analyzed as actions in these practical situations. Sustainable employability includes also the possibility of an employee to use his/her full potential at work and, at the same time, maintain health and well-being (van der Klink et al. 2016).

Work ability and employability have a lot in common as they both originate from individual characteristics. In work ability, individual characteristics are related to health and functional capacity. In employability, more emphasis is given to knowledge, skills, and attitudes (Saikku 2013). Work and work tasks play a role in work ability, whereas in employability the role of the labor market is more important. However, work ability cannot be based only on individual abilities but also on the availability of work and the employer's readiness to offer suitable work for the individual.

In the employability concept, disease or injury plays no particular role. Therefore, rehabilitation can be initiated based on prolonged unemployment or social exclusion, as well as on problems of getting employment or challenges related to disease or injury. The obstacles of employment among persons with disabilities or chronic medical conditions are mainly related to prejudices and societal structures. Everybody who wants to work should be considered to have work ability to conduct some work if this work is organized according to his/her situation and needs with necessary support.

As to the planning and contents of rehabilitation, the employability concept emphasizes the active role of the rehabilitee, clarification of the motivating factors, and active collaboration with the employers to find suitable work opportunities. For example in supported employment, the starting point is that if an individual wants to work, a suitable and motivating job will be looked for. After this, coaching will be given at work to meet the needs of this specific job. Support will be offered both to the individual and the employer to create possibilities of meeting the expectations for the work performance. This support can include adjustments in work organization or working hours, changes in physical work environment, as well as planning the work tasks. A work coach can reduce the insecurity related to employment of an individual who may have been outside of the labor market for an extended period.

The employability concept of work ability differs from ordinary rehabilitation in two respects. First, disease or injury as the criterion for rehabilitation is less important, and more attention is given to the practical problems in receiving or maintaining employment. Second, in the provision of rehabilitation, the assessment and coaching outside the workplace are replaced by coaching at work. In addition, support is directed to the employed person or his/her supervisor and the workplace. Separate assessment and coaching processes are replaced by supporting work participation at the workplace. The obstacles of being employed may be related to the individual's injury, and therefore various adjustments may be needed at the workplace. Some obstacles are often related to attitudes at the workplace, and this may require changes in personnel policy and recruitment practices of individual workplaces, as well as more comprehensive education and lobbying in work life.

Supported employment has been traditionally implemented in the vocational rehabilitation of challenging groups, i.e., individuals with severe mental disorder, intellectual disability, or brain damage. Among these groups, employment is substantially complicated by the stigma related to the disease or injury. In addition, negative attitudes hamper the rehabilitees' possibilities to demonstrate work ability. The concept of individual placement and support (IPS) has shown good results as part of psychiatric rehabilitation both in the USA and in Europe (Reme et al. 2018).

In the employability concept of work ability, health is only one part of the picture, and it does not have a central role. Collaboration with health care is secured when needed in rehabilitation.

Work Ability as a Social Construct of Various Systems

In this concept, work ability is primarily seen as a social construct based on norms, values, and goals of the society or system in each era. The criteria of work ability and work disability change according to the change in the socioeconomic context of the society and its various systems, e.g., labor market, health care, and social insurance. This means that norms in society have an influence on the decisions regarding an individuals' work ability.

In the analysis of work ability, employment, and RTW, a systemic perspective has been pointed out more strongly than earlier. The importance of various stakeholders and collaboration between organizations has been emphasized in maintaining and restoring work ability. The case management ecological concept (Loisel 2009) describes the employee inside and between his/her personal system, the workplace system, the health-care system, and the social security system. This concept highlights the collaboration between various organizations and the dependence of work ability on many stakeholders, but the concept does not include analyses of the interdependencies or relationships between the stakeholders.

This work ability concept emphasizes the fact how relative the work ability and work disability are and how employment and retirement depend on the circumstances in the society, as well as on the goals set by its various systems. Hence, the question is always about different interpretations in the service systems regarding the factors that should be included when assessing the prerequisites of work ability (Jansson 2014; Seing et al. 2012; Ståhl 2010). Decisions about work ability and rehabilitation are primarily based on negotiations between various stakeholders (workplaces, insurance systems, health care) and on fitting their divergent viewpoints.

Different stakeholders construct work ability differently leading to divergent concepts of rehabilitation, employment, and RTW. In Swedish studies, the rehabilitation process has been described as a negotiation between the stakeholders, where the employer has a kind of priority. If from the workplaces perspective the employee cannot work, the other stakeholders cannot influence the decision (Seing et al. 2012). The ethical principles behind vocational rehabilitation have been studied showing that the power relations of the stakeholders decide how the ethical questions are made visible during the process (Ståhl et al. 2014).

Successful collaboration between all stakeholders is crucial when trying to develop and integrate health and social services and to provide good vocational rehabilitation. Seven different concepts of collaboration have been reported: (1) exchange of information; (2) collaboration through a service coordinator in the organization; (3) meetings of the representatives of the organizations; (4) multi-professional working groups with participants from various organizations; (5) partnership based on agreements between the organizations; (6) use of shared facilities enabling, e.g., proving services together to the customers; and (7) shared budgeting of the projects. Flexible solutions seem to benefit the results of the activities (Andersson et al. 2011).

Emerging Concepts of Work Ability and Rehabilitation

The concepts of work ability typically either focus on some specific sector (disease-specific and many of the psychosocial concepts) or describe the nature of connections without specifying the different factors that may be important for work ability (Work Ability House, ICF). On one hand, multidimensional concepts cover many factors at the micro, meso, and macro level without paying special attention to any of them. The role of an active individual and his/her goal-oriented actions remain invisible in multidimensional concepts (Scobbie and Dixon 2015). On the other hand, the case management ecological concept (Loisel 2009) and the conceptual mapping of work ability (Lederer et al. 2014) are operational concepts with the credit for recognizing the key stakeholders in work ability promotion. These two concepts are based on scarce evidence of work ability in relation to the interaction between different stakeholders.

Costa-Black et al. (2013) state that there are no multidimensional concepts that could capture the multisystemic dynamics in the phenomenon of work ability including both individual and environmental interactions and the systemic factors that influence decision-making. In their opinion, only few concepts have managed in this to some extent. The concept by Faucett (2005) is related to work ability and RTW in musculoskeletal disorders, and that by Feuerstein et al. (2010) is related to cancer survivors. As a third example, Costa-Black et al. present the application of ICF framework emphasizing work ability (Heerkens et al. 2004).

From the rehabilitation point of view, it is important to consider the individual as an active player planning his/her future, as well as the development of work ability in the interaction of the working individual, his/her work, and the environment. Consequently, work ability is a process that must be assessed by monitoring the activities realized in practical work and various contexts. The concept of work ability should not be restricted only or primarily to employed individuals. Diminished work ability should also be assessed without the prerequisite of an existing disease or injury, i.e., without medicalization of the problems compromising work ability.

At the level of an individual, the basis of rehabilitation is his/her active role and goal-oriented actions from young to old age. That includes increasing competencies at various stages of the employment, activities at work and outside work, retraining, but also unemployment periods and disability. Work ability develops at work, by working, as well as in interactions with the social and physical environment. The special role of motivation in work ability is that it increases the possibilities of learning and developing. In rehabilitation, attention must be paid to factors related to getting immediate employment, continuing at work, or RTW. In addition to physical and mental health, education, competencies, and social skills, other relevant factors include the meaning of work, attitudes and beliefs, coping mechanisms, planning activities at work, and financial incentives. An individual must be encouraged to overcome prejudices and structural obstacles present in work life. The assessment of the need for rehabilitation can include factors related to the cultural background and language skills, age and the stage of the employment, as well as factors supporting well-being in various areas of life.

At the level of organization and work community, interventions are needed to focus on systemic obstacles. They are attitudes at the workplace, different practices related to recruitment, and personnel policy, which can prevent starting or continuing employment of a person with disability or long unemployment period. The challenge might be to address attitudes in the labor market and society. Moreover, better collaboration is required between the workplace and the rehabilitation providers. This requires multidisciplinary teams and rehabilitation professionals who are active in managing interest conflicts between organizations. In the future, work-related issues should be emphasized more than nowadays to provide rehabilitation to individuals who need diverse support to continue at work. The work-related challenges are, e.g., prolonged and recurrent changes at work, such as changes in the organization, work tasks, work processes, teams, supervisors, instability at work or recurrent overload at work, as well as decision latitude.

At the societal level, attention should be given to legislative issues, as well as social, health, education, and labor services. The concept of work ability applied in legislation most likely influences the solutions at the workplaces (e.g., discrimination of people with disabilities, attitudes toward immigrants, job security). An extensive concept of work ability has been developed that moves to earlier intervention and maintenance of work ability in rehabilitation. This development is due to the fact that various factors related to work ability are known better than earlier.

Managing the Process of Rehabilitation

In practice, work ability means how a person is capable of doing his/her job, how he/she returns to work after disability, and how he/she continues in working life. RTW can happen with or without rehabilitation activities. These described work ability concepts can assist to plan rehabilitation and to describe how rehabilitation should be delivered in ideal circumstances. So far, rehabilitation has not always resulted in the expected results.

Recently, the European Agency for Safety and Health at Work published a review on rehabilitation promoting RTW (Vandenbroeck et al. 2016). Based on the synthesis, guidelines were given at national, intervention, and workplace level. National governments and authorities are recommended to direct legislation and guidelines from disease and disability to promoting the possibilities of the individual to use the remaining capabilities according to the ICF framework so that factors related to work ability are widely considered. This means not only guiding the actions of health-care professionals but also clarifying the administrative practices related to working, as well as increasing the financial incentives of working instead of receiving social security benefits.

In rehabilitation interventions, individual tailoring and stepwise advancement are important so that rehabilitation starts already early in the beginning of disability with simple interventions and advances, if disability persists, to multidisciplinary and more demanding rehabilitation requiring more resources. The key players are the decision-makers in health care, i.e., general practitioners and occupational health physicians. At the level of workplaces, interventions to promote RTW should be integrated into the general strategy of well-being at work.

Another recent review covering vocational rehabilitation practices in 32 European countries (Belin et al. 2016) classifies countries according to how the implementation of rehabilitation is defined at the level of political decisions and legislation. The Nordic countries, the Netherlands, Germany, and Austria have adopted a policy covering all citizens so that rehabilitation is not restricted to special groups having a permanent impediment or injury or being on sickness absence for a long time. This enables rehabilitation already when an individual is still participating in work life, and, hence, rehabilitation is closer to secondary than to tertiary prevention. The view about rehabilitation is holistic, and the workplaces have clear obligations to participate in it. The legislation also obligates various stakeholders to collaborate with each other.

Other countries, like Italy, Switzerland, France, Belgium, Luxemburg, Great Britain, and Iceland, have good systems for rehabilitation, but they are implemented only after a long absence from work. They also lack a systematic collaboration and coordination of rehabilitation providers. The third group of countries (Bulgaria, Estonia, Ireland, Spain, Lithuania, Hungary, Portugal, and Romania) lack national coordination of rehabilitation, or rehabilitation is strictly restricted to those individuals who have a permanent handicap. Interestingly, all these countries have similar practices of short-term work disability and mainly also pension benefits related to permanent disability. The concept of work disability does not seem to guide the rehabilitation practices. Instead, the idea of promoting work ability seems to be crucial in the official practices of the first group of countries. This, however, does not guarantee that it takes place in practice.

The comprehensive concept of work ability requires collaboration of many stakeholders in rehabilitation. For the rehabilitation of back pain, the so-called Sherbrooke concept was developed in Canada (Loisel et al. 1994) with good results when combining medical rehabilitation with adjustments at the workplace. The concept has been developed to include even other stakeholders in health care and the workplace, and the concept has been used as a framework for rehabilitation in many parts of the world (Briand et al. 2007; Bültmann et al. 2009; Durand et al. 2003). The conclusion of the trials has been that the process did not flow as planned if the views of all stakeholders were not similar and if the processes did not support each other in favor of the shared goal (Bültmann et al. 2009). A qualitative meta-analysis including RTW interventions showed that despite good intentions the rehabilitation was not successful due to lack of proper coordination of collaboration among various stakeholders (Andersen et al. 2012).

Differences in viewpoints of various stakeholders influence also the way work ability is assessed. In Sweden, there is a statutory obligation to assess the degree of work ability and possibilities of RTW in a collective negotiation with not only the employee and employer but also participants from the social security agency and health care. The aim has been to increase their collaboration. Seing et al. (2012) analyzed the taped negotiations. The reasoning of the representatives from various organizations was influenced by divergent logics and rules that clearly complicated the finding of solutions related to the rehabilitation. The stakeholders often seemed to play with their own rules leading to a kind of power play in the collective negotiation.

A systematic review concluded that professionals often use various work capability assessment methods to assess work ability. These methods, however, do not seem to help to combine the assessed work capability to the profession and the characteristics of work so that it would help to plan comprehensive rehabilitation or to evaluate the results of rehabilitation (Cronin et al. 2013). In Finland and many other countries, rehabilitation is connected to the decisions related to disability pension so that rehabilitation should be attempted before disability pension can be granted (Belin et al. 2016). The situation is problematic from the rehabilitation point of view if rehabilitation is started after a long sickness absence. A person has already adapted the disabled role and waits for a positive disability pension decision. Rehabilitation requires an active role, whereas demonstrating disability encourages passive behavior.

Cross-References

▶ Concepts and Social Variations of Disability in Working-Age Populations
▶ Implementing Best Practice Models of Return to Work
▶ Shifting the Focus from Work Reintegration to Sustainability of Employment

References

Andersen MF, Nielsen KM, Brinkmann S (2012) Meta-synthesis of qualitative research on return to work among employees with common mental disorders. Scand J Work Environ Health 38(2):93–104

Andersson J, Ahgren B, Axelsson SB, Eriksson A, Axelsson R (2011) Organizational approaches to collaboration in vocational rehabilitation-an international literature review. Int J Integr Care 11:e137

Anner J, Brage S, Donceel P et al (2013) Validation of the EUMASS Core Set for medical evaluation of work disability. Disabil Rehabil 35(25):2147–2156

Baumberg B, Warren J, Garthwaite K, Bambra C (2015) "Incapacity needs to be assessed in the real world…". Rethinking the work capability assessment. Demos. Retrieved from https://www.demos.co.uk/files/Rethinking_-_web_1_.pdf?1426175121. Cited 2.2.2020

Belin A, Dupont C, Oulès L, Kuipers Y, Fries-Tersch E (2016) Rehabilitation and return to work: analysis report on EU and Member States policies, strategies and programmes. Publications Office of the European Union. Retrieved from https://osha.europa.eu/en/publications/rehabilitation-and-return-work-analysis-report-eu-and-member-states-policies-strategies. Cited 2.2.2020

Besen E, Young AE, Shaw WS (2015) Returning to work following low back pain: towards a concept of individual psychosocial factors. J Occup Rehabil 25(1):25–37

Briand C, Durand MJ, St-Arnaud L, Corbiere M (2007) Work and mental health: learning from return-to-work rehabilitation programs designed for workers with musculoskeletal disorders. Int J Law Psychiatry 30(4–5):444–457

Bültmann U, Sherson D, Olsen J et al (2009) Coordinated and tailored work rehabilitation: a randomized controlled trial with economic evaluation undertaken with workers on sick leave due to musculoskeletal disorders. J Occup Rehabil 19(1):81–93

Costa-Black KM, Feuerstein M, Loisel P (2013) Work disability concepts: past and present. In: Loisel P, Anema JR (eds) Handbook on work disability: prevention and management. Springer, New York, pp 71–93

Cronin S, Curran J, Iantorno J et al (2013) Work capacity assessment and return to work: a scoping review. Work 44(1):37–55

de Boer W, Donceel P, Brage S, Rus M, Willems J (2008) Medico-legal reasoning in disability assessment: a focus group and validation study. BMC Public Health 8:335

Durand MJ, Vachon B, Loisel P, Berthelette D (2003) Constructing the program impact theory for an evidence-based work rehabilitation program for workers with low back pain. Work 21(3):233–242

Engeström Y (1987) Learning by expanding: an activity-theoretical approach to developmental research. Orienta-Konsultit, Helsinki

Escorpizo R, Finger ME, Glassel A et al (2011a) A systematic review of functioning in vocational rehabilitation using the International Classification of Functioning, Disability and Health. J Occup Rehabil 21(2):134–146

Escorpizo R, Reneman MF, Ekholm J et al (2011b) A conceptual definition of vocational rehabilitation based on the ICF: building a shared global concept. J Occup Rehabil 21(2):126–133

European Foundation for the Improvement of Living and Working Conditions (1997) Preventing absenteeism at the workplace. Research summary. Office for Official Publications of the European Communities, Luxembourg

Fadyl JK, McPherson KM, Schluter PJ, Turner-Stokes L (2010) Factors contributing to work-ability for injured workers: literature review and comparison with available measures. Disabil Rehabil 32(14):1173–1183

Faucett J (2005) Integrating 'psychosocial' factors into a theoretical concept for work-related musculoskeletal disorders. Theor Issues Ergon Sci 6(6):531–550

Feuerstein M, Todd BL, Moskowitz MC et al (2010) Work in cancer survivors: a concept for practice and research. J Cancer Surviv 4(4):415–437

Finger ME, Escorpizo R, Glassel A et al (2012) ICF Core Set for vocational rehabilitation: results of an international consensus conference. Disabil Rehabil 34(5):429–438

Franche RL, Krause N (2002) Readiness for return to work following injury or illness: conceptualizing the interpersonal impact of health care, workplace, and insurance factors. J OccupRehabil 12(4):233–256

Heerkens Y, Engels J, Kuiper C, Van Der Gulden J, Oostendorp R (2004) The use of the ICF to describe work related factors influencing the health of employees. Disabil Rehabil 26(17):1060–1066

Ilmarinen J (2001) Aging workers. Occup Environ Med 58(8):546–552

Ilmarinen J (2017) Personal communication

Ilmarinen J, Gould R, Järvikoski A, Järvisalo J (2008) Diversity of work ability. Results of the Health 2000 Survey. In: Gould R, Ilmarinen J, Järvisalo J, Koskinen S (eds) Dimensions of work ability. Finnish Centre for Pensions, The Social Insurance Institution, National Public Health Institute, Finnish Institute of Occupational Health, Helsinki. Retrieved from http://www.julkari.fi/handle/10024/78055. Cited 2.2.2020

ILO (1983) C159 - Vocational Rehabilitation and Employment (Disabled Persons) Convention 1983 (No. 159), https://www.ilo.org/dyn/normlex/en/f?p=NORMLEXPUB:12100:0::NO::P12100_ILO_CODE:C159

Jansson I (2014) On the nature of work ability. Academic thesis. Jönköping University, Jönköping School of Health Sciences. Retrieved from http://www.diva-portal.org/smash/get/diva2:705046/FULLTEXT01.pdf. Cited 2.2.2020

Järvikoski A, Takala E-P, Juvonen-Posti P, Härkäpää K. Työkyvynkäsite ja työkykymallitkuntoutuksentutkimuksessa ja käytännöissä (The concept of work ability in the research and practice of rehabilitation) (in Finnish with English abstract). Social Insurance Institution of Finland, Social security and health reports 13, 2018, 86 pp. ISBN 978-952-284056-1 (pdf)

Kivimäki M, Vahtera J, Elovainio M, Virtanen M, Siegrist J (2007) Effort-reward imbalance, procedural injustice and relational injustice as psychosocial predictors of health: complementary or redundant concepts? Occup Environ Med 64(10):659–665

Kristman VL, Shaw WS, Reguly P et al (2017) Supervisor and organizational factors associated with supervisor support of job accommodations for low back injured workers. J Occup Rehabil 27(1):115–127

Lederer V, Loisel P, Rivard M, Champagne F (2014) Exploring the diversity of conceptualizations of work (dis)ability: a scoping review of published definitions. J Occup Rehabil 24(2):242–267

Loisel P (2009) Developing a new paradigm: work disability prevention. Occup Health Southern Africa 15(Special ICOH issue):56–60

Loisel P, Durand P, Abenhaim L et al (1994) Management of occupational back pain: the Sherbrooke concept. Results of a pilot and feasibility study. Occup Environ Med 51(9):597–602

Reme S, Monstad K, Fyhn T, Sveinsdottir V, Løvvik C et al (2018) A randomized controlled multicenter trial of individual placement and support for patients with moderate-to-severe mental illness. Scand J Work Environ Health 2019 45(1):33–41

Royal College of Physicians (2010) Medical rehabilitation in 2011 and beyond. Report of a working party. RCP, London

Saikku P (2013) Perspectives to work ability and its assessment among unemployed (in Finnish). In: Karjalainen V, Keskitalo E (eds) Kaikki työuralle! Työttömien aktiivipolitiikkaa Suomessa. THL, Helsinki, pp 120–149

Schultz IZ, Stowell AW, Feuerstein M, Gatchel RJ (2007) Concepts of return to work for musculoskeletal disorders. J Occup Rehabil 17(2):327–352

Schwegler U, Anner J, Boldt C et al (2012) Aspects of functioning and environmental factors in medical work capacity evaluations of persons with chronic widespread pain and low back pain can be represented by a combination of applicable ICF Core Sets. BMC Public Health 12:1088

Scobbie L, Dixon D (2015) Theory-based approach to goal setting. In: Siegert RJ, WMM L (eds) Rehabilitation goal setting: theory, practice and evidence. CRC Press, Boca Raton

Seing I, Stahl C, Nordenfelt L, Bulow P, Ekberg K (2012) Policy and practice of work ability: a negotiation of responsibility in organizing return to work. J Occup Rehabil 22(4):553–564

Ståhl C (2010) In cooperation we trust. Interorganizational cooperation in return-to-work and labour market reintegration. Academic dissertation. Linköping

Ståhl C, MacEachen E, Lippel K (2014) Ethical perspectives in work disability prevention and return to work: toward a common vocabulary for analyzing stakeholders' actions and interactions. J Bus Ethics 120(2):237–250

Stay at Work and Return to Work Process Improvement Committee (2006) Preventing needless work disability by helping people stay employed. J Occup Environ Med 48(9):972–987

Sullivan MJ, Feuerstein M, Gatchel R, Linton SJ, Pransky G (2005) Integrating psychosocial and behavioral interventions to achieve optimal rehabilitation outcomes. J Occup Rehabil 15(4):475–489

Turner-Stokes L, Fadyl J, Rose H et al (2014) The Work-ability Support Scale: evaluation of scoringaccuracy and rater reliability. J Occup Rehabil 24(3):511–524

van der Klink JJ, Bültmann U, Burdorf A et al (2016) Sustainable employability-definition, conceptualization, and implications: a perspective based on the capability approach. Scand J Work Environ Health 42(1):71–79

Vandenbroeck S, Verjans M, Lambreghts C, Godderis L (2016) Research review on rehabilitation and return to work. European Agency for Safety and Health at Work. Retrieved from https://osha.europa.eu/en/tools-and-publications/publications/research-reviewrehabilitation-and-return-work/view. Cited 2.2.2020

WHO (2001) International classification of functioning, disability and health: ICF. World Health Organization, Geneva

Young AE, Roessler RT, Wasiak R et al (2005) A developmental conceptualization of return to work. J Occup Rehabil 15(4):557–568

Facilitating Competitive Employment for People with Disabilities

31

Expanding Implementation of IPS Supported Employment to New Populations

Gary R. Bond, Robert E. Drake, and Jacqueline A. Pogue

Contents

Introduction	572
Origins of Supported Employment	573
Individual Placement and Support (IPS)	574
Classification of Disability Groups	575
IPS for People with Serious Mental Illness	576
IPS in Other Populations	578
Nonpsychotic Psychiatric Disorders	578
Common Mental Disorders	579
Affective Disorders	580
Moderate to Severe Mental Illness	580
Posttraumatic Stress Disorder (PTSD)	581
Borderline Personality Disorder	581
Substance Use Disorder	581
Opioid Use Disorder	582
Substance Use Disorders and Criminal Justice Involvement	582
Intellectual and Developmental Disorders	582
Intellectual and Developmental Disabilities	582
Autism Spectrum Disorders	583
Musculoskeletal and Neurological Disorders	583
Spinal Cord Injury	583
Chronic Pain	584
Traumatic Brain Injury	584
Discussion	584
Conclusions	585
Cross-References	585
References	585

G. R. Bond (✉) · R. E. Drake · J. A. Pogue
Westat, Lebanon, NH, USA
e-mail: garybond@westat.com; RobertDrake@westat.com; JackiePogue@westat.com

© Springer Nature Switzerland AG 2020
U. Bültmann, J. Siegrist (eds.), *Handbook of Disability, Work and Health*, Handbook Series in Occupational Health Sciences, https://doi.org/10.1007/978-3-030-24334-0_31

Abstract

Background: To review the history, effectiveness, and current use of Individual Placement and Support, also called IPS supported employment, with various disability groups.

Methods: Tertiary review of studies of IPS supported employment.

Results: IPS has developed and spread rapidly around the world over the past 30 years. Controlled research has strongly supported its effectiveness in improving employment outcomes. In long-term studies, the employment outcomes have been sustained. These positive outcomes have been demonstrated across a variety of clinical, demographic, and socioeconomic groups of the population of people with serious mental illness. Studies have also found IPS to be cost-effective. Recent research on other disability groups, including people with anxiety, depression, posttraumatic stress disorder, developmental disabilities, substance use disorder, and spinal cord injury, has shown promise.

Conclusions: IPS is a flexible approach to helping unemployed people with disabilities gain employment. Clients, practitioners, and program leaders understand its eight principles and find them appealing. IPS should be offered to all people with serious mental illness and to veterans with posttraumatic stress disorder who want to work competitively. Research on other disability groups shows promise, warranting rigorous replication studies.

Keywords

Supported employment · Individual Placement and Support · Employment · Common mental disorder · Posttraumatic stress disorder · Substance use disorder · Intellectual developmental disorder

Introduction

The opportunity to pursue meaningful employment is a human right. In the latter half of the twentieth century, nearly all wealthy countries accepted the notion that people with disabilities should have freedom from dehumanizing conditions such as institutionalization, segregation, sheltered employment, and paternalism, as well as opportunities to participate fully in the community. Yet compared to the general population, people with disabilities are employed at a much lower rate. Among people with serious mental illness, employment rates are less than 20% (Bond and Drake 2014). The rates are higher for other disorders, but typically substantially lower than for people without disabilities (EASPD 2016). People with disabilities want to work, and if given appropriate help and the opportunity, most can be successful.

In this chapter, we describe Individual Placement and Support (IPS), an employment service that helps people with disabilities achieve meaningful, competitive, mainstream employment (Drake et al. 2012). Although originally developed for people with serious mental disorders, service providers have in recent years been offering IPS services to other disability groups.

This chapter describes the history, effectiveness, and current use of IPS around the world. Consistent with the preferences of people with disabilities, we focus exclusively on integrated competitive employment (also called "open employment"), defined as regular community jobs that anyone can apply for, paying a comparable wage that others receive to perform the same work (at least minimum wage). Competitive jobs refer to jobs in integrated workplaces in which people both with and without disabilities work under the same conditions (e.g., supervisory arrangements). Competitive jobs differ from various types of noncompetitive work opportunities, such as transitional employment, which are time-limited jobs, intended to provide work experiences but which are not permanent; "set-aside" jobs, which are restricted to people with disabilities; and government-subsidized jobs for people out of the labor market.

Origins of Supported Employment

In the 1980s, rehabilitation researchers in the USA developed a new approach to vocational rehabilitation services to address the growing number of long-term clients in sheltered workshops who had little prospects of entering the competitive workforce, despite the justification given by workshop managers that sheltered work experiences served to prepare clients for community jobs. This new approach was called supported employment and was intended for people with the most severe disabilities (Wehman and Moon 1988). Historically, most vocational rehabilitation services for people with severe disabilities were stepwise: first, training clients in protected settings and then placing them in regular jobs, based on the assumption that people with severe disabilities were incapable of working in mainstream employment without prevocational training and preparation. "Train-and-place," the term for this stepwise approach, continues to be a common, if not the dominant, vocational model throughout the world.

Stepwise vocational rehabilitation programs vary widely. In some, clients participate in unpaid work experiences, sometimes for extended periods, on the assumption that these experiences will prepare them for competitive work. In other cases, training includes placement in jobs paying minimum wage and set aside for people with disabilities. Another type of traditional work program, often financed through government subsidies, is the sheltered workshop (sometimes called a social firm), typically providing menial work activities in segregated settings for minimum or subminimum wages. Research shows, however, that sheltered employment and other set-aside jobs do not lead to competitive work but are almost always an end point where some clients may remain indefinitely (Wehman and Moon 1988).

In contrast to the train-and-place model, early proponents of supported employment conceptualized a "place-and-train" approach, placing clients directly into competitive jobs and providing job coaching (as needed) and long-term support (Wehman and Moon 1988). Initially, supported employment programs mainly targeted people with intellectual disabilities, but subsequently extended more broadly to people with any severe disability.

Supported employment therefore describes employment services that eschew stepwise programs and provide direct assistance to clients to gain competitive work with support (and training) in the workplace. Throughout the world, vocational rehabilitation programs and practitioners offer supported employment services. The operational details of what constitutes supported employment, however, are not standardized, and practices vary widely.

Individual Placement and Support (IPS)

The IPS model of supported employment is a well-defined, standardized, evidence-based practice developed in the USA in the 1980s for people with serious mental illness (Becker and Drake 2003). IPS follows eight principles, all of which have empirical support:

(1) *Focus on the goal of competitive employment.* Agencies providing IPS services are committed to regular jobs in the community (competitive employment) as an attainable goal for clients with serious mental illness seeking employment.
(2) *Zero exclusion/eligibility based on client choice.* Every person who is interested in work is eligible for services regardless of "readiness," work experience, symptoms, or any other issue.
(3) *Attention to client preferences.* Services align with clients' preferences and choices, rather than practitioners' expertise or judgments. IPS specialists help clients find jobs that fit their preferences.
(4) *Rapid job search.* IPS programs help clients look for jobs right away, beginning the job search soon after a person expresses interest in working, rather than providing lengthy pre-employment assessment, training, and counseling. The rapid job search principle is contrary to the train-place stepwise philosophy widely adopted in traditional vocational rehabilitation programs.
(5) *Integration of employment services with mental health treatment.* IPS programs closely integrate with mental health treatment teams (comprised of mental health clinicians, care managers, psychiatrists, nurses, and other mental health professionals).
(6) *Personalized benefit counseling.* IPS specialists help clients obtain personalized, understandable, and accurate information about how working may impact their disability insurance and other government entitlements.
(7) *Targeted job development.* Based on clients' interests, IPS specialists build relationships with employers through repeated contact, learning about the business needs of employers and introducing employers to qualified job seekers.
(8) *Individualized long-term support.* Individualized, follow-along supports continue for as long as the client wants and needs the support to keep their job.

Table 1 A typology of employment interventions tailored to employment status

Employment status	Possible reasons	Goal	Interventions
Current employee but poor job performance and/or problems with absenteeism	Depression/anxiety; work stress; job dissatisfaction; poor job match	Retain employment with current employer with better job performance and higher job satisfaction	Work accommodations; psychological interventions (e.g., cognitive behavior therapy); reassign to a different position within existing work place; find new job with professional help (e.g., IPS)
Employee on sick leave or short-term/long-term disability	Injury; illness; depression/anxiety	Return to work	Same as above
Not employed	Lack of work experience, skills, or education; disability; displaced worker (e.g., factory closing); other external factors (e.g., single parent who cannot afford child care; transitions from prison or military)	Obtain meaningful employment that matches preferences; after starting work, maintain employment	IPS; training and education for a specific occupation

Unlike return-to-work programs for workers who are not coping well in their current employment or who are on sickness leave because of illness or injury, IPS generally helps people who are out of labor market, as schematized in Table 1. IPS programs do help clients who are applying for a job (and after they begin a job) with accommodations in the workplace and also help clients who are currently employed find a different job (if, e.g., their current job is a poor match).

Classification of Disability Groups

To organize the emerging literature on IPS studies with other populations, we sought a heuristic framework for classifying disability groups. No standardized method for classifying disabilities exists. We reviewed the literature to identify an appropriate framework. The World Health Organization classification of diseases is too granular (with a listing of 166 diseases) (Murray et al. 2012). A report commissioned by the European Union developed a simpler classificatory system: *Mental and Behavioral Disorders, Musculoskeletal Diseases, Neurological Conditions, Respiratory Diseases,* and *Cardiovascular Conditions.* A Swedish study developed a typology of disability groups consisting of six broad categories (communicative-hearing, communicative-speech-reading, communicative-vision, psychological disability, medical disability, and physical disability) (Boman et al. 2015). The US federal agency responsible for vocational rehabilitation services for people with disabilities uses a broad classification system indicating the following proportions of groups served: *Psychosocial and Psychological* (33%), *Intellectual and Learning Disability* (31%), *Physical Disability* (20%), *Auditory and Communication* (11%), and *Visual* (5%) (www2.ed.gov/programs/rsabvrs/resources/fy2016-vr-performance-chart.pdf).

For the current report, we identified four broad categories, *psychiatric disorders*, *substance use disorders*, *intellectual and learning disabilities*, and *musculoskeletal/ neurological disorders,* based on the conditions for which IPS programs have been developed. Our classification does not exhaust the entire range of disabling conditions. Further, it includes substance use disorders, even though US governmental agencies responsible for rehabilitation services often do not recognize substance use disorder as a disability. Nevertheless, people with substance use disorders are an important target group because substance use often results in difficulties in the workplace and job loss; conversely, employment often plays a critical role in the recovery process.

IPS for People with Serious Mental Illness

IPS began as an intervention for people with serious psychiatric disorders, also referred to as serious mental illness. Serious mental illness has not been defined consistently, either in practice or in the research literature (Schinnar et al. 1990). Most definitions include three elements: a ***diagnosis*** of a mental, behavioral, or emotional disorder, excluding substance use disorders; ***duration*** over a period of 6 months or more; and a functional ***disability*** that seriously interferes with or limits one or more major life activities (e.g., those relating to employment, self-care, self-direction, interpersonal relationships, learning and recreation, independent living, and economic self-sufficiency) (Goldman 1984). The most common diagnoses for people with serious mental illness are schizophrenia-spectrum disorders, bipolar disorder, and psychotic depression. Serious mental illness differs from common mental disorders, which include anxiety disorders and nonpsychotic depressive disorders.

Of the major disability groups, people with psychiatric disabilities have the lowest employment rates (EASPD 2016), and within this population, the employment rates are even lower for the subgroup with serious mental illness (Marwaha et al. 2007). Many professionals believe that people with serious mental illness are either incapable of working or, if they are able, that sheltered employment is the only viable option. Yet most people with serious mental illness want to work competitively (Bond and Drake 2014), and the research shows that the large majority have this capability if given the opportunity and adequate support through IPS services.

IPS has been shown effective in two dozen randomized controlled trials of programs serving people with serious mental illness, with competitive employment rates for IPS more than twice that for clients enrolled in standard services

(Drake et al. 2016; Modini et al. 2016). These controlled trials, conducted both inside and outside the USA, have included more than 5000 people who were followed for an average of 19 months. In most IPS studies, the competitive employment rate for IPS participants exceeds 50%, compared to less than 25% for participants receiving services as usual. The findings regarding the effectiveness of IPS compared to other vocational services have been consistently as strong in other countries as in the USA. However, the overall employment rates in studies conducted outside the USA are lower for both IPS and control groups (Bond et al. 2012). Two main factors influencing overall rates are labor laws and welfare policies (Metcalfe et al. 2018). Employment rates among people with disabilities are lower, for example, in Northern Europe (such as Sweden, Norway, and the Netherlands), where societal welfare benefits are especially generous. Conversely, US labor laws make it easier than in Europe to terminate workers, perhaps leading US employers to be more willing to make job offers to applicants with disabilities.

In addition to employment rates, IPS studies have documented the effectiveness of IPS across a range of employment outcomes, including time to starting employment, total weeks worked, hours worked, earnings, hours worked per week, and job satisfaction. Across many studies, the average time between enrollment in IPS and starting a competitive job is less than 5 months, and average job tenure in an initial job is about 10 months. Total employment earnings for IPS clients are more than double that for clients receiving usual vocational services (Bond et al. 2012; Drake et al. 2012). Over the long term (5–10 years), about half of clients who enroll in IPS become steady workers, defined as working on average at least 6 months every year of the follow-up period (Hoffmann et al. 2014).

Within different subgroups of the psychiatric population, defined by age, diagnosis, education level, severity of psychiatric symptoms, work history, hospitalization history, criminal justice history, and many other client factors, IPS has proven more beneficial than alternative vocational services (Campbell et al. 2011). For example, IPS has demonstrated better competitive employment outcomes for people with serious mental illness and co-occurring substance use disorders (Mueser et al. 2011).

People who obtain competitive employment through IPS have improved self-esteem, improved quality of life, and reduced symptoms (Luciano et al. 2014). Several IPS studies suggest that IPS is cost-effective compared to other vocational services, especially in the long term (Hoffmann et al. 2014). The main area of cost reduction for IPS clients is decreased use of psychiatric inpatient services compared to clients receiving services as usual (Drake et al. 2016).

IPS has spread throughout the USA and around the world. A 2016 US survey found over 500 IPS programs nationwide, and that number continues to grow (Johnson-Kwochka et al. 2017). IPS is also expanding in more than a dozen other countries. One major factor in the expansion of IPS has been an international learning community (Becker et al. 2014). Through the leadership of the IPS Employment Center (https://ipsworks.org), this learning community has helped to create state leadership, infrastructure, training, supervision, fidelity assessments, and routine outcome data collection and analysis. It has offered education and training online, an annual conference, and participation in numerous research studies aimed at improving services. IPS programs track their employment rates every quarter and with high regularity report them to the IPS Employment Center. Over an 18-year period since the inception of the learning community in 2002, IPS programs in the learning community have sustained an average employment rate exceeding 40%, even during the recession from 2007 to 2009 (Becker et al. 2014). By 2018, the learning community had grown to over 300 IPS programs in 24 states in the USA and many more in 6 countries outside the USA.

The literature on IPS for people with serious mental illness includes outcome evaluations, process and implementation studies, qualitative reports, and many other types of research inquiries. This work has continued for more than three decades, establishing IPS as one of the best researched of all vocational interventions. However, research on IPS for other populations is in its early stages of development.

IPS in Other Populations

A recent systematic review of studies evaluating the effectiveness of IPS in other populations (Bond et al. 2019). Drawing on that review, Table 2 summarizes the results from 13 studies and the designs of 3 studies in progress.

Nonpsychotic Psychiatric Disorders

Psychiatric populations other than serious mental illness include depression, anxiety disorders, and adjustment disorders, affective disorders, posttraumatic stress disorder, and personality disorders such as borderline personality disorder. These disorders rank near the top in global burden of disease and are among the most disabling of all conditions (EASPD 2016; Murray et al. 2012). Yet surprisingly, rehabilitation researchers have not extensively studied vocational rehabilitation approaches for people with nonpsychotic psychiatric disorders who are out of the labor market. Instead, most research has focused on accelerating return to work for the subgroup of this population who are currently employed but on sick leave (Joyce et al. 2016; Nieuwenhuijsen et al. 2014).

We identified eight IPS studies on people with nonpsychotic mental disorders, including six randomized controlled trials, one pre-post observational study, and one study that is still in progress. As we describe below, researchers have frequently modified or augmented IPS in applications in these other populations. Three studies evaluated IPS programs for people with *common mental disorders*, which refers to depression, anxiety disorders, and adjustment disorders (WHO 2017). The common mental disorder grouping appears frequently in the occupational health literature (Weich and Lewis 1998). The remaining studies include one that enrolled people with affective disorders, one for people with either moderate or severe psychiatric disorders, two focusing on veterans with posttraumatic stress disorders, and one study in progress for young adults with borderline personality disorder.

Table 2 Studies of IPS in other populations

Condition		Country	Investigator	Type of study
Psychiatric disorders	Common mental disorder	Norway	Reme (2015)	RCT
	Common mental disorder	Denmark	Hellström (2017)	RCT
	Common mental disorder	Sweden	Nygren (2011)	Pre-post
	Moderate/severe mental disorder	Norway	Reme (2019)	RCT
	Affective disorder	Sweden	Bejerholm (2017)	RCT
	PTSD	USA	Davis (2012)	RCT
	PTSD	USA	Davis (2018)	RCT
	Borderline personality disorder	Australia	Chanen (2019)	Protocol
Substance use disorders	Opioid users	USA	Lones (2017)	RCT
	Formerly incarcerated with substance use order	USA	LePage (2016)	RCT
Intellectual disabilities	Intellectual/developmental disabilities	USA	Noel (2018)	Program evaluation
	Autism spectrum disorders	USA	McLaren (2017)	Case study
Musculoskeletal/neurological disorders	Spinal cord injury	USA	Ottomanelli (2012)	RCT
	Chronic pain	Norway	Rødevand (2017)	Pilot
	Chronic pain	Norway	Linnemørken (2018)	Protocol
	Traumatic brain injury	Norway	Howe (2017)	Protocol

PTSD posttraumatic stress disorder, *RCT* randomized controlled trial

Common Mental Disorders

Reme et al. (2015) conducted a randomized, controlled, multicenter trial in Norway for 1193 participants with common mental disorders. Participants came from three subgroups: employees on sick leave, those at risk of going on sick leave, and those on long-term benefits. The intervention had two components: a work-focused cognitive behavior therapy aimed at helping employees on sick leave return to work and individual job support based on the IPS model. The control group received usual care. At 12-month follow-up, a significantly higher percentage of intervention participants were employed than control participants (44% vs. 37%). The effects of the intervention on the long-term disability group were stronger (24% vs. 12%). The intervention group also showed significant reductions in depression and anxiety symptoms and significant increases in health-related quality of life, compared to usual care. In a long-term follow-up after the intervention ended, Øverland et al. (2018) found that employment differences persisted for the long-term disability group, but not for the others.

Hellström et al. (2017) examined the effects of IPS modified for 326 people with mood and anxiety disorders in Denmark on work and education compared with a control group receiving usual services. After 24 months, 44% of IPS participants had returned to work or education, compared with 38% control participants, a non-significant difference. The groups also did not differ in number of weeks on employment or education, self-reported well-being, or interviewer-rated depression, anxiety, and global level of functioning.

The study was only a weak test of IPS in this population because modifications eliminated several critical ingredients of IPS. First, the researchers assumed that integration with treatment was impractical because people with mood and anxiety disorders were treated in many different settings in Denmark. Second, the participants looked for jobs themselves through ordinary job-seeking channels. Third, benefits counseling was provided on an ad hoc basis.

Nygren et al. (2011) conducted a pre-post study of IPS in Sweden for 65 people on sickness benefits. The sample had a mixture of diagnoses, mostly depression or anxiety disorder. Over a 1-year follow-up, 25% of the participants gained employment. Participants who worked showed reduced psychiatric symptoms and improved global functioning.

Affective Disorders

Bejerholm et al. (2017) conducted a randomized controlled trial in Sweden to evaluate an enhanced version of IPS incorporating motivational interviewing and cognitive strategies for 61 people with affective disorders. Over a 12-month period, 42% of IPS clients attained competitive employment, significantly more than 4% in the control condition who were offered traditional vocational rehabilitation. IPS clients also had significantly better outcomes for hours and weeks employed, time to employment, depression, and quality of life.

Moderate to Severe Mental Illness

Reme et al. (2019) conducted an 18-month, multisite, randomized controlled trial of IPS in Norway for 410 people with moderate to severe mental illness. The study compared IPS, implemented according to an IPS manual, to high-quality usual care (which included "work with assistance" and/or traineeship in a sheltered business). Significantly more of the IPS group than the control group were competitively employed at 18 months (37% versus 27%) with similar results for the participants with moderate mental illness. IPS also yielded significantly greater improvements compared to the control group, on psychological distress, symptoms of depression, subjective health complaints, functioning, health-related quality of life, and global well-being.

Posttraumatic Stress Disorder (PTSD)

Davis et al. (2012) conducted a randomized controlled trial of IPS for 85 military veterans with PTSD, comparing IPS to the usual vocational services (i.e., a stepwise transitional work program). The study was conducted at a Department of Veterans Affairs (VA) medical center in the USA. During the 12-month follow-up period, 76% of the IPS participants gained competitive employment, significantly more than 28% of control participants. IPS participants also worked significantly more weeks and earned significantly higher income than control participants.

In a replication study, Davis et al. (2018) conducted a multisite randomized controlled trial comparing IPS to the VA transitional work program for 541 unemployed veterans with PTSD. A higher proportion of IPS participants attained a competitive job (69% vs. 57%). Other competitive employment outcomes (total earnings from employment, days employed, time to first job, employed full time) significantly favored IPS. Change in posttraumatic stress disorder symptom ratings marginally favored IPS.

Borderline Personality Disorder

In preparation for a randomized controlled trial, Chanen (2019) conducted a pilot study at a clinic for young adults with borderline personality disorder in Melbourne, Australia (see Bond et al. 2019). Over an 18-month period, 11 (48%) of 23 youth receiving IPS gained competitive employment or started an educational program. In 2019 this research group initiated a randomized controlled trial of IPS in this clinic. The study will examine 12-month competitive employment and education outcomes for 108 youth.

Substance Use Disorder

Most published research on the effectiveness of employment and training services for people with substance use disorders is outdated (Magura et al. 2004; Platt 1995). The prevailing service models have been stepwise employment approaches, with generally poor outcomes.

People with substance use disorders often have legal problems. In the USA, people who use illegal drugs are likely to have criminal justice involvement, often leading to incarceration. Historically, vocational services for people with legal involvement have emphasized pre-vocational job readiness training, self-directed job searches, time-limited follow-along supports, and noncompetitive employment options. A recent review has suggested that transitional employment programs or other traditional approaches are ineffective both for preventing recidivism (i.e., repeat incarceration) and for helping people achieve long-term steady employment (Doleac 2018).

We identified two randomized controlled trials examining IPS for people with substance use disorder.

Opioid Use Disorder

Lones et al. (2017) conducted a randomized controlled trial of IPS for people with opioid use disorders enrolled in a methadone treatment program in Portland, Oregon. The researchers randomly assigned 45 participants to IPS or a 6-month waitlist. Over a 6-month follow-up, 50% of the IPS group obtained a competitive job, significantly more than 5% of the control group.

Substance Use Disorders and Criminal Justice Involvement

LePage et al. (2016) conducted a randomized controlled trial comparing IPS combined with a group-based vocational intervention to a control group consisting of the group intervention only. The study enrolled US military veterans with at least one felony conviction, 88% of whom had a substance use disorder. Over a 6-month period, significantly more of the IPS group obtained employment, compared to the control group (46% vs. 21%). The IPS group also worked significantly more hours and earned more wages than the control group.

Intellectual and Developmental Disorders

The World Health Organization defines intellectual and developmental disorders (formerly known as mental retardation) as "a group of developmental conditions characterized by significant impairment of cognitive functions, which are associated with limitations of learning, adaptive behavior and skills" (p. 175) (Salvador-Carulla et al. 2011). This group of disorders includes a diverse range of medical conditions affecting cognitive function, all of which have onset before the age of 18. Worldwide, people with intellectual and developmental disabilities have been referred to adult day programs (which may have sheltered work opportunities) with little prospect of graduating to competitive employment (Rusch and Braddock 2004).

We found two IPS studies for people with intellectual and developmental disabilities, one a program evaluation of a multisite demonstration study and the other a multiple case study of IPS for young adults with autism spectrum disorder.

Intellectual and Developmental Disabilities

Noel et al. (2018) conducted a program evaluation of a statewide implementation of IPS for high school students with intellectual and developmental disabilities and/or psychiatric disabilities in Illinois. The demonstration project involved collaboration between 10 community mental health centers and local school systems. The participating sites all initiated IPS services and successfully enrolled youth into their IPS programs. In the last quarter of the follow-up period, the mean quarterly employment rate for the ten sites was 36%. The main implementation barriers for these new IPS programs were a lack of collaboration between IPS and the schools, competing expectations, and stigma. In addition, at several sites, the IPS program was competing with existing stepwise programs that were firmly entrenched in the school systems.

Autism Spectrum Disorders

McLaren et al. (2017) described a pilot IPS program for five young adults with autism spectrum disorders who obtained competitive employment within 1 year. All five clients maintained their jobs over the study period. In addition to gaining employment, participants and their families also reported improvements in independence, self-confidence, and family relationships.

Musculoskeletal and Neurological Disorders

Musculoskeletal and neurological disorders include injuries or pain in the musculoskeletal system and/or neurological impairments affecting role functioning, including work functioning. This broad classification includes spinal cord injuries, pain syndromes, and traumatic brain injuries. Although rehabilitation programs for people with musculoskeletal and neurological disorders are widespread, most address physical rehabilitation (e.g., mobility and tasks of daily living), and few include vocational rehabilitation interventions.

Spinal Cord Injury

Ottomanelli et al. (2012) conducted a randomized controlled trial comparing IPS to treatment as usual for US military veterans with spinal cord injuries. The multisite study recruited veterans being treated at spinal cord injury clinics in 6 VA medical centers and randomly assigned 81 participants to IPS and 76 participants to treatment as usual. Over a 1-year follow-up period, the IPS group had a significantly higher rate of competitive employment than the control group (26% vs. 11%). The 2-year follow-up findings were even stronger, with more IPS clients obtaining employment (Ottomanelli et al. 2014a). Ottomanelli et al. (2013) found no improvements in health-related quality of life, disability, social integration, and mobility. However, participants who held a competitive job reported significantly better social integration and mobility.

The investigators made several modifications to the IPS model necessitated by the nature of spinal cord injury. For example, employment services were integrated with the medical treatment for spinal cord injury rather than with mental health care. Other modifications included different approaches to employers regarding requirements for workplace accommodations (Ottomanelli et al. 2014b).

Chronic Pain

Rødevand et al. (2017) conducted a pilot interview study of IPS for eight patients with chronic pain in a Norwegian hospital outpatient pain clinic. Over a 12-month period, three (38%) gained employment. Based on this pilot, Linnemørken et al. (2018) have launched a randomized controlled trial evaluating the effectiveness of IPS for unemployed Norwegians receiving treatment for chronic pain at a hospital outpatient clinic.

Traumatic Brain Injury

Howe et al. (2017), in another Norwegian study, described a protocol for a randomized controlled trial to evaluate the effects of a vocational intervention for patients with mild to moderate traumatic brain injury. The intervention integrates cognitive rehabilitation training with supported employment, based loosely on IPS fidelity standards. The study will examine the impact of the intervention on competitive employment outcomes, including work productivity, and changes in self-reported symptoms, emotional and cognitive functioning, and quality of life.

Discussion

Extensive research on IPS (including two dozen randomized controlled trials conducted throughout the world) validates the intervention for people with serious mental illness. This literature encompasses effectiveness, long-term outcomes, cost-effectiveness, cross-cultural implementation, and non-vocational as well as vocational outcomes. IPS research now extends to other populations seeking competitive employment, including people with anxiety, depression, posttraumatic stress disorder, substance use disorder, autism, and spinal cord injury. Recent randomized controlled trials show consistently higher competitive employment rates for IPS. The findings are particularly strong for veterans with PTSD. For these other populations, the initial studies are encouraging but need replication. Further, the findings regarding non-vocational outcomes show inconsistent measures and results. Several studies also augmented IPS with cognitive behavioral therapy, confounding any results for symptom reduction. Symptom control and quality of life improvements may accrue to those who become steadily employed, rather than to those assigned to IPS, consistent with studies of those with serious mental disorders (Luciano et al. 2014).

Current research does not clarify the need for modifications of IPS related to the characteristics of any specific disability or condition. People in all disability groups are heterogeneous and probably need an individualized approach like IPS, undergirded with a set of pragmatic principles that are not specific to any impairment or condition. The commonalities facing unemployed people as they choose the types of jobs, employers, and work settings that match their experiences, preferences, and abilities and as they strive to maintain employment may outweigh any specific deficits associated with their disability. Modifications to IPS fidelity standards may be necessary in some cases, but IPS principles thus far obtain across disabilities.

Conclusions

All people with disabilities deserve the opportunity to work. IPS research robustly demonstrates that most people with serious mental illness can succeed in competitive employment, which enhances their lives in many ways. Research on other disability populations, though just emerging, suggests potential to enhance their recoveries through employment as well. We conclude that IPS potentially benefits many disability groups and warrants additional rigorous research.

Cross-References

▶ Addictive Disorders: Problems and Interventions at Workplace

References

Becker DR, Drake RE (2003) A working life for people with severe mental illness. Oxford University Press, New York

Becker DR, Drake RE, Bond GR (2014) The IPS supported employment learning collaborative. Psychiatr Rehabil J 37:79–85

Bejerholm U, Larsson ME, Johanson S (2017) Supported employment adapted for people with affective disorders: a randomized controlled trial. J Affect Disord 207:212–220

Boman T, Kjellberg A, Danermark B, Boman E (2015) Employment opportunities for persons with different types of disability. ALTER, Eur J Disab Res 9:116–119

Bond GR, Drake RE (2014) Making the case for IPS supported employment. Adm Policy Ment Health Ment Health Serv Res 41:69–73

Bond GR, Drake RE, Becker DR (2012) Generalizability of the individual placement and support (IPS) model of supported employment outside the US. World Psychiatry 11:32–39

Bond GR, Drake RE, Pogue JA (2019) Expanding individual placement and support to populations with conditions and disorders other than serious mental illness. Psychiatr Serv. https://doi.org/10.1176/appi.ps.201800464

Campbell K, Bond GR, Drake RE (2011) Who benefits from supported employment: a meta-analytic study. Schizophr Bull 37:370–380

Chanen A (2019) Individualised vocational support for youth with borderline personality disorder: a randomised controlled trial investigating vocational outcomes with individual placement and support compared with usual vocational services. Clinical trial registration: ACTRN12619001220156. ANZCTR (Australain New Zealand clinical trials registry). www.ANZCTR.org.au/ACTRN12619001220156.aspx

Davis LL et al (2012) A randomized controlled trial of supported employment among veterans with posttraumatic stress disorder. Psychiatr Serv 63:464–470

Davis LL et al (2018) Effect of evidence-based supported employment vs transitional work on achieving steady work among veterans with posttraumatic stress disorder: a randomized clinical trial. JAMA Psychiat 75:316–324

Doleac JL (2018) Strategies to productively reincorporate the formerly-incarcerated into communities: a review of the literature. (http://jenniferdoleac.com/wp-content/uploads/2018/06/Doleac_Reentry_Review.pdf). Economics Department, Texas A&M University, College Station

Drake RE, Bond GR, Becker DR (2012) Individual placement and support: an evidence-based approach to supported employment. Oxford University Press, New York

Drake RE, Bond GR, Goldman HH, Hogan MF, Karakus M (2016) Individual placement and support services boost employment for people with serious mental illness, but funding is lacking. Health Aff 35:1098–1105

EASPD (2016) Report on the comparison of the available strategies for professional integration and reintegration of persons with chronic diseases and mental health issues. European Association of Service Providers to Persons with Disabilities (http://www.easpd.eu), Brussels

Goldman HH (1984) Epidemiology. In: Talbott JA (ed) The chronic mental patient: five years later. Grune & Stratton, Orlando, pp 15–31

Hellström L, Bech P, Hjorthøj C, Nordentoft M, Lindschou J, Eplov LF (2017) Effect on return to work or education of individual placement and support modified for people with mood and anxiety disorders: results of a randomised clinical trial. Occup Environ Med 74:717–725

Hoffmann H, Jäckel D, Glauser S, Mueser KT, Kupper Z (2014) Long-term effectiveness of supported employment: five-year follow-up of a randomized controlled trial. Am J Psychiatr 171:1183–1190

Howe EI et al (2017) Combined cognitive and vocational interventions after mild to moderate traumatic brain injury: study protocol for a randomized controlled trial. Trials 18:483. https://doi.org/10.1186/s13063-13017-12218-13067

Johnson-Kwochka AV, Bond GR, Drake RE, Becker DR, Greene MA (2017) Prevalence and quality of individual placement and support (IPS) supported employment in the United States. Adm Policy Ment Health Ment Health Serv Res 44:311–319

Joyce S, Modini M, Christensen H, Mykletun A, Bryant R, Mitchell P, Harvey S (2016) Workplace interventions for common mental disorders: a systematic meta-review. Psychol Med 46:683–697

LePage JP, Lewis AA, Crawford AM, Parish JA, Ottomanelli L, Washington EL, Cipher DJ (2016) Incorporating individualized placement and support principles into vocational rehabilitation for formerly incarcerated veterans. Psychiatr Serv 16:735–742

Linnemørken LT, Sveinsdottir V, Knutzen T, Rødevand L, Hernæs KH, Reme SE (2018) Protocol for the individual placement and support (IPS) in pain trial: a randomized controlled trial investigating the effectiveness of IPS for patients with chronic pain. BMC Musculoskelet Disord 19(47). https://doi.org/10.1186/s12891-12018-11962-12895

Lones CE, Bond GR, McGovern MP, Carr K, Leckron-Myers T, Hartnett T, Becker DR (2017) Individual placement and support (IPS) for methadone maintenance therapy patients: a pilot randomized controlled trial. Adm Policy Ment Health Ment Health Serv Res 44:359–364

Luciano AE, Bond GR, Drake RE (2014) Does employment alter the course and outcome of schizophrenia and other severe mental illnesses? A systematic review of longitudinal research. Schizophr Res 159:312–321

Magura S, Staines GL, Blankertz L, Madison EM (2004) The effectiveness of vocational services for substance users in treatment. Subst Use Misuse 39:2165–2213

Marwaha S et al (2007) Rates and correlates of employment in people with schizophrenia in the UK, France and Germany. Br J Psychiatry 191:30–37

McLaren J, Lichtenstein JD, Lynch D, Becker DR, Drake RE (2017) Individual placement and support for people with autism spectrum disorders: a pilot program. Adm Policy Ment Health Ment Health Serv 44:365–373

Metcalfe JD, Drake RE, Bond GR (2018) Economic, labor, and regulatory moderators of the effect of individual placement and support among people with severe mental illness: a systematic review and meta-analysis. Schizophr Bull 44:22–31

Modini M et al (2016) Supported employment for people with severe mental illness: a systematic review and meta-analysis of the international evidence. Br J Psychiatry 209:14–22

Mueser KT, Campbell K, Drake RE (2011) The effectiveness of supported employment in people with dual disorders. J Dual Disord 7:90–102

Murray CJ, Vos T, Lozano R, Naghavi M, Flaxman AD, Michaud C et al (2012) Disability-adjusted life years (DALYs) for 291 diseases and injuries in 21 regions, 1990–2010: a systematic analysis for the global burden of disease study. Lancet 380:2197–2223

Nieuwenhuijsen K et al. (2014) Interventions to improve return to work in depressed people. Cochrane database of systematic reviews: Issue 12. Art. No.: CD006237. https://doi.org/10.1002/14651858.CD006237.pub3

Noel VA, Oulvey E, Drake RE, Bond GR, Carpenter-Song EA, DeAtley B (2018) A preliminary evaluation of individual placement and support for youth with developmental and psychiatric disabilities. J Vocat Rehabil 48:249–255

Nygren U, Markström U, Svensson B, Hansson L, Sandlund M (2011) Individual placement and support – a model to get employed for people with mental illness – the first Swedish report of outcomes. Scand J Caring Sci 25:591–598

Ottomanelli L et al (2012) Effectiveness of supported employment for veterans with spinal cord injuries: results from a randomized multisite study. Arch Phys Med Rehabil 93:740–747

Ottomanelli L, Barnett SD, Goetz LL (2013) A prospective examination of the impact of a supported employment program and employment on health-related quality of life, handicap, and disability among veterans with SCI. Qual Life Res 22:2133–2141

Ottomanelli L, Barnett SD, Goetz LL (2014a) The effectiveness of supported employment for veterans with spinal cord injury: 2-year results. Arch Phys Med Rehabil 95:784–790

Ottomanelli L, Barnett SD, Toscano R (2014b) IPS in physical rehabilitation and medicine: the VA spinal cord injury experience. Psychiatr Rehabil J 37:110–112

Øverland S, Grasdal AL, Reme SE (2018) Long-term effects on income and sickness benefits after work-focused cognitive-behavioural therapy and individual job support: a pragmatic, multi-centre, randomised controlled trial. Occup Environ Med 75:703–708

Platt JJ (1995) Vocational rehabilitation of drug abusers. Psychol Bull 117:416–433

Reme SE, Grasdal AL, Løvvik C, Lie SA, Øverland S (2015) Work-focused cognitive–behavioural therapy and individual job support to increase work participation in common mental disorders: a randomised controlled multicentre trial. Occup Environ Med 72:745–752

Reme SE, Monstad K, Fyhn T, Sveinsdottir V, Løvvik C, Lie SA, Øverland S (2019) A randomized controlled multicenter trial of individual placement and support for patients with moderate to severe mental illness. Scand J Work Environ Health 45:33–41

Rødevand L, Ljosaa TM, Granan LP, Knutzen T, Jacobsen HB, Reme SE (2017) A pilot study of the individual placement and support model for patients with chronic pain. BMC Musculoskelet Disord 18:550. https://doi.org/10.1186/s12891–12017–11908-12893

Rusch FR, Braddock D (2004) Adult day programs versus supported employment (1988–2002): spending and service practices of mental retardation and developmental disabilities state agencies. Res Pract Pers Severe Disabil 29:237–242

Salvador-Carulla L et al (2011) Intellectual developmental disorders: towards a new name, definition and framework for "mental retardation/intellectual disability" in ICD-11. World Psychiatry 10:175–180

Schinnar A, Rothbard A, Kanter R, Jung Y (1990) An empirical literature review of definitions of severe and persistent mental illness. Am J Psychiatr 147:1602–1608

Wehman P, Moon MS (eds) (1988) Vocational rehabilitation and supported employment. Paul Brookes, Baltimore

Weich S, Lewis G (1998) Poverty, unemployment, and common mental disorders: population based cohort study. BMJ 317:115. https://doi.org/10.1136/bmj.317.7151.1115

WHO (2017) Depression and other common mental disorders: global health estimates (WHO/MSD/MER/2017.2). World Health Organization, Geneva

Implementing Best Practice Models of Return to Work

32

Vicki L. Kristman, Cécile R. L. Boot, Kathy Sanderson, Kathryn E. Sinden, and Kelly Williams-Whitt

Contents

Introduction	590
Return to Work Definition	591
Overview of Conceptual Models of Return to Work	592
Proposed New Practice-Oriented Model	592
Comparison of Practice-Oriented Models	597
Application of the Best Practices for RTW Implementation Model	601
Phase I: Stay-at-Work	603
Phase II: Early Return to Work	604
Phase III: Prolonged Return to Work and Recurrence	605
Applying the Best Practices for RTW Implementation Model	605
Summary	606
Best Practice Recommendations	606
Conclusion	609
Cross-References	610
References	610

V. L. Kristman (✉)
EPID@Work Research Institute, Department of Health Sciences, Lakehead University, Thunder Bay, ON, Canada
e-mail: vkristman@lakeheadu.ca

C. R. L. Boot
Department of Public and Occupational Health, Amsterdam Public Health Research Institute, Amsterdam UMC, VU University, Amsterdam, The Netherlands

K. Sanderson
EPID@Work Research Institute, Faculty of Business Administration, Lakehead University, Thunder Bay, ON, Canada

K. E. Sinden
EPID@Work Research Institute, School of Kinesiology, Lakehead University, Thunder Bay, ON, Canada

K. Williams-Whitt
Dhillon School of Business, University of Lethbridge, Calgary, AB, Canada

© Springer Nature Switzerland AG 2020
U. Bültmann, J. Siegrist (eds.), *Handbook of Disability, Work and Health*, Handbook Series in Occupational Health Sciences, https://doi.org/10.1007/978-3-030-24334-0_32

Abstract

Over the last few decades, we have seen a considerable number of models of return to work (RTW) and work disability. The majority of these are conceptual models developed from research on musculoskeletal disorders. The aim of this chapter is to develop a new practice-based model of RTW implementation, compare it to existing practice-based models, demonstrate the application of the new model using a case scenario, and indicate how it fits with recommendations for best practices from those engaged in RTW on a daily basis. The "Best Practices for RTW Implementation Model" has a holistic approach and identifies three stages involved in best practices for RTW, Stay-at-Work, early RTW, and prolonged RTW and takes into account the workplace's organizational culture and structure. Keys to staying at work are positive supervisor and co-worker relations to enable early identification and action to solve problems. For early RTW, the role of the RTW coordinator is key, and workplace adjustments that may be both formal and informal are an important mechanism to get absent workers back into the workplace as soon as possible. Prolonged RTW follows from an unsuccessful RTW, and optimizing the work environment to match the (remaining) capacities of the employee is central. The model has the capacity to be of value to both researchers and practitioners focusing on the RTW process regardless of reason for employee absence or jurisdiction.

Keywords

Return to work · Implementation · Practice models · Work disability

Introduction

Over the last few decades, we have seen a considerable number of conceptual models of return to work (RTW) and work disability. Many of these models were developed from research evidence on musculoskeletal disorders, in particular, low back pain (Costa-Black et al. 2013; Knauf and Schultz 2016). More recently, research evidence in the area of RTW for cancer survivors led to the development of a model specific to cancer (Feuerstein et al. 2010). Studies of RTW specific to other diseases and disorders, such as common mental health disorders, spinal cord injury, stroke, etc., have elucidated that many factors related to RTW, especially workplace factors, are generic across disorders (Shaw et al. 2013). Although we now have multiple conceptual models for RTW, only a handful of models exist to guide the practice and implementation of RTW (Bourbonnais et al. 2006; Dyck 2017; IWH 2007).

Therefore, the objective of this chapter is to review existing best practice models of RTW. First, we define RTW as conceptualized in this chapter. Next, we briefly review the conceptual literature on RTW and work disability to develop a new practice-oriented model of RTW. Then we compare our proposed new model to existing practice-oriented models to identify model strengths and limitations. The barriers and facilitators to the implementation of RTW are highlighted through the application of our new proposed model to a typical case of work absence. We conclude with best practice recommendations.

Return to Work Definition

Successful RTW is a key factor for the prevention of work disability in workers with chronic disease or disability. Although workers with chronic disease or disability are less likely to participate in work or employment, a large part of their work is in active paid work. Moreover, given the increase in the average age of the working population, the number of older workers with a chronic disease is likely to increase. Generally, work is considered to have a positive influence on health, as it gives meaning to life, social relationships, and opportunities for personal development, that is, when working conditions are healthy. A healthy work environment is even more important for the large and growing group of workers with chronic disease or disability as they have different requirements and their work capacity might differ from healthy co-workers. Working with a chronic disease or disability often goes along with difficulties in work functioning that may change over time depending on the progressive nature of the disease or changes in working conditions. This may lead to intermittent work absence. The key to preventing work disability is the RTW process.

In the field of work disability prevention, there has been a plethora of research conducted on RTW, both as an outcome and as a process. Although it may seem simple to distinguish RTW from not returning to work following an episode of work absence, the definition of RTW requires more than the answer to the question "Have you returned to work?". Young and colleagues described RTW as a developmental and dynamic process involving multiple phases (Young et al. 2005) from off work to reentry, maintenance, and advancement.

Important aspects of successful RTW vary by stakeholder perspective (Hees et al. 2012). Here, we mention a few of the common outcomes considered in defining successful RTW: (1) duration, (2) number of hours, (3) location, and (4) task. With regard to the duration of RTW, successful RTW is often defined as a minimum number of days between the 1st day of absence and the 1st day of RTW. For example, in the Netherlands, successful RTW is defined as RTW within at least 28 days which is in line with work disability compensation policies (a RTW episode of fewer than 28 days is considered as a continuation of the previous episode). The number of hours of RTW is another important aspect of the definition of successful RTW. Successful RTW may be considered working the same number of hours as before the episode of work absence. Location is of relevance as RTW in the workers' own job or at the same employer is considered more successful than RTW at a different employer or in a different job within the same employer. Tasks are also of relevance as they relate to changes compared to the job before the work absence episode as a change of tasks may promote RTW but may have consequences for career opportunities in the longer run.

Overall, many definitions of successful RTW include aspects of duration, number of hours and location, and seldom aspects of at-work productivity (Hees et al. 2012). Often, RTW is a process from being work disabled to taking up job tasks and maintenance of employment and sometimes even continuation of the working career path. Different stakeholders involved in the RTW process have different ideas about successful RTW (Hees et al. 2012). For an employer, successful RTW may relate to costs or duration until RTW, staff turnover, or at-work functioning (Hees et al. 2012). For employees, job satisfaction, work-home balance, and mental functioning have shown to be important outcomes of the RTW process (Hees et al. 2012), whereas professionals relate to restoration of functional abilities needed for specific tasks (Hees et al. 2012). This chapter focuses on best practices in the implementation of RTW with the objective of achieving RTW success and minimizing work disability. Differences in the definition of RTW may help to understand and explain differences between best practices in implementing RTW. These four aspects of defining successful RTW (i.e., duration, location, number of hours, and task) as outcomes can be used as targets for implementing best practices in the process of RTW.

Overview of Conceptual Models of Return to Work

Many books, book chapters (Costa-Black et al. 2013; Knauf and Schultz 2016; Schultz et al. 2015), and journal articles (Kristman et al. 2016; Schultz et al. 2007) have addressed conceptual models of RTW and work disability. Most models were developed from research findings related to musculoskeletal disorders. Over the last decade, research evidence suggests that many aspects of RTW are common to various diseases and disorders (Shaw et al. 2013). Yet, few models of RTW and work disability have taken a holistic approach to conceptualizing the problem.

In fact, there is no single parsimonious multivariable model that describes best practices in the implementation of RTW. Therefore, the purpose here is to briefly review theoretical models that contribute to RTW best practices. Table 1 highlights the features of relevant conceptual models and indicates their contribution to the implementation of best practices of RTW. In the next section, we use this information to develop a new practice-based model, based on these existing conceptual models.

Proposed New Practice-Oriented Model

Since existing theoretical models do not provide a holistic view of the implementation of the RTW process, we developed a new practice-oriented holistic RTW model (Fig. 1) based on the contributions of the conceptual models listed in Table 1: "Best Practices for RTW Implementation Model." Although return to work is traditionally accepted as the process involved following a work absence due to injury or illness,

Table 1 Conceptual models of RTW and work disability

Conceptual model	Model features	Contribution to implementation
Karasek job demand-control model (JDC) (Karasek Jr 1979)	Job demands should be balanced by control (e.g., social support) over how to do the work to avoid job strain	Suggests RTW is dependent on control over work, social support, and a reduction of job demands; high job demands or low control may be barriers to RTW
Biopsychosocial model (Waddell 1987)	Many factors can contribute to work disability including biology, behavioral, and social factors	Behavioral and social factors contribute to RTW
Biomedical model (Leibowitz 1991)	Focuses on the individual impairment and clinical response	The health issue is an important consideration in RTW
Feuerstein model (Feuerstein 1991)	RTW results from interactions between behavior, medical status, physical capabilities, and work demands	Considers psychological/behavioral resources as a modifier of the medical status, physical capabilities, and work demands on RTW
Effort-reward imbalance model (ERI) (Siegrist 1996)	Work stress occurs due to an imbalance between the employee efforts and rewards received	Efforts and rewards should be considered in RTW
International Classification of Functioning (ICF) (WHO 2001)	Social participation, including work, depends on biology and life activities and is influenced by environmental and personal factors	Health, psychosocial, and environmental factors are important considerations for RTW
Institute of Medicine (IOM 2001)	The workplace interacts with the person to explain health	It is important to consider both personal and workplace factors in RTW
Case-management ecological model (Loisel et al. 2001)	Identifies important systems and stakeholders in work disability: Insurance, workplace, healthcare, and personal system operate within a societal context	It is important to consider all stakeholders in the RTW process
Faucett's integrated model (Faucett 2005)	Disability is a result of the physical work environment and management that lead to worker strain; the model separates individual and external factors	Workplace management, the physical work environment, and worker perceptions of these are important factors to consider in RTW
Cancer and work model (Feuerstein et al. 2010)	This is a comprehensive model for disability in cancer survivors including influences of health, symptoms, function, work demands, and environment within an organizational, legal, and financial context; also provides considerations for characteristics of cancer survivors	Many important RTW factors overlap across health conditions; special considerations should be given to symptoms specific to some conditions, such as cancer, in the process of RTW

(continued)

Table 1 (continued)

Conceptual model	Model features	Contribution to implementation
Perceived uncertainty model (Stewart et al. 2012)	An awareness of not knowing what will happen in relation to health, work, and life in general can influence RTW	Worker perceived uncertainty, along with expectations, and coping ability can influence RTW
Workplace factors model (Kristman et al. 2016)	This model presents the three basic principles for workplace factors influencing RTW	Consider workplace factors at reentry, aversive, and appetitive workplace factors when attempting a RTW

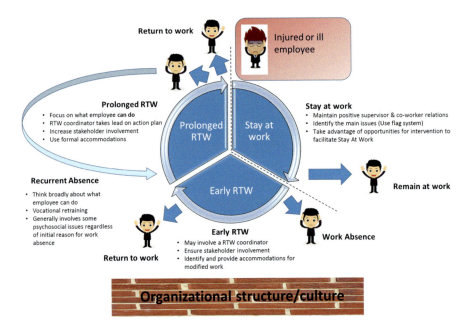

Fig. 1 Best Practices for RTW Implementation Model

there is emphasis by employers and insurers to encourage "Stay-at-Work." Stay-at-Work is initiated when a worker has reported an injury and/or illness. The employer is then tasked to engage with the employee in developing strategies that accommodate limitations resulting from the injury or illness with the goal of retaining the employee's status at work. Although timing in the employee absence is different, there is overlap in the methodological approaches as well as associated barriers and facilitators between return to work and Stay-at-Work. Consequently, our model highlights the stages involved in the best practices of RTW (Durand et al. 2014): (1) Stay-at-Work, (2) early RTW, and (3) prolonged RTW. The model also highlights the importance of the workplace's organizational structure and culture as the pillar upon which the implementation of RTW occurs. This final point is key, and the success or failure of RTW implementation hinges on the organizational structure and culture established at the workplace where the RTW is being attempted (Franche et al. 2005a; Friesen et al. 2001; MacEachen et al. 2006; Schultz et al. 2007). Organizational structure is the arrangement of authority, communication, rights, and duties of an organization (Ashkenas 1995). It often defines how activities in the workplace are coordinated and supervised to achieve the aims of the organization. For example, developing corporate policies and procedures that outline internal and external stakeholder roles and responsibilities as well as flow of information relative to the RTW is critical to success of RTW implementation. Organizational culture reflects the values and behaviors that contribute to the social and psychological environment of an organization (Schein 1984). Organizational cultures that are people- and safety-oriented are associated with improved RTW (Franche et al. 2005b).

In practice, the best way to ensure a RTW is to prevent an absence in the first place. We label this the Stay-at-Work stage. The primary goal is to identify the main issue(s) that a worker or workers may be facing that could lead to work disability and implement any changes that may allow the worker(s) to remain at work. Although RTW is often conceptualized as starting from an absence, in reality RTW is a process that does not necessarily have to start with an absence but rather begins with an illness or injury. Having a worker stay in the workplace to recover, rather than having the worker recover at home, will maximize some of the important "successful RTW" outcomes: duration, zero days lost; number of hours, workers may or may not be able to work the same number of hours as before the injury or illness, but a gradual return to normal hours may be accelerated if the employee is still at work; location, will help the worker maintain job with the same employer; and tasks, tasks may need to vary to accommodate the abilities of the injured or ill worker, but as the worker recovers, the tasks can gradually return to the pre-injured state.

The Stay-at-Work stage should involve an examination of the workplace to identify issues or changes that can help an injured or ill worker remain at the workplace. Within a people- and safety-oriented culture, maintaining positive supervisor and co-worker relations will ensure that everyone in the workplace is promoting worker well-being (Lysaght and Larmour-Trode 2008; Shaw et al. 2006). Issues that a worker or workers are dealing with can be identified early, and an attempt can be made to rectify any problems prior to an absence occurring. We recommend using the flag system to identify the main issues (Shaw et al. 2009). This system involves the identification of healthcare, psychosocial, and employee's perception of workplace factors and the actual workplace factors that may be leading to a possible work absence. Some solutions to keep a worker at work may involve allowing the worker time to attend healthcare appointments, repairing broken workplace relations, or rectifying employees' misguided perceptions. Workplace factors are broad and are often conceptualized into four categories including (1) physical job demands, (2) psychosocial job demands, (3) work organization and support, and (4) workplace beliefs and attitudes (Kristman et al. 2016; Shaw et al. 2013). Opportunities for workplace intervention include the use of informal accommodations that allow the employee to control work intensity or rest periods (Tjulin et al. 2010), the modification of job demands (Janssen 2000; Karasek Jr 1979), increasing the amount of control in the job (Gimeno et al. 2005), increasing the amount of reward related to the job (Janssen 2000), or the use of employee assistance programs (Jacobson Frey and Attridge 2010). Developing a written "Stay-at-Work" plan (SAWP) provides a reference document that all stakeholders can use throughout the process. This can become the cornerstone of the Stay-at-Work initiative. Often, relatively easy fixes addressing the worker's primary concerns can allow the worker to remain at work and prevent an absence altogether (Amick et al. 2000; Shaw et al. 2006).

The early RTW stage begins once the worker is absent from work, with or without compensation. In this stage, it is important to repeat all aspects of the Stay-at-Work stage, especially if these were not done before the worker went on leave. At this stage, it may be important to involve an individual with expertise in disability management and RTW such as a RTW coordinator (Franche et al. 2005a; Gardner et al. 2010; Pransky et al. 2010; van Oostrom et al. 2007) or an occupational health physician. In some jurisdictions, involving experts in disability management and RTW may only occur when the duration of work absence has exceeded a threshold of time. For example, in the Netherlands, a problem analysis has to be performed when work absence lasts more than 6 weeks. Employers arrange a meeting between the occupational physician and the worker before the 6th week of absence, often after 4 weeks (Bockting 2007) to facilitate a RTW solution. Additionally, RTW coordinators will often conduct a case review, including ergonomic and workplace assessments, social problem-solving, and workplace mediation (Shaw et al. 2008). Effective communication and collaboration between all stakeholders, including the worker, the supervisor, the healthcare provider, the worker's union (if existing), and any insurers, is vital (Franche et al. 2005a; Friesen et al. 2001; Young et al. 2005). This communication and collaboration is easier when the RTW process occurs in an organization where a strong organizational culture exists, an organizational culture that is understood to have particularly strong effects on the ways in which organization members think and behave; it is usually contrasted with competing influences on organization members other than culture, including direct supervisory oversight, rules such as job descriptions and budgets, and explicit contracts (Peterson and Fischer 2004). Stakeholders should discuss all the potential barriers and facilitators to RTW. These barriers may include access to appropriate healthcare, personal issues with the worker, aversive workplace factors, and difficulties working through the compensation process. A written return to work plan (RTWP) becomes critical to facilitate this process. A RTWP is similar to the SAWP in that it provides a cornerstone document that outlines stakeholder roles and responsibilities. It differs in that modifications to work, appointments, rehabilitation strategies, and gradual increases in modifications to work (i.e., duration and tasks) are clearly outlined. The RTWP should be developed in collaboration with all stakeholders including the worker, supervisor, RTW coordinator, and, where applicable, healthcare professional.

We have identified prolonged RTW as the period of time when a worker's absence results following an initial failed RTW attempt (Frank et al. 1996). Examples that may contribute to the failed RTW include recurrence/exacerbation of injury/illness, contextual barriers experienced by the worker requiring resolution before continued return to work, and/or a new injury/illness (Frank et al. 1996). During the prolonged RTW stage, the focus should be on what an employee can do (i.e., capabilities). The stakeholders should develop a RTWP (Tjulin et al. 2010), outlining the roles and responsibilities of all involved with timelines attached. Formal accommodations can help to remove or modify barriers (Franche et al. 2005b; Krause et al. 1998). The supervisor or workplace personnel involved in day-to-day operations should be involved (Franche et al. 2005a, b) and the absent worker. Depending on context and jurisdiction, it may be required to include additional employer stakeholders such as union, management, and other co-workers (MacEachen et al. 2006). The workplace should provide paid time for medical appointments, if needed (Pryce et al. 2007). Most importantly, continued communication and collaboration between all parties will help to achieve a timely and successful RTW (Nieuwenhuijsen et al. 2004; Yarker et al. 2010).

If RTW is not achieved according to the RTWP, this stage should be repeated with ideas for new interventions, increased social support, and increased participation. If this is still unsuccessful, the absence may become recurrent (ongoing long-term absence). At this stage, there are generally psychosocial issues regardless of the initial reason for work absence. Modifiable psychosocial risk factors associated with prolonged absence from work include fear of reinjury with movement, pain catastrophizing, personal beliefs regarding perceived degree of disability, and depressive disorders (Sullivan et al. 2005). Vocational retraining or assistance with a job search for a new position may need to be considered. Research has shown some evidence for the success of community-based psychosocial interventions (Sullivan et al. 2005). However, early, multidisciplinary, and time-contingent, activating interventions appear to be the most effective to support RTW (Hoefsmit et al. 2012), but more research is needed to evaluate interventions used at the recurrent stage.

Comparison of Practice-Oriented Models

Previously, the development of conceptual models highlighted the progression and growth of knowledge related to RTW factors and interventions. However, in order to facilitate RTW, supervisors or RTW coordinators need practical tools to guide the complex process of accommodating and reintegrating a worker following an absence.

The sheer variety of considerations for RTW make the development and implementation of a practice-oriented model difficult. Successful RTW is dependent upon an extensive list of factors, which include but are not limited to the structure and culture of the organization, industry, type of work, required modifications, social influences, and job demands. As a result, a fully comprehensive model becomes overwhelming to implement, and a simpler model does not capture the essential components of a RTW plan.

Implementing any type of RTW comes with a host of barriers. As each individual situation will eventually reveal, there is far more to a successful RTW than what can be easily captured in a "one-size-fits-all" solution. There are, however, some common barriers to RTW that are significant and should be addressed. First, RTW inherently begins once a worker has reported an injury or illness that results in absence from work; however, developing a strategy to facilitate the worker staying at work to enable recovery will enhance RTW outcomes. Consequently, current models that begin the RTW process once the worker has experienced absence result in suboptimal conditions for vital relationship development: conveying support, building trust, and negotiating expectations. Second, much of the RTW research has focused on physical conditions which require modified duties, and as a result, the mental and emotional aspects of RTW are often neglected or become secondary to the physical condition. While the models are intended to be inclusive, the specific needs of mental health in RTW considerations are lacking. This is important for two reasons: the absence frequency and duration for employees with stress and mental health concerns continue to increase (Mental Health Commission of Canada 2015), and many physical health issues are related, or compounded, by mental health issues (Scott et al. 2007). Third, the models assume a level of competence in RTW for the facilitator and/or supervisor. For many small- and medium-sized organizations, the RTWP is highly dependent upon the direct supervisor, due to lack of other organizational supports. The process of planning and implementing a RTWP can become overwhelming and confusing. Therefore, theoretical models themselves are often a barrier for organizations as they lack in lay-application, and the practical implications of the constructs within the model are unclear. Finally, RTW is rarely a linear process. Models need to include and anticipate trial and error, relapse, and regression.

Table 2 contains a description of three of the most widely used practice-oriented models, as well as a description of the newly proposed "Best Practices for RTW Implementation Model." This comparison is designed to highlight key aspects of the models without attempting to be exhaustive. However, comparing the models and the inherent strengths provides an overview of how the models are intended to guide the RTW facilitator.

While all of the three existing practice models have clear strengths, they also possess limitations, many of which are addressed within the Best Practices for RTW Implementation Model. The new model was designed with features to increase ease of use as well as including a process that encourages accommodation prior to the worker being absent from work due to injury or illness (i.e., Stay-at-Work). Also integral to the model is the recognition that organizational climate, context, and structure will influence and inform the RTW process. These factors are situational and company specific.

The process model, while extremely comprehensive, creates a series of steps that easily become overwhelming for the non-RTW specialist. For large organizations with RTW staff, this model may capture the complexity of RTW. However, without

Table 2 Comparison of Return to Work Practice Models

	Process model[a,b]	Participative model[c-g]	IWH 7 Principles[h]	Best Practices for RTW Implementation Model
Overview	Within a disability management framework, this graduated RTW process of shared responsibility considers social issues and fairness to all parties	A stepwise process from sick leave to return to work involving all stakeholders in the development of a RTW plan designed to fit specific workers or organizational needs	A set of steps which ensures an individualized RTW plan is developed to reintegrate workers in a safe and timely manner	A three-component model which is engaged prior to the work absence. Each phase builds upon the prior with a holistic biopsychosocial focus

Model in brief	1. Collaboration and cooperation between stakeholders
	2. Focus on a safe and timely RTW with early intervention
	3. Active involvement of supervisors and unions with clear roles
	4. One person responsible for case management
	5. Develop individual RTW plans:
	  1. Assess capabilities of employee
	  2. Tasks and duration suitable for RTW
	  3. Determine accommodation
	4. Monitor progress documentation
		1. Creating conditions: assign a process manager, check the key stakeholders, prepare the organization
		2. Problem analysis: aim to reach consensus about problems to be solved
		3. Solutions analysis: aim to reach consensus about solutions between key stakeholders
		4. Action plan: define a protocol for implementation
		5. Implementation: support the implementation process and plan an evaluation
		6. Evaluation: check if the targets are met, the solutions implemented, and that the
			1. Workplace committed to health and safety
			2. Accommodation offered to encourage early and safe RTW
			3. RTW planner as lead considers worker, supervisor, and co-worker needs
			4. Supervisors provided training on RTW planning and disability prevention
			5. Early and considerate contact with worker by supervisor
			6. RTW coordination assigned
			7. Communication between healthcare providers, worker, and supervisors essential
				1. Stay-At-Work – issue identification with informal supports, work modifications jointly decided with the worker and supervisor.
				2. Early RTW – formal case review with all stakeholders which identifies challenges and opportunities for RTW
				3. Gradual RTW – action plan developed with a focus on worker's capabilities and implementing a range of RTW strategies

(continued)

Table 2 (continued)

	Process model[a,b]	Participative model[c–g]	IWH 7 Principles[h]	Best Practices for RTW Implementation Model
		problems are solved. Advise about next steps if needed 7. Problems are prioritized		
Strengths	Comprehensive view of RTW Social aspects including supervisor and co-worker attitude recognized as factors effecting outcomes Clear connection with job description and duties Fits well with physical and mental disabilities	Focus is on worker voice Proactive approach Can be used to address both individual worker level and organizational level RTW issues Feasibility of implementing solutions is high as this is taken into account as prioritizing factor	Focus on safety commitment Early worker communication essential Highlights union involvement and role of collective agreement Red flags/green lights cards and guidelines to identify what to watch for and behaviors that enable RTW	Priority given to building relationships and communication expectations prior to work absence Views the worker as a whole person, instead of focusing on what is "wrong" Identifies other issues related to RTW such as organizational context and co-worker support Includes informal, formal, and creative interventions to address psychosocial needs
Situational strength	Physical disabilities and injuries with easily quantifiable measures	Highly applicable for RTW issues of psychological safety	Generic steps that could fit any model, however not enough as a stand-alone RTW solution	Any RTW situations with complex physical and/or mental/social needs

[a](Dyck 2017)
[b](Cullen et al. 2018)
[c](Bourbonnais et al. 2006)
[d](Driessen et al. 2010)
[e](Kraaijeveld et al. 2016)
[f](Rivilis et al. 2008)
[g](van Oostrom et al. 2009)
[h](IWH 2007)

significant dedicated resources, it becomes unmanageable. Small- to medium-sized organizations may struggle with the complexity of steps and procedures. While this model strongly addresses physical and mental health injury and illness, it lacks in psychosocial considerations. This is one of the key and unique strengths of the participative model.

Prioritizing the need for the employee's voice is one of the hallmarks of the participative model. As with the process model, a high degree of RTW competence is required, albeit in different areas. The participative model is built on a foundation of communication, inclusion, and cooperation, which requires an expertise in itself, as well as a parallel organizational culture. In situations where relationships are strained or the structure is more competitive, this model may not be an appropriate approach.

The IWH 7 Principles are perhaps less of a model and more of a practice guide. The principles set the philosophical base for a RTW plan that focuses on safety. The well-known red flags/green light cards are extremely approachable regardless of practitioner background, yet they do not present a flow or structure to the RTW plan. The cards do however raise many important considerations for overcoming roadblocks, which can easily be incorporated in the other three models. It therefore may be more accurate to classify the IWH 7 Principles as a toolkit, than a RTW model.

The design of the Best Practices for RTW Implementation Model (see Fig. 1) was deliberate in the recognition of the need to address the dynamics and accommodations resulting from injury or illness, before an absence occurs (i.e., Stay-at-Work). This allows practitioners to begin a dialogue on essential RTW factors: health interventions, supervisor/employee relationships, and proactive work modifications. This also sets the tone for a cooperative RTW planning process, should it be required. The new model also allows for flexibility in involvement, as it suggests, but does not require a RTW facilitator. This model presents a flow to the RTW activities that can be understood and implemented by various organizational members, which may be more feasible in smaller organizations. The importance of flexibility and the need to consider the psychosocial are essential as many RTW processes cannot follow a firm set of prescribed steps, due to the complexity of the RTW requirements and/or co-occurring injury and illness.

The method by which this new model can assist in RTW planning and implementation is illustrated in the following section.

Application of the Best Practices for RTW Implementation Model

The following provides an overview of the application of our newly formed conceptual model for facilitating RTW. The model is applied to a hypothetical clinical case (Box A). Application of the model begins in phase 1 with the injured worker and progresses through each subsequent phase to demonstrate feasibility of identified key constructs to resolve the RTW barriers and establish successful RTW.

Box A Case Scenario
Client: Male, 45 yo; married; one child
   DOI: January 6, 2018
   Injury: left upper extremity; depression
   Injury category: Work-related
   Occupation: Cafeteria worker
   RTW: Currently off work; two previous failed RTW
   Context: The injured person is a cafeteria worker; the cafeteria is located in an office building and is owned by a food service company.
   Current Status: The worker has experienced a left upper extremity injury (rotator cuff and biceps tear) while reaching overhead to obtain a large container of food product at work. He is unable to perform sustained work involving the upper extremity without experiencing increased, localized pain. In addition to musculoskeletal complaints, the worker was diagnosed with depression in September 2018 and has been receiving treatment under the supervision of a psychiatrist. It has been 10 months since the initial incident, and the worker is reporting increased pain and is uncertain about his ability to RTW.
   In addition to the issues related to implementation of developing a suitable RTW plan for the injured worker, the organization has failed to establish a corporate Return-to-Work program including policies and procedures that clearly outlines roles/responsibilities and process for the involved stakeholders (i.e., injured worker, supervisor, co-workers). This has left all workplace parties including the injured worker feeling lost in the process. The primary contact for the RTW is the company's HR Manager; this person has been tasked to establish a suitable RTW plan that is agreed upon by all stakeholders.
   Capabilities. The injured workers' abilities from their family physician include minimal lifting overhead and minimal repetitive movements involving the left upper extremity. The psychiatrist has recommended a graduated RTW starting at 2 h per day in a supported environment.
   Medication: A series of medications for both pain and anxiety. Gabapentin (400 mg 3×/day), Flexeril (10 mg/day), and Paxil (20 mg/day).
   History: The worker was injured on January 6, 2018, while lifting a 20 lb. container of food product. The injury report indicates the container was on a high shelf, and, while reaching up to pick up the container to carry to their workstation, he felt a twinge in his low back and left upper extremity in the area of their shoulder and upper arm.
   When the worker reported the injury to the supervisor, the supervisor attempted to create a Stay-at-Work plan by providing modified duties. However, the worker felt the duties were not meaningful and were demeaning. Furthermore, co-workers who were considered friends by the worker openly questioned the worker's integrity and pointedly asked when he would be back

(continued)

to "helping the team" again. The worker did not RTW the following day, and the plan failed.

Two weeks later, the supervisor attempted to implement an early RTW plan. The supervisor contacted the worker and obtained information about his capabilities to better identify appropriate modified duties. However, the duties extended beyond the worker's outlined functional capabilities and exacerbated their condition. The worker tolerated the plan for 1 week before "calling in sick." During a follow-up telephone conversation with the worker, he mentioned that the 30-min commute was too long and exacerbated his shoulder pain. The supervisor indicated that he was frustrated and suggested that the worker try another form of work because it seems like this work is too difficult for him. This left the worker feeling isolated and unwelcome in the workplace; gradually the worker began feeling depressed and experiencing episodic anxiety. The supervisor didn't know how to proceed after this, and although attempted to contact the worker a couple of times following the failed RTW, there was no response. The worker has remained off work but is now in a position where both the insurer and employer are seeking an update and asking for a RTW plan to be implemented.

Treatment History: After the first day of work, the worker followed up with their family physician. He was referred and initially treated by a chiropractor with no improvement; the worker was then referred to orthopedic specialist and was not found to be a surgical candidate. MRI revealed a bulging disc at L5-S1 and a rotator cuff w/ biceps tear. The worker completed two rounds of physical therapy, first in February 2018, was released to work, then progressively got worse, and was referred to physical therapy again in May 2018. During August 2018, the worker became more frustrated with ongoing pain and became despondent; family members suggested follow-up with his family physician who recommended that he seeks treatment from a psychiatrist. He has been receiving appropriate treatment under a psychiatrist for depression since the beginning of September 2018 and has reported benefit from same.

Phase I: Stay-at-Work

What Happened: Despite lacking a formal, corporate RTW policy and procedure, the worker's supervisor developed a SAWP immediately following the incident to support the worker following his injury. However, the duties provided were unsuitable and considered demeaning by the worker. Furthermore, co-workers were unsupportive of the RTW and questioned the worker about the length of the modified RTW. Subsequently the worker terminated the RTW plan and remained off work for an additional 6 months.

Applying the Best Practices for RTW Implementation Model: The following three constructs reflect critical steps in facilitating Stay-at-Work: (i) maintaining positive supervisor and co-worker relations, (ii) identifying the main issues, and (iii) taking advantage of opportunities to facilitate Stay-at-Work. Failure of the initial Stay-at-Work plan might have been avoided if the workplace had facilitated a coordinated RTW with all stakeholders, ensured ongoing monitoring and collaboration with the injured worker, and educated workplace parties about the RTW. In particular, the supervisor should have better coordinated the plan with the worker and ensured the worker was returning to a positive, supportive environment among his colleagues. Furthermore, developing a clear SAWP that articulated roles, responsibilities, and duties would have ensured a cohesive approach. These activities are critical to supporting RTW and would also have been enforced had the organization established stakeholder roles and responsibilities with a clear RTW policy and procedures aligned with a positive, worker-centered environment.

Phase II: Early Return to Work

What Happened: The worker remained off work for 2 weeks before the supervisor attempted contact. Although the supervisor obtained updated capability information, the provided modified work was not appropriate and reinjured the worker. The RTW was successful for 1 week after which the worker terminated the plan. The supervisor followed up with the worker but became frustrated and suggested the worker seek alternative employment. This isolated the worker who eventually became anxious and depressed.

Applying the Best Practices for RTW Implementation Model: The following three constructs are critical to supporting early RTW and have been reviewed in the context of the case scenario: (1) involve a RTW coordinator, (2) ensure stakeholder engagement, and (3) identify and provide suitable accommodations for modified work.

A RTW coordinator is an individual with expertise in facilitating RTW and expertise in disability management; examples of professions that often become RTW coordinators include occupational therapists, kinesiologists, physical therapists, and nurses (Pransky et al. 2010). Furthermore, the RTW coordinator is a designated individual who can provide an unbiased perspective on the RTW strategy, independent from workers' direct supervisor and/or workplace. Within the context of the case scenario, the supervisor should have recognized personal limitations associated with supporting the worker through their recovery and involved a RTW coordinator. The RTW coordinator would have provided a more supportive interaction between the worker and their supervisor resulting in a RTWP that was more suitable based on functional abilities information. Furthermore, the RTW coordinator would have developed a RTWP based on the capability information which clearly outlined required modifications to tasks/duties and duration to ensure suitability of the work.

Phase III: Prolonged Return to Work and Recurrence

What Happened: The worker remained off work for over 10 months, and although the supervisor attempted intermittent contact, the worker avoided contact. The worker continued to receive treatment for both his musculoskeletal injury and depression; however the efforts to coordinate a RTW were less robust. Parties subsequently came together to facilitate a RTWP for the worker based on his newly acquired functional ability information from both his family physician and psychiatrist.

Applying the Best Practices for RTW Implementation Model

The following four constructs are critical to supporting RTW after a prolonged absence from work: (1) focus on employee capabilities not limitations, (2) RTW coordinator assuming lead on developing the RTWP, (3) increased stakeholder engagement, and (4) use of formal accommodations for modified work.

Because the organization did not establish a corporate return to work policy to establish stakeholder roles and responsibilities, this became a barrier in developing suitable modified duties. For example, the supervisor and worker lacked processes to provide updated information and responsibilities within the RTW planning phase, which resulted in the worker experiencing a prolonged absence from work. In this prolonged absence phase, as the RTW coordinator assumes a lead role in negotiating the RTW plan, the roles and responsibilities of each member including the worker and supervisor would become more clearly established which will facilitate development of a suitable RTWP. For example, standard practice would require that the worker's responsibilities would include providing updated functional ability information when requested, providing feedback on suitability of modified work, and immediately identifying barriers associated with the RTWP. The supervisor would be responsible for requesting updates from the worker regarding the RTWP and discussing identified barriers with the worker and the RTW coordinator to facilitate solutions.

Within this phase, it is critical to focus on facilitating workers' capabilities. For example, updated information regarding the workers' functional abilities was provided from the treatment team. A graduated RTW was supported by the worker's family physician and psychiatrist, and clear information about the worker's capabilities was provided including:

- Lifting above shoulder (restricted to 5 kg to start).
- Avoid repetitive movements involving the left upper extremity (first 2 weeks).
- Start a graduated RTW at 2 h per day in a supportive environment.
- Flexible break times during high emotion.

Within the context of the model, the RTW coordinator would take the lead and organize a meeting between the supervisor and worker to develop a RTWP based on the worker's capabilities and establish an implementation strategy. The implementation strategy would include (i) a communication plan that ensures regular communication between the worker and supervisor and (ii) development of a formal, written RTWP based on worker's capabilities, job demands, and input from the worker and supervisor. The RTWP should act as a contract between all stakeholders where all members agree to and subsequently sign to the terms of the plan. The RTWP would clearly delineate the formal accommodations agreed upon by all stakeholders. Examples of formal accommodations may include (i) modification to duration of tasks to accommodate lifting and repetitive movement limitations; (ii) modification to workday length to accommodate the starting RTW duration of 2 h per day; (iii) modification to tasks performed at work to accommodate the lifting restriction; and (iv) modification to workflow to accommodate flexible break times. It is important to note that the RTWP should include a gradual progression of these formal accommodations over the duration of the RTWP to facilitate a return-to-full hours/duties within the parameters of the RTW goal. Furthermore, treatment strategies including exercises and modifications to work environment (i.e., ergonomic interventions) should also be included within the development and implementation of the plan.

Summary

Several recommendations can be made following application of the model that would have reduced exposure to a prolonged absence and facilitated the worker's RTW in the initial Stay-at-Work phase:

1. Establish a corporate policy that clearly outlines individual roles and responsibilities.
2. Develop a formal RTWP based on worker's capabilities and job requirements.
3. Identify a convenient time for all stakeholders (injured worker, RTW coordinator supervisor) to meet for an initial RTW meeting to review roles/responsibilities and proposed RTWP.
4. Ensure a transparent communication strategy between all stakeholders.

Best Practice Recommendations

The purpose of this chapter has been to review scientific models of RTW and develop a process-based approach that can guide stakeholders who want to decrease work disability and improve the success of their RTW/Stay-at-Work programs. Therefore, it is important to understand not only how this process model fits with the scientific literature but also how it fits with recommendations for best practices that have been developed by those who are engaged in RTW on a daily basis. Recommendations for RTW best practices can be found on government websites (e.g., https://www.ccohs.ca/products/webinars/best_practices_rtw.pdf (Pomaki et al. 2010), https://www.worksafemt.com/media/WSMT_SAW-RTW_Best_Practices.pdf (WorkSafeMT)), insurer-provided toolkits (e.g., Morneau Shepell 2016), and in educational materials developed for training RTW coordinators or human resources professionals (e.g., The Conference Board of Canada 2013), among other places. These nonacademic sources are referred to as gray literature. A summary of some key recommendations from the stakeholder literature is provided in Box B.

A review of the publicly available best practices for RTW suggests there is consistency between our model (the "Best Practices for RTW Implementation Model" based in the scientific literature) and recommendations arising from field experience. For example, both the model and best practice recommendations:

- Identify key stakeholders.
- Explore opportunities for job accommodations.
- Highlight the importance of respectful and systematic communication.
- Recognize the impact of organizational culture and providing a supportive environment for employees with health challenges.
- Suggest steps to take during the RTW process.

But there are also important differences. First, the best practice recommendations from the gray literature tend to target employer practices and include organization-wide recommendations, while the model we have developed is more focused on individual cases and is useful to any stakeholder involved in RTW. The gray literature advises employers to create organization-wide systems that include employee training, work disability data analysis, and job demands analysis. There are also specific recommendations about how to create a culture that supports RTW by developing a vision/value system and demonstrating a commitment to health and safety. While these may be the appropriate steps to change culture, they are not necessarily based on empirical research in RTW. There are many reasons for this, including the difficulty of conducting research that can isolate the impact of culture interventions on RTW outcomes (Williams-Whitt et al. 2016; Woodman 2014) and questions about whether organizational culture can be engineered (Fitzgerald 1988; Harris and Ogbonna 2011) and how long it may take for a culture change initiative to become embedded in an organization (Schaubroeck et al. 2012). Organizational culture is not only the visible manifestations of a system of beliefs, like policies and procedures, but also the unconscious assumptions that influence how people in organizations solve problems (Schaubroeck et al. 2012; Schein 1984). So, it is particularly difficult to measure and to change. In other words, we know scientifically that organizational culture is important to RTW success, but we do not necessarily know how to create the right culture. This is why our model rests on a foundation of organizational culture but focuses more on specific RTW processes, barriers, and facilitators.

A second important difference is that our model incorporates different stages of RTW and demonstrates its iterative nature. It shows who should be involved at different stages or for different levels of RTW complexity. The best practice recommendations tend to be linear and do not account for the informal accommodations that often occur in smaller workplaces, or when the injury or illness has not resulted in time off work. It also accounts for situations where there are multiple or recurring absences, as we might see with chronic illnesses or mental health conditions. The model is flexible, allowing for experimentation and gradually increasing duties.

Finally, our model incorporates the flag system as a tool to help stakeholders systematically identify potential barriers and facilitators to RTW success. There is a greater focus on employee capabilities rather than medical restrictions as well as the goal of achieving success from the perspective of multiple stakeholders (e.g., workers compensation boards, employees, healthcare providers).

> **Box B Stakeholder Recommended Best Practices**
> 1. **Include stakeholders in planning, communications, and coordination of RTW activities.**
> 2. **Build an organizational culture that supports RTW:**
>   (a) Develop a vision, values, principles, and policies based on people-centered human resources management.
>   (b) Communicate with workers in a way that shows concern, empathy, and willingness to help. Treat them as more than their illness or injury.
>   (c) Demonstrate a strong commitment to health and safety.
>   (d) Emphasize that safe and timely RTW benefits the organization and the employee.
>   (e) Acknowledge and address normal human reactions to difficult situations.
>   (f) Investigate and address social and workplace realities.
>   (g) Encourage supportive co-worker relationships.
>   (h) Deal with discrimination and bad faith behavior.
> 3. **Develop a RTW system:**
>   (a) Assign responsibilities and empower supervisors and RTW coordinators.
>   (b) Train RTW coordinators, supervisors, and workers.
>   (c) Create a communication plan.
>
> - Simple, standardized forms for employees and healthcare workers.
> - Information sheet that can be given to workers at the start of a health-related work absence, including a description of the RTW process and contact information.
>   (d) Track organization-wide statistics on injuries, illnesses, and work disability costs.
>   (e) Conduct physical and psychological job demands analyses that can be shared with stakeholders.
>   (f) Identify jobs and tasks that are easily modified or suitable for common injuries or illnesses/work limitations.
>   (g) Develop a process for resolving disagreements or complaints about the RTW process.
>
> (continued)

(h) Monitor systems and outcomes.

4. **Develop a RTW Process:**

STEP 1: Make early and considerate contact to arrange a joint meeting when it is safe and appropriate to discuss limitations and possible accommodations.
STEP 2: Gather information about the duties and demands of the employee's current job.
STEP 3: Facilitate a discussion among the relevant stakeholders (employee, supervisor, human resources, OHS, etc.) to identify the tasks/duties the employee can safely perform, any barriers to performance, and other skills and abilities that may allow the employee to work outside of their current job.
STEP 4: Brainstorm how the employee's current job might be modified to enable the employee to continue in that role, or if that is not possible, consider other jobs within the organization that match the employee's medical restrictions and other abilities.
STEP 5: Evaluate options considering suitability, safety, length of accommodation, complexity, impact on other workers, resources, and costs.
STEP 6: Collaboratively reach agreement on an appropriate solution or seek additional expertise if needed.
STEP 7: Create a progressive plan for the RTW with goals, accountabilities, and review dates.
STEP 8: Monitor and manage the RTW process through regular communication, addressing social issues and adjustments as needed.

Conclusion

This chapter focuses on the implementation of best practice models of RTW. We reviewed existing best practice models of RTW. In contrast to the large body of evidence on RTW, models focusing on guiding the practice and implementation of RTW are sparse. Previous work has indicated that many aspects of RTW are similar for different chronic diseases and disorders, which support a generic approach regardless of the cause of RTW and a holistic approach.

Based on the existing models, we developed a new practice-oriented model for RTW. Compared to the existing models, the new model has a holistic approach and identifies three stages involved in best practices for RTW, Stay-at-Work, early RTW, and prolonged RTW and takes into account the workplace's organizational culture and structure. Keys to staying at work are positive supervisor and co-worker relations to enable early identification and action to solve problems. For early RTW, the role of the RTW coordinator is key and workplace adjustments that may be both formal and informal. Prolonged RTW follows from an unsuccessful RTW, and optimizing the work environment to match the (remaining) capacities of the employee is central. Formal workplace adjustments are more common.

We applied our model to a case and compared it with recommendations for best practices that have been developed over time by those involved in guiding RTW. This comparison showed many similarities that strengthened the base for our model. Some differences were identified; e.g., we chose a strong basis of organizational culture because we do not (yet) know how to create the right culture for RTW.

We conclude that the Best Practices for RTW Implementation Model has the potential to be of added value for both researchers and practitioners focusing on the RTW process as it takes into account barriers identified from scientific research and is in line with recommendations for best practices.

Cross-References

- ▶ Concepts of Work Ability in Rehabilitation
- ▶ Employment as a Key Rehabilitation Outcome
- ▶ Investing in Integrative Active Labour Market Policies

References

Amick BC, Habeck RV, Hunt A, Fossel AH, Chapin A, Keller RB, Katz JN (2000) Measuring the impact of organizational behaviors on work disability prevention and management. J Occup Rehabil 10:21–38

Ashkenas R (1995) The Boundaryless organization: breaking the chains of organizational structure. The Jossey-Bass Management Series. Jossey-Bass, Inc., Publishers, 350 Sansome Street, San Francisco, CA 94104

Bockting A (2007) Changes in legislation on disability in the Netherlands. Inclusion in Working Life. Paper presented at the ISSA European Regional Meeting, Oslo, pp 15–16

Bourbonnais R, Brisson C, Vinet A, Vézina M, Lower A (2006) Development and implementation of a participative intervention to improve the psychosocial work environment and mental health in an acute care hospital. Occup Environ Med 63:326–334

Costa-Black KM, Feuerstein M, Loisel P (2013) Work disability models: past and present. In: Handbook of work disability. Springer, New York, pp 71–93

Cullen KL, Irvin E, Collie A, Clay F, Gensby U, Jennings PA, ... Newnam S (2018). Effectiveness of workplace interventions in return-to-work for musculoskeletal, pain-related and mental health conditions: an update of the evidence and messages for practitioners. J Occup Rehabil 28(1):1–15

Driessen MT, Groenewoud K, Proper KI, Anema JR, Bongers PM, van der Beek AJ (2010) What are possible barriers and facilitators to implementation of a participatory ergonomics programme? Implement Sci 5:64

Durand M-J, Corbière M, Coutu M-F, Reinharz D, Albert V (2014) A review of best work-absence management and return-to-work practices for workers with musculoskeletal or common mental disorders. Work 48:579–589

Dyck D (2017) Disability management: theory, strategy and industry practice, 6th edn. LexisNexis, Toronto, ON Canada

Faucett J (2005) Integrating 'psychosocial' factors into a theoretical model for work-related musculoskeletal disorders. Theor Issues Ergon Sci 6:531–550

Feuerstein M (1991) A multidisciplinary approach to the prevention, evaluation, and management of work disability. J Occup Rehabil 1:5–12

Feuerstein M, Todd BL, Moskowitz MC, Bruns GL, Stoler MR, Nassif T, Yu X (2010) Work in cancer survivors: a model for practice and research. J Cancer Surviv 4:415–437

Fitzgerald TH (1988) Can change in organizational culture really be managed? Organ Dyn 17:5–15

Franche R-L, Baril R, Shaw W, Nicholas M, Loisel P (2005a) Workplace-based return-to-work interventions: optimizing the role of stakeholders in implementation and research. J Occup Rehabil 15:525–542

Franche R-L et al (2005b) Workplace-based return-to-work interventions: a systematic review of the quantitative literature. J Occup Rehabil 15:607–631

Frank JW, Brooker AS, DeMaio SE, Kerr MS, Maetzel A, Shannon HS, Sullivan TJ, Norman RW, Wells RP (1996) Disability resulting from occupational low back pain: Part II: What do we know about secondary prevention? A review of the scientific evidence on prevention after disability begins. Spine 21(24):2918–2929

Friesen MN, Yassi A, Cooper J (2001) Return-to-work: the importance of human interactions and organizational structures. Work 17:11–22

Gardner BT, Pransky G, Shaw WS, Nha Hong Q, Loisel P (2010) Researcher perspectives on competencies of return-to-work coordinators. Disabil Rehabil 32:72–78

Gimeno D, Amick B, Habeck R, Ossmann J, Katz J (2005) The role of job strain on return to work after carpal tunnel surgery. Occup Environ Med 62:778–785

Harris LC, Ogbonna E (2011) Antecedents and consequences of management-espoused organizational cultural control. J Bus Res 64:437–445

Hees HL, Nieuwenhuijsen K, Koeter MW, Bültmann U, Schene AH (2012) Towards a new definition of return-to-work outcomes in common mental disorders from a multi-stakeholder perspective. PLoS One 7(6):e39947

Hoefsmit N, Houkes I, Nijhuis FJ (2012) Intervention characteristics that facilitate return to work after sickness absence: a systematic literature review. J Occup Rehabil 22:462–477

IOM (2001) Musculoskeletal disorders and the workplace: low back and upper extremities. National Academy Press, Washington, DC

IWH (2007) Seven "Principles" for successful return to work. Institute for Work & Health. https://www.iwh.on.ca/tools-and-guides/seven-principles-for-successful-return-to-work. Accessed 7 June 2018

Jacobson Frey J, Attridge M (2010) Employee assistance programs (EAPs): an allied profession for work/life. Work and family encyclopedia. Sloan Work and Family Research Network. Available online: https://workfamily.sas.upenn.edu/wfrn-repo/object/6ot29wy5fk9m9z2v

Janssen O (2000) Job demands, perceptions of effort-reward fairness and innovative work behaviour. J Occup Organ Psychol 73:287–302

Karasek Jr RA (1979) Job demands, job decision latitude, and mental strain: implications for job redesign. Adm Sci Q 285–308

Knauf MT, Schultz IZ (2016) Current conceptual models of return to work. In: Handbook of return to work. Springer, Boston, MA, pp 27–51

Kraaijeveld R, Schaafsma F, Ketelaar S, Boot C, Bültmann U, Anema J (2016) Implementation of the participatory approach for supervisors to prevent sick leave: a process evaluation. Int Arch Occup Environ Health 89:847–856

Krause N, Dasinger LK, Neuhauser F (1998) Modified work and return to work: a review of the literature. J Occup Rehabil 8:113–139

Kristman VL, Shaw WS, Boot CR, Delclos GL, Sullivan MJ, Ehrhart MG (2016) Researching complex and multi-level workplace factors affecting disability and prolonged sickness absence. J Occup Rehabil 26:399–416

Leibowitz G (1991) Organic and biophysical theories of behavior. J Dev Phys Disabil 3:201–243

Loisel P et al (2001) Disability prevention. Dis Manag Health Out 9:351–360

Lysaght RM, Larmour-Trode S (2008) An exploration of social support as a factor in the return-to-work process. Work 30:255–266

MacEachen E, Clarke J, Franche RL, Irvin E (2006) Workplace-based Return to Work Literature Review Group. Systematic review of the qualitative literature on return to work after injury. Scand J Work Environ Health 1:257–269

Mental Health Commission of Canada (2015) Informing the future: Mental health indicators for Canada. Mental Health Commission of Canada, Ottawa

Nieuwenhuijsen K, Verbeek J, De Boer A, Blonk R, Van Dijk F (2004) Supervisory behaviour as a predictor of return to work in employees absent from work due to mental health problems. Occup Environ Med 61:817–823

Peterson MF, Fischer R (2004) Organizational culture and climate. In: Spielberger CD (ed) Encyclopedia of applied psychology. Elsevier Science & Technology, Oxford, UK. Retrieved from http://ezproxy.lakeheadu.ca/login?url=https://search.credoreference.com/content/entry/estappliedpsyc/organizational_culture_and_climate/0?institutionId=7307

Pomaki G, Franche R-L, Khushrushahi N, Murray E, Lampinen T, Mah P (2010) Best practices for return-to-work/stay-at-work interventions for workers with mental health conditions. Occupational Health and Safety Agency for Healthcare in BC (OHSAH), Vancouver, BC

Pransky G, Shaw WS, Loisel P, Hong QN, Désorcy B (2010) Development and validation of competencies for return to work coordinators. J Occup Rehabil 20:41–48

Pryce J, Munir F, Haslam C (2007) Cancer survivorship and work: symptoms, supervisor response, co-worker disclosure and work adjustment. J Occup Rehabil 17:83–92

Rivilis I, Van Eerd D, Cullen K, Cole DC, Irvin E, Tyson J, Mahood Q (2008) Effectiveness of participatory ergonomic interventions on health outcomes: a systematic review. Appl Ergon 39:342–358

Schaubroeck JM et al (2012) Embedding ethical leadership within and across organization levels. Acad Manag J 55:1053–1078

Schein EH (1984) Coming to a new awareness of organizational culture. Sloan Manag Rev 25:3–16

Schultz IZ, Stowell AW, Feuerstein M, Gatchel RJ (2007) Models of return to work for musculoskeletal disorders. J Occup Rehabil 17:327–352

Schultz IZ, Gatchel RJ (eds) (2015) Handbook of return to work: from research to practice (vol. 1). Springer, New York, NY

Scott KM et al (2007) Depression–anxiety relationships with chronic physical conditions: results from the World Mental Health Surveys. J Affect Disord 103:113–120

Shaw WS, Robertson MM, McLellan RK, Verma S, Pransky G (2006) A controlled case study of supervisor training to optimize response to injury in the food processing industry. Work 26:107–114

Shaw W, Hong Q-n, Pransky G, Loisel P (2008) A literature review describing the role of return-to-work coordinators in trial programs and interventions designed to prevent workplace disability. J Occup Rehabil 18:2–15

Shaw WS, Van der Windt DA, Main CJ, Loisel P, Linton SJ (2009) Early patient screening and intervention to address individual-level occupational factors ("blue flags") in back disability. J Occup Rehabil 19:64–80

Shaw WS, Kristman VL, Vézina N (2013) Workplace issues. In: Handbook of work disability. Springer, New York, NY, pp 163–182

Morneau Shepell (2016) Best practices in absence and disability management: the complete guide for today's people leaders. Morneau Shepell Ltd. http://www.morneaushepell.com/permafiles/83778/morneau-shepells-best-practices-absence-management.pdf. Accessed 26 Oct 2018

Siegrist J (1996) Adverse health effects of high-effort/low-reward conditions. J Occup Health Psychol 1:27

Stewart AM, Polak E, Young R, Schultz IZ (2012) Injured workers' construction of expectations of return to work with sub-acute back pain: the role of perceived uncertainty. J Occup Rehabil 22:1–14

Sullivan MJ, Ward LC, Tripp D, French DJ, Adams H, Stanish WD (2005) Secondary prevention of work disability: community-based psychosocial intervention for musculoskeletal disorders. J Occup Rehabil 15:377–392

The Conference Board of Canada (2013) Creating an effective workplace disability management program. The Conference Board of Canada. http://www.sunlife.ca/static/canada/Sponsor/About%20Group%20Benefits/Group%20benefits%20products%20and%20services/The%20Conversation/Disability/CreatingAnEffectiveWorkplace_SUNLIFE_EN.PDF. Accessed 26 Oct 2018

Tjulin Å, MacEachen E, Ekberg K (2010) Exploring workplace actors experiences of the social organization of return-to-work. J Occup Rehabil 20:311–321

van Oostrom SH, Anema JR, Terluin B, Venema A, de Vet HC, van Mechelen W (2007) Development of a workplace intervention for sick-listed employees with stress-related mental disorders: Intervention Mapping as a useful tool. BMC Health Serv Res 7:127

van Oostrom SH, van Mechelen W, Terluin B, de Vet HC, Anema JR (2009) A participatory workplace intervention for employees with distress and lost time: a feasibility evaluation within a randomized controlled trial. J Occup Rehabil 19:212–222

Waddell G (1987) 1987 Volvo award in clinical sciences. A new clinical model for the treatment of low-back pain. Spine 12:632–644

WHO (2001) International classification of functioning, disability and health: ICF. World Health Organization, Geneva

Williams-Whitt K, Bültmann U, Amick B, Munir F, Tveito TH, Anema JR (2016) Workplace interventions to prevent disability from both the scientific and practice perspectives: a comparison of scientific literature, grey literature and stakeholder observations. J Occup Rehabil 26:417–433

Woodman RW (2014) The role of internal validity in evaluation research on organizational change interventions. J Appl Behav Sci 50:40–49

WorkSafeMT Stay At Work /Return to Work best practices. WorkSafe Montana. https://www.worksafemt.com/media/WSMT_SAW-RTW_Best_Practices.pdf. Accessed 26 Oct 2018

Yarker J, Munir F, Bains M, Kalawsky K, Haslam C (2010) The role of communication and support in return to work following cancer-related absence. Psycho-Oncology 19:1078–1085

Young AE, Wasiak R, Roessler RT, McPherson KM, Anema J, Van Poppel MN (2005) Return-to-work outcomes following work disability: stakeholder motivations, interests and concerns. J Occup Rehabil 15:543–556

IGLOO: A Framework for Return to Work Among Workers with Mental Health Problems

33

Karina Nielsen, Joanna Yarker, Fehmidah Munir, and Ute Bültmann

Contents

Introduction	616
Developing a Framework for RTW: IGLOO	617
Individual-Level Resources	618
Group-Level Resources	620
Leader-Level Resources	621
Organizational-Level Resources	623
Overarching Resources: Work and Non-work Related Legislation and Social Welfare Policy	624
Discussion	625
Interaction Between Resources	627
Conclusions	628
Cross-References	628
References	629

Abstract

It is important for society and for organizations to support workers returning to work following mental health-related absence. Recent evidence points to an increase in mental health problems among the general population, with approximately 38.2% of the EU population suffering from a mental disorder each year

---

K. Nielsen (✉)
Institute for Work Psychology, University of Sheffield, Sheffield, UK
e-mail: k.m.nielsen@sheffield.ac.uk

J. Yarker
Birkbeck, University of London, London, UK

F. Munir
Loughborough University, Loughborough, UK

U. Bültmann
Department of Health Sciences, Community and Occupational Medicine, University of Groningen, University Medical Center Groningen, Groningen, The Netherlands
e-mail: u.bultmann@umcg.nl

(European Commission 2008, 2016). Of those who take a period of sick leave, 55% of workers make unsuccessful attempts to return to work (RTW), and 68% of those who do return have less responsibility and are paid less than before (Matrix Insight 2013). A number of challenges have been reported by workers following a period of long-term sickness absence; however current research has been somewhat limited by a focus on the initial return and a siloed approach where work and non-work contexts are considered separately.

In this book chapter, we apply the IGLOO (individual, group, leader, organizational and overarching contextual factors that may support sustainable RTW) model (Nielsen et al. 2018). In doing so, we focus on the sickness absence before return to work and consider the factors that could support return to work following long-term sickness absence. We provide an overview of the resources that may facilitate return to work among workers who are on sick leave with mental health problems. Based on the IGLOO framework, we identify and discuss resources, i.e., factors that facilitate return to work at five levels: the individual (e.g., beliefs about being able to manage a successful return to work, health behaviors), the group (work groups, friends, and family), the leader (line managers and healthcare provides who take the lead in supporting workers return), the organizational (Human Resource policies and external organizations such a charities), and the overarching context (social security systems). We discuss these resources that pertain to the work context but also the non-work context and highlight the importance of understanding how resources apply at different levels. We argue that there is a need to understand how societal factors, such as legislation, culture, and national policies, impact return to work outcomes. We propose a holistic approach that focuses on integrating the resources in and outside work and is needed to facilitate successful and sustainable return to work for workers with mental health problems.

Keywords

Return to work · Multi-level interventions · Sickness absenteeism · Mental health

Introduction

Recent evidence points to an increase in mental health problems among the general population (European Commission 2008, 2016). Mental disorders are highly prevalent in Europe and present a major burden on individuals, organizations, society, and the economy of the European Union (EU). Approximately 38.2% of the EU population suffer from a mental disorder each year, most frequently anxiety disorders (14%), insomnia (7%), major depression (6.9%), somatoform disorders (6.3%), and alcohol and drug dependence (4%) (Wittchen et al. 2011). One quarter of the EU working population is expected to experience a mental health problem during their lifetime (EU-OSHA 2014).

Work, employment, and mental health are closely intertwined for at least four reasons. First, it has been found that having a good quality job protects against poor mental health (Paul and Moser 2009). Second, workers with mental health problems are 6–7 times more likely to be unemployed suggesting that more could be done to promote good working lives for these workers (OECD 2014). Third, importantly not all jobs are good, and there is significant evidence that poor working conditions are linked to poor mental health (Madsen et al. 2017; Stansfeld and Candy 2006), which in turn can be related to long-term sickness absence (Melkevik et al. 2018). Fourth, it has been found that 55% of workers with mental health problems make unsuccessful attempts to return to work (RTW) following an episode of long-term sick leave caused by poor mental health. Of those who do return, 68% have less responsibility and are paid less than before (Matrix Insight 2013). The costs of medical expenses, increased need of healthcare, and social care costs due to mental ill-health exceed 4% of GDP in the OECD countries (OECD 2014). Together, these findings make it important for society and for organizations to manage mental health and support employees in the RTW process.

Although work is often mentioned as the main cause for sickness absence due to poor mental health (Løvvik et al. 2014a), helping workers with mental health problems return to work is important because work can have a positive impact on mental health problems for at least six reasons (Ekbladh and Sandqvist 2015; Harnois et al. 2000). First, work means earning an income. Second, work provides a time structure to the day, and a lack of structure has been found to be a major psychological burden. Third, work enables social interaction and prevents isolation. Fourth, work provides an identity as employment is an important element in defining oneself. Fifth, work presents an opportunity for collective effort and purpose. It can give the worker a sense of making a meaningful contribution to a greater whole, and this is achieved in collaboration with others. Finally, work offers the opportunity of regular activity and thus prevents individuals from overthinking and linking back to the old saying of idle hands are the devil's workshop. It is thus important to understand how we can create conditions that help workers with mental health problems return to work and to stay at work.

In the present book chapter, we apply the IGLOO (individual, group, leader, organizational, and overarching contextual factors that may support sustainable RTW) model (Nielsen et al. 2018) to the RTW domain and review the literature on how this approach may support workers with mental health problems to return to work after long-term sickness absence. We thus focus on the sickness absence period *before* RTW. We know of no agreed definition of long-term sickness absence but suggest that the long-term sickness absence can be defined as the period beyond which the organization pays the worker a salary and social benefits take over which is the case in many developed countries. This period is different across national contexts due to the variations in national social security systems.

Developing a Framework for RTW: IGLOO

As an analysis tool, we use the IGLOO framework to classify/order the resources that may support workers return to work. We draw on conservation of resources

(COR) theory (Hobfoll 1989) as our underlying theoretical framework. COR theory suggests that individuals are motivated to protect and accumulate resources. Resources are defined as "anything perceived by the individual to help attain his or her goals" (Halbesleben et al. 2014, p.6), in this case RTW. According to COR, both positive and negative spirals may occur. In a situation where individuals do not have sufficient resources to cope with the demands of the situation, resource depletion may be the result, and workers may not feel they have the necessary resources to return to work. Positive gain spirals, on the other hand, occur when individuals get the opportunity to engage in resource caravans: individuals invest resources to build additional resources and thus resources at multiple levels in and outside the workplace may create synergistic effects (Hobfoll 1989), for example, when workers with mental health problems get support to build their resources this may make them confident that they can successfully return to work.

The IGLOO framework for RTW takes a broad view on resources. We consider the individual's resources, the social resources (the resources inherent in social interactions, both vertically, interactions with leaders/line managers and horizontally, interactions with colleagues, and outside work friends and family), and the organizational resources relating to the way work is organized, designed, and managed.

In the field of work psychology, recent developments have focused on the need to identify resources at multiple levels and called for interventions to strengthen resources at four levels: the individual, the group, the leader, and the organizational level, also termed the IGLO model (Day and Nielsen 2017; Nielsen et al. 2017). More recently, the model has been extended with an additional level, the overarching context, i.e., the wider national legislation and culture (Nielsen et al. 2018), which may influence RTW. The IGLO(O) model suggests that the antecedents of worker health and well-being can be classified according to these five levels. We propose that this understanding of resources may be transferred to the RTW domain where resources can promote RTW among workers with mental health problems (Table 1).

Individual-Level Resources

Cognitive, Affective, and Behavioral Resources Related to Work

At the individual-level, RTW is influenced by a range of factors encompassing cognitive, emotional, and behavioral responses related to work. The cognitive aspect relates to the individual's own belief about their mental health status, their assessment of their symptoms, and their confidence (i.e., self-efficacy) in their own abilities and skills in managing their job demands upon RTW (de Vries et al. 2018). Combined with emotional responses to their illness (e.g., presence of and level of emotional distress), these illness perceptions (Leventhal et al. 1997) influence an individual's own expectations of RTW and, in turn, their actual behavior in returning to, delaying, or not returning to work. Thus, RTW expectations have been found to be a strong predictor of actual RTW (Løvvik et al. 2014b). Furthermore,

Table 1 Overview of resources that support workers' return to work

	Work domain	Outside work domain
Individual-level resources	Self-perceptions Attribution of mental health problems Goal orientation Coping strategies	Self-efficacy Self-esteem Motivation Resilience Self-care (exercise and healthy eating)
Group-level resources	Peer support Ongoing contact with colleagues Positive work climate Colleagues' understanding of mental health problems Collaborative work structure	Marital status Understanding family and friends Practical and emotional support from family and friends
Leader-level resources	Supervisor support Ongoing communication	Experienced healthcare providers Understanding the workers as a person, not a client/patient Trusting relationship with healthcare providers Continued and ongoing contact with the same healthcare provider Access to therapy
Organizational-level resources	Human resource practices and policies Occupational health services	Access to voluntary and third sector support services
Overarching context resources	Sickness benefit compensation Health insurance Surveillance Work disability policies	Financial support, e.g., childcare provision Cultural values regarding mental health, e.g., prevalence and nature of debates in media

beliefs about the causal attribution for the sick leave also impact RTW outcomes. Many individuals with mental health problems attribute the cause of their perceptions and beliefs about their problems to work. These include the work itself such as high job demands, to perceptions of attitudes and behaviors of supervisors and colleagues toward their illness (Løvvik et al. 2014a; Corbière et al. 2016). Ability to attain work-related goals and worry about work-related factors is also associated with longer sickness absence (Norrmen et al. 2010). The causal attribution component of illness perceptions may influence various health behaviors and the sorts of strategies individuals use to control and cope with their illness (e.g., Olsen et al. 2015). For example, adopting avoidance coping strategies may prolong sick leave as the individual is reluctant to face the work issues, he or she believes caused their illness.

Proposition 1 Individuals' work-related cognitive, affective, and behavioral resources influence individuals' readiness to RTW.

Individual Resources at Play in the Non-work Domain

Psychological factors such as low motivation to return, severity of depressive symptoms, perceptions of illness, and personality traits (perfectionism) are reported to be strong predictors of long-term sick leave and low RTW rates (Lagerveld et al. 2010; Huijs et al. 2012; Nigatu et al. 2017). However, self-efficacy in RTW is a key factor in RTW itself and individuals who have higher RTW self-efficacy are more likely to RTW (Nigatu et al. 2017). Being willing to utilize healthy strategies to support both physical and mental well-being are therefore of great importance for RTW. These include exercising and eating healthily and regularly (Jansson et al. 2014), focusing on self-care and leisure (Cowls and Galloway 2009), and building resilience toward work-related stress (Netterstrøm et al. 2013). These all contribute toward regaining a sense of a capable self (Nielsen et al. 2013) and a sense of control, which in turn contribute to RTW. However, encouraging an individual to engage with health restoring strategies is challenging if the individual perceives being on sick leave as beneficial to their mental health, continues to adopt reactive-passive coping strategies (Van Rhenen et al. 2008), and continues to perceive there is no work-related solution.

Proposition 2 Cognitive, affective, and behavioral resources will influence an individuals' drive and ability to achieve RTW.

Group-Level Resources

Social Support at Work During Sick Leave

A number of group-level resources may influence RTW. Support from peers and colleagues may be crucial for successful RTW (de Vries et al. 2014); however, it must be carefully considered how and which nature of support is needed. One underlying framework for understanding the role of social support for supporting workers with mental health problems return to work is the social identity theory (SIT, Tajfel and Turner 1979; Tajfel 2010). According to SIT (Tajfel and Turner 1979), individuals also have a social identity beyond their individual identity. Having a social identity means that an individual feels she/he belongs to a wider social group, e.g., a group of colleagues at work. This belongingness partly determines the individual's behavior. Transferring this to the RTW context, the extent to which workers feel part of a social network at their place of work, will influence their RTW. Colleagues can do simple things to maintain the sense of belongingness to the work group, such as sending a card, chocolate, or flowers, sending the occasional email, and inviting them to social events. Although the worker on sick leave may not feel like attending events, they are reminded that the work group still sees them as part of the group.

Holmgren and Ivanoff (2004) found that workers who are on sick leave from a workplace with inherent conflicts found it difficult to return. Examples of such conflicts could revolve around being a female in a male-dominated workplace or being the only worker with a higher education. The nature of these conflicts meant that they were not easily solved. Workers on sick leave found themselves being questioned by their workmates and felt the odd one out. Workers reported that colleagues who demonstrated an understanding of their problems were a major resource that helped them believe they could and would return (Dunstan and MacEachen 2013; Noordik et al. 2011).

Stigma is a prevalent problem and colleagues may have little understanding of the recovery process (Harnois et al. 2000). Workers on long-term sick leave may also fear they will not be welcomed back at work. If workers returned to a high-performance environment where pay for performance forms part of the reward structure, colleagues may be perceived to be less accepting of reduced work functioning (Saint-Arnaud et al. 2006; Noordik et al. 2011). In summary, current research has focused on the negative aspects of groups, but we propose that being part of a supportive group environment may be related to RTW.

Proposition 3 Workers with mental health problems who feel part of a supportive work group are more likely to return to work.

Social Resources in the Non-work Domain

There is limited research focusing on the importance of the social context outside work. In their scoping review, de Vries et al. (2018) concluded that there was insufficient evidence to conclude whether factors such as family history of depression, the size of the social network, and support from family and friends had a positive influence on RTW. Individual studies have found that married employees are more likely to return to work (Norder et al. 2015) and understanding friends and family members are also important (Holmgren and Ivanoff 2004; Noordik et al. 2011). Furthermore, there is indicative evidence that emotional and practical support from family and friends is important to RTW (Reavley et al. 2012); however, support from colleagues and family was not found to be related to shorter RTW (<3 months) (Ekberg et al. 2015). Although we found no research supporting this notion, being a member of religious or church groups may also provide an important social network outside work, which can help supporting the individual RTW.

Proposition 4 Employees with mental health problems are more likely to return to work if they have a supportive network outside work.

Leader-Level Resources

Line Manager Resources

Line managers' behaviors have been associated with employee health and well-being (Arnold 2017; Harms et al. 2017; Inceoglu et al. 2018; Montano et al. 2017; Skakon et al. 2010). Previous research has found that line managers play an important role in supporting workers with mental health problems return to work (Aas et al. 2008; Munir et al. 2012). A good relationship and ongoing communication during sick leave is crucial, and studies indicate that line managers often do communicate with workers on sick leave (Negrini et al. 2018; Nieuwenhuijsen et al. 2004). Interestingly, these conversations were rarely about RTW as most line managers were aware of the importance of not forcing the worker to return (Negrini et al. 2018; Nieuwenhuijsen et al. 2004). Only 22% of line managers supported return before symptoms of mental health had fully disappeared. Good communication between workers on sick leave and line managers resulted in full RTW when workers no longer reported depressive symptoms. Line managers were found to communicate better when return had an impact on the department's performance (Nieuwenhuijsen et al. 2004). This suggests that financial incentives may be important to motivate line managers supporting workers returning; however, there may also be at risk that it incentivizes line managers to coerce workers to return to work before they are ready.

Proposition 5 Employees with mental health problems who experience supportive line management are more likely to return to work.

Links to Healthcare Service Providers

Outside the work context, healthcare service providers may be as important as line managers in supporting RTW. De Vries et al. (2014) found that healthcare providers who lacked expertise in mental health problems, provided inadequate treatment for mental health disorders and paid insufficient attention to the importance of returning to work delayed RTW. General practitioners or healthcare professionals may facilitate RTW when they acknowledge the worker on sick leave as an individual rather than as a patient/client (Andersen et al. 2014). Similarly, Sturesson et al. (2014) found that trust in the relationship, i.e., that workers on sick leave felt they had a say in decision-making and that they were believed and felt listened to and were important for RTW, together with healthcare providers being seen as dedicated to support workers. Equally a relationship between the worker on sick leave and the healthcare provider that was characterized by professionalism, continuity, and seeing the person as a whole has been found to be important for RTW. In contrast, being in contact with specialized medical staff was found to be negatively associated with full RTW (Nigatu et al. 2017), possibly because such healthcare professionals may not see return as a crucial outcome but focus more on treating the illness.

Healthcare service providers may also provide access to wider services. Access to therapy may also play an important role. A recent meta-analysis showed that cognitive behavior therapy, stress reduction programs, and problem-solving therapy can reduce the number of sick leave days in the intervention group compared to the control group (Nigatu et al. 2016) but do not lead to improved RTW rates over the control group.

Proposition 6 Healthcare providers with the necessary expertise in mental health issues and who provide adequate support may support workers with mental health issues return to work.

Organizational-Level Resources

Organizational Resources

Noordik et al. (2011) noted that there was a gap between solutions and intentions to return to work and their implementation at work for employees returning to work after mental ill-health sickness absence. It is important that organizational structures and processes are in place if intentions are to be translated into practice. Exploring the factors related to length of sickness absence, Ekberg et al. (2015) found that important resources supporting those returning after 3 months were fair procedures and reduced demands at work. In the group of workers who returned between 3–12 months, reduced demands, also in terms of a reduced physical load, were important. Lacking resources in the form of an employer signalling wanting to get rid of the worker on sick leave or not providing guidance as to how to return was found to delay RTW (de Vries et al. 2014). In a study of women returning to work after long-term sickness absence due to poor mental health, Holmgren and Ivanoff (2004) showed that women found it challenging to return to an organization where many changes had taken place and their job descriptions were no longer valid. De Vries et al. (2014) found that workers reported a poor fit with the organization after RTW. These findings suggest that an important resource at the organizational level is that Human Resources ensure job descriptions are reflective of the returning worker's tasks and are amended if needed.

The ability, motivation, and opportunity (AMO) model proposed by Appelbaum et al. (2001), frequently used within Human Resource practices, offers a useful framework for ensuring that appropriate supports are in place for the returning worker. For example, considering whether there is there still a good fit between the role and the returner's abilities to do the job, their motivation for the task and the opportunities afforded to them to regain their skills and knowledge and develop new skills could help to mitigate problems experienced during the return that may lead to relapse. Occupational health professionals are well positioned to support this process.

Proposition 7 Employees with mental health problems who experience well-organized work with clear and fair policies and practices are more likely to return to work.

Organizational Resources in the Non-work Domain

Voluntary, third sector or community led support services operate outside the traditional formal mental health services (e.g., Mind in the UK and Denmark, Beyond Blue in Australia). These services may address gaps in formal service provision, which often outstrips demand or complement existing services. To the authors' knowledge, there is no evidence to explore the impact of these complementary services; however, it is reasonable to suggest that those who are able to access these additional services, over and above therapeutic services, such as responsive telephone support, online e-health guidance resources, drop in sessions, or workshops, are more likely to feel better supported during their absence and the initial RTW, thereby increasing the likelihood of a successful return.

Proposition 8 Employees with mental health problems who are able to access good quality advice from community and voluntary services to complement therapeutic treatments are more likely to return to work.

Overarching Resources: Work and Non-work Related Legislation and Social Welfare Policy

Mental health problems are the leading cause of disease burden worldwide (Whiteford et al. 2015). Mental health problems affect not only individuals, their families, and workplaces but also communities and society. Therefore, means to promote the mental health and well-being of people of all ages are becoming increasingly important as well as effective national policies and practices to help people to return to work and to stay at work – both to extend working careers and to prevent labor market marginalization, i.e., work disability, economic inactivity, unstable working career, downward occupational mobility, or status as "working poor" (OECD 2014; European Commission 2010).

RTW policies and practices and measures to prevent work disability operate within a national legislative and health and social welfare policy context, e.g., sickness benefit compensation, health insurance, and surveillance. Many different systems are involved in work disability prevention and the RTW process, such as the legislative, health, and insurance system, i.e., the society's safety net with provincial and federal laws, regulations of jurisdiction, and compensation (Loisel et al. 2005). All these systems and their stakeholders must be considered, preferably in an integrated approach, when looking at RTW resources in the overarching, societal context, in which they are embedded. However, RTW policies and practices often do not acknowledge system influences.

When looking at work-related musculoskeletal disorders and work injuries, attempts have been made to compare different countries, i.e., Canada and Australia (Macpherson et al. 2018), or eight different workers compensation systems within one country (Australia, Collie et al. 2016). As the majority of studies on RTW after mental health problems have been conducted in one jurisdictional context (Lagerveld et al. 2010), the impact of RTW resources from the contribution of overarching legislation, policies, and practices cannot be separated out. A recent systematic review and meta-analyses on predictors of RTW after depression (Ervasti et al. 2017) has not only shown a significant heterogeneity between studies but also concluded that there is a dearth of observational studies and called particularly for more research focusing on the role of labor market factors. Another recent review by Nigatu et al. (2017) on prognostic factors for RTW in workers with common mental disorders, reported on two studies from Australia and the Netherlands addressing the contact with a medical specialist (Prang et al. 2016; Nieuwenhuijsen et al. 2004). De Vries et al. (2018) identified only one article focusing on system impacts of mental health coverage, fringe benefits, and disability management (Salkever et al. 2003) in a scoping review on determinants of sickness absence and RTW in workers with common mental disorders. Clearly, more research is needed on legislative, health, and insurance system influences on RTW in workers with mental health problems – preferably by using a comparative approach to identify resources in the overarching context.

Uneven foci of work disability policy research across cause-based and comprehensive social security systems were identified in a recent scoping review by MacEachen et al. (2018). Articles on cause-based systems dwelled on system fairness and policies of proof of entitlement, while those on comprehensive systems focused more on system design complexities relating to worker inclusion and scope of medical certificates. Overall, a clear difference in the nature of problems examined in the different systems was observed. For research to better inform policy making, the authors call for cross-pollination of research topics across the systems and more international comparison studies that are attuned to these policy differences (MacEachen et al. 2018).

Proposition 9 Employees with mental health problems who live and work in countries within an overarching context whose labor legislation and practices support RTW are more likely to RTW.

To date, research on the impact of welfare policies and cultural values for RTW after mental health problems is sparse. It can be speculated that countries with good systems for childcare or eldercare could alleviate additional external pressures. For example, in countries where childcare is readily available and reasonably priced, workers on sick leave may still be able to afford childcare and thus be able to get relief from childcare during the day. Similarly, in countries where the elder care burden is placed on society rather than the children of the elderly, having to deal with the care of the elderly in the family (such as cooking and cleaning in two homes, making hospital appointments, transporting the elderly and managing the elderly's finances), may alleviate the pressure. A culture accepting of people with mental health problems may mean organizations are more likely to employ workers with mental health problems as recruiters are less prejudiced. National public health campaigns on mental health are likely to reduce stigma and increase the understanding that workers with mental health problems do not just "need to get on with it" and are not scroungers on society.

Proposition 10 Employees with mental health problems who live and work in countries within an overarching context where welfare policies reduce potential external/additional strain on workers on sick leave and where the culture values are supportive of people with mental health problems are more likely to RTW.

Discussion

In this chapter we present a case for considering resources at multiple levels to support employees with mental health problems to return to work. Building on the work of Day and Nielsen (2017) and Nielsen et al. (2017), we identify resources at five levels: the individual, the group, the leader, the organizational level, and the overarching context, i.e., the wider national legislation and culture (Nielsen et al. 2018), which may influence RTW after mental health problems. In a recent review of RTW interventions, Dibben et al. (2018) found weak and contradictory evidence for either achieving employment outcomes or cost effectiveness. We propose that considering resources within and across the multiple levels may help us to develop more effective RTW interventions that accrue health, employability, and financial gains for individuals, organizations, and society.

For individual resources, the causal attributions of illness perceptions, RTW self-efficacy, and RTW expectations are key psychological resources that influence the outcome of other individual resources and behaviors including the form of coping strategies utilized, ability to manage stress, and motivating oneself to engage in healthy behaviors such as exercise which has an antidepressant effect (Schuch et al. 2016). Thus, causal attributions of illness, RTW self-efficacy, and RTW self-expectations are of great importance in returning to work.

Although there is plenty of research suggesting that social support from colleagues is important, research has paid less attention to what this social support may look like, while the worker is on sick leave. There are important issues concerning breaches of confidentiality and stigma that may prevent colleagues from keeping in touch with even close friends, while they are on sick leave. More research needs to be conducted to understand the importance of keeping in touch, perhaps even visiting or taking the person on sick leave out for dinner or the movies. We know very little about whether this is done or whether it helps the RTW process. We need more research to understand how social networks outside work can support workers' return. As concluded by de Vries et al. (2018), there is insufficient knowledge about which group-level factors may support RTW. They suggest that previous history of mental health problems in the family may be important. This could work both ways. On the one hand, having previous history of mental health problems may mean that workers may be more prone to experience long-term issues. On the other hand, and on a more positive note, previous history may present opportunities for vicarious learning. The concept of vicarious learning (Bandura 1986) suggests that friends and family who have previous history of mental health and have recovered may act as role models and may share information and advice on how to manage the RTW process.

Despite growing acknowledgement that line managers play a vital role in supporting the returning worker, there is limited evidence to guide best practice. While maintaining communication during absence has been found to promote RTW (Aas et al. 2008), less is known about what should be done where the manager contributed to or was the cause of absence. Some research points to managers supporting returners more proactively when there are clear gains to performance (Nieuwenhuijsen et al. 2004); however, more research is needed to understand how managers can be incentivized to support the returning employee. Such incentives are particularly salient given that the majority of managers are reluctant to support a return unless the employee is fully recovered and symptom-free (Negrini et al. 2018). Finding ways to encourage line managers to support employees back to work when they feel ready but are not yet at full capacity, presenting some symptoms, will be an important part of the RTW solution.

While there is an understanding that good job design and well-managed work demands can help employees return to work following mental health sick leave (Ekberg et al. 2015), surprisingly little is known about the range of work adjustments that could be put in place to support returning employees. Despite the wide spread use of staged or phased RTW programs to support returning employees, there is little evidence to guide practice and help allied professionals and employers make informed, evidence-based decisions about how to structure the return or the length of time the phased return should be implemented. Importantly, despite increasing reliance on additional support from third sector services, the authors could not find any evidence for the benefits accrued from support provided by voluntary or charity sectors. This is not to suggest that these services have no important role to play, but rather to suggest that as yet we have little understanding of what supports are helpful, are effective, or provide a return on investment. Further research is needed, examining resources provided at work and outside work to understand what needs to be in place to support returning employees.

For the overarching societal context, work-related and non-work-related national legislative, health, and social welfare policy measures, e.g., sickness benefit compensation, health insurance, and culture, may support RTW after mental health problems. We need to conduct more studies focusing on the impact of these overarching societal factors on RTW, separately, but also jointly with the resources available at other levels to better understand how these factors collectively shape the RTW trajectories of workers with mental health problems. Research has to address the complex interplay between the systems and stakeholders, i.e., the family, the workplace, the insurer, and the healthcare provider, who are interacting with the patient/worker in the RTW process.

Addressing this systemic and multidimensional RTW challenge requires adopting a transdisciplinary perspective. In addition, to better understand the impact of the societal context on RTW, more knowledge must be developed in cross-national or cross-jurisdictional, comparative approach. As is clear from our brief review much research has focused on the barriers to RTW and the lack of resources, less attention has been paid to the positive factors, which may help workers return. There is a need to explore and identify which resources may have a positive impact and shorten sickness absence periods.

Interaction Between Resources

In the present framework, we outline the resources at five different levels; however, it is equally important to understand how resources at these levels interact. For example, the study by Nieuwenhuijsen et al. (2004) found that line managers often interacted with others, e.g., occupational health professionals, and were particularly motivated to do so when return influenced financial outcomes in their department. Furthermore, upper-level resources may influence lower-level resources. For example, national sickness benefit systems that put the onus on RTW and provide financial incentives for organizations to support workers return to work are more likely to result in organizations developing and implementing HR policies that proactively support workers returning. Likewise, organizational policies, programs, and practices, such as training line managers in how to manage difficult conversations and policies for peer interaction with the person on sick leave, are likely to influence the behaviors of line managers and colleagues. Also, whether GPs and healthcare providers provide access to additional services such as therapy depends on the social systems and the national strategies to provide funding for such services. Understanding the interaction between resources at different levels and in and outside the work domain becomes especially important in light of the studies by de Vries et al. (2014) that showed that occupational physicians and line managers did not agree on the factors that are important for RTW and Hees, Nieuwenhuijsen, Koeter, Bültmann, and Schene (2012) that showed that employees found a "good work-home balance" important for a successful RTW (next to sustainability, job satisfaction, and mental functioning) while occupational physicians and line managers regarded "sustainability" and "at-work functioning" to be of importance. These divergences in opinion may well influence how they each support workers returning and may at times counteract each other. Finally, it is important that the different stakeholders at work and outside work on the different levels are aware of the expectations and resources of all involved stakeholders in the process toward RTW.

Conclusions

In the present book chapter, we employed the IGLOO framework to provide a broad overview of the resources, which may help workers with mental health problems return to work. Using the IGLOO model as our analytical framework helped us identify areas where we still lack knowledge on how to support RTW. In particular, there is a lack of understanding of how societal factors may support RTW. We need to develop our knowledge of how legislation, culture, and national policies translate into RTW trajectories. At other levels, plentiful research has been conducted, e.g., there is a plenitude of research that shows the importance of peer support; however, despite the quantity of research, there is still much to be learned about the nature of this research.

In summary, we argue that a more holistic approach is required that includes a strong focus on integrating the resources in and outside the work domain to facilitate a timely RTW for workers with mental health problems.

Cross-References

- ▶ Common Mental Disorders and Work
- ▶ Investing in Integrative Active Labour Market Policies

▶ Implementing Best Practice Models of Return to Work
▶ Occupational Determinants of Affective Disorders

References

Aas RW, Ellingsen KL, Lindøe P, Möller A (2008) Leadership qualities in the return to work process: a content analysis. J Occup Rehabil 18(4):335–346

Andersen MF, Nielsen K, Brinkmann S (2014) How do workers with common mental disorders experience a multidisciplinary return-to-work intervention? A qualitative study. J Occup Rehabil 24(4):709–724

Appelbaum E, Bailey T, Berg P, Kalleberg AL (2001) Do high performance work systems pay off? In: Vallas SP (ed) The transformation of work. Emerald Group, Oxford, pp 85–107

Arnold KA (2017) Transformational leadership and employee psychological well-being: a review and directions for future research. J Occup Health Psychol 22(3):381–396

Bandura A (1986) The explanatory and predictive scope of self-efficacy theory. J Social Clin Psychol 4:359–373

Collie A, Lane TJ, Hassani-Mahmooei B, Thompson J, McLeod C (2016) Does time off work after injury vary by jurisdiction? A comparative study of eight Australian workers' compensation systems. BMJ Open 6(5):e010910. https://doi.org/10.1136/bmjopen-2015-010910

Corbière M, Samson E, Negrini A, St-Arnaud L, Durand MJ, Coutu MF, Lecomte T (2016) Factors perceived by employees regarding their sick leave due to depression. Disabil Rehabil 38(6):511–519

Cowls J, Galloway E (2009) Understanding how traumatic re-enactment impacts the workplace: assisting clients' successful return to work. Work 33(4):401–411

Day A, Nielsen K (2017) What does our organization do to help our well-being? Creating healthy workplaces and workers. In: Chmiel N, Fraccaroli F, Sverke M (eds) An introduction of work and organizational psychology. Wiley Blackwell, Sussex: UK. pp 295–314

de Vries G, Hees H, Koeter MW, Lagerveld SE, Schene AH (2014) Perceived impeding factors for return-to-work after long-term sickness absence due to major depressive disorder: a concept mapping approach. PLoS One 9(1):e85038

de Vries H, Fishta A, Weikert RSA, Wegewitz U (2018) Determinants of sickness absence and return to work among employees with common mental disorders: a scoping review. J Occup Rehabil 28(3):393–417

Dibben P, Wood G, O'Hara R (2018) Do return to work interventions for workers with disabilities and health conditions achieve employment outcomes and are they cost effective? A systematic narrative review. Empl Relat 40(6):999–1014

Dunstan DA, MacEachen E (2013) Bearing the brunt: Co-workers' experiences of work reintegration processes. J Occup Rehabil 23:44–54

Ekberg K, Wåhlin C, Persson J, Bernfort L, Öberg B (2015) Early and late return to work after sick leave: predictors in a cohort of sick-listed individuals with common mental disorders. J Occup Rehabil 25(3):627–637

Ekbladh E, Sandqvist J (2015) Psychosocial factors' influence on work ability of people experiencing sick leave resulting from common mental disorders. Occup Ther Ment Health 31(3):283–297

Ervasti J, Joensuu M, Pentti J, Oksanen T, Ahola K, Vahtera J, Kivimäki M, Virtanen M (2017) Prognostic factors for return to work after depression-related work disability: A systematic review and meta-analysis. J Psychiatr Res 95:28–36

EU-OSHA (2014) Psychosocial risks in Europe: prevalence and strategies for prevention. Publications Office of the European Union, Luxembourg

European Commission (2008) EU high-level conference "Together for mental health and well-being" – European pact for mental health and well-being. Retrieved from: http://ec.europa.eu/health/ph_determinants/life_style/mental/docs/mh_conference_mi_en.pdf

European Commission (2010) Why socio-economic inequalities increase? Facts and policy responses in Europe. Directorate-general for research socio-economic sciences and humanities. Retrieved from: https://ec.europa.eu/research/social-sciences/pdf/policy_reviews/policy-review-inequalities_en.pdf

European Commission (2016) European framework for action on mental health and wellbeing. Retrieved from: http://www.mentalhealthandwellbeing.eu/publications

Halbesleben JRB, Neveu JP, Paustian-Underdahl SC, Westman M (2014) Getting to the "COR": understanding the role of resources in conservation of resources theory. J Manag 40(5):1334–1364

Harms PD, Credé M, Tynan M, Leon M, Jeung W (2017) Leadership and stress: a meta-analytic review. Leadersh Q 28(1):178–194

Harnois G, Gabriel P, World Health Organization (2000) Mental health and work: impact, issues and good practices. WHO, Geneva

Hees HL, Nieuwenhuijsen K, Koeter MW, Bültmann U, Schene AH, Botbol M (2012) Towards a new definition of return-to-work outcomes in common mental disorders from a multi-stakeholder perspective. PLoS One, 7:e39947

Hobfoll SE (1989) Conservation of resources: a new attempt at conceptualizing stress. Am Psychol 44(3):513–524

Holmgren K, Ivanoff SD (2004) Women on sickness absence—views of possibilities and obstacles for returning to work. A focus group study. Disabil Rehabil 26(4):213–222

Huijs JJ, Koppes LL, Taris TW, Blonk RW (2012) Differences in predictors of return to work among long-term sick-listed employees with different selfreported reasons for sick leave. J of Occup Rehabil 22:301–311

Inceoglu I, Thomas G, Chu C, Plans D, Gerbasi A (2018) Leadership behavior and employee well-being: an integrated review and a future research agenda. Leadersh Q 29(1):179–202

Jansson I, Perseius K, Gunnarsson AB, Bjorklund A (2014) Work and everyday activities: experiences from two interventions addressing people with common mental disorders. Scand J Occup Ther 21(4):295–304

Lagerveld SE, Bultmann U, Franche RL, van Dijk FJ, Vlasveld MC, van der Feltz-Cornelis CM, Nieuwenhuijsen K (2010) Factors associated with work participation and work functioning in depressed workers: a systematic review. J Occup Rehabil 20(3):275–292

Leventhal H, Benyamini Y, Brownlee S, Diefenbach M, Leventhal EA, Patrick-Miller L, Robitaille C (1997) Illness representations: theoretical foundations. In: Petrie KJ, Weinman JA (eds) Perceptions of health and illness: current research and applications. Harwood Academic Publishers, Amsterdam, pp 19–45

Loisel P, Buchbinder R, Hazard R, Keller R, Scheel I, Tulder MV et al (2005) Prevention of work disability due to musculoskeletal disorders: the challenge of implementing evidence. J Occup Rehabil 15(4):507–524

Løvvik C, Øverland S, Hysing M, Broadbent E, Reme SE (2014a) Association between illness perceptions and return-to-work expectations in workers with common mental health symptoms. J Occup Rehabil 24(1):160–170

Løvvik C, Shaw W, Øverland S, Reme SE (2014b) Expectations and illness perceptions as predictors of benefit recipiency among workers with common mental disorders: secondary analysis from a randomised controlled trial. BMJ Open 4(3):e004321

MacEachen E, Varatharajan S, Du B, Bartel E, Ekberg K (2018) The uneven foci of work disability research across cause-based and comprehensive social security systems. Int J Health Serv 20731418809857. https://doi.org/10.1177/0020731418809857

Macpherson RA, Lane TJ, Collie A, McLeod CB (2018) Age, sex, and the changing disability burden of compensated work-related musculoskeletal disorders in Canada and Australia. BMC Public Health 18(1):758. https://doi.org/10.1186/s12889-018-5590-7

Madsen IE, Nyberg ST, Hanson LM, Ferrie JE, Ahola K, Alfredsson L, ... Chastang JF (2017) Job strain as a risk factor for clinical depression: systematic review and meta-analysis with additional individual participant data. Psychol Med 47(8):1342–1356

Matrix Insight (2013) Economic analysis of workplace mental health promotion and mental disorder prevention programmes and of their potential contribution to EU health, social and economic policy objectives, Matrix Insight, Research commissioned by the European Agency for Health and Consumers

Melkevik O, Clausen T, Pedersen J, Garde AH, Holtermann A, Rugulies R (2018) Comorbid symptoms of depression and musculoskeletal pain and risk of long term sickness absence. BMC Public Health 18(1):981

Montano D, Reeske A, Franke F, Hüffmeier J (2017) Leadership, followers' mental health and job performance in organizations: a comprehensive meta-analysis from an occupational health perspective. J Organ Behav 38(3):327–350

Munir F, Yarker J, Hicks B, Donaldson-Feilder E (2012) Returning employees back to work: developing a measure for supervisors to support return to work (SSRW). J Occup Rehabil 22 (2):196–208

Negrini A, Corbière M, Lecomte T, Coutu MF, Nieuwenhuijsen K, St-Arnaud L, ... Berbiche D (2018) How can supervisors contribute to the return to work of employees who have experienced depression? J Occup Rehabil 28(2):279–288

Netterstrøm B, Friebel L, Ladegaard Y (2013) Effects of a multidisciplinary stress treatment programme on patient return to work rate and symptom reduction: results from a randomised, wait-list controlled trial. Psychother Psychosom 82(3):177–186

Nielsen MBD, Rugulies R, Hjortkjaer C, Bültmann U, Christensen U (2013) Healing a vulnerable self: exploring return to work for women with mental health problems. Qual Health Res 23 (3):302–312

Nielsen K, Nielsen MB, Ogbonnaya C, Känsälä M, Saari E, Isaksson K (2017) Workplace resources to improve both employee well-being and performance: a systematic review and meta-analysis. Work Stress 31(2):101–120

Nielsen K, Yarker J, Munir F, Bültmann U (2018) IGLOO: an integrated framework for sustainable return to work in workers with common mental disorders. Work Stress 32(4):1–18

Nieuwenhuijsen K, Verbeek JHAM, De Boer AGEM, Blonk RWB, Van Dijk FJH (2004) Supervisory behaviour as a predictor of return to work in employees absent from work due to mental health problems. Occup Environ Med 61(10):817–823

Nigatu YT, Liu Y, Uppal M, Mckinney S, Rao S, Gillis K, Wang J (2016) Interventions for enhancing return to work in individuals with a common mental illness: systematic review and meta-analysis of randomized controlled trials. Psychol Med 46(16):3263–3274

Nigatu YT, Liu Y, Uppal M, McKinney S, Gillis K, Rao S, Wang JL (2017) Prognostic factors for return to work of employees with common mental disorders: a meta-analysis of cohort studies. Soc Psychiatry Psychiatr Epidemiol 52(10):1205–1215

Noordik E, Nieuwenhuijsen K, Varekamp I, van der Klink JJ, van Dijk F (2011) Exploring the return-to-work process for workers partially returned to work and partially on long-term sick leave due to common mental disorders: a qualitative study. Disabil Rehabil 33(17–18):1625–1635

Norder G, Bültmann U, Hoedeman R, Bruin JD, van der Klink JJ, Roelen CA (2015) Recovery and recurrence of mental sickness absence among production and office workers in the industrial sector. Europ J Public Health 25:419–423

Norrmen G, Svardsudd K, Andersson DK (2010) The association of patient's family, leisure time, and work situation with sickness certification in primary care in Sweden. Scand J Prim Health Care 28(2):76–81

OECD (2014) Making mental health count: the social and economic costs of neglecting mental health care. OECD health policy studies. OECD Publishing, Paris

Olsen IB, Øverland S, Reme SE, Løvvik C (2015) Exploring work-related causal attributions of common mental disorders. J Occup Rehabil 25(3):493–505

Paul KI, Moser K (2009) Unemployment impairs mental health: meta-analyses. J Vocat Behav 74 (3):264–282

Prang K, Bohensky M, Smith P, Collie A (2016) Return to work outcomes for workers with mental health conditions: a retrospective cohort study. Injury 47(1):257–265

Reavley NJ, Ross A, Killackey EJ, Jorm AF (2012) Development of guidelines to assist organisations to support employees returning to work after an episode of anxiety, depression or a related disorder: a Delphi consensus study with Australian professionals and consumers. BMC Psychiatry 12(1):135

Saint-Arnaud L, Saint-Jean M, Demasse J (2006) Towards an enhanced understanding of factors involved in the return- to-work process of employees absent due to mental health problems. Can J Commun Ment Health 25(2):303–315

Salkever DS, Shinogle JA, Goldman H (2003) Return to work and claim duration for workers with long-term mental disabilities: impacts of mental health coverage, fringe benefits, and disability management. Ment Health Serv Res 5(3):173–186

Schuch FB, Vancampfort D, Richards J, Rosenbaum S, Ward PB, Stubbs B (2016) Exercise as a treatment for depression: a meta-analysis adjusting for publication bias. J Psychiatr Res 77:42–51

Skakon J, Nielsen K, Borg V, Guzman J (2010) Are leaders' well-being, behaviours and style associated with the affective well-being of their employees? A systematic review of three decades of research. Work Stress 24(2):107–139

Stansfeld S, Candy B (2006) Psychosocial work environment and mental health—a meta-analytic review. Scand J Work Environ Health 32:443–462

Sturesson M, Edlund C, Falkdal AH, Bernspång B (2014) Healthcare encounters and return to work: a qualitative study on sick-listed patients' experiences. Prim Health Care Res Dev 15(4):464–475

Tajfel H (ed) (2010) Social identity and intergroup relations. Cambridge University Press, Cambridge

Tajfel H, Turner JC (1979) An integrative theory of intergroup conflict. In: Austin WG, Worchel S (eds) The social psychology of intergroup relations. Brooks/Cole, Monterey, pp 7–24

van Rhenen W, Schaufeli WB, van Dijk FJH, Blonk RWB (2008) Coping and sickness absence. Int Arch Occup Environ Health 81(4):461–472

Whiteford HA, Ferrari AJ, Degenhardt L et al (2015) The global burden of mental, neurological and substance use disorders: an analysis from the global burden of disease study 2010. PLoS One 10:e0116820

Wittchen HU, Jacobi F, Rehm J, Gustavsson A, Svensson M, Jönsson B, . . . & Fratiglioni L (2011) The size and burden of mental disorders and other disorders of the brain in Europe 2010. Eur Neuropsychopharmacol 21(9):655–679

Shifting the Focus from Work Reintegration to Sustainability of Employment

34

The Case of Spinal Cord Injury and Acquired Brain Injury

Monika E. Finger and Christine Fekete

Contents

Introduction	634
Case Examples	634
Sustainable Employment and Return to Work in Persons with Physical Disabilities	636
Two Neurological Conditions: Spinal Cord Injury and Acquired Brain Injury	638
Return to Work and Vocational Rehabilitation in SCI and ABI	640
Employment and Return to Work Rates	641
What Predicts Successful Return to Work in SCI?	642
What Predicts Successful Return to Work in ABI?	642
From Work Reintegration to Sustainability of Employment	643
Sustained Employment in the Context of SCI and ABI Research	643
Facilitators and Barriers to Sustained Employment of Persons with SCI: The Persons Perspective	644
Facilitators and Barriers to Sustained Employment of Persons with ABI: The Persons Perspective	647
Challenges and Implications for Research	653
Implications for Practice	654
Conclusions	655
Cross-References	656
References	656

Abstract

Given the various functional limitations, work participation is a critical and fluctuating outcome in persons with acquired neurological conditions, such as spinal cord injury (SCI) or acquired brain injury (ABI). While there is an impressive body of research on factors related to return to work after SCI and ABI, evidence on *sustained employment* applying a life course approach is scarce

---

M. E. Finger (✉) · C. Fekete
Swiss Paraplegic Research, Nottwil, Switzerland

Department of Health Sciences and Medicine, University of Lucerne, Lucerne, Switzerland
e-mail: monika.finger@paraplegie.ch; christine.fekete@paraplegie.ch

© Springer Nature Switzerland AG 2020
U. Bültmann, J. Siegrist (eds.), *Handbook of Disability, Work and Health*, Handbook Series in Occupational Health Sciences, https://doi.org/10.1007/978-3-030-24334-0_33

and mainly available from qualitative research. Long-term work trajectories of persons with SCI and ABI are complex, and sustainability may depend on various factors, such as motivation, new employment identities, and supporting family members, employers, and coworkers. Flexible work schedules and adapted task profiles, an accessible workplace, and technical devices were reported as facilitators for sustained employment on the organizational level. To properly accommodate the often changing abilities after the initial RTW period and therefore to prevent premature labor market exit, a continuous "person-job-match" monitoring is recommended. The better understanding of how persons with SCI or ABI can be sustainably integrated in the labor market remains methodologically challenging, and large-scale longitudinal studies applying a life course approach are needed to gain more insights.

Keywords

Sustained employment · Return to work · Vocational rehabilitation · Neurological conditions · Acquired brain injury · Spinal cord injury

Introduction

Case Examples

Alexander, 35 Years, Acquired Brain Injury
Alexander was 29 years old when he was hit by a car while driving with the motorbike home from work. He sustained facial fractures, a closed head injury, and multiple orthopedic fractures on his left leg and pelvis. At that time, he worked as a sales clerk in a bike shop and lived with his wife and his one-year-old daughter in a three room flat on the third floor in an apartment building.

Alexander arrived at the hospital with a continuously deteriorating value on the Glasgow Coma Scale (GCS). In an emergency surgery, the bleeding in the skull cavity was removed. In the following days, Alexander's orthopedic injuries also had to be surgically treated. He was admitted to rehabilitation 4 weeks after the accident. At that time, Alex was alert, with short-term memory difficulties, subtle difficulties with word finding and higher level tasks, such as planning and managing the daily routine. He showed slightly impaired muscle strength in the right arm, and was not allowed to bear more than 10 kg weight on the right leg due to the orthopedic fractures. His wife was relieved to see him steadily recovering, but was also slightly concerned because he was unusually impatient with his daughter and very sensitive to noise.

Ten weeks after the accident Alex was discharged home, fully ambulatory but still with some restrictions in short-term memory and troubles in higher

(continued)

level tasks, such as writing business letters on the computer. Work on the computer was also difficult, because of his increased fatigability. A community-based rehabilitation program was denied by the insurer as perceived not further beneficial to the patient. Instead, a 50% return to work with an increase to 100% within 8 weeks was recommended.

Because Alex feared stigmatization, he returned to his former workplace without telling his employer that he still suffered from leftovers of his brain injury. Instead he referred to pain in face and leg, to justify the needed additional brakes. When returning home, he was exhausted and needed rest. In the following weeks, Alex's performance at work stabilized also due to his continuing great interest in motorcycles and his technical knowhow. At home his family learned to deal with his grown need for rest and tried to give him room.

Nevertheless, Alex felt himself constantly burdened to his limits. Therefore he declined when his boss offered to send him on a management course to forgo the associated job promotion. Although he kept up his performance as a sales clerk, when his employer retired 5 years later, and a new boss restructured the business, Alexander could no longer meet the requirements despite his best efforts. He collapsed and his physician diagnosed a burnout.

Charlotte, 49 Years, Traumatic Spinal Cord Injury
Charlotte was 45 years old when she slipped from the ladder while helping her mother cleaning the windows. The fall ended up in a rib fracture and a traumatic injury of the spinal cord at the thoracic level T6. As the emergency team immediately recognized the severity of the accident, she was admitted to the university hospital of the next larger town. Charlotte underwent a spinal surgery the same day and was diagnosed with a complete paraplegia, indicating a complete lesion of motor and sensory functions below the lesion level of the sixth thoracic vertebra (T6). She spent the acute phase in the university hospital and was then transferred to first rehabilitation in a specialized clinic, offering a broad range of therapies to manage the consequences of her spinal cord injury. Besides physiotherapy, bladder and bowel management, occupational therapy, and psychological support to adapt to the new life situation, Charlotte had the opportunity to participate in vocational rehabilitation.

Given her wheelchair dependency, returning to the previous job as a real estate broker was hardly possible. The job coach contacted her previous employer and invited him to discuss potential alternatives that would fit her special needs. However, it turned out difficult and the pre-injury employer could not offer her an adequate solution as there were no vacancies and no

(continued)

> budget to create new jobs in the company. Charlotte was deeply disappointed but quickly understood that flexibility and openness for new possibilities would be necessary strategies to deal with the new situation. Together with her job coach, she identified a retraining program for accounting in real estate management.
>
> After discharge from 28 weeks of first rehabilitation, Charlotte was optimistic and with the help of her network, she found a wheelchair accessible apartment and soon started the retraining, which she could finance by her private savings. It was a tough job as getting ready in the morning took her almost 2 h, the catheterization to empty the bladder, the mobility limitations, and the added burden for self-care presented a substantial burden in her daily life. Luckily, Charlotte was at stable mental health and the injury did not affect her energy and drive level. After 2 years, she received her diploma and finally found a part-time job nearby. The new colleagues and the employer were supportive and Charlotte received an adapted workplace. The supportive environment and her ability to quickly adapt to new situations helped her keeping the job.

Sustainable Employment and Return to Work in Persons with Physical Disabilities

Persons with physical disabilities are less likely to participate in paid work, which places nonworking individuals at increased risk of poverty, ill health, as well as reduced integration and participation (OECD 2010; Bickenbach et al. 2013). Empirical evidence documents for example that persons with physical disabilities who are excluded from paid work report worse physical and mental health, higher rates of psychological distress, lower self-worth, and lower well-being as compared to persons engaged in paid work. Besides the negative consequences for the individual, excluding persons with disabilities from the labor market also has enormous societal consequences, such as increased expenses on social benefits or disability pensions, decreased tax revenues, or loss of social cohesion, diversity, and creativity (OECD 2018). To reduce individual and societal costs of labor market exclusion of persons with disabilities, work reintegration of persons with disabilities is of crucial importance. A recent synthesis of systematic reviews identified major prognostic factors for successful work reintegration across different health and injury conditions (Cancelliere et al. 2016). Although many factors were disease-specific, higher socioeconomic status, self-efficacy, optimistic expectations for recovery and work reintegration, and lower health condition severity were reported be associated with successful work reintegration across conditions. In contrast, older age, being female, pain, depression, high physical work demands, previous sick leave, unemployment, or activity limitations were negatively related to work integration. Importantly, coordinated and multidisciplinary work reintegration interventions predicted successful return to work (RTW) (Cancelliere et al. 2016). In persons with a sudden onset of a physical disability (e.g., due to an accident, a disease, or violence), vocational rehabilitation interventions early after disability occurrence have proven to be effective to support work reintegration (Hoefsmit et al. 2012). However, successful RTW after disability onset may only demark a starting point with regard to life course work trajectories. A closer look into the literature reveals that RTW rates shortly after injury onset and vocational rehabilitation are often overestimated and do not reflect long-term employment rates in persons with disabilities (OECD 2010; Cuthbert et al. 2015).

Longitudinal studies identified considerable temporal instability of post-disability employment. DiSanto et al. (2018) defined, for example, four typical trajectories for persons with moderate to severe traumatic brain injury (TBI): (1) stable employment over time, (2) no paid employment, (3) unstable employment that relates to diverse on-off-on work situations, and (4) delayed employment, where participants returned to work after 2 years (DiSanto et al. 2018). Comparable trajectories were observed for persons with nontraumatic brain injury and spinal cord injury (SCI) (Marti et al. 2017). However, most longitudinal studies that evaluate the post-disability employment status only include short follow-up periods of 3–12 months after rehabilitation or vocational interventions. While these studies evaluate the short-term success of RTW interventions, they are unable to assess the sustainability of work integration from a life course perspective. The narrow time frame of these studies does, for example, not adequately capture persons who need more time for RTW as described in the "delayed employment trajectory" group (DiSanto et al. 2018).

Evaluating sustained employment after the initial RTW period in persons with disabilities is crucial to better understand the prerequisites in terms of work conditions and support to stay and thrive at work over time. In other words, information on predictors of *sustainable* employment in persons with disabilities is needed to tailor interventions that aim to integrate those vulnerable groups in the long term. In medical research, employment is mainly seen as one outcome after vocational rehabilitation and the follow-up time frame of interest is often restricted to a maximum of 6 month after RTW (Vogel et al. 2011). Occupational health research just recently shifted the focus on the construct of sustainable employability, taking into account an individual's ability to function at the workplace and in the labor market throughout the working age (van der Klink et al. 2016). This research stream is mainly driven by the interest of National Labour and Social Security Departments to improve the likelihood of persons who were successfully reintegrated after disability onset to sustain their employment rather than switch between employment, unemployment, and social benefits. Human resource management (HRM) policies and actions on the other hand aim to shape work and the workplace in a way that employees are enabled to provide constant performance over time. HRM measures largely aim at preparing the work environment for demographic changes (i.e., the aging society) and include adaptations to accommodate workers who age into disability (Kramar 2014). For persons with disabilities resulting from illness or injury, the sustainability of employment after RTW is as crucial as for aging workers and depends not only on individual adjustments and organizational and environmental adaptations but also on matching their skills, abilities, competences, and interests to the work requirements (Nützi et al. 2017). According to a conceptual job matching framework for RTW of persons with SCI, the match of stable factors (e.g., abilities, vocational interests, work stiles), modifiable factors (e.g., education, experiences and needs of the person, work contexts), the organizational context, and the workplace are seen as predictive for job satisfaction, work stress, and job performance, which in turn are likely to impact on the sustainability of employment (Nützi et al. 2019).

While most recent attempts to capture relevant predictors for work sustainability are focused on specific dimensions, such as the work environment or an individual's characteristics, an integrated framework for sustainable employment taking into account the interaction of different dimensions has only recently been developed (Nielsen et al. 2018). With the IGLOO framework, Nielsen et al. (2018) presented an integrated approach to assess relevant resources for sustainability at the individual (e.g., cognition, behavior), group (e.g., support, attitudes from others), leader (e.g., supervisors support), organizational (e.g., the HRM's practices and policies), and the overarching contextual level (e.g., the social welfare policies). Interestingly, this framework not only integrates resources from different levels but also from the work and the nonwork context. This points to the fact that sustainable employment might only be fostered if the individuals' situation is captured in a comprehensive way, including the home and the work sphere as well as environmental and societal circumstances (Nielsen et al. 2018). Given that resources on the diverse levels are interacting and labor markets are rapidly changing due to globalization, societal changes, and technological advances, these larger scale changes may also impact upon the individual level with consequences on work demands, abilities, and needs of employees. Hence, sustainability of employment has to be monitored continuously throughout the life course.

Integrating the perspective of occupational health psychology (Fleuren et al. 2016) and the theory of work adjustment from vocational psychology (Dawis 2005), we understand *sustainable employment* as a *person–job–workplace match that enables a person to stay healthy and satisfied at work over time, with a work performance that meets the expectations of the person and the employer.*

Two Neurological Conditions: Spinal Cord Injury and Acquired Brain Injury

SCI and ABI are primary examples of acquired neurological injuries that are major causes of years of healthy life lost as a result of disability worldwide. SCI affects the spinal cord and ABI affects the brain, and while they affect different structures of the nervous system, both can impair the biological, psychological, and social functioning of a person, resulting in chronic disability. SCI and ABI significantly impact on mobility, self-care, work abilities, community, and social life. Affected individuals also face challenges caused by complex medical, cognitive, and emotional problems and together, these two health conditions represent prototypically a wide range of challenges occurring in persons with neurological disorders. In addition, the literature reports that over 39% of persons with traumatic SCI are also diagnosed with TBI (Budisin et al. 2016), which makes the effects of both disorders exponentially burdensome.

Spinal Cord Injury (SCI)

An SCI is a life-altering condition and one of the most devastating injuries that an individual can experience. In most cases, it not only impacts on all aspects of the individuals functioning, but goes along with numerous long-term physical, psychological, social, and financial implications (Bickenbach et al. 2013). Up to 90% of injuries in working age population are of traumatic etiology, mostly caused by traffic accidents followed by falls and assaults. The nontraumatic etiologies of SCI include an underlying pathology (e.g., tumor, infection, musculoskeletal disease) that causes an injury to the spinal cord. Given the demographic changes related to aging societies, the prevalence of nontraumatic SCI is steadily increasing. The estimated annual global incidence of SCI is 40–80 cases per million population, and it is assumed that 250,000 to 500,000 persons are newly injured with SCI yearly, with males having a threefold risk of becoming spinal cord injured than women (Bickenbach et al. 2013). Although SCI is rather rare, SCI is one of the most costly chronic health conditions. Recent estimates of annual healthcare costs for persons with tetraplegia in Canada amount to 150,900 Can$ in the first year and about 53,600 Can$ annually for the following years, while paraplegia costs are about 104,600 Can$ in the first and 24,700 Can$ in the following years (Bickenbach et al. 2013), not including indirect costs.

The injury severity can be classified according to the location on the spinal cord (level of injury, paraplegia vs. tetraplegia) and the completeness of the lesion (complete vs. incomplete), which indicates whether symptoms include partial or complete loss of sensory function or motor control of arms, legs, and/or body. Severe SCI may also affect the systems that regulate bowel or bladder control, breathing, heart rate, and blood pressure. These primary physical impairments are often associated with secondary complications, such as pressure ulcers, urinary tract infections, pneumonia, and orthostatic problems. Moreover, chronic pain is reported as highly prevalent among persons with SCI (Brinkhof et al. 2016).

Appropriate medical care, rehabilitation, and social support can help persons with SCI lead a fulfilling and productive life (van Leeuwen et al. 2012). Rehabilitation with the aim to optimize functioning in the interaction with the environment aims to reintegrate the individuals after the SCI into the community, but also intends to enable individuals to self-management and to prevent secondary health conditions. Vocational rehabilitation as part of the rehabilitative process after onset of SCI has been proven to be effective to integrate persons with SCI into the labor market.

Acquired Brain Injury (ABI)

An ABI is defined as a damage to the brain that occurs from a traumatic or nontraumatic etiology and is not related to a congenital disorder or a degenerative disease, such as Alzheimer's disease, multiple sclerosis, or Parkinson's disease. Traumatic brain injury can be caused by various events, such as a blow to the head, a fall, a traffic accident, or a sports-related injury. Nontraumatic brain injury is caused by illness such as meningitis or encephalitis, oxygen deprivation (anoxia), or stroke. Estimates of incidence and prevalence of ABI vary considerably depending on the source and methods of calculation. Data from a systematic review suggest an overall incidence rate of 262 cases per 100,000 persons for Europe (Peeters et al. 2015). The majority of cases are diagnosed as mild injury, while the incidence rate for severe injuries is estimated annually at 10.6 per 100,000 persons. Comparable to the case of SCI, the consequences of ABI can be devastating and expensive for the individual, family, and society. For instance, direct medical costs for patients with severe ABI in Australia were estimated at AUD 250,000, not including lifelong disability benefits.

Individuals who sustain an ABI may encounter a wide range of problems, with various degrees of expression: observable consequences may include movement and balance disorders, paralysis or changed facial expression, altered voice or dysarthria, whereas nonobservable "silent" problems may include reduced attention, concentration and memory, increased fatigability, planning problems, diminished self-control and social behavior, emotional instability, and communication problems (Stocchetti and Zanier 2016). The initial Glasgow Coma Score and the duration of post-trauma amnesia (Teasdale et al. 2014) are standards used to classify the severity of ABI into mild, moderate, and severe. Similar to SCI, the spectrum of the severity of injury and its consequences is rather broad, and persons who sustain a mild form of ABI may not encounter any limitations, while severe injuries often lead to severe lifelong disability.

Structured multidisciplinary rehabilitation is found to be valuable to improve both physical and neuropsychological outcomes. Nevertheless, most problems identified in the subacute phase tend to persist over time, although the degree of the remaining symptoms may vary substantially and is not always linked to initial severity (Ponsford et al. 2014).

Return to Work and Vocational Rehabilitation in SCI and ABI

Given the various functional limitations, work participation is a critical and fluctuating outcome in persons with acquired neurologic disabilities, such as SCI or ABI. Paid work is not only important to maintain economic self-sufficiency but also presents a source for psychological well-being, mental health, social integration, and participation (van Velzen et al. 2009b). Therefore, returning to work after the injury has been identified as a major rehabilitation goal in persons with neurological conditions, and an impressive body of research addresses the topic of RTW in SCI and ABI (Escorpizo et al. 2014; van Velzen et al. 2009b). It is however important to note that RTW is not just a dichotomous outcome indicating whether a person has successfully returned to work or not. Returning to work after a major injury should be understood as a dynamic process involving different stages in potentially different settings, which may result in success, failure, or changes of the strategy. For example, the RTW process can include first attempts to work in supported work places, the return to an adapted work place at the pre-injury employer, the change of the job and therefore the change of the employer, or the complete resumption of work without any alterations. To better understand the complex process of RTW and to adequately capture the individuals' work ability, it has been suggested to describe RTW outcomes along the lines of four criteria (Vogel et al. 2011): (1) RTW attempts (no; failed; successful attempt), (2) current working status (working; not working), (3) time to RTW, and (4) number of working hours (less; same; more hours than before injury). Beyond the pure description of objective indicators of RTW as suggested by Vogel et al. (2011), we suggest to add job performance during working hours as fifth criterion to gather insights into qualitative characteristics of an individuals' RTW trajectory. Job performance describes an individuals' ability to execute job tasks and seems important as persons with neurological conditions often have severe performance constraints. Again, job performance might not be stable during the working life course and is affected by health complications or contextual factors.

Employment and Return to Work Rates

Employment rates describe the ratio of the employed persons to the working age population of a country. Employment rates of persons with SCI or ABI vary considerably across countries (Young and Murphy 2009; van Velzen et al. 2009a), largely due to differences in national economies, labor market characteristics, official statistics, and social welfare state policies. The average global employment rate for persons with SCI is estimated at 37%, with rates ranging from 12% to 74% (Lidal et al. 2007). Data on employment rates for persons with ABI are even less reliable and sound epidemiological data is lacking. However, available data on RTW rates for persons with moderate to severe ABI or stroke range from 30% to 65% at 1 year after injury, with mean employment rates of around 40% that remain largely stable in the period of 5–10 years after injury. For persons with mild ABI, employment rates range from 46% to 100% 1 year after injury, with large variations across studies and settings (Iverson et al. 2012). Besides economic country specificities, the vast differences in estimates may further arise because of different definitions of employment (e.g., full- vs. part-time work, sheltered employment, or even unpaid work) and the risk of selection bias in study samples.

In addition, a universal definition of RTW is missing, and given the fact that RTW is a dynamic process including different individual trajectories, the reported employment rates are difficult to compare. With 70% of persons with ABI (Bahadur et al. 2017) and 68% of persons with SCI (Young and Murphy 2009), a rather high proportion of affected persons reports having worked at least at some point after disability onset. Around 40–50% of persons with SCI or ABI succeed to return to work within 2 years after injury (van Velzen et al. 2009a; Reinhardt et al. 2016), with a majority of persons working in part-time positions (Reinhardt et al. 2016). Importantly, these RTW rates may be overestimated (Cuthbert et al. 2015; Krause and Reed 2011), as employment status is usually determined at the end of the medical treatment or rehabilitation, and many individuals who initially returned to work are unable to sustain in employment over time (Lidal et al. 2007). Given the potentially fluctuating success of short-term work integration, the work life courses of persons with chronic disabilities need continuous monitoring after initial rehabilitation and work reintegration.

What Predicts Successful Return to Work in SCI?

Current evidence describes RTW in SCI as the result of various interrelated factors, including functioning, contextual factors (i.e., personal and environmental factors), and health conditions. For example, male gender, younger age at injury, longer time since injury, Caucasian origin, high pre-injury education, high personal value to work, or employment at injury in a low intensity job have been identified as personal factors that increase the likelihood for successful RTW (Escorpizo et al. 2014). Furthermore, accesses to assistive devices, independent use of transportation, social support, job accommodation, and flexible schedules (e.g., reduced work hours) have been observed to be predictive for successful RTW. In contrast, persons with severe injuries, secondary health conditions, such as bowel incontinence, urinary tract infections, pain, depression, or pressure sores, are at risk of labor market exclusion (Marti et al. 2016). Studies on the effect of the work environment reported that supported employment programs (Ottomanelli et al. 2013; Roels et al. 2016; Escorpizo et al. 2018) and vocational rehabilitation counseling improve the employment rates after disability onset (Jang et al. 2005; Jongbloed et al. 2007; Marini et al. 2008).

What Predicts Successful Return to Work in ABI?

Similar to the case of SCI, many factors may be involved in the successful RTW after an ABI. However, evidence on predictors for RTW cannot be generalized for ABI, but needs to be reported separately by etiology (traumatic or nontraumatic) or injury severity (mild to severe). For example, a systematic review on factors that predict RTW in persons with *nontraumatic* brain injuries found, against expectations, that age, gender, the injury location, and pre-injury education were not predictive for successful RTW, and results concerning the predictive value of cognitive or physical functioning, such as muscle strength, were inconclusive (van Velzen et al. 2009b). Another review including 42 studies on *traumatic* brain injury synthesized evidence for predictors for work-related difficulties, defined as job instability over 5-years post injury or unemployment (Scaratti et al. 2017). Age above 34 years, female gender, low educational level, pre-injury unemployment, higher Glasgow Coma Scale scores and injury severity, length of stay in acute and rehabilitation care, lower functional independence, and cognitive impairments were identified as predictors for work-related difficulties, such as lower work participation, reduced working hours, or enhanced job cessation (Scaratti et al. 2017). Social support also seems predictive for work-related difficulties, for example, married individuals had a higher probability of stable employment than unmarried individuals (Scaratti et al. 2017). A review on four studies including persons with *mild traumatic* brain injuries found that persons with mild injuries had no significantly increased risk for long-term work disability (Cancelliere et al. 2014). However, low pre-injury education was strongly related to reduced RTW rates and increased work instability, and persons with low educational levels more often reported delayed RTW (>6 month after injury) compared to persons with higher education. Furthermore, the authors concluded that nausea or vomiting at hospital admission, extracranial injuries, severe head or bodily pain early after injury, and limited job independence and decision-making latitude were associated with reduced success in RTW in persons with mild traumatic brain injury (Cancelliere et al. 2014).

Vocational rehabilitation interventions in persons with moderate to severe ABI have been proven effective to improve RTW outcomes (Donker-Cools et al. 2016). Vocational rehabilitation may include work directed interventions in combination with education, training of work-related and social skills, and job coaching. Due to the heterogeneity of problems in ABI patients, it is recommended to apply a patient-centered approach in which relevant stakeholders (e.g., family members, employers) are involved early after injury (Donker-Cools et al. 2016).

From Work Reintegration to Sustainability of Employment

Sustained Employment in the Context of SCI and ABI Research

While there is an impressive body of research on factors related to RTW after SCI and ABI, empirical evidence on the factors related to *sustained employment* is scarce. Obviously, investigating sustained employment urges a shift in research designs taking into account a long observation period reflected by a life course approach. Results of longitudinal studies from the United States, such as the National Institute on Disability and Rehabilitation Research's *Traumatic Brain Injury Model Systems National Database*, may allow first insights into work integration patterns and employment trajectories. An important finding of this work trajectory research is that work participation of persons with TBI markedly declines 5–10 years post injury (Cuthbert et al. 2015). This finding again underlines the necessity of a long-term perspective on work integration as the initial RTW rates in ABI obviously not correspond to long-term work outcomes which are likely to decrease over time. Similarly, findings from a longitudinal cohort study of persons with SCI in Canada showed that long-term work participation strongly depended on age, as younger and middle-aged persons had a lower risk to receive disability benefits than those aged 55–64 years (Jetha et al. 2014). However, these two longitudinal studies intended to provide basic epidemiological data on labor market participation and were not specifically designed to investigate predictors for sustained employment. Therefore, information on resources that support sustainability of employment, for example, as defined in the IGLOO model (Nielsen et al. 2018), remains largely unstudied in these cohorts.

Several important concerns led to new research priorities in research on labor market participation in persons with disabilities. The shift from work reintegration to sustainable employment was mainly due to the growing interest from multiple stakeholders in ensuring that people with disabilities remain at work throughout their working lives, the awareness that work participation is a complex phenomenon including a variety of factors that predict the work trajectories, and finally, the recognition of the importance of a patient-centered, individual approach to rehabilitation and long-term support of affected persons.

Facilitators and Barriers to Sustained Employment of Persons with SCI: The Persons Perspective

Given that large-scale epidemiological studies on predictors for sustained employment in persons with SCI are widely lacking, qualitative research might be a good starting point to identify facilitators and barriers of sustainability. We identified three qualitative studies (Marti et al. 2017; Meade et al. 2016; Wilbanks and Ivankova 2015) in which participants discussed relevant factors or resources at different levels of the IGLOO model (Nielsen et al. 2018). Persons with SCI were asked about the supporting factors and the challenges to stay at work as well as about their subjective meaning of work. These studies only included persons who were either full- or part-time employed or had at least 7 years of work experience after SCI before age-related retirement (Table 1).

At the *individual level*, two major topics were repeatedly discussed as important: secondary health conditions and personal motivation. Participants often cited secondary health conditions, such as pain, pressure sores, or bladder and bowel incontinence as the biggest challenges to stay at work. Given that these health complications are widely prevalent in persons with SCI, their management should also take priority in work sustainability discussions. On a psychological level, the achievement of personal independence, a new work identity, satisfaction and pleasure, being part of a team, the feeling to contribute to society and to move forward were mentioned as intrinsic motivators. In relation to extrinsic motivation, financial security, acquiring health insurance, and encouragements from family members or relevant others were declared as important motivators to stay in employment.

Social relationships emerged as important issue at the *group level*. Good personal relationships and interactions with colleagues at work, but also with family or personal supporters were mentioned as conducive, whereas stigmatization and

Table 1 Qualitative studies on facilitators and barriers of sustained employment in persons with spinal cord injury (k = 3)

First author, year; country	Sample size (gender)	Diagnosis; time post injury	Method	Study objective	Outcome facilitators	Barriers
Marti, 2017; Switzerland	n = 15 (3 f, 12 m)	n = 10 paraplegia, n = 5 tetraplegia; >13 y	Semi-structured interviews, thematic analysis	To explore long-term employment pathways	Developing new employment identity Need for recognition, job satisfaction Desire to RTW Combining skills from pre-SCI job and VR Support of pre-SCI employer	Trapped in pre-SCI employment identity Problem finding new job interest, orientation Frustration with job search Competing responsibilities, e.g., housework, child care VR as missed opportunity as not used for new orientation
Meade, 2016; United States	n = 44 (14 f, 30 m) (6 focus groups)	n = 24 paraplegia, n = 10 tetraplegia; >10 y	Focus group study, thematic analysis	To explore the relationship of employment with physical health and functioning	Develop daily routine supportive for employment Prevention of health complications Good interaction with personal caregivers Ability to communicate and self-advocate (e.g., asking for job accommodations)	Letting go of previous employment Time needed to do basic health maintenance Secondary conditions and aging (physical decline, fatigue, osteoporosis leading to fractures, shoulder degeneration due to wheel chair propulsion)

(continued)

Table 1 (continued)

First author, year; country	Sample size (gender)	Diagnosis; time post injury	Method	Study objective	Outcome facilitators	Barriers
Wilbanks, 2015; United States	n = 4 (1 f, 3 m)	n = 3 paraplegia, n = 1 tetraplegia; 24–37 y	Semi-structured interviews, thematic analysis	To identify factors that facilitate adults with SCI rejoining the workforce	Understanding employers Supportive work environment Accessibility of workplace Home health aide paid by state resources Assistive technology, e.g., office space, car *Intrinsic motivators*: Ambition, work ethic, wanting to be normal and fit with society, challenge stigma, making an impact *Extrinsic motivators*: Rehab-professionals, role models, family members, financial benefits, health insurance	Stamina to keep fixed schedule Physical health (e.g., bladder and bowel control, shoulder problems, pain) Prejudices, fight against myth that persons with physical disabilities also encounter mental or cognitive limitations

Abbreviations: *SCI* Spinal cord injury, *RTW* Return to work, *y* Years prejudice against persons with disabilities were revealed as barriers for successful long-term employment (Meade et al. 2015; Wilbanks and Ivankova 2015).

At the *leader level*, a good relationship with the employer and the direct supervisor and their commitment to engage a person with SCI were revealed as important prerequisites for sustained employment (Marti et al. 2017; Meade et al. 2015; Wilbanks and Ivankova 2015). In order to develop an understanding of the needs of persons with disabilities, an open exchange among work specialists, the employer, and the person with SCI were also acknowledged as helpful in the initial RTW phase. In the long term, participants emphasized the importance of recognition and options for further professional developments and job promotion. Furthermore, accessibility to the workplace (e.g., wheelchair accessible offices, toilets) and a supportive work environment (e.g., availability of assistive technology, adapted devices) are prerequisites for productive work. However, long working hours without the possibility of reducing hours or adapting tasks are difficult for many persons in the long term (Meade et al. 2015).

At the *societal level*, a majority of study participants stressed the importance of good health care and an adequate health insurance system. In Switzerland, some participants expressed concerns about the social security legislation as there is a risk of losing the disability pension if working hours are increased (Marti et al. 2017).

Facilitators and Barriers to Sustained Employment of Persons with ABI: The Persons Perspective

Returning to work is often an enormous challenge for persons with ABI, as work reintegration is dependent on a certain level of recovery and progress in healing, or even with the expectation of returning to normality. As persons with ABI are often confronted with cognitive, physical, emotional, and social demands at work that are difficult to fulfill, RTW therefore might be associated with disappointments, frustrations, and unfulfilled expectations of oneself, the employer, and colleagues. In order to better understand the needs and challenges persons with ABI face, a number of qualitative studies were performed to complement results from longitudinal studies (Table 2). Although results need careful interpretation as the time at which the study participants were interviewed largely varies, ranging from a few months to many years after RTW, these findings may nevertheless provide valuable information with regard to sustainability of employment.

At the *individual level*, participants and relatives identified so-called invisible consequences of the injury as one of the major challenges for long-term work integration. Invisible problems, such as diminished memory functions, difficulties in concentrating in a restless environment, or difficulties in interacting in a conversation with several people due to impaired speech functions, were found to cause insecurity or fear. Symptoms such as increasing fatigue, visual problems, or problems to control feelings were also perceived as very disturbing (Balasooriya-Smeekens et al. 2016). In relation to these invisible consequences of the brain injury, participants reported that they no longer recognized themselves, and were often

Table 2 Qualitative studies on facilitators and barriers of sustained employment in persons with acquired brain injury (k = 5)

First author, year; country	Sample size (gender)	Diagnosis; time post injury	Method	Study objective	Outcome facilitators	Barriers
Balasooriya-Smeekens, 2016; UK	$n = 60$ (23 f, 37 m)	Stroke; $n = 31 < 2$ y post-stroke, time post-stroke unknown for $n = 29$	Content analysis of online forum blog entries mentioning "back at work"	To explore facilitators and barriers of work after stroke	Having had stroke at workplace increases visibility and understanding Improving of employer's knowledge about stroke enhances support Involving occupational health specialists to adapt work plan Supportive employer and coworkers Family support Change of demanding job to manageable job Adequate coping strategies	Invisibility of impairments leading to misunderstanding/misinterpretation of behavior and performance (cognitive problems, fatigue) Lack of knowledge about consequences and temporal course of ABI Unfulfilled expectations (of person, employer, and colleagues) Lack of self-awareness Lack of support at work (not feeling understood, not meeting performance expectations) Secondary health conditions (fatigue, psychological problems, memory or cognitive problems, language or speech problems, physical problems) Stress, fear, negative feelings toward work

Bush, 2016; United States	$n = 5$ TBI; $n = 6$ family members; $n = 1$ job supervisor	TBI; 2–16 y	Semi-structured interviews	To evaluate post-injury work experiences in TBI and significant others	Motivation to work (independent of job) Job satisfaction Regular contact to employer Job modifications Coping strategies (e.g., making notes) Family support Convenient working hours Good salary Feeling as credible community member	Coworkers and employers behavior (avoiding contact) Limited computer literacy Difficulty to find new job Uncontrolled emotions, low frustration tolerance Need of supervision to complete tasks Insufficient work quality Difficulty to keep track of changes at work Display tangential speech Chaotic, loud environment in open space office Visual and spatial problems Lack of awareness of impairments and its consequences
Cogné, 2017; France	$n = 39$ TBI; $n = 18$ stroke (19 f, 38 m); $n = 57$ (relatives)	TBI or stroke; 5 y follow-up of persons in VR program	Semi-structured telephone interviews with patients and relatives	To report outcomes of VR and predictors of RTW	74% performed less demanding job than before injury	Decreased income Unavailability of adequate jobs

(continued)

Table 2 (continued)

First author, year; country	Sample size (gender)	Diagnosis; time post injury	Method	Study objective	Outcome facilitators	Barriers
Grigorovich, 2017; Canada	n = 14 (for interviews); n = 58 for record analysis (18 f, 40 m)	Mild to severe TBI	Thematic interviews Quantitative data analysis from records	To evaluate employment support services	Practice recommendations for community based services were formulated: Time dedicated for assistance in goal planning Focus on developing job-finding skills and support them on securing the job On the job support and training Long-term support for person and employer Good relationships with employer and coworkers	Difficulty to find suitable jobs or convince employers to hire a person with ABI No financial support for employer as incentive

| Libeson, 2018; Australia | n = 15 (7 f, 8 m) | TBI (n = 10 severe, n = 4 moderate, n = 1 mild); 1–8 y | Face-to-face semi-structured interviews | To understand the RTW experience | Family support
Personal motivation
Employer support (flexibility, adapted work)
Financial incentives | Lack of family support
"Over-motivated" unable to cope with work demands
Lack of employer support (negative attitude, unrealistic demands and expectations)
End of incentives leads employer to stop support
Nature of job (complex, demanding work tasks) |

Abbreviations: *ABI* Acquired brain injury, *TBI* Traumatic brain injury, *RTW* Return to work, *y* Years disappointed by their own performance, whereas relatives reported that a lack of self-awareness led to conflicts in daily life (Balasooriya-Smeekens et al. 2016). Therefore, study participants stressed the importance of receiving support from competent health or work professionals who help understanding the consequences of the injury and developing appropriate coping strategies (Bush et al. 2016).

Another important factor mentioned by persons with ABI was their motivation to succeed at work. Studies revealed that factors like feelings of being a credible community member and job satisfaction were the most important intrinsic motivators, whereas work adapted to personal performance levels, suitable working hours, and adequate salary were mentioned as relevant for sustainability of the work situation (Cogne et al. 2017). Barriers to sustained employment were predominantly fear of not being able to fulfill expectations of employers and coworkers and psychosocial work stress (Balasooriya-Smeekens et al. 2016).

At the *group level*, the invisible problems of ABI not only impact the affected person but also lead to negative interactions with coworkers who are not aware of the consequences of the ABI. Study participants described that coworkers who recognized slower or error-prone work performance reacted by stigmatizing the persons with ABI as lazy or odd by ignoring or even treating them with open hostility (Bush et al. 2016; Libeson et al. 2018). Due to fear of stigmatization and subsequent job loss, persons with ABI reported the tendency to hide their limitations at the workplace. In the home environment, family members tended to release persons with ABI from chores they could no longer carry out correctly. The responsibility to support the family member with ABI in performing his or her job tasks was perceived as burden in some relationships, especially if the person with ABI was unaware of own deficits (Bush et al. 2016). Studies have shown that an informed and supportive employer and a good social network at the workplace were even more important for long-term work participation than the original severity of the brain injury.

At the *leader level*, evidence and experiences of persons with ABI equally stressed the importance of a supportive, understanding employer for stable work integration. Integrating the employer throughout the RTW process was described as helpful as a better understanding of the health condition and its consequences in terms of job performance and social behavior was essential to avoid unrealistic demands and expectations of employers (Libeson et al. 2018). Employers' commitment to support employees with ABI also increased if they had competent contact persons or services to provide long-term support (Grigorovich et al. 2017). However, persons with ABI and vocational rehabilitation professionals also complained that most employers were not interested or willing to employ persons with ABI at all.

At the *societal level*, longitudinal studies illustrated the variability of work trajectories after sustaining a brain injury and that an accurate prediction of whether a particular ABI patient would successfully return to and sustain work (Cuthbert et al. 2015). One major barrier that participants and providers encountered was a lack of employers who were willing to provide or create suitable jobs for persons with ABI. Therefore, it is debated if incentives, such as public compensation of parts of the salary, would help to convince potential employers to hire a person with ABI.

The comparison of individuals with SCI and ABI reveals that work participation has a high subjective importance for persons with both neurological conditions as labor market participation is strongly related to social integration and offers the possibility to experience a certain "normality." It also becomes clear that relationships with employers and colleagues at work are decisive for the success of long-term work integration in both conditions. As a consequence of their mobility limitations, persons with SCI obviously encounter more difficulties in workplace accessibility and in the organization and timing of work and healthcare needs than persons with ABI. In SCI, secondary health conditions, such as chronic pain, urinary tract infections, or pressure sores, are prevalent problems and challenges for work sustainability; however, given that many persons with SCI are not affected in their cognitive functioning, career opportunities and promotion are also of concern. In contrast, persons with ABI tend to struggle with performance limitations due to cognitive, emotional, and behavioral problems that may linger and appear when they are exposed to stressful situations in the work environment.

Challenges and Implications for Research

To better understand how persons with SCI or ABI can be included in the labor market in the long term remains a methodological challenge as for example cross-sectional observations or longitudinal studies with short follow-up time frames will not provide sufficient information to study sustainability. Obviously, investigating sustained employment urges the availability of data that traces the persons' employment history as well as potential determinants of sustainability over the life course of employable age.

Prospective cohort studies may only be valuable sources of information if the time frame is adequate. Given the fact that SCI and ABI are rather rare conditions, prospective cohort studies might not be effective in addressing issues of sustainability as it is challenging to attain adequate sample sizes to draw meaningful conclusions. The Europeans' largest community survey on persons with an SCI, the Swiss Spinal Cord Injury (www.swisci.ch) survey, provides a good example for the challenge to achieve sufficient power. In 2012, 1458 persons with SCI participated in the community survey, and thereof, 771 (53%) were involved in paid work and thus eligible to study sustained employment (Reinhardt et al. 2016). In 2017, 405 of the employed baseline participants completed the follow-up survey and 362 of them were in employable age. Of this employable age group, 53 persons prematurely left the labor market during the 5 year follow-up period. This example demonstrates the need of a rather large initial sample to attain an adequate sample size to study predictors of change. Including research questions on factors related to sustained employment in large-scale epidemiological cohorts on persons with SCI or ABI would therefore be a prerequisite to obtain sufficient statistical power to quantitatively analyze data.

Retrospective designs might be valuable alternatives to large-scale prospective studies. Retrospective designs have the advantage that trajectories of labor market participation can be assessed in detail based on a person's curriculum. Also, key information on the etiology, disability-related diagnosis, or other time invariant factors (e.g., age, gender, time of occurrence of injury) might be easily assessed. However, the major challenge of retrospective studies is the evaluation of time-varying factors that may impact on the labor market participation. For example, the assessment of personal or environmental factors or health-related problems at the time of the labor market drop-out may be prone to recall bias.

Identifying determinants of sustained employment remains an additional challenge. Current research on labor market participation and RTW has shown that successful integration depends on an interaction between biomedical, personal, and environmental factors. In view of the complexity of information required, qualitative studies may provide a valuable starting point to identify how persons with SCI or ABI can successfully manage sustainable employment. Such studies may provide the basis to inform large-scale epidemiological studies, and ultimately the planning of targeted interventions, to facilitate long-term employment in persons with neurological conditions.

Implications for Practice

We found convincing evidence on the importance of RTW in terms of health benefits and social integration and detected good arguments why it is essential for rehabilitation specialists and affected persons to look beyond the RTW phase. Although only a few qualitative studies with small sample sizes evaluated factors relevant for sustainable work, results seem to point in a same direction: RTW is a starting point, but sustaining work participation is an endeavor that encompasses the entire working life course. Its success is largely dependent on the availability of resources from various levels and the support from different stakeholders. The grounds for a successful work trajectory after SCI or ABI are already laid in the first rehabilitation phase and need to be monitored throughout the life course. Problems arising along the path have to be addressed at various levels until retirement age is reached. Although specific measures to resolve potential problems need to be defined, depending on respective health conditions, settings, and social legislations, general implications for practice can be formulated along the IGLOO model (Nielsen et al. 2018).

A main practical implication at the *individual level* is that persons with acquired neurological disabilities need time, information, and guidance from rehabilitation professionals during the acute and first rehabilitation phase to prepare for the work reintegration phase. The support of health professionals in this phase is needed to overcome the challenging adaptations to altered physical and/or cognitive and emotional abilities. Moreover, some individuals may need specific support to prevent secondary health conditions (e.g., pressure sores, urinary tract infections in SCI) and to manage potentially chronic health issues such as pain in SCI or fatigue in ABI. Strengthening communication and self-advocacy is another crucial part in first rehabilitation, and if affected persons are unable to represent themselves, relatives or significant others should be involved whenever possible. It is furthermore critical that affected persons develop realistic plans on their professional future, including the clear knowledge on their needs to successfully return and sustainably remain at work after injury.

At the *group level*, social support and acceptance by colleagues has to be seen as the most important support factors for employees with SCI or ABI. Whenever possible, rehabilitation specialists should involve coworkers of affected persons early in the reintegration process with the aim to familiarize them with the persons' needs, the clinical picture of the injury, and the remaining strengths of the employee with the disability. A better understanding of the health condition and its consequences is likely to help to create mutual understanding, prevent fear, and reduce prejudices what is likely to lead to an inclusive work atmosphere.

A good relationship between the employee with the disability and the employer was identified as a crucial resource at the *leader level*. The employers should support the integration not only during the RTW phase but also in the long run. A good and trustful relationship can be fostered by the rehabilitation professional during initial vocational rehabilitation. After completion of the initial rehabilitation phase, public services (e.g., state rehabilitation services, or employers' associations) should be sensitized to support persons with disabilities in retaining jobs or, in case of labor market exit, in finding new jobs. Given their restricted opportunities, finding a new job is often challenging and needs negotiating and building relationships with employers. In the long run, rehabilitation professionals are important partners to provide guidance and information if problems arise after the RTW phase, which is especially needed in small companies. Larger organizations often have an occupational health and human resource (HR) department that accommodate working conditions, such as flexible work models, and monitor the work-health performance of disabled employees.

At the *contextual level*, persons with ABI and SCI should be granted access to health services, additional education, or skills training if required. It is highly recommended that this constant support and development of own abilities is not limited to the rehabilitation phase, but continues over the working age course. The constant availability of resources at the contextual level presupposes that ABI and SCI are recognized as chronic conditions in respective social security and healthcare systems.

Conclusions

Although work participation is an important personal goal early after injury for most persons with SCI or ABI, it is a critical and fluctuating outcome. Being engaged in paid work is not only important to maintain financial self-sufficiency and social inclusion but also affects health and well-being and provides the opportunity to experience a sense of "normality" after injury. Return to work is therefore one of the primary rehabilitation goals, and the success of rehabilitation is often measured by the work status early after community reintegration. While an impressive body of research has documented modifiable facilitators and barriers for RTW in ABI and SCI, evidence on sustainability of employment is rare and mainly available from qualitative research.

Evidence from qualitative studies on sustained employment reported that besides personal motivation from the person's side, work conditions such as flexible work schedules and adapted task profiles and a supporting work environment including an engaged employer and understanding coworkers are decisive for long-term work participation. In addition to intense rehabilitation efforts to support persons with disabilities, the RTW process should be accompanied by an experienced rehabilitation professional to moderate the communication between the affected person, the employer, and other stakeholders, such as insurers, coworkers, and family members. Such a return-to-work rehabilitation may be a starting point of successful work integration. In order to ensure sustained employment in the long term, the need for continuous monitoring of a person-job-match thereafter becomes apparent. Monitoring structures need to be improved, strengthening existing services (e.g., company physicians, HR specialists), to develop continuous person-job-match information. These improvements could serve to accommodate employees with other chronic health conditions as well, thus contributing to better health and well-being at work.

Cross-References

- IGLOO: A Framework for Return to Work Among Workers with Mental Health Problems
- Implementing Best Practice Models of Return to Work
- Occupational Determinants of Cognitive Decline and Dementia
- Return to Work After Spinal Cord Injury

References

Bahadur S, McRann J, McGilloway E (2017) Long-term employment outcomes following rehabilitation for significant neurological impairment in UK military personnel: a 3-year study. J R Army Med Corps 163:355–360. https://doi.org/10.1136/jramc-2016-000703

Balasooriya-Smeekens C, Bateman A, Mant J et al (2016) Barriers and facilitators to staying in work after stroke: insight from an online forum. BMJ Open 6(4):e009974. https://doi.org/10.1136/bmjopen-2015-009974

Bickenbach J, Officer A, Shakespeare T et al (2013) International perspectives on spinal cord injury. World Health Organization and The International Spinal Cord Society, Geneva

Brinkhof MW, Al-Khodairy A, Eriks-Hoogland I et al (2016) Health conditions in people with spinal cord injury: contemporary evidence from a population-based community survey in Switzerland. J Rehabil Med 48(2):197–209. https://doi.org/10.2340/16501977-2039

Budisin B, Bradbury CC, Sharma B et al (2016) Traumatic brain injury in spinal cord injury: frequency and risk factors. J Head Trauma Rehabil 31(4):E33–E42. https://doi.org/10.1097/htr.0000000000000153

Bush EJ, Hux K, Guetterman TC et al (2016) The diverse vocational experiences of five individuals returning to work after severe brain injury: a qualitative inquiry. Brain Inj 30(4):422–436. https://doi.org/10.3109/02699052.2015.1131849

Cancelliere C, Kristman VL, Cassidy JD et al (2014) Systematic review of return to work after mild traumatic brain injury: results of the international collaboration on mild traumatic brain injury prognosis. Arch Phys Med Rehabil 95(3 Suppl):S201–S209. https://doi.org/10.1016/j.apmr.2013.10.010

Cancelliere C, Donovan J, Stochkendahl MJ et al (2016) Factors affecting return to work after injury or illness: best evidence synthesis of systematic reviews. Chiropr Man Therap 24(1):32. https://doi.org/10.1186/s12998-016-0113-z

Cogne M, Wiart L, Simion A et al (2017) Five-year follow-up of persons with brain injury entering the French vocational and social rehabilitation programme UEROS: return-to-work, life satisfaction, psychosocial and community integration. Brain Inj 31(5):655–666. https://doi.org/10.1080/02699052.2017.1290827

Cuthbert JP, Pretz CR, Bushnik T et al (2015) Ten-year employment patterns of working age individuals after moderate to severe traumatic brain injury: a national institute on disability and rehabilitation research traumatic brain injury model systems study. Arch Phys Med Rehabil 96(12):2128–2136. https://doi.org/10.1016/j.apmr.2015.07.020

Dawis RV (2005) The Minnesota theory of work adjustment. In: Brown S, Lent R (eds) Career development and counseling: putting theory and research to work. Wiley, Hoboken, pp 3–23

DiSanto D, Kumar RG, Juengst SB et al (2018) Employment stability in the first 5 years after moderate-to-severe traumatic brain injury. Arch Phys Med Rehabil 100(3):412–421. https://doi.org/10.1016/j.apmr.2018.06.022

Donker-Cools BH, Daams JG, Wind H et al (2016) Effective return-to-work interventions after acquired brain injury: a systematic review. Brain Inj 30(2):113–131. https://doi.org/10.3109/02699052.2015.1090014

Escorpizo R, Miller W, Trenaman L et al (2014) Work and employment following spinal cord injury. In: Eng JJ, Teasell R, Miller W et al (eds) Spinal cord injury rehabilitation evidence. Version 5.0., SCIRE Project, Vancouver. https://www.scireproject.com/rehabilitation-evidence/work-and-employment. Accessed 1 Oct 2019

Escorpizo R, Smith EM, Finger ME, Miller WC (2018) Work and employment following spinal cord injury. In: Eng JJ, Teasell RW, Miller WC, Wolfe DL, Townson AF, Hsieh JTC, Connolly SJ, Noonan VK, Loh E, McIntyre A, Sproule S, Queree M, Benton B (eds) Spinal cord injury rehabilitation evidence. Version 6.0. Vancouver: p 1–35

Fleuren BB, de Grip A, Jansen NW et al (2016) Critical reflections on the currently leading definition of sustainable employability. Scand J Work Environ Health 42(6):557–560. https://doi.org/10.5271/sjweh.3585

Grigorovich A, Stergiou-Kita M, Damianakis T et al (2017) Persons with brain injury and employment supports: long-term employment outcomes and use of community-based services. Brain Inj 31(5):607–619. https://doi.org/10.1080/02699052.2017.1280855

Hoefsmit N, Houkes I, Nijhuis FJ (2012) Intervention characteristics that facilitate return to work after sickness absence: a systematic literature review. J Occup Rehabil 22(4):462–477. https://doi.org/10.1007/s10926-012-9359-z

Iverson GL, Lange RT, Waljas M et al (2012) Outcome from complicated versus uncomplicated mild traumatic brain injury. Rehabil Res Pract 2012:415740. https://doi.org/10.1155/2012/415740

Jang Y, Wang Y, Wang J (2005) Return to work after spinal cord injury in Taiwan: the contribution of functional independence. Arch Phys Med Rehabil 86(4):681–686

Jetha A, Dumont FS, Noreau L et al (2014) A life course perspective to spinal cord injury and employment participation in Canada. Top Spinal Cord Inj Rehabil 20(4):310–320. https://doi.org/10.1310/sci2004-310

Jongbloed L, Backman C, Forwell SJ et al (2007) Employment after spinal cord injury: the impact of government policies in Canada. Work 29(2):145–154

Kramar R (2014) Beyond strategic human resource management: is sustainable human resource management the next approach? Int J Hum Resour Manag 25(8):1069–1089. https://doi.org/10.1080/09585192.2013.816863

Krause JS, Reed KS (2011) Barriers and facilitators to employment after spinal cord injury: underlying dimensions and their relationship to labor force participation. Spinal Cord 49(2):285–291. https://doi.org/10.1038/sc.2010.110

Libeson L, Downing M, Ross P et al (2018) The experience of return to work in individuals with traumatic brain injury (TBI): a qualitative study. Neuropsychol Rehabil:1–18. https://doi.org/10.1080/09602011.2018.1470987

Lidal IB, Huynh TK, Biering-Soerensen F (2007) Return to work following spinal cord injury: a review. Disabil Rehabil 29(17):1341–1375

Marini I, Lee GK, Chan F et al (2008) Vocational rehabilitation service patterns related to successful competitive employment outcomes of persons with spinal cord injury. J Vocat Rehabil 28(1):1–13

Marti A, Boes S, Lay V et al (2016) The association between chronological age, age at injury and employment: is there a mediating effect of secondary health conditions? Spinal Cord 54(3):239–244. https://doi.org/10.1038/sc.2015.159

Marti A, Escorpizo R, Schwegler U et al (2017) Employment pathways of individuals with spinal cord injury living in Switzerland: a qualitative study. Work 58(2):99–110. https://doi.org/10.3233/wor-172617

Meade MA, Reed KS, Saunders LL et al (2015) It's all of the above: benefits of working for individuals with spinal cord injury. Top Spinal Cord Inj Rehabil 21(1):1–9. https://doi.org/10.1310/sci2101-1

Meade MA, Reed KS, Krause JS (2016) The impact of health behaviors and health management on employment after SCI: physical health and functioning. Top Spinal Cord Inj Rehabil 22(1):39–48. https://doi.org/10.1310/sci2201-39

Nielsen K, Yarker J, Munir F et al (2018) IGLOO: an integrated framework for sustainable return to work in workers with common mental disorders. Work Stress 32(4):400–417. https://doi.org/10.1080/02678373.2018.1438536

Nützi M, Trezzini B, Medici L et al (2017) Job matching: an interdisciplinary scoping study with implications for vocational rehabilitation counseling. Rehabil Psychol 62(1):45–68. https://doi.org/10.1037/rep0000119

Nützi M, Schwegler U, Staubli S et al (2019) Factors, assessments and interventions related to job matching in the vocational rehabilitation of persons with spinal cord injury. Work 64(1):117–134. https://doi.org/10.3233/WOR-192975

Ottomanelli L, Barnett SD, Goetz LL (2013) A prospective examination of the impact of a supported employment program and employment on health-related quality of life, handicap, and disability among veterans with SCI. Qual Life Res 22(8):2133–2141. https://doi.org/10.1007/s11136-013-0353-5

Peeters W, van den Brande R, Polinder S et al (2015) Epidemiology of traumatic brain injury in Europe. Acta Neurochir 157(10):1683–1696. https://doi.org/10.1007/s00701-015-2512-7

Ponsford JL, Downing MG, Olver J et al (2014) Longitudinal follow-up of patients with traumatic brain injury: outcome at two, five, and ten years post-injury. J Neurotrauma 31(1):64–77. https://doi.org/10.1089/neu.2013.2997

Reinhardt JD, Post MW, Fekete C et al (2016) Labor market integration of people with disabilities: results from the Swiss spinal cord injury cohort study. PLoS One 11(11):e0166955. https://doi.org/10.1371/journal.pone.0166955

Roels E, Aertgeerts B, Ramaekers D et al (2016) Hospital-and community-based interventions enhancing (re) employment for people with spinal cord injury: a systematic review. Spinal Cord 54(1):2

Scaratti C, Leonardi M, Sattin D et al (2017) Work-related difficulties in patients with traumatic brain injury: a systematic review on predictors and associated factors. Disabil Rehabil 39(9):847–855. https://doi.org/10.3109/09638288.2016.1162854

Stocchetti N, Zanier ER (2016) Chronic impact of traumatic brain injury on outcome and quality of life: a narrative review. Crit Care 20(1):148. https://doi.org/10.1186/s13054-016-1318-1

Teasdale G, Maas A, Lecky F et al (2014) The Glasgow coma scale at 40 years: standing the test of time. Lancet Neurol 13(8):844–854. https://doi.org/10.1016/s1474-4422(14)70120-6

The Organisation for Economic Co-operation and Development (2010) Sickness, disability and work: breaking the barriers: a synthesis of findings across OECD countries. OECD, Paris.

https://read.oecd-ilibrary.org/social-issues-migration-health/sickness-disability-and-work-breaking-the-barriers_9789264088856-en#page8. Accessed 1 Oct 2019

The Organisation for Economic Co-operation and Development (2018) Good jobs for all in a changing world of work: the OECD job strategy. OECD Publishing, Paris. https://www.oecd-ilibrary.org/content/publication/9789264308817-en. Accessed 1 Oct 2019

van der Klink J, Bültmann U, Burdorf A et al (2016) Sustainable employability – definition, conceptualization, and implications: a perspective based on the capability approach. Scand J Work Environ Health 42(1):71–79

van Leeuwen CMC, Post MWM, van Asbeck FWA et al (2012) Life satisfaction in people with spinal cord injury during the first five years after discharge from inpatient rehabilitation. Disabil Rehabil 34(1):76–83. https://doi.org/10.3109/09638288.2011.587089

van Velzen JM, van Bennekom CA, Edelaar MJ et al (2009a) How many people return to work after acquired brain injury?: a systematic review. Brain Inj 23(6):473–488. https://doi.org/10.1080/02699050902970737

van Velzen JM, van Bennekom CA, Edelaar MJ et al (2009b) Prognostic factors of return to work after acquired brain injury: a systematic review. Brain Inj 23(5):385–395. https://doi.org/10.1080/02699050902838165

Vogel AP, Barker SJ, Young AE et al (2011) What is return to work? An investigation into the quantification of return to work. Int Arch Occup Environ Health 84(6):675–682. https://doi.org/10.1007/s00420-011-0644-5

Wilbanks SR, Ivankova NV (2015) Exploring factors facilitating adults with spinal cord injury rejoining the workforce: a pilot study. Disabil Rehabil 37(9):739–749. https://doi.org/10.3109/09638288.2014.938177

Young AE, Murphy GC (2009) Employment status after spinal cord injury (1992–2005): a review with implications for interpretation, evaluation, further research, and clinical practice. Int J Rehabil Res 32(1):1–11

Investing in Integrative Active Labour Market Policies

35

Finn Diderichsen

Contents

Introduction: Why Active Labour Market Policies Are Important 662
Policy Entry Points of Relevance for Employment of Those with Limited Workability 664
Labour Market Policies in Europe 665
The Tools of Active Labour Market Policies 667
Flexibility and Security in Labour Market Policies 669
Effect of ALMP on Employment 670
Effects on Employment of the Disabled 671
Effects on Income and Health 671
Cross-References 673
References 673

Abstract

This chapter explains why active labour market policies (ALMPs) are of increasing relevance in EU countries. It details the policy entry points in a model based on ICF. It describes the spending and different profiles of ALMP in European countries and recent developments toward more focus on activation and motivation and less focus on protection. ALMPs are aiming at both supply and demand of labour and at the matching between workplaces and employee workability. Labour market policies apply several tools to increase motivation, qualification, socialization, and networking. Tools that aim at combining different types of flexibility and security are described including "flexicurity." The literature on effects of ALMP on employment, income, and health is described shortly. The chapter shows that there might be room for policies to meet both economic and social objectives, but the challenge of ALMP is to enhance individual choice while at the same time maintaining adequate social protection, healthy workplaces, and incentives to work there.

F. Diderichsen (✉)
Department of Public Health, University of Copenhagen, Copenhagen, Denmark
e-mail: fidi@sund.ku.dk

© Springer Nature Switzerland AG 2020
U. Bültmann, J. Siegrist (eds.), *Handbook of Disability, Work and Health*, Handbook Series in Occupational Health Sciences, https://doi.org/10.1007/978-3-030-24334-0_34

Keywords

Active labour market policy · Protection · Activation · Integration · Health · Employment

Introduction: Why Active Labour Market Policies Are Important

Labour markets policy (LMP) is the public regulation of the labour market to ensure high employment rates, low unemployment, healthy and developing working conditions, ensure labour supply with relevant qualifications, and incentives to work for the unemployed.

There is in the OECD countries a broad political consensus about the purposes of LMP mentioned above, but the actual means to achieve them is subject to considerable controversy and varies strongly between countries and over time. One school argues that the labour markets primarily need a *supportive* policy that helps employers to find and afford the labour force with the qualifications they need. Another tradition fears that unregulated labour markets will produce high unemployment and inequalities, suggesting a *corrective* policy that aims at regulating work hours and environment, supports the unemployed economically, legislates against discrimination, etc. Labour market policies can be *passive* (PLMP), i.e., support those not working economically, and *active* (ALMP) in order to increase both supply and demand of labour and improve matching of individuals to available jobs (OECD 2010). National labour market policies create the environment in which clinical rehabilitation and employment services work and may strongly modify their effectiveness.

Labour market policies are needed since labour markets do not work very well if left to themselves. There are numerous market failures such as barriers for people to find and move between jobs; discrimination related to sex, race, and health; disincentives to take a work; etc. Hence few markets are so regulated as labour markets, and no country leaves the labour markets completely unregulated. Well-functioning labour markets are crucial for boosting economic growth, generating tax revenues, and limiting inequalities. But they are also – as we shall see – important for population health including the incidence and social consequences of ill-health. The last issue is about how people with ill-health and disabilities manage on the labour market.

> **Do Active Labour Markets Policies (ALMPs) Make a Difference?**
> In 1980–1995 first Britain and later Sweden were hit by economic crisis and high unemployment. Britain spent a small fraction on ALMP compared to Sweden and deregulated the labour market (including employment protection) during that period. Table 1 show employment rates in the working ages – 25–59 years. Employment rates are lower in Britain, and while their over times

(continued)

were only small reductions in employment in Sweden independently of health and education, Britain experienced a sharp decline – in particular among those with limiting illness and few qualifications. The table illustrates the importance of macroeconomic conditions and individual education and health as determinants of employment and how labour market policies can modify these associations.

Employment rates (employed in % of the population) in the age group 15–64 years have for the last 25 years on average been around 65% in the OECD countries. In addition, 5–10% (with large variations between countries and periods) are economically active but unemployed and job seeking. This means that 25–30% are inactive on the labour market. With the prospect of an aging population with growing needs for pensions, care, etc., there has been an increasingly strong focus on active labour market policies to increase the employment rates (OECD 2010). But not all of the 25–30% inactive are able to take a job and comply with the demands of modern labour markets. 4–10% of the population in OECD countries are on disability benefits with large variations across nations. That proportion has slowly been increasing over the years in many countries. That is surprising since many indicators of the overall health development show positive trends in these countries. Surveys indicate that 15% of the working age population report disability, i.e., chronic health problems with activity limitations. That prevalence has not changed much, and the same is true for the proportion reporting no good self-rated health. The prevalence of self-reported disability, however, shows remarkable international variations from 5% in Korea and 20% in Denmark (OECD 2010). Many factors may influence these numbers. The exact meaning of disability in different languages might be different, and countries with more generous definition of disability in the eligibility criteria for disability benefits might make more people report disability. The growing prevalence of people on disability benefits might be influenced by growing work demands related to globalization, increased productivity, constant restructuring and reorganization, etc. An additional problem is that 40% of the disabled have very short

Table 1 Employment rates (%) among men in Britain and Sweden 1979–1995. (Source: Burström et al. 2000)

Men aged 25–59% employed		Britain		Sweden	
		1978–1985	1989–1995	1979–1985	1989–1995
Professional/ managerial	Limiting illness	88	79	92	89
	No lim. illness	96	94	99	97
Unskilled manual	Limiting illness	56	43	82	78
	No lim. illness	83	80	98	95

education (less than upper secondary school education), a proportion that is increasing over time, in particular for the younger age groups. The association between education, employment, and health is gradually becoming stronger which is a challenge for the active labour market policies that aim at increasing employment by improving education and health (Diderichsen 2016).

Many European countries are experiencing demographic changes with declining numbers of people in working ages and are facing a pressure to limit the number of economically inactive. Since definitions of disabilities are vague and modifiable by the context in terms of labour demands and disability policies including eligibility criteria, labour market policies try to strike a balance between securing the social protection of the disabled and making employment possible and attractive for more people. It has for some years now been argued by OECD (OECD 2010) and others that there is a substantial scope for bringing people currently in the inactive groups including the sick and disabled, lone parents, elderly, and other not categorized groups into employment. There might thus be room for policies to meet both economic and social objectives. Indeed, part of the challenge is to enhance individual choice while at the same time maintaining adequate social protection, healthy workplaces, and incentives to work there.

Policy Entry Points of Relevance for Employment of Those with Limited Workability

Labour market policies apply many tools that are working at different steps in a process from a disorder to disability. Figure 1 illustrates a process based on WHO's ICF model of disability (WHO 2001; Vornholt et al. 2018). ICF is a theoretical framework defining disability as a relationship between functions, activities, participation, and the interacting environmental and individual factors. Diseases, injuries, and aging might impair mental and somatic structure and *functions*. This might lead to limitations in basic *activities* (such as mobility, communication, memory, etc.). Depending on the context, i.e., the prevailing labour market, work demands, etc., some of these functional limitations will influence the ability to comply with work demands. *Workability* is this interaction between function and work demands (van den van den Berg et al. 2009). Workability is also influenced by *qualifications*, skills, and social competences and to what extent they correspond to the demands of the labour market. People with full or some workability congruent with existing jobs might still have difficulties in finding a job (*participation*) on the labour market due to lack of jobs (low *supply*), lack of networks or ability to find the right work that matches their workability, as well as lack of *motivation* and incentives to work. Job demands might be *flexible* with a potential to be adapted to individual abilities. Finally, depending on coverage and levels of benefits for the unemployed and disabled, the lack of employment might lead to *social exclusion* and poverty.

The key issue of the ICF model is that disability is created by an *interaction* between capacity to perform activities and the environmental and individual context. This approach attempts to directly assess disability as the interaction between

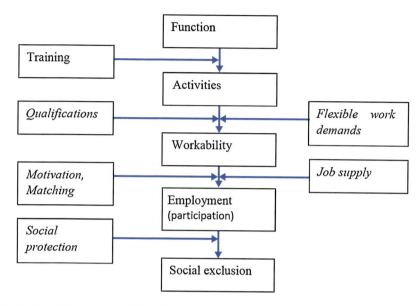

Fig. 1 The ICF concepts of disability (function, activities, and participation) expanded with relevant individual and contextual factors to be modified with labour market policies

medical, functional, environmental, and personal factors, rather than indirectly infer disability from a proxy of impairment or functional capacity assessments. In reality this is not easy, and, in many countries, there has in practice been a tendency to choose the more indirect approach and often gradually make the medical criteria more strict, without considering the changing work demands (see section "Effects on Employment of the Disabled").

The tools of the active labour market policies aim at influencing five of the *modifying factors* in Fig. 1: qualifications, work demands, motivation, matching, and job supply (see section "The Tools of Active Labour Market Policies").

Labour Market Policies in Europe

Labour market policies were originally not created primarily to increase employment among people with disabilities. When the first labour market policies were formulated in the 1940s by two Swedish economists Rehn and Meidner, they were together with wage policy, an integrated part of welfare state policies, that aimed at combining economic growth on a competitive global market with reduced inequalities, low inflation, and high employment (Erixon 2010). The purpose was not primarily to keep unemployment down, since it was already very low in postwar Sweden (1–3%). The model was created to promote structural transformation of Swedish industry and society in the 1960s–1970s and was a way of creating better well-paid jobs. The policy implied what has been called "creative destruction" by favoring productive companies that could keep up with wage rises and send those who could not out on the global market, i.e., to low-income countries. However, the model also promoted "security of the wings," by investing in active labour market policies, where the dismissed obtained possibilities to reskill and the generous unemployment benefits made transitions to the evolving new jobs less risky.

Labour market policies have changed a lot since then. Political changes have left the Rehn-Meidner model less relevant today, but the integration of labour markets policies into a broader range of welfare policies areas dealing with education, social protection, and health (rehabilitation) is more relevant than ever. As part of a general tendency to make the welfare state a "social investment state" that is more preparing than repairing, labour market policies have become more a question of activation than protection and with education still a central component (Morel et al. 2012).

Table 2 shows the spending on active and passive labour market policies in some European countries 1996–2016. In the mid-1990s, unemployment was high in many countries, and spending on labour markets policy, both active and passive were accordingly quite high – 1 to 5% of GDP. The Nordic countries were high spenders and the UK as an outlier with very low spending. As we saw in Table 1, this was associated with particularly low employment rates among the workforce with limited qualifications and health in the UK. The international pattern of LMP spending was changed 20 years later, and in particular spending on passive measures has been cut back substantially in Denmark, Finland, Germany, the Netherlands, and Sweden. The Nordic countries are still spending relatively more on active measures even today.

The amount of money spent on labour market policies however only provides a very simplified picture of cross-national differences. A more detailed analysis of the variations distinguishes three different dimensions of labour market policies for disabled (Tschanz and Staub 2017). The social *protection* dimension includes universality of entitlements, required work incapacity for eligibility, coverage,

Table 2 Public spending (% of GDP) on active labour market policy (LMP) including training, incentives, subsidies, and passive labour market policy including unemployment benefits and early retirement pension

	Active LMP		Passive LMP	
	1996	2016[a]	1996	2016[a]
Denmark	1.51	1.66	3.84	1.15
Finland	1.32	0.85	3.49	1.85
France	1.04	0.76	1.49	1.98
Germany	1.05	0.26	2.40	0.82
Italy	0.33	0.42	0.92	1.29
Netherlands	0.77	0.49	3.08	1.68
Sweden	1.79	0.90	1.94	0.55
UK	0.09	0.03	0.62	0.31

Sources: OECD (2018)
[a]UK:2011; France & Italy:2015

levels, and duration of benefits. The dimension of labour market *integration* is based in the existence of subsidized or sheltered employment, employers' obligations, vocational rehabilitation, and work incentives. The third dimension of *civil rights* is based on anti-discrimination laws, equality laws, building codes, and regulations with regard to public transport and communication. An empirical analysis with data from around 2007 shows that one cluster consist of the Southern European catholic countries characterized by high levels of protection, low levels of integration, and moderate levels of civil rights. The second cluster consists of mostly Eastern European countries with moderate levels of protection and integration and few civil rights. The third cluster of central European countries has little social protection, high level of activation, and average levels of rights. The fourth cluster consists of the Nordic countries and Germany with high levels of both protection, integration, and rights.

The Tools of Active Labour Market Policies

Active labour market policies include many different strategies (see Table 3). It can be oriented toward both the employed and unemployed workforce to improve the *supply* of qualified labour through counselling, education, retraining, and subsidized mobility. It can also be oriented toward the employers in order to create a stronger *demand* for labour. That can be achieved through committing employers to more social responsibility, use of quotas and certifications, and legislation against discrimination that oblige to employ at last some people that are less in demand, such as immigrants and disabled. It may finally be oriented to achieve a better matching through employment services, job training, adult apprentice arrangements, and subsidized flex-jobs where demands are matching the workability of the employee. General workplace regulation of the work environment is also a way of ensuring workplaces where even people with limited workability can work (Muntaner et al. 2010).

The passive labour market tools are primarily there to ensure decent material living conditions of those without jobs and to protect them from poverty and social exclusion. The main types of benefits are unemployment benefits, early retirement pensions, sickness benefits, and disability pensions. For those with no access or who are not qualifying to any of these, most countries have a system of low-level means tested welfare benefits. Changing the coverage, benefit levels, and eligibility criteria has often been used in order to increase labour supply and motivation. This has been shown to have strong effects not only on the numbers of welfare recipients but also on their living conditions (Jensen et al. 2019) (see section "Effects on Income and Health").

Since the late 1990s, strategies focusing on motivation have been a dominating element in ALMP. Increasing demands on the unemployed for searching and accepting the jobs available, reducing benefit levels, and shortening length of benefits are all regulations put in place to provide incentives for people to accept the available jobs. Benefits can be withdrawn if people do not participate in

Table 3 Purposes, strategies, actions, and target groups for different elements of general labour market policies. (Modified after Bredgaard et al. 2017)

Labour market policy					
	Passive	Active			
Strategy	Economic support	Motivation	Qualification	Socialization	Network creation
Problem	Lack of income	Lack of incentives and motivation	Lack of professional qualifications	Lack of social competences	Lack a relevant network
Action examples	Unemployment benefits, early retirement and disability pension	Reduced benefits, demands of job-seeking and acceptance	Education, retraining, skills upgrading	Counselling, employment projects	Job training, wage subsidies mentors
Target groups	Citizens without self-support	Labour market ready on benefits	Unskilled, or with outdated skills	Not labour market ready on benefits	Long-term unemployed, immigrants
Purpose	Improve material living condition	Quick return to work	Improved employability	Improved workability	Create employer contact, reduce stigmatization

activation programs or retraining. Using these economic incentives has turned out to be effective (see section "Effect of ALMP on Employment") but is not without complications in relation to health. Unemployment increases, for example, the risk of depression (Kim and von dem Knesebeck 2016), which reduces motivation and activity. If unemployment then through these incentives is combined with economic stress, the health effect might be stronger and motivation even lower.

The strategy of qualification has been part of ALMP since the 1960s in most countries and is based on the assumption that education, skills, and competences are constantly changing and unemployed might need to update their skills to be able to comply with new jobs or to compensate for reduced workability due to illness. Retraining, programs for lifelong learning, and skills upgrading are tools in this strategy. The effectiveness of this strategy is more controversial. Macroeconomic studies seem to confirm a positive effect on employment, while many microeconomic evaluations have not been able to confirm an improved employability (Martin 2015; Card et al. 2018).

The strategy of socialization is built on the assumption that lack of social competences is an obstacle for some people. The strategy is typically the most relevant for people with mental disorders, addiction, criminality, and other social problems that have excluded them from participating in the labour markets for long periods and made them unfamiliar with working life. Young people who have been unemployed since school is another target group. The aim is often set to be a long-term improvement of workability and quality of life.

The networking strategy is a way to establish networks that provide employers with trustworthy information about skills among groups they have little experience from hiring and knowledge about – such as immigrants and refugees. The tools might be to create subsidized jobs, positions as trainees, etc., and this strategy has turned out to be quite effective.

Flexibility and Security in Labour Market Policies

An important aspect of labour market policies is the combination of security and flexibility. There are however different dimensions of both security and flexibility, and different LMP tools may promote different combinations of these dimensions (see Table 4). Income security is primarily ensured by passive labour market policies with income support during unemployment and disability. Employment security is primarily achieved by shortening the periods until an unemployed finds another job. Subsidized jobs and jobs with flexible demands are another way of securing employment even when workability is changing. Labour education is another way of ensuring employment when new skills are demanded. Job security is a question of whether people can stay in a certain type of job even when labour demands are declining or the specific job type demands new skills. Family/job security is a question to what extent family formation and childbirth influence security or whether legislation or agreements make it possible to have flexible work hours and whether they protect (paid) maternity leave and return to work later.

"Flexicurity" is a combination of three labour market conditions most famously existing in Denmark but found with different variations in other countries. It combines (1) a high level of *numerical flexibility*, i.e., low level of job security where it is easy to be fired and hired; (2) a high level of *income security* due to

Table 4 Policies to ensure combinations of flexibility and security. (Modified after Bredgaard et al. 2017)

	Job security	Income security	Employment security	Family/job security
Numerical flexibility	Shared workforce pools for employers	Economic compensation when unemployed	Active LMP	Maternity leave
Functional flexibility	Internal retraining	Job rotation	Labour education, lifelong learning	Flexible work demands and workplaces
Work hour flexibility	Employment service	Supplementary benefits	Combination jobs	Flexible work hours
Wage flexibility	Wage reduction in periods of crisis	Degree of income compensation	Subsidized jobs, flex-jobs	Payment during maternity leave

generous universal benefit systems; and (3) a high level of *employment security* due to active labour markets policies including retraining and lifelong learning. It has been praised for bringing Denmark relatively safe through the 2008 crisis and its ability to keep youth unemployment low when other countries could not. It is not primarily helpful for people with a weak position on the labour markets, i.e., unskilled or people with disabilities, and recent comparative studies on employment levels among these groups indicate that a Swedish model with higher job security is more effective in terms of ensuring high employment among people with short education and ill-health (McAllister et al. 2015).

Recent years have seen reductions in the security dimension in Denmark and other countries. Shortening of the allowed benefit periods of unemployment insurance has, for example, a shortening effect on length of unemployment periods with a faster return to work (Svarer 2015). The same happens when allowed length of sickness insurance periods is shortened. Recently some countries have changed eligibility criteria for disability pension to much stronger medical criteria of impairment and function (far from the disability view discussed in section "Policy Entry Points of Relevance for Employment of Those with Limited Workability"). These reforms have strong effects on the number of people with the different types of benefit but might also push people from one type of benefit to another or out in poverty (Waddington et al. 2016; Jensen et al. 2019)

Effect of ALMP on Employment

There have been made numerous reviews on effectiveness of active labour market policies (Martin 2015; Card et al. 2018). They include both microeconomic evaluations of specific programs and macroeconomic cross-country studies. In addition, OECD has done several reviews of single countries (OECD 2010).

The systematic reviews made on microeconomic evaluations seem overall to conclude that job search assistance and monitoring of the behavior of jobseekers tend to be effective particularly for women and disadvantaged. Some training programs, especially those tied to local labour market needs and private employers, are also effective particularly for the long-term unemployed. Targeted hiring subsidies can also work, while public sector job creation or subsidies do not work and are often found to have negative effects on later employment. In general, the effectiveness is better in the long run of several years than within few years (Card et al. 2018).

Macroeconomic studies show that activation regimes differ greatly in their scope and intensity across countries reflecting their different starting points, policy environments, and institutional cultures. They all involve different combinations of job search monitoring, benefit conditionality, and referral to activation programs. The overall conclusion is that activation regimes have proven effective to get recipients on unemployment benefits back into employment but have also worked for recipients of sole-parent benefits by providing affordable child care. The results are however much less encouraging for recipients of other benefits such as sickness and disability benefits (Martin 2015). That indicates a much lower effect among people with ill-health.

Effects on Employment of the Disabled

The question is then what we know about activation and return-to-work policies in relation to people with disabilities. Recent reviews (Sabariego et al. 2018; Vogel et al. 2017; Scharle and Csillag 2016) including large-scale trials with very strong designs mostly from Scandinavian countries (Rehwald et al. 2017; Poulsen et al. 2014) indicate that efforts to implement multidisciplinary coordinated interventions for long-term sick listed are not very effective, but graded return is. The use of partial sick leave increases the length of time spent in regular employment and also reduces the time spent in unemployment and in early retirement. Traditional active labour market programs and the use of physical therapy and training to reduce the effect of impaired functioning (see Fig. 1) appear to have no effect at all, or even adverse effects. But it might depend on local and national context and in a context where both generous benefits and ALMP coexist the chance of returning to work is higher (Sabariego et al. 2018).

Activation policies originally designed for unemployed have increasingly been used for people with disabilities who have partially reduced workability. This broader implementation of activation policies implies a change of the balance between rights and duties for the population and the state. The introduction of ALMP originally meant that the *state* should be more active and take a larger responsibility in procuring for citizens. The more recent focus on the individual ability to work (through prevention, rehabilitation, retraining, etc.) means that the responsibility to be employable now increasingly rests on the citizen. It is a shift in emphasis where the term "active" used to refer to actions taken by the state and now refers to actions taken by the citizen. In brief, the state now "activates instead of being active" (Hultqvist and Nørup 2017). Little knowledge exists so far regarding the effects and consequences of activation policies targeting these groups of disabled – a group that has previously been considered unable to take up ordinary work within European welfare states.

Some studies indicate that sanctioning recipients as an incentive to employment has a problematic effect on the disabled. It may push them away from employment benefits into low means-tested welfare benefits or inactivity and not into reemployment (Reves 2017; Andersen et al. 2016).

Effects on Income and Health

Reviews of existing evidence suggest that participation in ALMP programs, specifically government training programs, can have a positive effect on the well-being (psychological health) of the participants compared to those who remain unemployed or economically inactive. ALMPs can therefore have effect on well-being and health indirectly through their positive effect on employment chances but also directly by participation in programs and activation prior to the labour market entry (Vuori and Silvonen 2005; Sage 2013; Coutts et al. 2014). These reviews find reduced risk of depression, improved self-efficacy, social support, and motivation as a result of ALMP.

European surveys show that people with disability have a risk of poverty around 30% on average for EU countries, while those without disability have a risk of 21%, i.e., an excess risk of 9%. That difference has not changed much the last 10 years in most EU countries, but in Sweden and Germany where the cuts both in labour market spending and also in sickness benefits were particularly strong (see Table 2), the excess risk of poverty among the disabled compared to the non-disabled has increased – from 7% to 17.0% in Sweden and from 9% to 16% in Germany.

Even if evaluation of specific ALMP programs and interventions have shown positive health effects, cross-national macro-studies have not reproduced similar results, i.e., that countries with more ALMP spending should have smaller effects of unemployment on health. Studies have however shown that generous unemployment benefits can buffer the negative effects of unemployment on well-being and self-rated health (O'Campo et al. 2015; Voßemer et al. 2018), while policy effects among those working in insecure jobs is less clear. These studies seem to indicate that the negative effect of unemployment is weaker in countries with a stricter protection of labour market insiders with a more secure employment. Deregulation at the margins of the labour market might therefore increase the inequality between insiders and outsiders at the labour market.

Stuckler et al. analyzed the relation between per capita spending on ALMPs and suicide rates over different economic cycles. Countries with very low per capita expenditure on ALMP showed a strong tie between economic decline and rising suicide rates, while countries with high per capita spending showed no correlation (Stuckler et al. 2009).

It is however important to keep in mind that these effects of ALMP might be very heterogenous across different groups. Little is however known about the effects in different socioeconomic groups, and some studies indicate that the effects on people with extensive health problems and disabilities might be negative. A study from England illustrates how bad the effects of a more extreme version of activation can be: Many countries including the Scandinavian, UK, and Netherlands have introduced more stringent functional assessment for eligibility to disability benefits. Most countries have applied the new criteria to new benefit claimants, but the UK and Netherlands have gone further – reassessing all existing person with disability benefits. Barr et al. (2016) have evaluated population health effects of this activation policy and found a strong dose-response relationship between the number of disability reassessments per capita in a local community and reported cases of mental disorders including rising suicide rates and use of antidepressant drugs.

Cross-References

▶ Policies of Reducing the Burden of Occupational Hazards and Disability Pensions
▶ Reducing Inequalities in Employment of People with Disabilities
▶ The Changing Nature of Work and Employment in Developed Countries

References

Andersen I, Brønnum-Hansen H, Kriegbaum M et al. (2016) Increasing illness among people out of labor market – A Danish register-based study. Soc Sci Med 156:21–8. https://doi.org/10.1016/j.socscimed.2016.03.003

Barr B, Taylor-Robinson D, Stuckler D et al (2016) 'First, do no harm': are disability assessments associated with adverse trends in mental health? A longitudinal ecological study. J Epidemiol Community Health 70:339–345. https://doi.org/10.1136/jech-2015-206209

Bredgaard T, Jørgensen H, Madsen PK, Rasmussen S (2017) Dansk Arbejdsmarkedspolitik. 2. udgave. Jurist- og Økonomforbundets Forlag, København

Burström B, Whitehead M, Lindholm C, Diderichsen F (2000) Inequality in the social consequences of illness. Int J Health Serv 30(3):435–451. https://doi.org/10.2190/6PP1-TDEQ-H44D-4LJQ

Card D, Klive J, Weber A (2018) What works? A meta-analysis of recent active labour market policies. J Eur Econ Assoc 16(3):894–931. https://doi.org/10.1093/jeea/jvx028

Coutts AP, Stuckler D, Cann DJ (2014) The health and wellbeing effects of active labor market programs, Chapter 13. In: Cooper CL (ed) Wellbeing, vol 6. Wiley, Chichester, pp 465–482. https://doi.org/10.1002/9781118539415.wbwell048

Diderichsen F (2016) Health inequalities – a challenge for the social investment welfare state. Nordic Welfare Res 1(1):43–54. https://doi.org/10.18261/ISSN.2464-4161-2016-01-05

Erixon L (2010) The Rehn-Meidner model in Sweden: its rise, challenges and survival. J Econ Issues 44(3):677–715. https://doi.org/10.2753/JEI0021-3624440306

Hultqvist S, Nørup I (2017) Consequences of activation policy targeting young adults with health-related problems in Sweden and Denmark. J Poverty Soc Justice 25(2):147–161. https://doi.org/10.1332/175982717X14940647262909

Jensen NK, Brønnum-Hansen H, Andersen I et al (2019) Too sick to work – too healthy to qualify. J Epidemiol Community Health 73(8):717–722. https://doi.org/10.1136/jech-2019-212191

Kim TJ, von dem Knesebeck O (2016) Perceived job insecurity, unemployment and depressive symptoms: a systematic review and meta-analysis of prospective observational studies. Int Arch Occup Environ Health 89(4):561–573. https://doi.org/10.1007/s00420-015-1107-1

Martin JP (2015) Activation and active labour market policies in OECD countries: stylised facts and evidence on their effectiveness. IZA J Labor Policy 4:4. https://doi.org/10.1186/s40173-015-0032-y

McAllister A, Nylén L, Backhaus M et al (2015) Do 'flexicurity' policies work for people with low education and health problems? Int J Health Serv 45(4):679–705. https://doi.org/10.1177/0020731415600408

Morel N, Palier B, Palme J (eds) (2012) Towards a social investment welfare state? Ideas, policies and challenges. The Policy Press, Bristol

Muntaner C, Benach J, Chung H et al (2010) Welfare state, labour market inequalities and health. In a global context: an integrated framework. Gac Sanit 24(Suppl 1):56–61. https://doi.org/10.1016/j.gaceta.2010.09.013

O'Campo P, Molnar A, Ng E et al (2015) Social welfare matters: a realist review of when, how, and why unemployment insurance impacts poverty and health. Soc Sci Med 132:88–95. https://doi.org/10.1016/j.socscimed.2015.03.025

OECD (2010) Sickness, disability and work: breaking the barriers. A synthesis of findings across OECD countries. OECD, Paris. www.oecd.org/publications/sickness-disability-and-work-breaking-the-barriers-9789264088856-en.htm

OECD (2018) Public spending on labour markets (indicator). https://doi.org/10.1787/911b8753-en. Accessed 5 Nov 2018

Poulsen OM, Aust B, Bjørner JB et al (2014) Effect of the Danish return-to-work program on long-term sickness absence: results from a randomized controlled trial in three municipalities. Scand J Work Environ Health 40(1):47–56. https://doi.org/10.5271/sjweh.3383

Reves A (2017) Does sanctioning disabled claimants of unemployment insurance increase labour market inactivity? An analysis of 346 British local authorities between 2009 and 2014. J Poverty & Social Justice 25(2):129–46. https://doi.org/10.1332/175982717X14939739331029

Rehwald K, Rosholm M, Svarer M (2017) Do public or private providers of employment services matter for employment? Evidence from a randomized experiment. Labour Econ 45:169–187. https://doi.org/10.1016/j.labeco.2016.11.005

Sabariego C, Coene M, Ito E et al (2018) Effectiveness of integration and re-integration into work strategies for persons with chronic conditions: a systematic review of European strategies. Int J Environ Res Public Health 15(3):552. https://doi.org/10.3390/ijerph15030552

Sage D (2013) Activation, health and well-being: neglected dimensions? Int J Sociol Soc Policy 33(1/2):4–20. https://doi.org/10.1108/01443331311295145

Scharle Á, Csillag M (2016) Disability and labour market integration. European Commission. https://doi.org/10.2767/26386

Stuckler D, Basu S, Suhrcke M, Coutts A, McKee M (2009) The public health effect of economic crises and alternative policy responses in Europe: an empirical analysis. Lancet 374:315–323. https://doi.org/10.1016/S0140-6736(09)61124-7

Svarer M (2015) Labour market policies in Denmark. In: Andersen TM, Bergman UM, SEH J (eds) Reform capacity and macroeconomic performance in the Nordic countries. OUP, Oxford

Tschanz C, Staub I (2017) Disability-policy models in European welfare regimes: comparing the distribution of social protection, labour-market integration and civil rights. Disabil Soc 32(8):1199–1215. https://doi.org/10.1080/09687599.2017.1344826

van den Berg TIJ, Elders LAM, de Zwart BCH, Burdorf A (2009) The effects of work-related and individual factors on the work ability index: a systematic review. Occup Environ Med 66(4):211e220. https://doi.org/10.1136/oem.2008.039883

Vogel N, Schandelmaier S, Zumbrunn T et al (2017) Return-to-work coordination programmes for improving return to work in workers on sick leave. Cochrane Database Syst Rev 30(3). https://doi.org/10.1002/14651858.CD011618.pub2

Vornholt K, Villotti P, Muschalla B et al (2018) Disability and employment – overview and highlights. Eur J Work Organ Psy 27(1):40–55. https://doi.org/10.1080/1359432X.2017.1387536

Voßemer J, Gebel M, Täht K et al (2018) The effects of unemployment and insecure jobs on well-being and health: the moderating role of labor market policies. Soc Indic Res 138(3):1229–1257. https://doi.org/10.1007/s11205-017-1697-y

Vuori J, Silvonen J (2005) The benefits of a preventive job search program on re-employment and mental health at 2-year follow-up. J Occup Organ Psychol 78(1):43–52. https://doi.org/10.1348/096317904X23790

Waddington L, Pedersen M, Liisberg MV (2016) Get a Job! active labour market policies and persons with disabilities in Danish and European Union Policy. Dublin Univ Law J 39(1):1–8. https://ssrn.com/abstract=2833790

WHO (2001) International classification of functioning, disability and health (ICF). World Health Organization, Geneva. https://www.who.int/classifications/icf/en/

Index

A

Ability, motivation and opportunity (AMO) model, 623
Absenteeism, 159, 253, 259, 261, 263, 266, 510
Abstinence, 518, 519
Accessibility, 334
　of workplaces, 316
Accident prevention, 107
Accommodation, 335
Acquired brain injury (ABI), 12, 634, 635
　contextual level, 655
　degrees of expression, 640
　employment and RTW rates, 641, 642
　group level, 652, 655
　individual level, 647, 654
　leader level, 652, 655
　RTW, 642, 643
　societal level, 652
　structured multidisciplinary rehabilitation, 640
　sustained employment, 643, 644, 647–654
　traumatic/non-traumatic aetiology, 640
Activation policies, 378, 379, 671
Activation strategies, 310
Active labor market policies (ALMPs), 13, 29–30, 94, 310, 662
　effect on employment, 670–671
　effect on income and health, 671–672
　employment rates, 663
　tools of, 665, 667–669
Activities of daily living (ADL), 57–60
Activity limitations, 59
Activity requirements, 93
Addictive disorders
　acute treatment, 516
　brief interventions, 515, 516
　detection, 507, 508
　diagnosis, 506, 507
　epidemiologic data, 509–510
　post-acute treatment, 516–520
　risk factors, 510, 511
　unemployment, 506
　working life, 506
　workplace interventions, 511–514
Adverse working conditions, 62
Affective disorders
　definition and diagnosis, 209–210
　etiology, 213–216
　prevalence, 211–213
　psycho-physiological mechanism, 214
Age-related functional decline, 56
Aging, 386, 496–498
Agriculture, 113
Airflow obstruction, 158
Alcohol at-risk drinking, 506
Alcohol intoxication, 511
Alcohol use disorder(s), 509
Alcohol Use Disorder Identification Test (AUDIT), 508, 509, 512
Allergic rhinitis, 160
Alzheimer's disease (AD), 640
　cognitive decline, 236
　cognitive reserve, 238
　longitudinal studies, 238
　prevalence, 236
Americans with Disabilities Act (ADA), 378
Anti-discrimination laws, 96
Anti-discrimination legislation, 94, 96
Anti-stigma interventions, 296
Anxiety, 211, 228, 440
Asbestos, 143–144
Asthma, 156–157
At-work functioning, 628
Autism spectrum disorders, 583

B

Back pain, 484, 496
Barriers to employment and coping efficacy scale (BECES), 542
Behavioral motivation, 542–543
Benefit conditionalities, 98
Benefit suspension, 94
Biomechanical exposures, 173
Biomedical model of disability, 93
Bio-psychosocial model, 510
Borderline personality disorder, 581
Brief interventions, 515, 516
Bullying, 255
    prevention, 293
Burden of disability, 60
Burden of injuries, 107–111
Burnout, 260
Business organizations, 267
Byssinosis, 41

C

Cadmium and cadmium compounds, 144
Cancer
    attributable fraction, 147–148
    employment, 403–410
    epidemiology, 130
    etiology, 129
    occupational cancer research, 148–149
    occupational chemical and lung cancer, 130
    occupational epidemiology, 148
    population attributable fraction, 147
    return to work, 403–411
    risks among female workers, 146
    survivorship and burden of health, 400–402
Cancer survivorship
    informal costs, 400
    life expectancy, 400
    mental comorbidity, 401
    middle and long-term survival, 401
    occupational aspects, 403
    physical and psychosocial consequences, 400
    research, 401
    and work model, 404
Cannabis Use Disorder Identification Test, 508
Capability approach, 387
Carbohydrate-deficient transferrin (CDT), 508, 512
Carcinogenesis, mechanisms of, 132
Carcinogenicity
    animal experimentation, 131–132
    high risk group, 141

Cardiac rehabilitation (CR)
    checklists, 444
    chemical and physical hazards, 438
    effectiveness, 432
    expert knowledge, 434
    gradual RTW during, 442
    job demands, 437
    job strain, 437
    lack of support, 438
    left ventricular ejection factor, 435
    multidisciplinary guideline, 433
    negative perceptions, 441
    occupational physician, 443
    privacy laws, 443
    psychological screening instruments, 434
    reduced heart function, 435
    re-integration plan, 441
    risk stratification, 442
    RTW interventions, cardiac patients, 441
    unhealthy lifestyle, 439
    vulnerable social-demographic status, 439
Cardiovascular diseases, 63
Carpal tunnel syndrome, 179
Causation hypothesis, 76
    working career impact after retirement, 79–80
    working life course perspective, 77–79
Cervical radiculopathy, 180
Chemical job exposure, 194
Chronic diseases, 74, 386
Chronic disorders, 6
Chronic illness
    integration of people with, 349
    workers with, 353
Chronic lung allograft dysfunction, 164
Chronic obstructive pulmonary disease (COPD), 158–159
Chronic pain, 584
Citizen, 671
Civil rights, 667
Cochrane review, 527
Cognition
    CONSTANCES cohort, 246–247
    educational attainment, 244
    lifetime exposure to solvents, 245
    neuropsychological exams, 245
    occupational complexity, 239
    in retirement, 245
    social health inequalities, 246
    solvent exposure on, 244
Cognitive behavioral therapy, 457
Cognitive decline, *see* Alzheimer's disease (AD)

Cognitive function, job strain and, 240
Cognitive reserve (CR), 238
Common mental disorders, 468
  barriers and opportunities of return to work, 471–477
  compensation system and societal perspective, 476–477
  healthcare perspective, 474–475
  individual perspective, 471–474
  workplace perspective, 475–476
Community based rehabilitation program, 635
Community reinforcement program, 519
Companies, 7
Compensation systems, 476
Competitive employment, 573
Competitive job, 544
Concept of work, 367
Confirmatory factor analysis, 58
Conflicts, 620
Conservation of resources (COR) theory, 617
Constructive pressure principle, 515
Consultation, 278
Contextual conditions, 371
Contingent employment, 376
Continuous positive airway pressure, 162
Continuous vocational education and training, 27
Convention on the Rights of Persons with Disabilities (CRPD), 333
  Article 27, 336–339
Coping strategies, 619
Core human competences, 20
Coronary bypass graft surgery (CABG), 432
Coronary heart disease, 10, 433
Costs
  of absenteeism and presenteeism, 261
  burden of, 256
  disability, 254
  health care, 252
  to workers, 261
  work-related disability, 257
Cumulative disadvantage model, 64, 65
Cystic fibrosis, 161

D

Demand-and supply side factors, 372
Demand for labor, 667
Demand-side approach, 94, 98
Dementia
  burden of, 236
  cause of, 236
  cognitive decline and, 236
  incidence, 236
  mental and physical stimulation, 239
  occupation vs., 238
  risk of AD and, 241
  social criteria of, 236
  socioeconomic burden of, 236
Depression, 668, 672
  prevention, 294
  symptoms, 440
Depressive disorders
  effort-reward imbalance and job insecurity, 221
  in epidemiological studies, 218
  future studies, 225–230
  genetic risk factors and gene-environment interaction, 215
  job strain and control, 221
  long working hours, 222
  magnitude of estimates in psychosocial work environment studies, 222
  monoamine hypothesis, 213
  psychological and sociological theories, 214
  publication bias, 222
  self-report of working condition, 223
  study design considerations, 217–218
  workplace bullying, 222
Developing countries, 35
  informal work, 46–48
  labor force, 35–37
  structural transformation (see Structural transformation)
  unemployment rates, 37
Directive 2000/78/EC, 277
Disability, 3, 7, 664
  active national labor and social policy, 66
  benefits, 310, 553
  bodily functions and structures, 64
  costs of, 262
  definition, 256
  discrimination, 315
  employment gap, 88, 325
  extended perspective of functioning, 64
  human activities, 64
  human functioning, 54
  improving the work ability, 67
  incidence of, 59
  less-privileged occupational groups, 66
  minority/universal perspective, 55–56
  models of good practice, 65
  monitoring of health-damaging working conditions, 65
  national regulations, 65
  opportunity of change, 65

Disability (cont.)
  payments, 257
  policy implications, 65
  prevention, 624
  rapidly aging societies, 55
  reducing the burden of disability, 67
  retirement, 63, 556
  societies, 54
  work ability and, 552
  working-age populations, 56–65
Disability adjusted life years (DALY), 110, 252, 509
Disability benefits, 90, 97, 530–531
  adequacy of, 312
Disability Discrimination Act, 529
Disability pension (DP), 56, 61–63
Disability policy, 87
  compensation/integration, 87, 93–94
  labor force participation, 88–90
  poverty, 87–88
  prevention, 87, 92
  social regulation, 87, 94–95
Disability Services Act, 530
Disabled employees, 655
Disabled people, education, training and work placements for, 320
Discrimination, 94, 337, 378, 379
Disease-specific factors, 393
Disincentives to work, 322
Double burden, 66
Dupuytren's disease, 180

E
Early exit from workforce, 386
Early return to work interventions, 491
Earnings replacement benefits, 310
Economic burden, 254
Economic globalization, 39
Economic structure, 119
Education, 26–27, 58
  attainment, 58, 64, 159
  inequalities, 81
Effort-reward imbalance model, 63, 217–218, 221, 253, 456, 471
Eligibility criteria, 312, 672
Employability, 315, 371–374
  work ability and, 562
Employers
  behaviour of, 348
  and compensation authority, 352
  Danish, 357
  incentives for, 352
  retaliation by, 354

Employment
  access to, 341
  cancer survivors, 402, 407
  changes, 21
  changing labor market conditions, 376–378
  determinants of labor market participation, 424
  factors, 403–405
  outcomes, 626
  people with disabilities, 374–376
  policies and regulations, 378–380
  prevalence, 403
  prognosis, 400
  protection legislation, 95, 97, 98
  rates, 332, 423, 641, 642
  rehabilitation outcomes, 369–371
  return to normalcy, 401 (see also Return to work)
  return to work rates, 423
  transitions, 79
  value of work, 367–369
  work-related issues, 401
Engine emissions, 142–143
English Longitudinal Study on Ageing (ELSA), 57, 58
Environment 'disability-friendly, 315
Equality, 339
  of opportunity, 381
Ethnic minority, 535
Europe, 577
European Directives, 275
European Union, 116
Evidence-based practice, 486
Evidence synthesis, 490
Executive functions, 454, 461
Exposures to risks, 107
Extending working lives, 313
Extrinsic allergic alveolitis (EAA), 163

F
Fairness, 625
Fatal injuries, 107
Fidelity, 585
Financial incentives, 93, 96, 622
Financial remuneration, 402
Fitness for work, 461
Fit note, 458
Fixed-effects model, 76
Flexible forms of work, 23–24
Flexicurity model, 13, 95, 97, 669
Flexicurity systems, 373, 377
Framework Directive 89/391/EEC, 277

Friction-cost method, 263
Functional disability, 454
Future employability, 18–19
 flexible forms of work, 23–24
 job characteristics, tasks and skill requirements, 19–22

G

Gamma-glutamyl-transferase (GGT), 508
Gender, 535
 inequalities, 36
Genitourinary system, 404
Glasgow Coma Scale (GCS), 634, 643
Global Activity Limitation Indicator (GALI), 57
Global approach, 176
Global GDP, 121
Good work-home balance, 628

H

Hand-arm vibration syndromes, 180
Harmonization, 275
Harmonizing work and disease treatment, 463
Health and Retirement Study (HRS), 57, 58
Health-behavior, 389
Healthcare professionals, 622
Health-care providers
 access to, 359
 behavior of, 352
 support of, 355
Health condition/impairment management, 321
Health factors, 389
Health inequalities, 80, 311
Health outcomes, 368
Health promotion programs, 304, 514
Health-related work exit
 disabling health, 62
 DP, 61
 early exit from paid work, 63
 exit from labor market, 61
 imbalance between high efforts spent and low rewards received, 62
 job with low control, 62
 low control, 63
 low occupational position, 62
 low recognition, 63
 low socioeconomic status, 63
 physical and psychosocial working conditions, 61
 poor health, 62

Health, safety and well-being (HSW), 275
Health surveillance, 299
Health trajectories, 79
Higher brain dysfunction, 454
Higher brain function, 454
High-income countries, 109
Hip osteoarthritis, 183
Hodgkin's disease, 405
Homogeneity tests, 194
Human abilities, 19
Human capacities, 21
Human carcinogenicity, 133
Human Development Index, 400
Human needs, 332
Human resource management (HRM), 637
Human rights, 8, 333
Human work, 19, 21
Hypersensitivity pneumonitis, 163

I

Idiopathic pulmonary fibrosis, 162
IGLOO framework, 12, 617–618, 638
Illness perceptions, 626
Imbalanced job design, 471
Impaired productivity, 160
Impairment, 154–155, 162
Improvement of work ability, 66
Incentives, 317
Income differences, 60
Individual placement and support (IPS), 98, 100, 426, 574–575
 affective disorders, 580
 borderline personality disorder, 581
 common mental disorders, 579–580
 cost reduction, 577
 intellectual and developmental disorders, 582–583
 moderate to severe mental illness, 580
 musculoskeletal and neurological disorders, 583–584
 nonpsychotic psychiatric disorders, 578–581
 for people with serious mental illness, 576–578
 posttraumatic stress disorder, 581
 substance use disorder, 581
Individual support and advice, 319
Industrialization, 40
Industry, 113
Inequalities, 4
Inequity, 378
Informal caregiving, 393
Informal economy, 46

Informal work, 46–48
Insecure jobs, 672
Instrumental activities of daily living
    (IADL), 57–59
Integration, 667
    of resources, 373
    policies, 67
Intellectual and developmental disabilities, 582
Interdisciplinary solutions, 468
International Agency for Research on Cancer
    (IARC), 133
    Monographs, 135, 140
International Classification of Functioning,
    Disability and Health (ICF), 54, 387
    classification, 64
    model, 57–59
International Labour Organisation (ILO)
    conventions, 276
    recommendations, 280
    standards, 280
Intrinsic values, 380
Ischemic heart disease, 190
    accumulated job strain, 201
    bullying, 194
    carbon disulphide, 201
    case control design, 191
    chemical toxic substances, 191
    demand control model, 191
    effort reward imbalance model, 191, 192
    forest plot, job strain, 194
    goal-directed organization intervention, 203
    job strain, 192
    lack of social support, 202
    long working hours, 199
    low decision latitude, 193
    noise at work, 202
    operational definitions in advance, 199
    population attributable risk, 200
    positive bias, 194
    prospective design, 191
    psychological demands vs. low decision
        latitude, 198
    regenerative functions, 197
    shift work, 201
    social class, 200
    tobacco smoke at work, 202
    work organization changes, 203
ISO 45001, 280

J
Job change, 156
Job crafting, 298
Job demand-control model, 456

Job development, 574
Job exposure matrix, 174, 244
Job-Finding Club, 519, 520
Job insecurity, 377
Job security
    governing, 354
    labor legislation affecting, 359
    protections of, 351
    rules, 354
    workers, 357
Job self-efficacy, 405
Job strain, 62, 253
    and cognitive function, 240
    high, 240
    model, 217–218, 221, 240
Job tenure, 544

K
Knee hygromas, 183
Knee osteoarthritis, 183

L
Labor force, 35–37
    participation, 88–90
Labor market
    flexibilization policies, 48
    institutions, 25
    participation, 2, 4, 36
    redefinition of, 38
    regulation, 28–29
Labor inspectorates, 284
Labor market participation, 485, 494, 654
Labor market policies, 368, 372, 379
    in Europe, 665–667
    ICF model of disability, 664
    security and flexibility, 669–670
    types, 662
Lateral and medial epicondylitis, 178
Learning community, 577
Legal coverage, 114
Legislative changes, 477
Legislative frameworks, 528
Legislative, health and insurance system
    influences, 625
Life course, 653, 654
Life expectancy, 72
Lifetime perspective, 176
Line managers, 626
Line managers' behaviors, 621
Living environment characteristics, 239

Lost productive time (LPT), 264
Lower socioeconomic position, 59
Low social support, 255

M
Meaningful work, 401, 402
Medical profession, 267
Medical rehabilitation, 66
Medication, 75
Melanoma, 404
Mental disorders, 401, 510
Mental health, 323
Mental illness, 11
Mental wellbeing, 291
Meta-analysis, 221–223
Middle-income countries (MICs), 34, 38–39
Mindfulness, 295
Minority approach, 55–56
Model of illness flexibility, 387
Modern Western societies, 64
Modifiable factors, 543
Monoamine hypothesis, 213
Mortality, 469
Motivation, 667
Motivational interviewing (MI), 515
Multicomponent interventions, 301
Multidimensional and multilevel conceptual model, 176
Multidimensional interventions, 366
Multidisciplinary coordinated interventions, 671
Multifactorial conditions, 370
Multilevel evaluation, 545
Multilevel interventions, 618
Multimorbidity, 386
Multiple regression modeling, 161
Multiple sclerosis, 640
Musculoskeletal and neurological disorders
  chronic pain, 584
  spinal cord injuries, 583–584
  traumatic brain injury, 584
Musculoskeletal disorders (MSD), 5, 10, 63, 171
  aging, 496–498
  biomechanical risk factors, 174
  cervical spine disorders, 180
  definition, 484
  elbow disorders, 178
  factors associated with, 485
  hand diseases, 178–180
  intervention evidence, 489–492
  lower limb disorders, 182–183
  lumbar spine disorders, 181
  multidimensional conceptual model of work-related, 175
  non-occupational factors, 173
  non-specific low back pain, 181–182
  occupational factors, 173–174
  organizational factors, 174
  principles of return to work, 487–488
  prognostic factors, 489
  psychosocial factors, 174
  radicular disorders in the lumbar spine, 181
  research evidence, seven principles, 492–494
  scientific evidence, 486
  sex and gender, 494–495
  shoulder diseases, 176–177
  sitting and standing, 495–496
  work disability, 494–498
  workplace intervention for disability reduction, 486–493
Myocardial infarction (MI), 432

N
National Disability Strategy, 530
National surveillance, 278
Neck pain, 484, 490
Negative right, 337
Networking strategy, 669
Neurodegenerative disorders, development of, 242
Neurological conditions
  ABI, 638–640
  SCI, 638–640
Neurological disabilities, 640, 654
Neurotoxicants, 243
Non-discrimination, 339
Non-fatal injuries
  occupational accidents, 114
  surveys, 118–119
Non-specific low back pain, 181–182
Non-specific neck pain, 180
Non-standard employment, 23, 24
Non-traumatic brain injury, 640
Non-traumatic spinal cord injury, 420
Norway, 110

O
Obstructive sleep apnea, 162
Occupational asthma, 157
Occupational carcinogens, 128, 135
  challenges, 132
  classifications, 134

Occupational carcinogens (cont.)
  compensation, 149
  epidemiology, 130
  exposures, 136
  listing, 132–133, 135
  occupations, industries and occupational circumstances, 138
  prevention, 149
  risk factors among women, 146
Occupational counseling, 411
Occupational determinants, 5
Occupational exposures, 4, 132, 135, 148
  preventive action, 5
Occupational hazards, 253
Occupational health, 6
  psychology, 638
  and safety services, 65
Occupational hierarchies, 66
Occupational injuries, 107
  burden of, 120–121
  cost estimates, 121–123
  estimation method, 113
  global division of deaths, 115
  policies and practices for prevention, 121–124
  severity pyramid, 119
Occupational uncertainty, 471
Online interventions, 7
Open employment, 573
Open questions, Affirmation, Reflective listening, and Summarizing (OARS), 515
Opioid use disorders, 582
Organizational culture, 595, 596, 601
Organizational intervention, 297
Organizational justice, 475
Organizational policies, programs and practices, 628
Organizational structure, 594

P
Paradoxical vocal fold motion disorder, 160
Paralysis, 420
Paraplegia, 419
Parkinson's disease, 640
Participant characteristics, 302
Participation work, 341
Participatory approaches, 297
Participatory ergonomics, 489
Passive jobs, 241
Pathway' model, 64
Patient-centered approach, 643

Peer supported interventions, 513
People with disabilities, 332
Perceived obstacles, 542
Percutaneous coronary intervention (PCI), 432
Permanent disability, 468
Personal factors
  classification, 388
  environmental factors, 390
  examples of, 387
  health-related, 387
  level of education, 392
  occupational factors, 390
  psychological resources, 390
  self-management, 392
  sociodemographic factors, 388
  socioeconomic status, 389
  subcategory of, 389
  sustainable work participation, 391
Personal identity, 402
Personality, 473
Persons with disabilities, 656
Physical demands, 254
Physical disabilities, 636
  RTW, 637, 638
  sustained employment, 637, 638
Pneumoconioses, 163
Polarization, 18, 20, 21, 24, 26
Policy
  context, 285
  definition, 274
  enforcement, 283
  hard law, 274
  interventions, 324
  making, 625
  orientations, 313
  perspective, 261
  recommendations, 13
  soft law, 274
  stakeholders, 285
Polycyclic aromatic hydrocarbons (PAHs), 141–142
Population attributable fraction (PAF), 147
Population attributable risk, 255
Positive psychology, 295
Positive rights
  and CRPD, 334–336
  importance, 334
  to work and political equality, 339–340
Postindustrial society, 90
Posttraumatic stress disorder, 581
Poverty, 107, 672
Precarious employment, 158
Premature deindustrialization, 39, 41

Presenteeism, 46, 159, 253, 259–261, 263, 266, 379
Primary prevention, 95
Privatization, 44
Productivity, outcome, 255
Program failure, 475
Programme logic, 313
Proinflammatory cytokines, 197
Prolonged working, 386
Prospective cohort studies, 254
Protection, 666
Psychoactive substances, 510
Psychological demands, 254
Psychological factors, 620
Psychosocial epidemiology, 217
Psychosocial interventions, 512
Psychosocial skills training, 512
Psychosocial stress, 63
Psychosocial work conditions, 203
Psychosocial work environment, 263, 458
Psychosocial work stressors, 252, 259
Psychotropic substances, 514
Punitive approach, 323

Q
Qualification demands, 377
Quality of life
 activities, 410
 cancer-related disabilities, 409
 and emotional well-being, 400
 fatigue, 410
 psychosocial distress, 410
Quality of work, 3, 380
Quality-oriented early childhood education, 26
Quotas, 95, 96

R
Radicular disorders, in lumbar spine, 181
Randomized controlled-trials (RCTs), 411, 576
Rapid review methodology, 291
Reasonable accommodations, 534
Recovery, 299
Re-employment, 98, 405, 470
Reforms, 322
Regulation, types of, 359
Regulatory issues, 8
Rehabilitation, 318, 401, 403, 411, 552
 ability and capacity to work, 518
 abstinence, 518, 519
 drug-dependent patients, 506
 employment, 518

intra-and extramural trainings, 517
medical, 554
outcomes, 369–371
planning and contents of, 562
post-acute treatment, 517
process, 544
services, 56
sociodemographic data, 517
vocational, 555
Rehabilitation Act, 529
Research agenda, 121
Resilience, 296
Resource-generation, 373, 380
Respiratory tract disease, 155
 See also Respiratory work disability
Respiratory work disability
 asthma, 156–157
 COPD, 158–159
 cystic fibrosis, 161
 lung fibrosis, 162–163
 lung transplantation, 163–164
 obstructive sleep apnea, 162
Retirement, 158
 cognitive aging and, 246
 cognitive function in, 245
 early, 392
Return-to-work (RTW), 96, 553, 599
 ABI, 642, 643
 after stroke, 10
 after treatment completion, 401
 application of best practices for implementation, 601–606
 barriers and opportunities of, 10
 barriers to successful, 439–441
 best practices for implementation model, 594, 601
 breast cancer patients, 405
 career changes, 409, 597–601
 conceptual models of, 592–594
 and coronary heart disease, 10
 in CR, 442–443
 definition, 591–592
 diagnosis, 403
 employees with coronary heart disease, 435–440
 employer accommodation, 404
 (*see also* Employment)
 graded, 474
 interventions, 377, 411, 474
 job loss, 405, 406
 job matching framework, 638
 lacking within CR, 433
 length of absence, 407

Return-to-work (RTW) (*cont.*)
  motivation and willingness, 403
  outcome measures, 8
  in patients with cardiovascular disease, 434
  planning, 318
  post-disability employment, 637
  practice-based model, 12
  practice-oriented holistic model, 592–597
  psychosocial issues, 410
  psychosocial support, 402
  quality of life issues, 409–410
  rates, 641, 642
  resources, 12
  SCI, 642
  sick leave, 406
  support, 2, 9, 432, 468, 487–488, 578
  sustainable outcomes, 12
  wages, 408
  work ability, 408
  work changes, 407
  work hours, 407
  work reintegration, 637
Rhinitis, 159
Right to work, 337, 339
Risk observatory, 121
Rotator cuff tendinopathy, 177

S
Safety at work, 106, 123
Salutogenic aspects of work, 91
Sanctions, 93, 98
Schizophrenia spectrum, 536
Secondary prevention, 96
Sectoral policies, 281
Selection hypothesis
  health-driven exit from paid employment, 73–74
  health problems, 74–75
  return to paid employment, 75–76
Self-efficacy, 541
Self-esteem, 541, 577
Sensation, 420
Serotonin transporter gene, 215
Service(s), 113
  sector, 41–42
Severe mental illness
  adherence to medication, 538
  behavioral motivation, 542–543
  clinican support, 532
  cognitive deficits, 537
  comorbidities, 537–538
  demographic factors, 534–535

  disability benefits, 530–531
  employment specialist competencies, 533
  environmental factors, 530–534
  experience and skills, 538–539
  individual factors, 534–543
  job acquisition and tenure, 527
  job match, 540
  perceived barriers to employment, 542
  policies and legal framework, 528–530
  psychiatric and physical conditions, 536–538
  psychiatric symptoms, 536–537
  self and motivational factors, 541–543
  skills and competencies, 539
  social skills, social adjustment and social functioning, 540–541
  social support, 532
  stigma and disclosure, 531–532
  vocational services, 533–534
  work accommodations and natural support, 534
  work history, 539
  working alliance, 533–534
Sheltered employment, 340, 573
Shoulder diseases, 176
  non-specific disorders, 177
  rotator cuff tendinopathy, 177
Sick leave, 253, 256, 259, 260, 264, 406
Sickness absence, 56, 97, 157, 468, 472, 475, 617
Sickness insurance
  compensation and, 354
  systems, 354
Sick pay, 97
Silicosis, 41
Sleep disturbance, 410
Small enterprises, 121
Social barriers, 375
Social causation hypothesis, 470
Social context, 621
Social cooperatives, 529
Social determinants, 455
Social dialogue, 281
Social distribution of disability, 56
Social enterprises, 529
Social gradient, 61
Social identity theory, 620
Social inequalities, 58, 59, 61, 63, 65–67
Social integration, 653
Social investment approach, 26
Social investment state, 666
Socialization, 668
Socially unequal burden of disability, 65

Social model of disability, 86
Social participation, 55, 56, 64
Social partner agreements, 281
Social protection, 23, 24, 312
  and active labor market policies, 29–30
  programs, 256
Social psychiatry, 209–210
Social regulation, 94–95
Social Security Disability Insurance (SSDI), 531
Social selection hypothesis, 470
Social support, 471, 626
Social value, 367, 368
Societal costs, 264
Socioeconomically deprived population groups, 58
Socioeconomic inequalities, 79
Socioeconomic status, 9, 472
Sociologic theory of latent functions, 77
Solvent
  organic, 242
  uses, 242
Solvent exposure, 242
  on cognition, 244
  long-term effects of, 243
Spinal cord injury (SCI), 12, 583–584, 635, 636
  chronic health conditions, 639
  community survey, 653
  contextual level, 655
  description, 419
  employment and RTW rates, 641, 642
  epidemiology, 420
  group level, 644, 655
  impairments and activity limitations, 420–421
  individual level, 644, 654
  leader level, 647, 655
  non-traumatic aetiology, 639
  physical impairments, 639
  RTW, 642
  secondary health problems, 421–422
  severity, 419
  societal level, 647
  sustained employment, 643, 644–647, 654
  traumatic aetiology, 639
  vocational rehabilitation, 424, 639
Standardized numbers, 109
Stepwise vocational rehabilitation programs, 573
Stigma, 621
Stress-as-offense-to-self (SOS) theory, 228
Stressful psychosocial work environment, 62, 67

Stress management, 294
Stress prevention, 293
Stroke, 190
  IHD and, 191
  prevalence, 190
Structural transformation, 38
  declining employment in agriculture, 39
  industrial sector, 39–41
  service sector, 41–42
Styrene, 144–145
Substance use brief interventions, 512, 513
Substance use disorders (SUD), 506, 507, 511, 520
  and criminal justice involvement, 582
  opioid use disorders, 582
Successful return to work, 591, 597
Suicide prevention, 294
Supply of labor, 667
Supply-side approach, 94, 98
Supply-side services, 97
Supported employment, 12, 94, 98, 573
  programs, 527
Supportive group environment, 621
Support-side approach, 98
Support-side policy, 94
Survey of Health, Aging and Retirement in Europe (SHARE), 57, 59
Sustainability, 370, 374, 628
  of employment, 12
Sustained employment
  determinants of, 654
  disabilities, 637
  environmental and societal changes, 638
  facilitators and barriers, ABI, 647–653
  facilitators and barriers, SCI, 644–647
  occupational health research, 637
  qualitative studies, 656
  SCI and ABI research, 643, 644
  work environment, 638
Sustained work capacity, 371
Symptom severity, 473

T
Tailoring, RTW interventions, 433
Tax credit, 321
Team Awareness program, 512
Technological progress, 18, 19, 22, 25
Temporary contracts, 393
Temporary employment, 376, 377
Tendonitis and tenosynovitis of hand/fingers, 179
Tertiary education, 27

Tertiary prevention, 96
Tetraplegia, 419
Timely retirement, 79
Train-and-place, 573
Traumatic brain injury (TBI), 584, 637, 640
Traumatic spinal cord injury, 420
Tripartite, 278

U

Ulnar nerve entrapment at the elbow, 178
UN Convention on the Rights of Persons with Disabilities, 86, 95
Unemployment, 378, 379, 401, 403, 405, 406, 408, 411, 470, 506, 516, 519
    and health outcomes, 368
    long-term, 375
    rate, 37, 374
Unifying model of workplace risk factors, 472
Universal access, 26
    to health care, 61
Universal approach, 55–56
Universal human condition, 64
Universal perspective of disability, 56

V

Validation, 476
Value of work, 367–369
Vapors, gases, dust or fumes (VGDF), 159
Veterans, 581
Vinyl chloride, 145–146
Vitamin model, 77
Vocal cord dysfunction, 160
Vocational counseling, 426
Vocational education and training, 27
Vocational intervention, 403
Vocational rehabilitation, 66, 338, 456, 458, 461, 573, 635, 637, 639, 642, 643, 655
    assessment, 425
    definition, 424
    evidence-based VR interventions, 426–427
    as part of spinal cord injury rehabilitation, 425–426
    workplace environment, 425
Vulnerable employment, 42–46
Vulnerable groups, 80–81

W

Wage subsidies, 317
Wealth, 61
Web-based interventions, 513, 514
Welfare policies and cultural values, 625
Wellbeing interventions, 290
Western Pacific region, 117
Work ability, 11, 56, 403, 405, 407, 408, 410, 411, 453, 458, 462, 664
    balance concept of, 554–555
    bio-psycho-social concepts of, 557–560
    concepts of, 553
    employability concept of, 562–563
    medical concept of, 553–554
    psychosocial concepts of, 555–557
    and rehabilitation, 564–565
    in research and rehabilitation, 553
    as social construct of various systems, 563–564
    and work disability, 552
Work Ability House, 557, 558
Work accommodation, 11, 487
Work accommodation and natural support scale (WANSS), 534
Work adjustments, 627
Work capacity, 341, 421
Work disability, 171, 392, 424, 426, 469, 475, 484, 591, 592–593, 595, 606
    aging, 496–498
    duration, 487
    health outcomes, 490
    management, 492
    musculoskeletal disorders, 494–498
    pain, 490
    sex and gender, 494–495
    sitting and standing, 495–496
    workplace interventions, 491
Work disability prevention
    legal scholars in work, 350
    literature, 350
    rules of relevance, 353–359
    Sherbrooke model of, 351
Work environment, 95, 403, 506, 543, 642
    legislation, 92
Workers' compensation, 256
    claims and productivity losses, 253
    design of, 353
    doctors involved in, 352
    fund, 253
    insurance, 254
    mechanism of payment, 267
    North American, 355
    protections in, 354
    psychosocial work stressors, 258
Workers' return to work, 617, 619
    expectations, 618
    group level resources, 620–621

Index 687

  individual level resources, 618–620
  interaction between resources, 627–628
  leader level resources, 621–622
  organizational level resources, 623–624
  overarching resources, 624–625
Work incentives, 93, 94, 97
Working-age populations
  cohort studies on aging, 56
  disabling functional limitations, 64
  early old age, 64
  ELSA, 57
  health-related work exit, 61–63
  HRS, 57
  less advantaged conditions, 64
  midlife, 64
  physical and cognitive functioning, 56
  prevalence and social distribution, 58–61
  restricted social participation, 63
  restriction in activity and participation, 58
  severe bodily impairment, 63
  SHARE, 57
Working conditions, 6, 87, 90–91
Working life, 2
  expectancy, 78
Work participation, 9, 387, 422, 424, 426, 640, 643, 653, 655

Workplace accommodations, 461
Workplace bullying, 222, 476
Workplace disability management programs (WPDM), 490
Workplace discrimination, 409
Workplace factors, 475
Workplace inclusion, 471
Workplace interventions, 92, 96
Workplace policies, 497
Work reintegration, 353, 358, 636
Work related activity, 322
Work-relatedness, 115
Work-related symptoms, 508
Work-related traffic injuries, 108
Worksite medical screening, 65
Work status, 369, 370
Work stress, meta-analysis, 259
Work sustainability, 638
Work trajectories, 652

Z
Zero exclusion, 574
Zero harm, 124

Printed in the United States
By Bookmasters